MW00736524

ADVANCES IN NEUROLOGY
Volume 78

Advances in Neurology

INTERNATIONAL ADVISORY BOARD

ADVANCES IN NEUROLOGY
Volume 78

Dystonia 3

Editors

Stanley Fahn, M.D.
H. Houston Merritt Professor of Neurology
College of Physicians and Surgeons
Columbia University/Columbia-Presbyterian Medical Center
New York, New York

Charles David Marsden, D.Sc., F.R.C.P., F.R.S.
Dean and Professor of Neurology
University Department of Clinical Neurology
Institute of Neurology and the National Hospital for Neurology and Neurosurgery
London, United Kingdom

Mahlon R. DeLong, M.D.
Department of Neurology
Emory University School of Medicine
Atlanta, Georgia

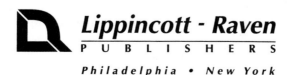

Lippincott - Raven
P U B L I S H E R S

Philadelphia • New York

Acquisitions Editor: Mark Placito
Developmental Editor: Gina Gerace
Manufacturing Manager: Kevin Watt
Supervising Editor: Kimberly Swan
Production Services: Hermitage Publishing Services
Cover Designer: Patty Gast
Indexer: Hermitage Publishing Services
Compositor: Compset, Inc.
Printer: Maple Press

Printed in the United States of America

9 8 7 6 5 4 3 2 1

ISBN: 0-7817-1538-5

ISSN: 0091-3952

Care has been taken to confirm the accuracy of the information presented and to describe generally accepted practices. However, the authors, editors, and publisher are not responsible for errors or omissions or for any consequences from application of the information in this book and make no warranty, express or implied, with respect to the contents of the publication.

 The authors, editors, and publisher have exerted every effort to ensure that drug selection and dosage set forth in this text are in accordance with current recommendations and practice at the time of publication. However, in view of ongoing research, changes in government regulations, and the constant flow of information relating to drug therapy and drug reactions, the reader is urged to check the package insert for each drug for any change in indications and dosage and for added warnings and precautions. This is particularly important when the recommended agent is a new or infrequently employed drug.

 Some drugs and medical devices presented in this publication have Food and Drug Administration (FDA) clearance for limited use in restricted research settings. It is the responsibility of the health care provider to ascertain the FDA status of each drug or device planned for use in their clinical practice.

Advances in Neurology Series

Contents

I. CLASSIFICATION AND PATHOPHYSIOLOGY

II. GENETICS OF PRIMARY TORSION DYSTONIA

V. DOPA-RESPONSIVE DYSTONIA

VI. OTHER DYSTONIA SYNDROMES

VII. PATIENT PERSPECTIVES

VIII. SUMMARY AND CONCLUSIONS

Contributing Authors

Laura Almasy, Ph.D.
Department of Genetics
Southwest Foundation for Biomedical
*   Research*
7620 North West Loop 410
San Antonio, Texas 78227-0531

Panagiotis Z. Anastasiadis, M.D.
William T. Gossett Neurology Laboratories
Henry Ford Hospital, 4D
One Ford Place
Detroit, Michigan 48202

Lauren A. Arnold, M.S.
Research Assistant
Institute of Metabolic Disease
Baylor University Medical Center
3812 Elm Street
Dallas, Texas 75226

R. A. E. Bakay, M.D.
Department of Neurosurgery
Emory University School of Medicine
The Emory Clinic, Building B
1365 Clifton Road
Atlanta, Georgia 30322

Oliver Bandmann, M.D.
Department of Neurology
MZ Nervenheilkunde
Neurologische Klinik mit Poliklinik
Rudolf-Bultmann-Str. 8
Marburg 35039
Germany

Michael P. Barnes, M.D., F.R.C.P.
Professor of Neurological Rehabilitation
University of Newcastle
Hunters Moor Rehabilitation Centre
Hunters Road
Newcastle upon Tyne
NE2 4NR
United Kingdom

Craig Bencsics, M.D.
Department of Neurology
University of Chicago
5841 South Maryland Avenue
Chicago, Illinois 60637

A. Berardelli, M.D.
Department of Neurological Sciences
University of Rome "La Sapienza"
Viale dell'Università 30
00185 Rome
Italy

Laurent Bezin, M.D.
William T. Gossett Neurology Laboratories
Henry Ford Hospital, 4D
One Ford Place
Detroit, Michigan 48202

Kevin J. Black, M.D.
Assistant Professor of Psychiatry and
*   Radiology*
Instructor in Neurology and Neurological
*   Surgery*
Washington University School of Medicine
Campus Box 8225
4525 Scott Avenue
St. Louis, Missouri 63110

Andrew Blitzer, D.D.S., M.D.
Head and Neck Surgical Associates
The Roosevelt Hospital
436 Third Avenue
New York, New York 10016

Allison Brashear, M.D.
Assistant Professor
Department of Neurology
Indiana University School of
*   Medicine/University Hospital*
550 University Boulevard, Room 6620
Indianapolis, Indiana 46202-5250

Xandra O. Breakefield, Ph.D.
Professor of Neurology
Massachusetts General Hospital
Building 149, 13th Street
Charlestown, Massachusetts 02129

Susan B. Bressman, M.D.
Neurological Institute
710 West 168th Street
New York, New York 10032

Mitchell F. Brin, M.D.
Associate Professor of Neurology
Director, Movement Disorder Center
Mount Sinai Medical Center
One Gustave L. Levy Place, Box 1052
New York, New York 10029

David J. Brooks, M.D.
Professor
Department of Neuroscience
Imperial College School of Medicine
Hammersmith Hospital
Du Cane Road
London W12 0NN
United Kingdom

Jonathan M. Brotchie, M.D.
Division of Neuroscience
School of Biological Sciences
University of Manchester
Manchester M13 9PT
United Kingdom

Anthony G. Butler, M.Sc.
Post-Graduate Research Associate
School of Clinical Neurosciences
The Medical School
University of Newcastle upon Tyne
NE2 4NR;
Hunters Moor Regional Rehabilitation
  Centre
Hunters Road
Newcastle upon Tyne
NE2 4NR
United Kingdom

Ian J. Butler, M.D.
Professor and Vice-Chairman
Department of Neurology
University of Texas Medical School-Houston
6431 Fannin Street
Houston, Texas 77030

Andrés O. Ceballos-Baumann, M.D.
Neurologische Klinik der Technischen
  Universität München
Möhlstr. 28
D-81675 München
Germany

Lorraine Clark, M.D.
Department of Neurology
University of California, San Francisco
Building 1, Room 101
1001 Potrero Avenue
San Francisco, California 94110

Alan R. Crossman B.Sc., Ph.D., D.Sc.
Professor of Anatomy
School of Biological Sciences
University of Manchester
Stopford Building, Oxford Road
Manchester M13 9PT
United Kingdom

Paul A. Cullis, M.D.
Clinical Associate Professor
Department of Neurology
Wayne State University School of Medicine
6E UHC DMC
Detroit, Michigan 48093

Antonio Currà, M.D.
Department of Neurological Sciences
Istituto Neurologico Mediterraneo
  Neuromed
Via Atinense 18
Pozzilli, I5, 86077
Italy

Muriel Dancoup, M.D.
Doctors Hospital
Iloilo City
Philippines

Deborah de Leon, M.S.
Genetic Counselor
Department of Neurology
Beth Israel Medical Center
10 Union Square East
New York, New York 10003

Mahlon R. DeLong, M.D.
Department of Neurology
Emory University School of Medicine
Woodruff Memorial Building, Suite 6000
Atlanta, Georgia 30322

William B. Dobyns, M.D.
Associate Professor
Division of Pediatric Neurology
Department of Neurology
University of Minnesota
Box 486
420 Delaware Street South East
Minneapolis, Minnesota 55455

Drake D. Duane, M.D.
Professor of Speech and Hearing Sciences
Director, Arizona Dystonia Institute
Arizona State University
10210 North 92nd Street, Suite 300
Scottsdale, Arizona 85258

Philip O.F. Duffey, M.B., B.S., M.R.C.P.
Specialist Registrar in Neurology
Newcastle General Hospital
Westgate Road
Newcastle upon Tyne NE4 6BE
United Kingdom

David Eidelberg, M.D.
Professor of Neurology
North Shore University Hospital
NYU School of Medicine
444 Community Drive, Suite 206
Manhasset, New York 11030

M. Evatt, M.D.
Department of Neurology
Emory University School of Medicine
1639 Pierce Drive, WMB 6000
Atlanta, Georgia 30322

S. Fabri, M.D.
Department of Neurological Sciences
University of Rome "La Sapienza"
Viale Università 30
Rome 00185
Italy

Stanley Fahn, M.D.
H. Houston Merritt Professor
  of Neurology
College of Physicians and Surgeons
Columbia University/Columbia-Presbyterian
  Medical Center
710 West 168th Street
New York, New York 10032

Martin R. Farlow, M.D.
Professor
Department of Neurology
Indiana University
541 North Clinical Drive, Suite 583
Indianapolis, Indiana 46202-5111

Terry D. Fife, M.D.
Assistant Professor
Department of Neurology
Barrow Neurological Institute
University of Arizona College
  of Medicine
222 West Thomas Road, Room 110
Phoenix, Arizona 85013

Blair Ford, M.D.
Assistant Professor
Department of Neurology
Columbia University
710 West 168th Street
New York, New York 10032

Yoshiaki Furukawa, M.D.
Visiting Professor
Human Neurochemical Pathology
  Laboratory
Clarke Institute of Psychiatry
250 College Street
Toronto, Ontario M5T 1R8
Canada

Gilberto L. Gamez, M.D.
Professor Emeritus
Departments of Neurology and Psychiatry
University of Santo Tomas
España Street
Manila 1008
Philippines

Thomas Gasser, M.D.
Privat dotent
Department of Neurology
Klinikum Großhadern
Ludwig-Maximilians-University
Marchioninistr. 15
München 81377
Germany

Robert R. Goodman, M.D., Ph.D.
Assistant Professor of Neurological Surgery
Columbia University
710 West 168th Street
New York, New York 10032

Paul E. Greene, M.D.
Assistant Professor
Department of Neurology
Columbia University
710 West 168th Street
New York, New York 10032

James F. Gusella, Ph.D.
Professor of Genetics and Bullard Professor of
   Neurogenetics
Director, Molecular Neurogenetics Unit
Harvard Medical School
Massachusetts General Hospital
13th Street, Building 149
Charlestown, Massachusetts 02129

Kei Hachimori, M.D.
Segawa Neurological Clinic for Children
2-8 Surugadai Kanda Chiyoda-ku
Tokyo 101 0062
Japan

Hiroaki Hagiwara, M.D.
Segawa Neurological Clinic for Children
2-8 Surugadai Kanda Chiyoda-ku

Tokyo 101-0062
Japan;
Department of Chemical Pharmacology
Faculty of Pharmaceutical Sciences
The University of Tokyo
7-3-1 Hongo, Bunkyo-ku
Tokyo 113
Japan

Mark Hallett, M.D.
Clinical Director, NINDS
NIH Building 10, Room 5N226
10 Center Drive, MSC 1428
Bethesda, Maryland 20892-1428

Takao Hashimoto, M.D., Ph.D.
Department of Neurology
Emory University School of Medicine
Woodruff Memorial Building
Suite 6000, P.O. Drawer V
Atlanta, Georgia 30322;
Third Department of Medicine
   (Neurology)
Shinshu University School of Medicine
3-1-1 Asahi
Matsumoto 390-8621
Japan

Maurice R. Hawthorne, B.S., F.R.C.S.
Consultant Otolaryngeal Surgeon
The North Riding Infirmary
Newport Road
Middlesbrough
Cleaveland TS1 5JE
United Kingdom

Brian Henry, B.Sc., Ph.D.
Division of Neuroscience
University of Manchester
Oxford Road
Manchester M13 9PT
United Kingdom

Jeffrey W. Hewett, M.D.
Molecular Neurogenetics Unit
Massachusetts General Hospital
13th Street, CNY Building 149, 6th floor
Charlestown, Massachusetts 00185-02129

Christopher J. Hille, M.D.
Division of Neuroscience
School of Biological Sciences
University of Manchester
Manchester M13 9PT
United Kingdom

Oleh Hornykiewicz, M.D.
Institute of Biochemical Pharmacology
University of Vienna
Borschkegasse 8a
Vienna A-1090
Austria

Michael Hutchinson, M.D., Ph.D.
Departments of Neurology and Radiology
New York University Medical Center
550 First Avenue
New York, New York 10016

Keith Hyland, Ph.D.
Associate Professor, Director of
*   Neurochemistry*
Institute of Metabolic Disease
Baylor University Medical Center
3812 Elm Street
Dallas, Texas 75226

Robert P. Iacono, M.D.
Associate Professor
Department of Neurosurgery
Loma Linda Medical University
101 West Mariposa Avenue
Redlands, California 92373

David Jacoby, M.D.
Molecular Neurogenetics Unit
Massachusetts General Hospital
13th Street, CNY Building 149, 6th floor
Charlestown, Massachusetts 02129

Joseph Jankovic, M.D.
Professor of Neurology,
Director, Parkinson's Disease Center and
*   Movement Disorders Clinic*
Baylor College of Medicine
6550 Fannin, Room 1801
Houston, Texas 77030

Beom S. Jeon, M.D., Ph.D.
Assistant Professor
Department of Neurology
Seoul National University Hospital
28 Yongon-dong, Chongno-gu
Seoul 110-744
Korea

Jae-Min Jeong, M.D.
Nuclear Medicine
College of Medicine
Seoul National University Hospital
28 Yongon-dong, Chongno-gu
Seoul 110-744
Korea

Un Jung Kang, M.D.
Assistant Professor
Department of Neurology
University of Chicago
5841 South Maryland Avenue, MC2030
Chicago, Illinois 60637

Stephen J. Kish, Ph.D.
Director
Human Neurochemical Pathology
*   Laboratory*
Clarke Institute of Psychiatry
250 College Street
Toronto, Ontario M5T 1R8
Canada

Martin Koller, M.D., M.P.H.
Director, Clinical Affairs
Clinical and Regulatory Departments
Athena Neurosciences, Inc.
800 Gateway Boulevard
South San Francisco, California 94080

Patricia L. Kramer, Ph.D.
Associate Professor of Neurology
Oregon Health Sciences University
3181 South West Sam Jackson Park Road,
*   L226*
Portland, Oregon 97201

Sandra M. Kuniyoshi, M.D.
Loma Linda University Medical Center
Movement Disorders Center
11234 Anderson Street, Room 2539
Loma Linda, California 92354

Anthony E. Lang, M.D., F.R.C.P.C.
Professor of Medicine
Department of Neurology
The Toronto Hospital/University of Toronto
399 Bathurst Street MP-11
Toronto, Ontario M5T 2S8
Canada

Mark S. LeDoux, M.D., Ph.D.
Assistant Professor
Department of Neurology
University of Tennessee College of Medicine
855 Monroe Avenue
Memphis, Tennessee 38163

Myung-Chul Lee
Nuclear Medicine
Seoul National University Hospital
28 Yongon-dong, Chongno-gu
Seoul 110-744
Korea

Frederick A. Lenz, M.D., Ph.D., F.R.C.S.
Associate Professor
Department of Neurosurgery
Johns Hopkins Hospital
Meyer Building 7-113
600 North Wolfe Street
Baltimore, Maryland 21287-7713

Robert A. Levine, Ph.D.
Director
William T. Gossett Neurology Laboratories
Henry Ford Health Sciences Center
One Ford Place, 4D Research
Detroit, Michigan 48202

Robert Lew, M.D.
Physiological and Pharmacological
  Sciences
University of Chicago
5841 South Maryland Avenue
Chicago, Illinois 60637

Dominique F. Lison, M.D., Ph.D., M.I.H.
Professor of Industrial Toxicology and
  Occupational Medicine
Catholic University of Louvain
Clos Chapelle-Aux-Champs, 30.54
Brussels 1200
Belgium

Joan F. Lorden, M.D.
University of Alabama at Birmingham
701 20th Street, Suite 770G
Birmingham, Alabama 35294-0107

Elan D. Louis, M.D., M.S.
Neurological Institute
710 West 168th Street
New York, New York 10032

Mario Manfredi, M.D.
Department of Neurosciences
University of Rome "La Sapienza"
Viale dell Università 30
Rome 00185
Italy

Joanne Markham, M.S.
Research Assistant Professor of Medicine
Department of Internal Medicine
Washington University School of Medicine
Institute for Biomedical Computing
700 South Euclid Avenue
St. Louis, Missouri 63110

Charles David Marsden, D.Sc., F.R.C.P., F.R.S.
Dean and Professor of Neurology
University Department of Clinical Neurology
Institute of Neurology and the National
  Hospital for Neurology and Neurosurgery
Queen Square
London WC1N 3BG
United Kingdom

John C. Mazziotta, M.D., Ph.D.
Professor of Neurology
Radiological Sciences and Medical and
  Molecular Pharmacology
UCLA School of Medicine
710 Westwood Plaza, Room 1240
Los Angeles, California 90095-1769

Lori McGee-Minnich, B.S.N.
Clinical Research Coordinator
Department of Neurology
Washington University School of Medicine
Box 8225, 4525 Scott Avenue
St. Louis, Missouri 63110

Klaus Mewes, Ph.D.
Assistant Professor
Department of Neurology
Emory University School of Medicine
1639 Pierce Drive, WMB 6000
Atlanta, Georgia 30322

Stephen M. Moerlein, M.D.
Mallinckrodt Institute of Radiology
Washington University School of Medicine
4525 Scott Avenue
St. Louis, Missouri 63110

Carol B. Moskowitz, M.D.
Neurological Institute
710 West 168th Street
New York, New York 10032

Michael Neystat, M.D.
Neurological Institute
710 West 168th Street
New York, New York 10032

Nobuyoshi Nishiyama, Ph.D.
Segawa Neurological Clinic for Children
2-8 Surugadai Kanda Chiyoda-ku
Tokyo 101 0062
Japan;
Assistant Professor
Department of Chemical Pharmacology
Faculty of Pharmaceutical Sciences
The University of Tokyo
7-3-1 Hongo, Bunkyo-ku
Tokyo 113
Japan

Yoshiko Nomura, M.D., Ph.D.
Segawa Neurological Clinic for Children
2-8 Surugadai Kanda, Chiyoda-ku
Tokyo 101 0062
Japan

Torbjoern G. Nygaard, M.D.
Neurological Institute
710 West 168th Street
New York, New York 10032

Christopher F. O'Brien, M.D.
Medical Director
Movement Disorders Center
Colorado Neurological Institute
701 East Hampden Avenue, Suite 530
Englewood, Colorado 80110-2776

Laurie J. Ozelius, Ph.D.
Instructor of Neurology
Molecular Neurogenetics Unit
Massachusetts General Hospital
13th Street, CNY Building 149 Room 6221
Charlestown, Massachusetts 02129

Orlino Pacioles, M.D.
Ricardo Limso Medical Center
Devao City
Philippines

Curtis E. Page, M.D.
The Molecular Neurogenetics Unit, Neurology
Massachusetts General Hospital
13th Street, CNY Building 149, 6th floor
Charlestown, Massachusetts 02129

Sung-Sup Park, M.D., Ph.D.
Assistant Professor
Department of Clinical Pathology
Seoul National University Hospital
28 Yongon-dong, Chongno-gu
Seoul 110-744
Korea

John Penney, M.D.
Molecular Neurogenetics Unit
Massachusetts General Hospital
Warren Building 408
32 Fruit Street
Boston, Massachusetts 02114

Martesio Perez, M.D.
University of the Philippines
Manila 1008
Philippines

Joel S. Perlmutter, M.D.
Associate Professor of Neurology and Radiology
Washington University School of Medicine
4525 Scott Avenue, Campus Box 8225
St. Louis, Missouri 63110

V. Perry, M.D.
Department of Neurosurgery
Meyer Building 7-113
Johns Hopkins Hospital
600 North Wolfe Street
Baltimore, Maryland 21287-7713

Deborah Raymond, M.S.
Genetic Counselor
Department of Neurology
Beth Israel Medical Center
10 Union Square East, Suite 2R, RACC
New York, New York 10003

Stephen G. Reich, M.D.
Associate Professor
Department of Neurology
Johns Hopkins University, School of Medicine
Suite 5070
601 North Caroline Street
Baltimore, Maryland 21287

Neil J. Risch, Ph.D.
Professor of Statistical and Population
  Genetics
Department of Genetics
Stanford University
300 Pasteur Drive
Stanford, California 94305

Sabine Rona, M.D.
Department of Neurosciences
University of Rome "La Sapienza"
Viale dell'Università, 30
Rome 00185
Italy

Raymond Rosales, M.D., Ph.D.
Associate Professor
Neurology and Psychiatry
University of Santo Tomas
3001MAB USTH Sampaloc
Manila 1008
Philippines

Saud Sadiq, M.D.
Neurological Institute
710 West 168th Street
New York, New York 10032

Tony Schoonenberg, C.R.T.T., C.P.F.T.
Loma Linda University Medical Center
Movement Disorders Center
11234 Anderson Street, Room 2539
Loma Linda, California 92354

Masaya Segawa, M.D., Ph.D.
Segawa Neurological Clinic for Children
2-8 Surugadai Kanda, Chiyoda-ku
Tokyo 101 0062
Japan

Christo Shalish, M.D.
The Molecular Neurogenetics Unit,
  Neurology
Massachusetts General Hospital
13th Street, CNY Building 149, 6th floor
Charlestown, Massachusetts 00185-02129

Mitsunobu Shimadzu, Ph.D.
Director
Department of Genetics
Mitsubishi Kagaku Bio-Clinical Laboratories,
  Inc.
3-30-1 Shimura
Itabashi-ku
Tokyo 174
Japan

Eufemio E. Sobrevega, M.D.
Doctors Hospital
Iloilo City
Philippines

Mikula K. Stambuk, M.D.
Department of Neurology and Neurological
  Surgery
Washington University School of
  Medicine
4525 Scott Avenue
St. Louis, Missouri 63110

Celia Stewart, Ph.D.
Assistant Professor
Department of Speech—Language Pathology
*   and Audiology*
New York University
719 Broadway, Suite 2
New York, New York 10003

Ritsuho Tanaka, M.D.
Segawa Neurological Clinic for Children
2-8 Surugadai Kanda Chiyoda-ku
Tokyo 108
Japan

Tatsuroh Tanaka, Ph.D.
Segawa Neurological Clinic for Children
2-8 Surugadi Kanda Chiyoda-ku
Tokyo 101 0062
Japan;
Department of Chemical Pharmacology
Faculty of Pharmaceutical Sciences
The University of Tokyo
7-3-1 Hongo, Bunkyo-ku
Tokyo 113
Japan

S. Triche, M.D.
Department of Neurology
Emory University School of Medicine
1639 Pierce Drive, WMB 6000
Atlanta, Georgia 30322

Joel M. Trugman, M.D.
Associate Professor of Neurology
University of Virginia Health System
Box 394
Charlottesville, Virginia 22908

Daniel D. Truong, M.D.
Parkinson's and Movement Disorder Institute
701 East 28th Street, Suite 401
Long Beach, California 90806

Kimiaki Uetake, M.D.
Segawa Neurological Clinic for Children
2-8 Surugadai Kanda Chiyoda-ku;
Hokkaido University School of Medicine
Department of Pediatrics
Tokyo 101 0062
Japan

Peter Y. K. Van den Bergh, M.D., Ph.D.
Professor
Service de Neurologie
Cliniques Universitaires St-Luc
10 Avenue Hippocrate
Brussels, B-1200
Belgium

Timothy P. Villegas, B.S.
University of Virginia School of Medicine
126-9 Turtle Creek Road
Charlottesville, Virginia 22901

Jerrold L. Vitek, M.D., Ph.D.
Associate Professor of Neurology
Director of the Program for Functional and
*   Stereotactic Neurology*
Emory University School of Medicine
1639 Pierce Drive
Atlanta, Georgia 30322

J. D. Wallace, M.D.
Athena Neurosciences, Inc.
800 Gateway Boulevard
South San Francisco, California 94080

Stephen Wachtel, M.D.
Department of Neurology
University of Chicago
5841 South Maryland Avenue
Chicago, Illinois 60637

Daniel E. Weeks, Ph.D.
Associate Professor of Human Genetics
University of Pittsburgh
A310 Crabtree Hall, 130 DeSoto Street
Pittsburgh, Pennsylvania 15261

Kirk C. Wilhelmsen, M.D., Ph.D.
Assistant Professor of Neurology in
*   Residence*
Ernest Gallo Clinic and Research Center at
*   University of California, San Francisco*
Building 1, Room 101
1001 Potrero Avenue
San Francisco, California 94110

Nicholas W. Wood, M.B., Ch.B., Ph.D., M.R.C.P.
Senior Lecturer in Clinical Neurology
Institute of Neurology
Queen Square
London WC1N 3BG
United Kingdom

Roger Woods, M.D.
Division of Brain Mapping
Department of Neurology
UCLA School of Medicine
710 Westwood Boulevard
Los Angeles, California 90024

Shoko Yukishita, M.D.
Segawa Neurological Clinic for Children
2-8 Surugadai Kanda Chiyoda-ku
Tokyo 101 0062
Japan

J. Zhang, M.D.
Department of Neurology
Emory University School of Medicine
1639 Pierce Drive, WMB 6000
Atlanta, Georgia 30322

T. A. Zirh, M.D.
Department of Neurosurgery
Johns Hopkins Hospital
Meyer Building 7-113
600 North Wolfe Street
Baltimore, Maryland 21287-7713

Preface

This is the third volume on dystonia published in *Advances in Neurology;* each volume represents the proceedings of an international symposium, approximately ten years apart. The first volume (Volume 14), entitled simply *Dystonia,* was published in 1976, and was a relatively slim 419 pages. It was an immediate, valuable resource and reference for the medical and scientific community for the dystonic disorders. Looking back, we find that this volume contained the early description of dopa-responsive dystonia (DYT5) and of lubag (X-linked dystonia-parkinsonism) (DYT3). It contained chapters on basal ganglia anatomy, physiology, and biochemistry; the bibliographic history of dystonia (especially DYT1 dystonia as it is called today); and descriptive clinical chapters on its natural history, dystonia in ethnic groups, and clinical variants, including the focal dystonias.

That volume might be said to have triggered an increased number of investigations on dystonia, but most of the credit for this heightened activity has to be given to the spurring of research by the Dystonia Medical Research Foundation (DMRF). The DMRF was founded and, in its formative years, virtually entirely supported by Samuel and Fran Belzberg. Research grants were awarded and dystonia centers created by the DMRF. The increase of knowledge and advances in therapy led to the Second International Symposium and the next volume, *Dystonia 2* in *Advances in Neurology* (Volume 50), published in 1988.

In *Dystonia 2* a better definition of the term dystonia was proposed, and there were sections on genetics (mainly DYT1), pathophysiology, biochemistry, imaging, animal models, epidemiology, variants of classical dystonia, focal dystonias, and treatment. The history of dystonia was covered as well, including the translation from German of Schwalbe's thesis of 1908 that described the disorder (DYT1) in three siblings. At the time of that volume, genetic linkage studies were underway for DYT1 dystonia, but the gene had not yet been mapped. The pattern of inheritance in the Ashkenazi Jewish population, however, was shown to be autosomal dominant (as in the non-Jewish population), and not recessive as previously proposed. The largest family of dopa-responsive dystonia was described, and the relationship of myoclonic-like jerks in patients with dystonia was discussed, leading to the understanding that such rapid movements can be present in DYT1 dystonia, but also in a new entity of myoclonic-dystonia. Secondary dystonias were covered, particularly tardive dystonia and psychogenic dystonia, which had been accepted by then. In the therapy section, there were many reports of the value of botulinum toxin injections for focal dystonias, and also covered were the effectiveness of anticholinergic and other agents. Surgery, including thalamotomy for generalized dystonia and peripheral denervation for torticollis, was reviewed. *Dystonia 2* covered 705 pages.

The Third International Dystonia Symposium took place in Miami, Florida, in October 1996. The decade between the second and third symposia was filled with tremendous advances, so much so that the organizers decided to make this a symposium open to all interested parties (unlike the previous two, which, because of space limitations, were by invitation only). In fact, the Third Symposium invited abstracts for both platform and poster presentations, in addition to the invited speakers. For the proceedings, the editors selected all the invited speakers and other presenters who made important contributions at the meeting.

Since *Dystonia 2,* the genes for DYT1 (Oppenheim's dystonia), DYT3 (lubag), and DYT5 (dopa-responsive dystonia) dystonia have been mapped, and DYT5's gene identified as the gene for GTP cyclohydrolase I, the first enzyme in the synthesis of tetrahydrobiopterin, the co-factor for tyrosine hydroxylase and other hydroxylases. Although not yet published at the time of the symposium, the DYT6 and DYT7 dystonias had been mapped and the DYT1 gene had been identified. The editors believed it important enough to delay the publication of the proceedings of the symposium by a few months in order to include the chapter describing the gene defect in DYT1 dystonia (see Chapter 10 by Breakefield et al.).

This volume reports on many other advances in dystonia besides genetic. The knowledge of the various new genetic discoveries and the pathology and biochemistry of dopa-responsive dystonia led to a major revision of the previous etiologic classification of dystonia; whereas that former classification merely divided etiology into simply primary and secondary dystonias, the new classification presented in this volume expands that greatly (see Chapter 1 by Fahn et al.). The pathophysiology of dystonia has also advanced from animal models and from PET scans in patients. Some understanding of the abnormal physiology in basal ganglia and cerebral cortex is described in this volume (see chapters by Hallett, Crossman, and Eidelberg and their respective colleagues). Other strains of botulinum toxin have been evaluated for treating focal dystonias, and surgical procedures for generalized dystonia are expanding. These topics and the different varieties of dystonia are covered in this volume.

While we can clearly see the considerable progress that has been made, we anticipate even greater developments on the road to conquering dystonia as scientists take advantage of the new genetic information. We hope this volume will serve as a stimulus to promote future research.

Acknowledgments

The Dystonia Medical Research Foundation was again the inspiring instrument to suggest the need for another international symposium on dystonia and a monograph of its proceedings. President Dennis Kessler and Treasurer Martin B. Sloate were key individuals in initiating the idea for the symposium, and Executive Director Dr. Valerie F. Levitan, its execution. The logistics in local arrangements were handled by Dr. Levitan. We are grateful to the National Institutes of Health for a symposium grant, 1R13NS35836-01, which was vital to financially support the symposium. Many pharmaceutical companies also contributed generously, without which the symposium would not have been successful. We thank the generosity of Allergan, Inc., Athena Neurosciences, Inc., Du Pont Merck Pharmaceutical Company, Roche Laboratories, SmithKline Beecham Pharmaceuticals, Pharmacia & Upjohn, and Medtronic Neurological.

There were also individuals and foundations who contributed, and to them we also acknowledge our appreciation. They are (in alphabetical order) Linda Dinkes, The Hermione Foundation, Harvey Hyman, Robert Konigsberg, Elsie K. Sloate, and Martin B. Sloate.

The organizers particularly thank the contributors and participants who took time from their busy schedules to meet, share information, and generate the excitement that took place during the Third International Dystonia Symposium.

Dystonia 3: Advances in Neurology, Vol. 78,
edited by S. Fahn, C. D. Marsden, and M. DeLong.
Lippincott–Raven Publishers, Philadelphia © 1998.

1

Classification of Dystonia

*Stanley Fahn, *Susan B. Bressman, and †Charles David Marsden

*Department of Neurology, Columbia-Presbyterian Medical Center, New York, New York 10032;
and †Department of Neurology, National Hospital for Neurology and Neurosurgery,
London, United Kingdom.

Dystonia has been defined as a syndrome of sustained muscle contractions, frequently causing twisting and repetitive movements, or abnormal postures (20,26). These involuntary movements are often exacerbated during voluntary movements, so-called action dystonia. The current and widely accepted classification of dystonia describes each patient with dystonia in three separate categories: age at onset, distribution, and etiology (20,26). Age at onset of primary dystonia is useful because it represents the best prognostic indicator as to whether there will be spread to other body parts (19,31,40). Distribution of dystonia is a partial indicator of severity of dystonia and is helpful in planning therapeutic strategy (24). Awareness of etiology is an ultimate aim in the clinical evaluation of dystonia, not only for treatment and genetic counseling, but also because it should lead to understanding the pathophysiology of the illness and how to prevent dystonia.

The current classification for etiology divides the dystonias into just two major categories, namely idiopathic (familial and sporadic) and symptomatic (20). This previous simplified scheme for etiology should now be expanded to encompass the recent discoveries in the genetics of dystonia, which indicate that more than one gene can cause idiopathic dystonia. This knowledge, plus the mapping of some

of these genes, expands our classification of idiopathic dystonia.

There has been greater awareness of forms of dystonia previously considered to be variants of idiopathic dystonia (21), such as dopa-responsive dystonia and myoclonic dystonia. Because these types include symptoms and signs other than dystonia, namely parkinsonism and myoclonus, respectively, we propose that the presence of these other types of abnormal movements argues for their being classified as distinct from idiopathic dystonia. In other words, we suggest that the major factors for listing a disorder as an idiopathic dystonia should be the phenotypic expression of dystonia and nothing but dystonia, and the exclusion of known symptomatic causes. The only exception would be the presence of tremor. Tremor in the idiopathic dystonias may be due to a dystonic tremor (17), which results from rhythmic group action potentials that occur in dystonia (56). It remains to be elucidated whether tremor that mimics essential tremor, which can be seen in many patients with dystonia as well as in members of their families (9,13,57,58), is actually a component of idiopathic dystonia (i.e., dystonic tremor) or the coexistence of the entity "essential tremor." At present, we suggest that such tremor can be part of the phenotypic expression of idiopathic dystonia.

TERMINOLOGY

We recommend using the term *primary* instead of *idiopathic* because the latter term indicates an unknown etiology, whereas for many of these primary dystonias, abnormal genes have now been discovered as the cause. To keep the symmetry, we prefer to use the term *secondary* instead of *symptomatic*.

In our proposed scheme for subdividing the etiologies into four distinct categories (see below), we need to distinguish between neurodegenerative and neurochemical disorders in order to separate dystonia-plus disorders from heredodegenerative disorders as described below. Here we define them as follows: A *neurodegenerative disease* is a neurologic disorder due to progressive dying and loss of neurons in the central nervous system (CNS), visible by light microscopy, and often accompanied by intracellular inclusions and gliosis; many neurodegenerative diseases are inherited, and some are known to have specific metabolic causes; but all produce visible pathologic changes in the brain. A *neurochemical disease* is a neurologic disorder due to a primary biochemical defect that alters CNS function and is not associated with a loss of neurons.

As will be seen, we suggest placing neurochemical diseases in the dystonia-plus category and neurodegenerative diseases in the heredodegenerative category.

SUBDIVIDING THE ETIOLOGIC CLASSIFICATION

In searching for a better way to handle the etiologic classification of the dystonias, we have taken a cue from the classification of parkinsonism. A useful approach has been to divide parkinsonian disorders into primary (usually called Parkinson's disease), secondary (due to environmental or structural causes), Parkinson-plus syndromes (in which other neurologic features in addition to parkinsonism also are present), and heredodegenerative syndromes (such as Hallervorden-Spatz disease, Wilson's disease, and Huntington's disease), which can present with a parkinsonian picture (25).

Thus, with our current understanding of the dystonias, we recommend that the original three categories remain for describing patients, namely age at onset, distribution, and etiology, and that the etiologic category be expanded to include four subcategories, primary, dystonia-plus, secondary, and heredodegenerative diseases, in which dystonia can be manifested as a prominent feature. Each of these etiologic subcategories contains currently recognized entities that appear to be distinct, and each may be enlarged in the future as further genetic, pathologic, and biochemical advances are made. Below, we describe the etiologic subcategories.

Primary Dystonia

Primary dystonia is defined as syndromes in which dystonia is the sole phenotypic manifestation with the exception that tremor can be present as well. Within this category is DYT1 dystonia in which the abnormal gene is located on chromosome 9q34.1 (36). This distinct genetic disorder was well characterized by Oppenheim in 1911, and it was Oppenheim who coined the term *dystonia musculorum deformans* to describe this disorder (45). To avoid ambiguity with other primary dystonias, we suggest that DYT1 dystonia also be known as Oppenheim's dystonia. The clinical phenotype as demonstrated by Bressman et al. (6) based on genetic assessment is that the onset is early in life, usually in childhood, and virtually always before the age of 40 years; one of the limbs is affected first in 90% of cases and the dystonia spreads to other body parts in the great majority; the cranial structures such as the face, pharynx, and tongue tend to be spared. Oppenheim's dystonia is inherited in an autosomal-dominant pattern with incomplete penetrance. The penetrance rate is 30% in Ashkenazi Jewish families (5,50) and about 40% in non-Jewish families (30).

The other primary familial dystonias listed in Table 1 have been definitively shown not to be caused by the DYT1 gene, and some of them are currently being genetically mapped into distinct entities. Several families with

TABLE 1. *Primary dystonias*

Oppenheim's dystonia (DYT1) (6,36,45)
  Autosomal dominant; incomplete penetrance; gene at 9q34.1
Adult-onset familial torticollis
  Autosomal dominant; gene at 18p (DYT7) in some families (38) and other families with genes not yet mapped (8)
Adult-onset familial cervical-cranial predominant
  Autosomal dominant
Childhood and adult onset, familial cranial and limb (DYT6)
  Autosomal dominant; gene at 8p21-q22 (2)
Other familial types to be identified as distinct entities
Sporadic, usually adult-onset

adult-onset familial torticollis have been reported, with one of them recently mapped to chromosome 18p, this locus being designated DYT7 (38). Other families with torticollis have been excluded from the DYT7 and the DYT1 regions (8); their genetic localizations have yet to be identified.

Cervical-cranial predominant dystonia is another form of autosomal-dominant primary dystonia; it has been seen in non-Jewish families that do not link to DYT1 (3,7). The site of onset is usually in the neck, which continues to dominate, but dystonia often spreads to involve the cranial structures as well, and occasionally the arm. Onset may be in childhood (3) or as an adult (7).

In two Mennonite families, a mixed type of autosomal-dominant dystonia has been seen in which onset can be either in childhood or adulthood, with involvement of limbs, and cervical and cranial regions. Dysphonia and dysarthria are often the most disabling feature. The abnormal gene has been mapped to 8p21-q22 (2). The locus has been designated as DYT6.

Undoubtedly, as other families with dystonia are reported, and their genes mapped, we will encounter additional genetic types. The most common forms of primary dystonia are the sporadic, adult-onset cases, most of which are focal or segmental. Once the genes for the primary dystonias are characterized, it is likely that many of them will be associated with a genetic etiology. Otherwise, their etiologies remain unknown.

Based on present knowledge Table 1 lists the currently recognized disorders among the primary dystonias.

Because the primary dystonias in their various genetic forms so far show no consistent pathologic change, it seems plausible and even likely that many or all of the primary dystonias may be neurochemical in origin, rather than a neurodegenerative disorder with neuronal loss.

Dystonia-Plus

The purpose of creating the subcategory of dystonia-plus in the etiologic classification of dystonia is to distinguish a group of diseases that are (a) distinct from the heredodegenerative dystonias and (b) also distinct from the primary dystonias.

1. While most neurodegenerative diseases are due to biochemical abnormalities, there are also biochemical disorders that do not result in structural neuronal degeneration. To distinguish this latter group, we refer to them as *neurochemical disorders,* the result of which is a neurophysiologic dysfunction without neuronal degeneration. The categories of primary dystonia and dystonia-plus are reserved for these neurochemical disorders.

2. The primary dystonias are characterized as pure dystonia disorders. For other neurochemical disorders in which the clinical phenotype includes neurologic features in addition to dystonia, we need a new designation, hence dystonia-plus. At present there are two such dystonia-plus conditions: dystonia with parkinsonism and dystonia with myoclonus (Table 2).

The hereditary dystonic-parkinsonian syndrome of dopa-responsive dystonia (DRD) (DYT5) was initially recognized because it often has marked diurnal variation of symptoms, with the patient being relatively free of symptoms in the morning and afflicted with severe symptoms late in the day (10,12,51). The response to levodopa was independently described by Segawa et al. (52) and Allen and Knopp (1), with the latter also pointing out the

TABLE 2. *Dystonia-plus syndromes*

Dystonia with parkinsonism
  Dopa-responsive dystonia
    GTP cyclohydrolase I deficiency (DYT5)
      1st step in BH_4 synthesis;
      Autosomal-dominant; gene at 14q22.1
    Tyrosine hydroxylase deficiency
      Autosomal-recessive; gene on chromosome 21
    Other biopterin deficient diseases
      a. 6-pyruvoyltetrahydropterin synthase deficiency
        2nd step in BH_4 synthesis;
        Autosomal-recessive
      Pterin-4a-carbinolamine dehydratase
        deficiency
      b. BH_4 regeneration after oxidation;
        Autosomal-recessive
        dihydropteridine reductase deficiency
      c. BH_4 regeneration after oxidation;
        Autosomal-recessive
  Dopamine-agonist responsive dystonia
    Autosomal-recessive; aromatic amino acid
      decarboxylase deficiency
Dystonia with myoclonic jerks that respond to alcohol
  Dystonia-myoclonus
    Autosomal-dominant; gene not mapped

parkinsonian component of the syndrome. Because not all patients with this syndrome have diurnal variation (41), but all are responsive to levodopa, the term *dopa-responsive dystonia* seems to us to be a more appropriate designation; this terminology also emphasizes the treatable nature of this disorder. Segawa and his colleagues (51) initially referred to this disorder, and still do, as progressive hereditary dystonia with diurnal fluctuations. But DYT1 dystonia is clearly a progressive hereditary dystonia, and apparently much more progressive than Segawa's disorder, so the term preferred by this group seems very ambiguous and therefore unsatisfactory. The fact that some patients, particularly those with adult onset, may present as pure parkinsonism with an excellent response to levodopa and nonprogressive course ("benign parkinsonism") (42) does not necessarily detract from the label of dopa-responsive dystonia.

Compared to Parkinson's disease, which usually requires increasingly higher doses of levodopa to get a satisfactory response, DRD markedly improves with low doses of levodopa. In part this is because DRD is nonprogressive

and nondegenerative. Both the dystonia and the parkinsonian signs that are present (bradykinesia, loss of postural reflexes, rigidity) respond well. The disease ordinarily begins in childhood with involvement of legs and gait; a peculiar feature is a tendency to walk on the toes, instead of heel-striking. Onset in adults can occur, and can be as a focal dystonia with cranial, neck, or arm involvement. Biopterin concentration is markedly reduced in the cerebrospinal fluid, and fluorodopa positron emission tomography (PET) is normal, fitting with the lack of degeneration of dopamine-containing neurons in the substantia nigra.

DRD is an autosomal-dominant disorder with reduced but gender-influenced penetrance; it is more common in women. Many cases are caused by identified mutations of the gene for guanosine triphosphate (GTP) cyclohydrolase I located at 14q22.1 (33,43). The enzyme coded by this gene catalyzes the first step in the biosynthesis of tetrahydrobiopterin (BH_4), the cofactor required for the enzymes tyrosine hydroxylase, phenylalanine hydroxylase, and tryptophan hydroxylase. These hydroxylase enzymes add an -OH group to the parent amino acid, and are required for the synthesis of the biogenic amines. The pathologic investigation of DRD revealed no loss of neurons within the substantia nigra pars compacta, but these neurons are immature with little neuromelanin (49). Neuromelanin synthesis requires dopamine (or other monoamines) as the initial precursor. Biochemically, there is marked reduction of dopamine concentration within the striatum in DRD (49). These pathologic and biochemical results clearly demonstrate that this disorder is best classified as a neurochemical disease rather than a neurodegenerative disease.

In addition to mutations of GTP cyclohydrolase I gene, other genetic disorders have now been shown to produce similar phenotypes, characterized by a response to levodopa or a dopamine agonist (Table 2).

A mutation of the tyrosine hydroxylase gene was discovered in an infant manifesting the phenotype of DRD and responding to levodopa

(35,39). Tyrosine hydroxylase activity was reduced to about 15% of normal; no autopsy has yet been reported. This is an autosomal-recessive disorder, in contrast to the more common DRD due to GTP cyclohydrolase I deficiency, which is an autosomal-dominant disorder. There has been no published neuropathologic report on this patient with tyrosine hydroxylase deficiency, so it is not known if this is a neurodegenerative disorder or a neurochemical disorder. For now, we will place it as a neurochemical one.

A variation of DRD is the clinical syndrome presenting in infancy with dystonia-parkinsonism, hypotonia, hyperhidrosis, miosis, and ptosis, with episodes of oculogyria and paroxysmal movements and later with bouts of deep sleep; these symptoms respond to dopamine agonists (32). There is reduced concentration of the metabolites of dopamine and serotonin in urine, namely homovanillic acid and 5-hydroxyindoleacetic acid, respectively. The enzymatic defect is a reduction of aromatic amino acid decarboxylase, which converts DOPA to dopamine and 5-hydroxytryptophan to 5-hydroxytryptamine (serotonin). Although there is no autopsy in these two affected twin boys and their older sibling who died, the dramatic and complete response to a dopamine agonist and a monoamine oxidase inhibitor makes it likely that this is a neurochemical rather than a neurodegenerative disease; hence it is placed in the dystonia-plus category.

A similar clinical presentation occurs with several pterin disorders (see Hyland et al., Chapter 30 of this volume). The autosomal-recessive biopterin deficiency states listed in Table 2, in addition to dystonia and parkinsonism, also manifest features of decreased norepinephrine and serotonin. The clinical features include miosis, oculogyria, rigidity, hypokinesia, chorea, myoclonus, seizures, temperature disturbance, and hypersalivation. These enzyme deficiencies cause hyperphenylalaninemia, and they may respond partially to levodopa. Without neuropathologic observations, we have arbitrarily listed these biopterin deficiency states as dystonia-plus syndromes rather

than as neurodegenerations because of their similar biochemical features to classic DRD. When postmortem analysis becomes available, we will reassess this classification.

Although muscle jerks (myoclonus) can be part of the clinical spectrum of primary dystonia, especially Oppenheim's dystonia (14,18, 44), there exists a separate hereditary disorder of dystonia with striking quick myoclonus that is a distinct entity (53). It has been called myoclonic dystonia and also hereditary dystonia with lightning jerks responsive to alcohol (37,48). Its distinction from hereditary essential myoclonus is not clear because the latter condition may have elements of dystonia (27,47). The genetic defect and pathology of myoclonic dystonia has yet to be reported, but it may well turn out to be a neurochemical disorder, and thus we place it in the dystonia-plus category. During the discussion of this presentation at the Third International Dystonia Symposium it was suggested that having one of the words being an adjective renders it subservient to the noun component of the name of the disorder; the preference appeared to be to call the disorder with both components being a noun, namely dystonia-myoclonus. The myoclonic jerks mainly affect the upper part of the body, usually sparing the legs. The pathology of dystonia-myoclonus remains unknown; it is transmitted as an autosomal-dominant disorder.

Another dystonia-Parkinson syndrome that might be considered in this category is rapid-onset dystonia-parkinsonism (4,15), for which the gene defect and the neuropathology remain to be determined. However, it seems likely that this disorder will prove to be neurodegenerative and therefore, for now, is better placed in that category. If, when the neuropathology becomes available, this disease shows no degenerative changes, we recommend that it be moved from the neurodegenerative category to the dystonia-plus category.

There also exist a variety of parkinsonian syndromes in which dystonia is a common feature. These include Parkinson's disease, progressive supranuclear palsy, and cortical-basal ganglionic degeneration. We suggest that these

entities be placed within the category of heredodegenerative diseases.

Secondary Dystonia

Secondary dystonia is defined as a dystonic
disorder that develops mainly as the result of
environmental factors that provide insult to the
brain. Spinal cord injury and peripheral injury
are also recognized as contributors to dystonia.
Other examples include levodopa-induced dystonia in the treatment of parkinsonism; acute
and tardive dystonia due to dopamine receptor
blocking agents; and dystonias associated with
cerebral palsy, cerebral hypoxia, cerebrovascular disease, cerebral infectious and postinfectious states, brain tumor, and toxicants such as
manganese, cyanide, and 3-nitroproprionic acid.
A more complete listing is presented in Table 3.
A number of disorders in this group, such as the

infectious and toxicant-induced neurodegenerations, do not present as a pure dystonia, but with
a mixture of other neurologic features, often
parkinsonian features of bradykinesia and rigidity. It should be mentioned that tardive dystonia
can mimic primary dystonia by being a pure
dystonia, but often tardive dystonia is associated
with features of classic tardive dyskinesia and
sometimes tardive akathisia (34), which helps
make the correct diagnosis.

Heredodegenerative Diseases

Heredodegenerative diseases is a category
where neurodegenerations produce dystonia
as a prominent feature; usually other neurologic features, especially parkinsonism, also are
present and can even predominate. In some patients with these disorders, dystonia may fail to
appear, and other neurologic manifestations
may be the presenting feature, for example,
chorea in Huntington's disease, in which dystonia may be a late-stage feature (28). Tremor
or juvenile parkinsonism may be the mode of
presentation in Wilson's disease, and dystonia
may fail to appear in such patients.

Because many of these neurodegenerations
are due to genetic abnormalities, the term *here-
dodegeneration* is applied to this category. But
some of the diseases listed here are of unknown etiology, and it is not clear what the role
of genetics might be. For convenience, we
place all the neurodegenerations in this category. These are listed in Table 4 in which we
organize the heredodegenerative disorders that
can cause dystonia by the nature of their genetics whenever the genes are known, followed by
other neurodegenerations in which the etiology
remains unknown.

The major X-linked recessive dystonic disorder is lubag, also called X-linked dystonia-
parkinsonism. Its gene locus, designated as
DYT3, is near the centromere on the X chromosome. The abnormal gene is a mutation that
appears to have occurred on the island of
Panay in the Philippines. The disease usually
begins in young boys and develops into either
generalized dystonia or segmental mandibular-
lingual dystonia. In some affected individuals,

TABLE 3. *Secondary dystonias*

Perinatal cerebral injury
  Athetoid cerebral palsy
  Delayed onset dystonia
  Pachygyria
Encephalitis, infectious and postinfectious
  Reye's syndrome
  Subacute sclerosing leukoencephalopathy
  Wasp sting
  Creutzfeldt-Jakob disease
  Human immunodeficiency virus
Head trauma
Thalamotomy
Cervical cord injury or lesion
Peripheral injury
Brainstem lesion, including pontine myelinolysis
Primary antiphospholipid syndrome
Focal cerebral vascular injury
Arteriovenous malformation
Hypoxia
Brain tumor
Multiple sclerosis
Central pontine myelinolysis
Drug-induced
  Levodopa
  Dopamine D2 receptor blocking agents
    Acute dystonic reaction
    Tardive dystonia
  Ergotism
  Anticonvulsants
Toxicants: Mn, CO, carbon disulfide, cyanide,
  methanol, disulfiram, 3-nitroproprionic acid
Metabolic: hypoparathyroidism
Psychogenic

TABLE 4. *Heredodegenerative dystonias*

X-linked recessive
  Lubag (X-linked dystonia-parkinsonism) (DYT3)
    Gene located at Xq13
  Pelizaeus-Merzbacher disease
Autosomal-dominant
  Rapid-onset dystonia-parkinsonism (RDP)
  Juvenile parkinsonism (presenting with dystonia)
  Huntington's disease (usually presents as chorea)
    Gene: IT15 for Huntington located at 4p16.3
  Machado-Joseph disease (SCA3)
  Dentato-rubro-pallido-luysian atrophy
  Other spinocerebellar degenerations
Autosomal-recessive
  Wilson's disease
    (Can also present with tremor or parkinsonism)
    Gene: Cu-ATPase located at 13q14.3
  Niemann-Pick type C (dystonic lipidosis) (sea-blue
    histiocytosis)
    Defect in cholesterol esterification; gene mapped
      to chromosome 18 (11,46)
  GM1 gangliosidosis
  GM2 gangliosidosis
  Metachromatic leukodystrophy
  Lesch-Nyhan syndrome
  Homocystinuria
  Glutaric acidemia
  Triose-phosphate isomerase deficiency
  Methylmalonic aciduria
  Hartnup's disease
  Ataxia telangiectasia
  Hallervorden-Spatz disease
  Juvenile neuronal ceroid-lipofuscinosis
  Neuroacanthocytosis
  Intranuclear hyaline inclusion disease
  Hereditary spastic paraplegia with dystonia
Probable autosomal recessive
  Familial basal ganglia calcifications
  Progressive pallidal degeneration
  Rett's syndrome
Mitochondrial
  Leigh's disease
    Genes: nuclear and mitochondrial DNA
  Leber's disease
    Gene: mitochondrial DNA
  Other mitochondrial encephalopathies
Associated with parkinsonian syndromes
  Parkinson's disease
  Progressive supranuclear palsy
  Multiple system atrophy
  Cortical-basal ganglionic degeneration

tum and no or little decrease of dopa uptake (16), compatible with the pathology that reveals a mosaic pattern of gliosis in the striatum with neuronal loss (54).

We recognize uncertainties in placing some of the disorders listed in Table 4 as being neurodegenerative without concrete evidence. Rapid-onset dystonia-parkinsonism may well prove to be a neurochemical disorder rather than a neurodegenerative one; there is no postmortem report. We chose placing this disorder in Table 4 rather than in Table 2 because the sudden onset suggests a toxic-metabolic-immunologic disorder, and this type is often associated with pathologic changes in the CNS. Dystonia and parkinsonism occurs between 14 and 45 years of age. The onset is either acute with the abrupt onset of symptoms over the course of several hours, or subacute with evolution over several days or weeks. Thereafter, progression of symptoms is usually very slow. It does not respond to levodopa, and it has been shown not to be linked to the DYT1 gene (15).

OTHER DYSKINESIA SYNDROMES WITH DYSTONIA PRESENT

Dystonia can appear in disorders not ordinarily considered to be a part of torsion dystonia (Table 5). These include dystonic tics (22), which are more conveniently classified with tic disorders; paroxysmal dyskinesias, which are more conveniently classified with paroxysmal dyskinesias (23); and hypnogenic dystonia, which can be either paroxysmal dyskinesias or seizures (29).

it may begin as a parkinsonian disorder, or parkinsonism can appear during its course. The freezing phenomenon may be a prominent feature. Occasional Filipino female heterozygotes can manifest mild dystonia or chorea (55). Fluorodeoxyglucose and fluorodopa PET scans show decreased striatal metabolism in the stria-

TABLE 5. *Other dyskinesia syndromes with dystonia present*

Tic disorders with dystonic tics
Paroxysmal dyskinesias with paroxysmal dystonia
  Paroxysmal kinesigenic choreoathetosis
  Paroxysmal dystonic choreoathetosis
  Intermediate paroxysmal dyskinesia
  Benign infantile paroxysmal dyskinesias
Hypnogenic dystonia
  (Sometimes these are seizures)

TABLE 6. *Pseudodystonia (not classified as dystonia, but can be mistaken for dystonia because of sustained postures)*

Sandifer syndrome
Stiff-man syndrome
Isaacs' syndrome
Satoyoshi syndrome
Rotational atlanto-axial subluxation
Soft tissue nuchal mass
Bone disease
Ligamentous absence, laxity, or damage
Congenital muscular torticollis
Congenital postural torticollis
Congenital Klippel-Feil syndrome
Posterior fossa tumor
Syringomyelia
Arnold-Chiari malformation
Trochlear nerve palsy
Vestibular torticollis
Seizures manifesting as sustained twisting postures

TABLE 8. *Classification of dystonia*

By age at onset
　Childhood onset, 0–12 years
　Adolescent onset, 12–20 years
　Adult onset, >20 years
By distribution
　Focal
　Segmental
　Multifocal
　Generalized
　Hemidystonia
By etiology
　Primary
　　Familial
　　Sporadic
　Dystonia-plus syndromes
　Secondary
　Heredodegenerative diseases

PSEUDODYSTONIA

To complete the revised classification, we think it important to list disorders that can mimic torsion dystonia, but are not generally considered to be a true dystonia (Table 6). These disorders typically manifest themselves as sustained muscle contractions or abnormal postures, which is why they are often mistaken for dystonia. But these contractions are secondary to either a peripheral or reflex mechanism or as a reaction to some other problem. For example, Sandifer's syndrome is due to gastroesophageal reflux, with apparent reduction of the gastric contractions when the head is tilted to the side; Isaacs' syndrome is due to continuous peripheral neural firing; orthopedic disease causes a number of postural changes; and seizures can result in sustained twisting postures.

TABLE 7. *Gene nomenclature for the dystonias*

DYT1 = 9q34.1, AD, early- and limb-onset
DYT2 = autosomal-recessive dystonia
DYT3 = Xq13, lubag
DYT4 = a whispering dysphonia family
DYT5 = 14q22.1, dopa-responsive dystonia, GTP cyclohydrolase I gene
DYT6 = 8p21-q22, mixed type dystonia
DYT7 = 18p, familial torticollis

CONCLUSION

The genetic forms of dystonia that have been given designated labels are listed in Table 7. The primary dystonias are DYT1, DYT2, DYT4, DYT6, and DYT7. DYT5 is classified as a dystonia-plus disorder, and DYT3 as a heredodegenerative dystonia.

The overall classification scheme as described here is presented in abbreviated form in Table 8. We believe this revised classification for etiology represents a useful update over the older scheme in keeping with current knowledge. We hope that progress from research on dystonia will cause the proposed scheme to be outdated soon.

REFERENCES

1. Allen N, Knopp W. Hereditary parkinsonism-dystonia with sustained control by L-dopa and anticholinergic medication. *Adv Neurol* 1976;14:201–213.
2. Almasy L, Bressman SB, Raymond D, et al. Idiopathic torsion dystonia linked to chromosome 8 in two Mennonite families. *Ann Neurol* 1997; 42:670–673.
3. Bentivoglio AR, Delgrosso N, Albanese A, Cassetta E, Tonali P, Frontali M. Non-DYT1 dystonia in a large Italian family. *J Neurol Neurosurg Psychiatry* 1997; 62:357–360.
4. Brashear A, DeLeon D, Bressman SB, Thyagarajan D, Farlow MR, Dobyns WB. Rapid-onset dystonia-parkinsonism in a second family. *Neurology* 1997;48: 1066–1069.
5. Bressman SB, de Leon D, Brin MF, et al. Idiopathic torsion dystonia among Ashkenazi Jews: evidence for

autosomal dominant inheritance. *Ann Neurol* 1989;26: 612–620.

6. Bressman SB, de Leon D, Kramer PL, et al. Dystonia in Ashkenazi Jews: clinical characterization of a founder mutation. *Ann Neurol* 1994;36:771–777.

7. Bressman SB, Heiman GA, Nygaard TG, et al. A study of idiopathic torsion dystonia in a non-Jewish family: evidence for genetic heterogeneity. *Neurology* 1994; 44:283–287.

8. Bressman SB, Warner TT, Almasy L, et al. Exclusion of the DYT1 locus in familial torticollis. *Ann Neurol* 1996;40:681–684.

9. Bundey S, Harrison MJG, Marsden CD. A genetic study of torsion dystonia. *J Med Genet* 1975;12:12–19.

10. Burns CLC. The treatment of torsion spasm in children with trihexyphenidyl (Artane). *Med Press* 1959; 241:148–149.

11. Carstea ED, Polymeropoulos MH, Parker CC, et al. Linkage of Niemann-Pick disease type C to human chromosome 18. *Proc Natl Acad Sci USA* 1993;90: 2002–2004.

12. Corner BD. Dystonia musculorum deformans in siblings: treated with Artane (trihexyphenidyl). *Proc Roy Soc Med* 1952;45:451–452.

13. Couch J. Dystonia and tremor in spasmodic torticollis. *Adv Neurol* 1976;14:245–258.

14. Davidenkow S. Auf hereditar-abiotrophischer Grundlage akut auftretende, regressierende und episodische Erkrankungen des Nervensystems und Bemerkungen uber die familiare subakute, myoklonische Dystonie. *Z Ges Neurol Psychiat* 1926;104:596–622.

15. Dobyns WB, Ozelius LJ, Kramer PL, et al. Rapid-onset dystonia-parkinsonism. *Neurology* 1993;43:2596–2602.

16. Eidelberg D, Wilhemsen K, Takikawa S, et al. Positron emission tomographic findings in Filipino X-linked dystonia-parkinsonism. *Ann Neurol* 1993; 34:185–191.

17. Fahn S. Atypical tremors, rare tremors, and unclassified tremors. In: Findley LJ, Capildeo R, eds. *Movement disorders: tremor.* New York: Oxford University Press, 1984:431–443.

18. Fahn S. The varied clinical expressions of dystonia. *Neurol Clin* 1984;2:541–554.

19. Fahn S. Generalized dystonia: concept and treatment. *Clin Neuropharmacol* 1986;9[Suppl 2]:S37–S48.

20. Fahn S. Concept and classification of dystonia. *Adv Neurol* 1988;50:1–8.

21. Fahn S. Clinical variants of idiopathic torsion dystonia. *J Neurol Neurosurg Psychiatry Special Supplement* 1989;96–100.

22. Fahn S. Motor and vocal tics. In: Kurlan R, ed. *Handbook of Tourette's syndrome and related tic and behavioral disorders.* New York: Marcel Dekker, 1993:3–16.

23. Fahn S. Paroxysmal dyskinesias. In: Marsden CD, Fahn S, eds. *Movement disorders 3.* Oxford: Butterworth-Heineman, 1994:310–345.

24. Fahn S. Medical treatment of dystonia. In: Tsui JJCT, Calne DB, eds. *Handbook of dystonia.* New York: Marcel Dekker, 1995:317–328.

25. Fahn S. Parkinsonism. In: Rowland LP, ed. *Merritt's textbook of neurology,* 9th ed. Baltimore: Williams & Wilkins, 1995:713–730.

26. Fahn S, Marsden CD, Calne DB. Classification and investigation of dystonia. In: Marsden CD, Fahn S, eds. *Movement disorders 2.* London: Butterworths, 1987: 332–358.

27. Fahn S, Sjaastad O. Hereditary essential myoclonus in a large Norwegian family. *Mov Disord* 1991;6:237–247.

28. Feigin A, Kieburtz K, Bordwell K, et al. Functional decline in Huntington's disease. *Mov Disord* 1995;10: 211–214.

29. Fish DR, Marsden CD. Epilepsy masquerading as a movement disorder. In: Marsden CD, Fahn S, eds. *Movement disorders 3.* Oxford: Butterworth-Heineman, 1994:346–358.

30. Fletcher NA, Harding AE, Marsden CD. A genetic study of idiopathic torsion dystonia in the United Kingdom. *Brain* 1990;113:379–395.

31. Greene P, Kang UJ, Fahn S. Spread of symptoms in idiopathic torsion dystonia. *Mov Disord* 1995;10:143–152.

32. Hyland K, Surtees RAH, Rodeck C, Clayton PT. Aromatic L-amino acid decarboxylase deficiency: clinical features, diagnosis, and treatment of a new inborn error of neurotransmitter amine synthesis. *Neurology* 1992;42:1980–1988.

33. Ichinose H, Ohye T, Takahashi E, et al. Hereditary progressive dystonia with marked diurnal fluctuation caused by mutations in the GTP cyclohydrolase I gene. *Nat Genet* 1994;8:236–242.

34. Kang UJ, Burke RE, Fahn S. Natural history and treatment of tardive dystonia. *Mov Disord* 1986;1:193–208.

35. Knappskog PM, Flatmark T, Mallet J, Ludecke B, Bartholome K. Recessively inherited L-dopa-responsive dystonia caused by a point mutation (Q381K) in the tyrosine hydroxylase gene. *Hum Mol Genet* 1995; 4:1209–1212.

36. Kramer PL, Heiman GA, Gasser T, et al. The DYT1 gene on 9q34 is responsible for most cases of early limb-onset idiopathic torsion dystonia in non-Jews. *Am J Hum Genet* 1994;55:468–475.

37. Kurlan R, Behr J, Medved L, Shoulson I. Myoclonus and dystonia: a family study. *Adv Neurol* 1988;50: 385–389.

38. Leube B, Rudnicki D, Ratzlaff T, Kessler KR, Benecke R, Auburger G. Idiopathic torsion dystonia: assignment of a gene to chromosome 18p in a German family with adult onset, autosomal dominant inheritance and purely focal distribution. *Hum Mol Genet* 1996;5:1673–1677.

39. Ludecke B, Knappskog PM, Clayton PT, et al. Recessively inherited L-dopa-responsive parkinsonism in infancy caused by a point mutation (L205P) in the tyrosine hydroxylase gene. *Hum Mol Genet* 1996;5: 1023–1028.

40. Marsden CD, Harrison MJG, Bundey S. Natural history of idiopathic torsion dystonia. *Adv Neurol* 1976; 14:177–187.

41. Nygaard TG, Marsden CD, Duvoisin RC. Dopa-responsive dystonia. *Adv Neurol* 1988;50:377–384.

42. Nygaard TG, Trugman JM, de Yebenes JG, Fahn S. Dopa-responsive dystonia: the spectrum of clinical manifestations in a large North American family. *Neurology* 1990;40:66–69.

43. Nygaard TG, Wilhelmsen KC, Risch NJ, et al. Linkage mapping of dopa-responsive dystonia (DRD) to chromosome 14q. *Nat Genet* 1993;5:386–391.

44. Obeso JA, Rothwell JC, Lang AE, Marsden CD. Myoclonic dystonia. *Neurology* 1983;33:825–830.

45. Oppenheim H. Uber eine eigenartige Krampfkrankheit des kindlichen und jugendlichen Alters (Dysbasia lordotica progressiva, dystonia musculorum deformans). *Neurol Centrabl* 1911;30:1090–1107.

46. Pentchev PG, Coml ME, Kruth HS, et al. A defect in cholesterol esterification in Niemann-Pick disease (type C) patients. *Proc Natl Acad Sci USA* 1985;82: 8247–8251.

47. Quinn NP. Essential myoclonus and myoclonic dystonia. *Mov Disord* 1996;11:119–124.

48. Quinn NP, Rothwell JC, Thompson PD, Marsden CD. Hereditary myoclonic dystonia, hereditary torsion dystonia and hereditary essential myoclonus: an area of confusion. *Adv Neurol* 1988;50:391–401.

49. Rajput AH, Gibb WRG, Zhong XH, et al. DOPA-responsive dystonia: pathological and biochemical observations in a case. *Ann Neurol* 1994;35:396–402.

50. Risch N, Bressman SB, de Leon D, et al. Segregation analysis of idiopathic torsion dystonia in Ashkenazi Jews suggests autosomal dominant inheritance. *Am J Hum Genet* 1990;46:533–538.

51. Segawa M, Hosaka A, Miyagawa F, Nomura Y, Imai H. Hereditary progressive dystonia with marked diurnal fluctuation. *Adv Neurol* 1976;14:215–233.

52. Segawa M, Ohmi K, Itoh S, Aoyama M, Hayakawa H. Childhood basal ganglia disease with remarkable response to L-dopa, "hereditary basal ganglia disease with marked diurnal fluctuation." *Shinryo* (Therapy-Tokyo) 1971;24:667–672.

53. Wahlstrom J, Ozelius L, Kramer P, et al. The gene for familial dystonia with myoclonic jerks responsive to alcohol is not located on the distal end of 9q. *Clin Genet* 1994;45:88–92.

54. Waters CH, Faust PL, Powers J, et al. Neuropathology of Lubag (X-linked dystonia-parkinsonism). *Mov Disord* 1993;8:387–390.

55. Waters CH, Takahashi H, Wilhelmsen KC, et al. Phenotypic expression of X-linked dystonia-parkinsonism (lubag) in two women. *Neurology* 1993;43:1555–1558.

56. Yanagisawa N, Goto A. Dystonia musculorum deformans: analysis with electromyography. *J Neurol Sci* 1971;13:39–65.

57. Yanagisawa N, Goto A, Narabayashi H. Familial dystonia musculorum deformans and tremor. *J Neurol Sci* 1972;16:125–136.

58. Zeman W, Kaelbling R, Pasamanick B. Idiopathic dystonia musculorum deformans. II. The formes frustes. *Neurology* 1960;10:1068–1075.

Dystonia 3: Advances in Neurology, Vol. 78,
edited by S. Fahn, C. D. Marsden, and M. DeLong.
Lippincott–Raven Publishers, Philadelphia © 1998.

2

Physiology of Dystonia

Mark Hallett

NINDS, Bethesda, Maryland 20892.

How the central nervous system produces the dramatic motor abnormalities in dystonia has been mysterious. It seems appropriate to start by looking at the involuntary movements themselves. A number of observations over many years have shown that dystonic movements are characterized by an abnormal pattern of electromyographic (EMG) activity with co-contraction of antagonist muscles and overflow into extraneous muscles. Cohen and Hallett (12) reported detailed observations on 19 patients with focal dystonias of the hand, including writer's cramp and cramp in piano, guitar, clarinet, and organ players. Five features, identified by physiologic investigation, were indicative of impaired motor control. The first was co-contraction, which could be in the form of a brief burst or continuous. In repetitive alternating movements at a single joint, antagonist muscles typically alternate firing. The dystonia patients might co-contract even with such quick movements. The second feature was prolongation of EMG bursts. In movements made as quickly as possible, EMG bursts normally last no longer than about 100 milliseconds. The patients had bursts of 200 or 300 milliseconds as well as very prolonged spasms. A third feature was tremor. A fourth was lack of selectivity in attempts to perform independent finger movements. The fifth feature was occasional failure of willed activity to occur. Rothwell and colleagues (52) reasoned that the important problem of excessive co-contraction could be due to deficient reciprocal inhibition, a funda-mental process represented at multiple levels of the central nervous system.

SPINAL AND BRAINSTEM REFLEXES

Reciprocal inhibition is represented even in the spinal cord and can be studied as a spinal reflex. Reciprocal inhibition can be evaluated in humans by studying the effect of stimulating the radial nerve at various times prior to producing an H-reflex with median nerve stimulation. The radial nerve afferents come from muscles that are antagonist to median nerve muscles. Via various pathways, the radial afferent traffic can inhibit motoneuron pools of median nerve muscles. Normal subjects show three periods of inhibition, reaching peaks at delays of 0, 10, and 75 milliseconds. The first period of inhibition is caused by disynaptic Ia inhibition, the second period of inhibition is explained as a presynaptic inhibition, and, unfortunately, very little is known about the third period of inhibition, but the long latency (75 to 200 milliseconds) requires a polysynaptic pathway. The first relative facilitation (at about 2-millisecond delay) is a function of Ib fiber actions, and indirect evidence indicates that the second facilitation (at about 50-millisecond delay) can be a function of cutaneous group II action. Reciprocal inhibition is reduced in patients with dystonia, including those with generalized dystonia, writer's cramp, spasmodic torticollis, and blepharospasm (11,14,38,43, 44,52). In the studies of Panizza et al. (43,44) and Chen et al. (11), reduction of inhibition is seen in all three periods, and in similar studies of Rothwell et al. (52) and Nakashima et al. (38) the first period was normal, whereas the second period was reduced (the third period was not studied). It should be noted that reciprocal inhibition can be abnormal even in asymptomatic arms, as in the situation of blepharospasm. In patients with generalized dystonia and spasmodic torticollis, the third period of inhibition was converted from inhibition to potentiation, an inversion of a physiologic phenomenon.

Other spinal and brainstem reflexes have been studied, and a common result is that inhibitory processes are reduced. Another example that has been extensively studied is the blink reflex. Abnormalities of blink reflexes were first identified for blepharospasm (3). In this disorder, eyelid closure can be spontaneous, but is often aggravated by light or somatosensory stimulation around the eyes, implicating involvement of reflex mechanisms. EMG of orbicularis oculi during a spasm, as in other dystonias, shows an interference pattern of activity similar to a voluntary contraction that typically lasts 200 milliseconds or more. The blink reflex obtained in the usual manner in patients with dystonia appears normal with normal latencies of the R1 and R2 components (although the R2 may seem large in amplitude or duration), but there are clear abnormalities with the blink reflex recovery cycle. In normal subjects, if a second blink reflex is produced at an interval of less than 3 seconds after a first blink reflex, the R2 component of the second blink reflex is reduced in amplitude compared with that of the first blink reflex. The amount of inhibition is proportional to the interval between the two stimuli for production of the blink reflexes. The curve relating the amplitude of the second R2 to the interval between the stimuli is called the *blink reflex recovery cycle*. Normal values can be determined, and patients with blepharospasm show less inhibition than normal. Abnormalities of blink reflex recovery have been demonstrated also in generalized dystonia, spasmodic torticollis, and spasmodic dysphonia (13). In the last two conditions, ab-

normalities can be found even without clinical involvement of the eyelids. Similarly, abnormalities are seen with perioral reflexes (56) and exteroceptive silent periods (39).

Several observations, therefore, suggest that reduction of spinal cord and brainstem inhibition is an important mechanism in dystonia. Superficially, this would seem to be a good explanation for co-contraction in voluntary movement and increased tone in this disorder. The fundamental disturbance, however, would more likely be an abnormal supraspinal command signal than disordered spinal circuitry.

From a clinical point of view, it is noteworthy that these reflexes may help with the diagnosis of dystonia. Abnormalities may be seen outside the clinically involved territory. For example, an abnormality in blink reflex recovery may be seen in a patient with spasmodic torticollis even without blepharospasm.

An important difficulty to keep in mind is that reduction in inhibition is not limited to patients with dystonia. Abnormalities of blink reflex and reciprocal inhibition are also seen in Parkinson's disease (33). The similarity of reflex behavior in dystonia and Parkinson's disease parallels many clinical similarities. Both have increased tone and bradykinesia, and, indeed, many times it is difficult to tell the diseases apart. Some patients can present with an apparent mild dystonia and go on to more obvious Parkinson's disease. Perhaps it is not strange that there are physiologic similarities. On the other hand, the physiology is clearly not identical. For example, there are clear differences in long-latency stretch reflex behavior, since the amplitude of these reflexes is increased in Parkinson's disease and normal in dystonia (53).

SENSORY DYSFUNCTION

Although we think of dystonia as a movement disorder, there are a number of phenomena relating to the sensory system that might suggest that dystonia could be primarily a sensory disorder (21). Sensory tricks can relieve a dystonic spasm. The most commonly noted is the *geste antagonistique* in spasmodic torticollis where, for example, a finger placed lightly on the face will neutralize the spasm. Such tricks are seen in all forms of dystonia. Pressure on the eyelids might improve blepharospasm, a toothpick in the mouth might relieve tongue dystonia, and sensation applied to parts of the arm might improve a writer's cramp. The physiology of sensory tricks is unknown.

Sensory symptoms may well precede the appearance of dystonia. By attending to this issue carefully, Ghika et al. (18) found that sensory symptoms were present in 11 successive patients with cranial dystonia. Symptoms included ill-defined pain, discomfort, distortion of sensation, and "phantom" kinetic or postural sensations. Common examples would be a gritty sensation in the eye preceding blepharospasm and irritation of the throat preceding spasmodic dysphonia. Photophobia is an example of distorted sensation. In none of the cases, however, could the investigators find an objective substrate. In some cases, their patients said that they made voluntary repetitive movements in order to relieve the sensory symptom, but the movements eventually got out of voluntary control.

Abnormal sensory input might well be a trigger for dystonia. Trauma to a body part is often a precedent to dystonia of that part (28). A blow to the head might precede torticollis, irritations of the eye are common in blepharospasm, and a deep cut of the hand might occur just before writer's cramp develops. Such trauma might also cause a syndrome of pain and sympathetic changes, controversially called *reflex sympathetic dystrophy* (RSD). Dystonia can be a feature of RSD. Even when trauma is not grossly apparent it may play a role. Repeated use of a body part, such as frequent writing, might be a precedent of dystonia of that part, such as writer's cramp. Frequent use can lead to trauma, sometimes painful and appreciated as the overuse syndrome. The relationship between the overuse syndrome and dystonia is not clear, but this feature may suggest that frequent movement may lead to dystonia via a sensory mechanism.

There may be an important problem with the processing of muscle spindle input. In patients with hand cramps, vibration can induce the patient's dystonia (30). Vibration activates many types of sensory fibers, but is particularly potent for Ia spindle afferents. In normal subjects, muscle vibration may cause a contraction of the muscle vibrated. This phenomenon, called the *tonic vibration reflex* (TVR), is a polysynaptic spinal cord reflex. In patients, the typical pattern of the action dystonia is reproduced by the vibration. Cutaneous input similar to that which produces the sensory trick can reverse the vibration-induced dystonia. Conversely, both action-induced and vibration-induced dystonia can be improved with lidocaine block of the muscle. Lidocaine's action is likely to be block of the gamma motor neurons, relaxation of the muscle spindles, and reduction in afferent discharge. Vibration induces presynaptic inhibition as well as the TVR. Because there is evidence for reduction of presynaptic inhibition from the reciprocal inhibition studies, this could explain how the TVR might be pathologically increased in dystonia. A possible conclusion is that spindle activity may play a special role in the neural networks that produce dystonia. On the other hand, vibration may improve spasmodic torticollis (32). Additionally, facial muscles do not have any muscle spindles (or, at most, very few), and the face is certainly subject to dystonia. Thus, muscle spindle afferent activity may not be always bad or even relevant.

The brain response to somatosensory input is abnormal in dystonia. Tempel and Perlmutter (54,55) have examined the rCBF response to vibration of the hand in patients with hand dystonia. Both the response in the primary sensory cortex region and the supplementary motor area (SMA) region was diminished compared with that of normal subjects. The somatosensory evoked potentials (SEPs) to median nerve stimulation may be abnormal in some late components. In particular, the amplitude of the N30 has been shown to be increased in some patients with hand dystonia whereas its latency and topography are normal (49). The N30 component of the median nerve SEP is a variable component with a controversial site of origin. It is clearly influenced by motor behavior and in most studies, is decreased in amplitude in patients with Parkinson's disease. Some other studies have also found an increased N30, whereas others have found it normal. For example, Nardone et al. (40) found a normal N30 in patients with spasmodic torticollis (although it must be noted that these patients have no apparent upper limb involvement). Using a very slow rate of stimulation, Grissom et al. (19) have found a decrease in the N30 in patients with focal hand dystonia. Studies of sensory receptive fields of neurons in the thalamus in humans with dystonia show expanded regions where cells all respond to the same passive movement (34).

A possible animal model of dystonia has been created in nonhuman primates who have experienced simultaneous sensory stimulation to the hand (4). Two adult owl monkeys were trained at a behavioral task that required them to maintain an attended grasp on a hand grip that repetitively opened and closed. The animals performed 300 trials per day, and over a period of months, the motor performance deteriorated. Although there was no task specificity and no involuntary muscle spasms, there was a definite motor dysfunction. After the development of the movement disorder, the primary somatosensory cortex was mapped with microelectrode recording. Receptive fields in area 3b were 10 to 20 times larger than normal, and many receptive fields emerged that extended across the surface of two or more digits, a phenomenon not seen in normal monkeys. A similar motor problem with altered sensory maps was seen in monkeys with a largely passive sensory task (58). These findings have led to the concept that synchronous sensory input over a large area of the hand can lead to remapping of the receptive fields and subsequently to a movement disorder. Of course, it can be noted that these tasks also have repetitive movements and such movements can lead to remapping of the motor system (45).

A recent study has even suggested some elemental sensory deficits in patients with hand dystonia (5). Graphesthesia and stereognosis were abnormal bilaterally even though the dystonia was unilateral. On the other hand, finger identification, localization of sensory stimuli, and kinesthesia were normal.

It is difficult to put all these clues about sensory dysfunction together, but since the sensory system is the primary driver of the motor system, it is clearly important to keep all these findings in mind.

CORTICAL MOTOR DYSFUNCTION

There are a number of defined abnormalities of the cortical motor system. Movement-related cortical potentials associated with self-paced finger movement in patients with hand dystonia show deficiency of the NS' component (thought to be generated in the motor cortex) (15). A focal abnormality of the contralateral central region was confirmed with an analysis of event-related desynchronization of the electroencephalogram (EEG) prior to movement, which showed a localized deficiency in dysynchronization of beta frequency activity (57). These results are consistent with a reduced excitability of the primary sensorimotor region.

Feve et al. (17) studied movement-related cortical potentials in patients with symptomatic dystonia including patients with lesions in the striatum, pallidum, and thalamus. With bilateral lesions, patients showed deficient gradients for the bereitschaftspotential and NS' bilaterally and lack of vertex predominance for the bereitschaftspotential and contralateral predominance for NS'. With unilateral lesions, the problem was worse for the symptomatic hand. These results confirm a reduced excitability of primary sensorimotor cortex, but are more extensive than what Deuschl et al. (15) found for their more mildly affected patients with idiopathic dystonia.

The contingent negative variation (CNV) is the EEG potential that appears between a warning and a go stimulus in a reaction time task. The CNV shows deficient late negativity with head turning in patients with torticollis (29) and for hand movement in patients with writer's cramp (25). The late negativity represents motor function similar to the movement-related cortical potential.

Ceballos-Baumann et al. (7) have studied voluntary movement in patients with dystonia using blood flow positron emission tomography (PET). The motor task was a freely chosen direction of joystick movement with pacing tones every 3 seconds. Depressed activity compared with normal was seen in caudal supplementary area (SMA) and bilateral primary sensorimotor cortex. (The location of caudal SMA was −26 mm, further back than its usual position.) Significant overactivity compared with normal was seen in many sites including the contralateral premotor cortex, the rostral SMA (or pre-SMA), the anterior cingulate area, the ipsilateral dorsolateral prefrontal cortex, and the contralateral lentiform nucleus (primarily the putamen). Preliminary studies by this same group with handwriting in patients with focal hand dystonia have produced similar results (8).

Ibanez (24) has looked at several manual tasks in patients with focal hand dystonia using blood flow PET. There was a normal pattern with simple finger tapping. With a strong sustained contraction, dystonic patients showed deficient rCBF in the contralateral sensorimotor area. With handwriting, there was deficient rCBF of the premotor cortex bilaterally, both the rostral and caudal SMA, and the anterior cingulate cortex.

On the other hand, studies with transcranial magnetic stimulation (TMS) show increased excitability of motor cortex (27). There was no change in the motor threshold, nor was there any abnormality of the motor evoked potential (MEP) size with increase in the level of background contraction. There was, however, an abnormal increase in the MEP size with increasing stimulus intensity. Ikoma et al. (26) have also found enlarged motor maps for dystonic muscles.

Inhibition in motor cortex is also deficient in patients with hand dystonia. Ridding et al. (50) studied intracortical inhibition with the "double pulse paradigm." MEPs are inhibited when conditioned by a prior subthreshold TMS stimulus to the same position at intervals of 1 to 5 milliseconds. Inhibition was less in both hemispheres of patients with focal hand dystonia.

Inhibition can also be evaluated with double pulses at longer intervals with the muscle under study either at rest or contracted. Chen et al. (10) investigated this type of inhibition in patients with writer's cramp and found a deficiency only in the symptomatic hand and only with background contraction. This abnormality is particularly interesting since it is restricted to the symptomatic setting, as opposed to many other physiologic abnormalities in dystonia that are more generalized.

Chen et al. (10) also found that the silent period following an MEP was slightly shorter for the symptomatic hemisphere in patients with focal hand dystonia. A nonsignificant trend had been seen by Ikoma et al. (27) earlier. This also indicates a deficiency of inhibition.

Summarizing the motor pathophysiology, there is a decrease in amplitude of the movement-related cortical potential and CNV and a decrease in blood flow with voluntary movement in motor cortex and premotor cortex. On the other hand, there is increased excitability of the motor cortex to TMS demonstrated by increased MEP amplitudes, increased MEP map size, decreased inhibition, and a shortened silent period. How to link these motor abnormalities into a coherent theory is not certain. One possible speculation is that the motor cortex is hyperexcitable and that the deficient activation with movement is a compensation. Another possibility is that the deficiencies recognized by the EEG and PET studies are deficiencies of inhibition rather than deficiencies of excitation. This would easily explain the increased motor cortex excitability and be a suitable explanation for the excessive movement seen in patients with dystonia.

The hypothesis of lack of inhibition in the cortex is interestingly compatible with the earlier conclusion made about the spinal cord and brainstem where lack of inhibition appears to be the primary disturbance.

HOW THE BASAL GANGLIA CAN BE RESPONSIBLE

Although defective functioning of the cortex is a likely mechanism for the motor disturbance in dystonia, it is unlikely that the primary abnormality is in the cortex. Considerable evidence from secondary dystonia suggests the primary abnormality is in the basal ganglia circuitry. Lesions in the putamen, caudate, and thalamus can give rise to dystonia (2, 36,47). We also know from the entity of dopa-responsive dystonia that dopamine deficiency in the basal ganglia can lead to dystonia, at least at an early age.

PET has been used to try to find abnormalities of metabolism in the brain of patients without known lesions. Findings using glucose metabolism of patients at rest have been difficult to interpret because the abnormalities have not been reproducible. For example, some studies report an increased metabolism in the striatum (9), some a decrease (31), and others no change (42). Using a principal components method, there is some evidence for a relative putaminal hypermetabolism (16).

Using imaging to assess dopamine and dopamine receptors, three preliminary studies concur that there is a loss of D2 receptors in the putamen (23,41,46). The meaning of this is not clear, but it could indicate that there is a reduction in the influence of the indirect pathway.

The basal ganglia can influence the motor system by its two output pathways from the internal division of the globus pallidus (GPi). One goes to the thalamus and then to the cortex. The other goes to the brainstem and spinal cord via the pedunculopontine nucleus (PPN). The output of the GPi to the thalamus is inhibitory, and the thalamocortical output is excitatory. The full effect of the basal ganglia upon the cortex is not known, but there is some evidence that the basal ganglia do affect cortical inhibition.

The first line of evidence of basal ganglia influence on inhibition is the effect of basal ganglia disorders on the silent period following TMS. In Parkinson's disease the silent period is shorter than normal and can be improved with dopaminergic treatment (6,48). In Huntington's disease, the silent period is longer than normal (51). Moreover, the clinical assessment of amount of chorea correlates with silent period length. The second line of evidence is the

dopaminergic control of short interval, intracortical inhibition. Bromocriptine given to normal subjects will increase the amount of inhibition (59).

It is not unreasonable to think, therefore, that if cortical inhibition is diminished in dystonia the basal ganglia could be responsible.

A SPECULATION ABOUT THE PATHOPHYSIOLOGY

In order to have a clear understanding of the pathophysiology, it is necessary to know the normal role of the basal ganglia in movement, and this is not well known. A model that I have advocated, which continues to have heuristic value, proposes that the function of the basal ganglia motor circuit is to help in the process of selection and inhibition of specific motor synergies to carry out a desired action (20,22). The direct path is select and the indirect path is to inhibit these synergies. The circuitry acts to enhance one motor action and inhibit others similar to the process of surround inhibition in sensory systems. This idea of center-surround organization was one of the possible functions of the basal ganglia circuitry suggested by Alexander and Crutcher (1).

Theoretical considerations (20) and animal models (37) have suggested that overactivity of the direct pathway might play a role. Eidelberg et al. (16) have interpreted their PET findings in the same way. Overactivity of the direct pathway should lead to excessive activation of the cortex. On the other hand, underactivity of the indirect pathway, suggested for example by the loss of D2 receptors, could also lead to excessive cortical activation. Another way of looking at it would be an imbalance of the two pathways in the direction of underactivity of the indirect pathway.

A net underactivity of indirect pathway influence has appeal for an explanation of dystonia for several reasons. First, it could result from a lesion of the basal ganglia. Second, it could result from a deficit of dopamine, thereby explaining dopa-responsive dystonia and the physiologic similarities between dystonia and Parkinson's disease. Third, considering a possible role for the indirect pathway in control of surround inhibition, loss of this type of inhibition should lead to overflow of the movement command, which is a principal characteristic of dystonic movement. Thus, surround inhibition would be diminished in the GPi, and this in turn would lead to loss of inhibition both at the cortical level and brainstem and spinal cord (the latter potentially via the PPN route).

Fourth, if dystonia results from loss of inhibition, then there is a way of thinking about how dystonia results in a number of different circumstances. There can be a significant loss of inhibition caused by genetic makeup or a brain lesion that will inevitably lead to dystonia. There can be a genetic tendency to loss of inhibition that can be pushed over the edge by some environmental factor such as repetitive exposure to a sensory stimulus or repetitive action. Both sensory and motor repetition lead to larger cortical representation areas, and at least in some circumstances this is mediated by a reduction in inhibition (35). Thus, the normal processes of brain plasticity may be pushed too far, and dystonia may result.

ACKNOWLEDGMENTS

Some of the material in this chapter has been modified from previous reviews (20,21).

REFERENCES

1. Alexander GE, Crutcher MD. Functional architecture of basal ganglia circuits: neural substrates of parallel processing. *Trends Neurosci* 1990;13:266–271.
2. Bathia KP, Marsden CD. The behavioural and motor consequences of focal lesions of the basal ganglia in man. *Brain* 1994;117:859–876.
3. Berardelli A, Rothwell JC, Day BL, Marsden CD. Pathophysiology of blepharospasm and oromandibular dystonia. *Brain* 1985;108:593–608.
4. Byl N, Merzenich MM, Jenkins WM. A primate genesis model of focal dystonia and repetitive strain injury: I. Learning-induced dedifferentiation of the representation of the hand in the primary somatosensory cortex in adult monkeys. *Neurology* 1996;47:508–520.
5. Byl N, Wilson F, Merzenich MM, et al. Sensory dysfunction associated with repetitive strain injuries of tendinitis and focal hand dystonia: a comparative study. *J Orthop Sports Phys Ther* 1996;23:234–244.
6. Cantello R, Gianelli M, Bettucci D, Civardi C, De Angelis MS, Mutani R. Parkinson's disease rigidity: mag-

netic motor evoked potentials in small hand muscles. *Neurology* 1991;41:1449–1456.
7. Cebellos-Baumann AO, Passingham RE, Warner T, Playford ED, Marsden CD, Brooks DJ. Overactive prefrontal and underactive motor cortical areas in idiopathic dystonia. *Ann Neurol* 1995;37:363–372.
8. Cebellos-Baumann AO, Sheean G, Passingham RE, Marsden CD, Brooks DJ. Botulinum toxin does not reverse the cortical dysfunction associated with writer's cramp. A PET study. *Brain* 1997; 120:571–582
9. Chase TN, Tamminga CA, Burrows H. Positron emission tomographic studies of regional cerebral glucose metabolism in idiopathic dystonia. *Adv Neurol* 1988; 50:237–241.
10. Chen R, Wassermann EM, Hallett M. Impairment of cortical inhibition in focal dystonia. *Ann Neurol* 1996; 40:536.
11. Chen RS, Tsai CH, Lu CS. Reciprocal inhibition in writer's cramp. *Mov Disord* 1995;10:556–561.
12. Cohen LG, Hallett M. Hand cramps: clinical features and electromyographic patterns in a focal dystonia. *Neurology* 1988;38:1005–1012.
13. Cohen LG, Ludlow CL, Warden M, et al. Blink reflex excitability recovery curves in patients with spasmodic dysphonia. *Neurology* 1989;39:572–577.
14. Deuschl G, Seifert G, Heinen F, Illert M, Lücking CH. Reciprocal inhibition of forearm flexor muscles in spasmodic torticollis. *J Neurol Sci* 1992;113:85– 90.
15. Deuschl G, Toro C, Matsumoto J, Hallett M. Movement-related cortical potentials in writer's cramp. *Ann Neurol* 1995;38:862–868.
16. Eidelberg D, Moeller JR, Ishikawa T, et al. The metabolic topography of idiopathic torsion dystonia. *Brain* 1995;118:1473–1484.
17. Feve A, Bathien N, Rondot P. Abnormal movement related potentials in patients with lesions of basal ganglia and anterior thalamus. *J Neurol Neurosurg Psychiatry* 1994;57:100–104.
18. Ghika J, Regli F, Growdon JH. Sensory symptoms in cranial dystonia: a potential role in the etiology? *J Neurol Sci* 1993;116:142–147.
19. Grissom J, Toro C, Trettau J, Hallett M. The N30 and N140-P190 median somatosensory evoked potential waveforms in dystonia involving the upper extremity. *Neurology* 1995;45[Suppl 4]:A458.
20. Hallett M. Physiology of basal ganglia disorders: an overview. *Can J Neurol Sci* 1993;20:177–183.
21. Hallett M. Is dystonia a sensory disorder? *Ann Neurol* 1995;38:139–140.
22. Hallett M, Khoshbin S. A physiological mechanism of bradykinesia. *Brain* 1980;103:301–314.
23. Horstink CA, Booij J, Berger HJC, van Royen EA, Horstink MWIM. Striatal D2 receptor loss in writer's cramp. *Mov Disord* 1996;11[Suppl 1]:209.
24. Ibanez V, Sadato N, Karp B, Deiber M-P, Hallett M. Investigation of cortical activity in writer's cramp patients: a PET study. *Neurology* 1996;46[Suppl 2]: A260.
25. Ikeda A, Shibasaki H, Kaji R, et al. Abnormal sensorimotor integration in writer's cramp: study of contingent negative variation. *Mov Disord* 1996;11:638– 690.
26. Ikoma K, Samii A, Mercuri B, Wassermann EM, Hallett M. Mapping of motor cortex by transcranial magnetic stimulation in dystonia. *Electroencephalogr Clin Neurophysiol* 1995;97:S194.

27. Ikoma K, Samii A, Mercuri B, Wassermann EM, Hallett M. Abnormal cortical motor excitability in dystonia. *Neurology* 1996;46:1371–1376.

28. Jankovic J. Post-traumatic movement disorders: central and peripheral mechanisms. *Neurology* 1994;44: 2006–2014.

29. Kaji R, Ikeda A, Ikeda T, et al. Physiological study of cervical dystonia. Task-specific abnormality in contingent negative variation. *Brain* 1995;118:511–522.

30. Kaji R, Rothwell JC, Katayama M, et al. Tonic vibration reflex and muscle afferent block in writer's cramp: implications for a new therapeutic approach. *Ann Neurol* 1995;38:155–162.

31. Karbe H, Holthoff VA, Rudolf J, Herholz K, Heiss WD. Positron emission tomography demonstrates frontal cortex and basal ganglia hypometabolism in dystonia. *Neurology* 1992;42:1540–1544.

32. Leis AA, Dimitrijevic MR, Delapasse JS, Sharkey PC. Modification of cervical dystonia by selective sensory stimulation. *J Neurol Sci* 1992;110:79–89.

33. Lelli S, Panizza M, Hallett M. Spinal cord inhibitory mechanisms in Parkinson's disease. *Neurology* 1991; 41:553–556.

34. Lenz FA, Seike SE, Jaeger CJ, et al. Single neuron analysis of thalamic activity in patients with dystonia. *J Neurophysiol,* submitted.

35. Liepert J, Classen J, Cohen L, Hallett M. Task-dependent changes of intracortical inhibition. *Exp Brain Res* 1998; 118:421–426.

36. Marsden CD, Obeso JA, Zarranz JJ, Lang AE. The anatomical basis of symptomatic hemidystonia. *Brain* 1985;108:463–483.

37. Mitchell IJ, Luquin R, Boyce S, et al. Neural mechanisms of dystonia: evidence from a 2-deoxyglucose uptake study in a primate model of dopamine agonist-induced dystonia. *Mov Disord* 1990;5:49–54.

38. Nakashima K, Rothwell JC, Day BL, Thompson PD, Shannon K, Marsden CD. Reciprocal inhibition in writer's and other occupational cramps and hemiparesis due to stroke. *Brain* 1989;112:681–697.

39. Nakashima K, Thompson PD, Rothwell JC, Day BL, Stell R, Marsden CD. An exteroceptive reflex in the sternocleidomastoid muscle produced by electrical stimulation of the supraorbital nerve in normal subjects and patients with spasmodic torticollis. *Neurology* 1989;39:1354–1358.

40. Mazzini L, Zaccala M, Balzarini C. Abnormalities of somatosensory-evoked potentials in spasmodic torticollis. *Mov Disord* 1994; 9:426–430

41. Naumann M, Pirker W, Reiners K, Brücke T. Imaging the pre- and postsynaptic side of striatal dopaminergic synapses in idiopathic focal dystonia: a SPECT study using β-CIT and epidepride. *Mov Disord* 1996;11 [Suppl 1]:206.

42. Otsuka M, Ichiya Y, Shima F, et al. Increased striatal 18F-dopa uptake and normal glucose metabolism in idiopathic dystonia syndrome. *J Neurol Sci* 1992;111: 195–199.

43. Panizza M, Lelli S, Nilsson J, Hallett M. H-reflex recovery curve and reciprocal inhibition of H-reflex in different kinds of dystonia. *Neurology* 1990;40:824–828.

44. Panizza ME, Hallett M, Nilsson J. Reciprocal inhibition in patients with hand cramps. *Neurology* 1989; 39:85–89.

45. Pascual-Leone A, Cammarota A, Wassermann EM, Brasil-Neto JP, Cohen LG, Hallett M. Modulation of motor cortical outputs to the reading hand of Braille readers. *Ann Neurol* 1993;34:33–37.

46. Perlmutter JS, Stambuck M, Markham J, Moerlein S. Quantified binding of [F18]spiperone in focal dystonia. *J Neurosci* 1997; 17:843–850.

47. Pettigrew LC, Jankovic J. Hemidystonia: a report of 22 patients and review of the literature. *J Neurol Neurosurg Psychiatry* 1985;48:650–657.

48. Priori A, Berardelli A, Inghilleri M, Accornero N, Manfredi M. Motor cortical inhibition and the dopaminergic system. Pharmacological changes in the silent period after transcranial brain stimulation in normal subjects, patients with Parkinson's disease and drug-induced parkinsonism. *Brain* 1994;117:317–323.

49. Reilly JA, Hallett M, Cohen LG, Tarkka IM, Dang N. The N30 component of somatosensory evoked potentials in patients with dystonia. *Electroencephalogr Clin Neurophysiol* 1992;84:243–247.

50. Ridding MC, Sheean G, Rothwell JC, Inzelberg R, Kujirai T. Changes in the balance between motor cortical excitation and inhibition in focal, task specific dystonia. *J Neurol Neurosurg Psychiatr* 1995;59:493–498.

51. Roick H, Giesen HJ, Lang HW, Benecke R. Postexcitatory inhibition in Huntington's disease. *Mov Disord* 1992;7:27.

52. Rothwell JC, Obeso JA, Day BL, Marsden CD. Pathophysiology of dystonias. *Adv Neurol* 1983;39:851–863.

53. Tatton WG, Bedingham W, Verrier MC, Blair RD. Characteristic alterations in responses to imposed wrist displacements in parkinsonian rigidity and dystonia musculorum deformans. *Can J Neurol Sci* 1984;11:281–287.

54. Tempel LW, Perlmutter JS. Abnormal vibration-induced cerebral blood flow responses in idiopathic dystonia. *Brain* 1990;113:691–707.

55. Tempel LW, Perlmutter JS. Abnormal cortical responses in patients with writer's cramp. *Neurology* 1993;43:2252–2257.

56. Topka H, Hallett M. Perioral reflexes in orofacial dyskinesia and spasmodic dysphonia. *Muscle Nerve* 1992;15:1016–1022.

57. Toro C, Deuschl G, Hallett M. Movement-related EEG desynchronization in patients with hand cramps: evidence for cortical involvement in focal dystonia. *Neurology* 1993;43[Suppl 2]:A379.

58. Wang X, Merzenich MM, Sameshima K, Jenkins WM. Remodelling of hand representation in adult cortex determined by timing of tactile stimulation. *Nature* 1995;378:71–75.

59. Ziemann U, Tergau F, Bruns D, Baudewig J, Paulus W. Changes in human motor cortex excitability induced by dopaminergic and anti-dopaminergic drugs. *Electroencephalogr Clin Neurophysiol* 1997; 105:430–437.

Dystonia 3: Advances in Neurology, Vol. 78,
edited by S. Fahn, C. D. Marsden, and M. DeLong.
Lippincott–Raven Publishers, Philadelphia © 1998.

3

Pathophysiology of Dystonia

Alan R. Crossman and Jonathan M. Brotchie

*School of Biological Sciences, Division of Neuroscience, University of Manchester,
Manchester M13 9PT, United Kingdom.*

Dystonia is the least well understood of all movement disorders associated with the basal ganglia, in terms of the underlying pathophysiology. Dystonia does not fit easily into either the hypokinetic or the dyskinetic category of basal ganglia disorders, but has some features of both. This appears to be something of a paradox, because recent research has shown that hypokinetic and dyskinetic disorders are mediated by quite different mechanisms. It is concluded that it is the precise temporal (and possibly spatial) characteristics of basal ganglia output activity that dictates the appearance of dystonia. It is argued that the best available model in which to study the mechanisms of dystonia is levodopa-induced dystonia in *N*-methyl-4-phenyl-1,2,3,6-tetrahydropyridine (MPTP) primates, and that findings here are likely to have relevance to other forms of dystonia for which no animal models exist. Evidence is reviewed implicating the neuropeptide cotransmitters dynorphin and enkephalin in the generation of dystonia.

Disorders of movement due to basal ganglia dysfunction are a major problem in contemporary neurology with considerable socioeconomic implications. They occur as a consequence of inherited or acquired disease or idiopathic neurodegeneration, or they may be iatrogenic. The spectrum of conditions is extraordinarily diverse, but they are generally categorized into those associated either with poverty of movement and hypertonia (exemplified by Parkinson's disease) or with abnormal involuntary movements (Huntington's disease, levodopa-

induced dyskinesia, ballism). For more than 30 years Parkinson's disease has remained the only condition for which effective, rational treatment has been available based on knowledge of the underlying neurochemical pathology, but even here major problems remain due to the long-term development of complications, such as drug-induced dyskinesias. Recent advances in understanding the neural mechanisms of both akinetic and dyskinetic syndromes, however, have led to the introduction of new treatment strategies for Parkinson's disease and for the complications of therapy.

Of all movement disorders associated with basal ganglia dysfunction, the least well understood, in terms of underlying pathophysiology, is dystonia. There are several reasons for this. One is that the possible mechanisms of dystonia are difficult to conceptualize against the background of current knowledge of basal ganglia function and dysfunction. Dystonia does not fit neatly into either the hypokinetic or the dyskinetic category. Rather, it has features of both. For example, dystonia can be observed in parkinsonian patients in the "off" phase and in other akinetic/rigid syndromes. Patients with dopa-responsive dystonia (Segawa's disease) may have dystonia as the only presenting sign and the pharmacology of this disorder suggests a close mechanistic relationship to Parkinson's disease. On the other hand, dystonia may be observed as part of the dyskinetic syndrome, which develops in many parkinsonian patients as a complication of long-term dopaminergic therapy.

Another factor that inhibits progress is the general lack of good animal models of dystonia of basal ganglia origin, which replicate both the human pathology or precipitating factor and clinical manifestation, in which the neural mechanisms can be investigated experimentally. There are two exceptions: levodopa- or dopamine agonist-induced dystonia and acute dystonic reactions to neuroleptic drugs, although only the former has been subjected to any degree of mechanistic analysis.

It thus appears from the foregoing that dystonia may share pathophysiologic mechanisms in common with both parkinsonism and dyskinesia, although how this can be so is far from clear, in that these are thought to be mediated by quite distinct mechanisms, representing opposite poles of a continuum of dysfunction, as described below.

FUNCTIONAL ANATOMY OF THE BASAL GANGLIA

The basal ganglia consist of the striatum (caudate nucleus and putamen) and globus pallidus (medial and lateral segments) to which there are a number of closely related nuclei of the diencephalon (thalamus, subthalamic nucleus) and mesencephalon (substantia nigra, pedunculopontine nucleus). The striatum may be regarded as the "input" portion of the basal ganglia because it receives the majority of afferents from other regions of the brain, notably the cerebral cortex, thalamus, and substantia nigra pars compacta (SNc). The medial globus pallidus (GPm) and substantia nigra pars reticulata (SNr) are regarded as the "output" regions because they give rise to the majority of fibers projecting to other levels of the neuraxis, principally the thalamus and pedunculopontine nucleus (PPN). The following account of abnormalities in these connections in movement disorders focuses on the GPm, although homologous connections and changes in activity are also thought to exist for the SNr. The striatum gives rise to two distinct inhibitory, GABAergic projections to the globus pallidus: the so-called direct pathway to the GPm and the indirect pathway to the lateral pallidal segment (GPl). Each pathway is associated with specific peptide neuromodulators, dynorphin and substance P being colocalized in the direct pathway and enkephalin in the indirect pathway. The indirect pathway is so called because it permits striatal control of the GPm via the intermediary of the subthalamic nucleus (STN). This structure is itself in receipt of GABAergic pallidosubthalamic fibers from GPl and the origin of excitatory, glutamatergic fibers to the pallidum. Activation of the direct pathway thus inhibits basal ganglia output cells whereas activation of the indirect pathway causes their excitation. The cells of origin of the direct and indirect pathways are apparently under the differential control of the dopaminergic nigrostriatal pathway, such that the direct pathway is excited, and the indirect pathway inhibited, by dopamine. Additionally, a GABAergic connection that links GPl and the output regions of the basal ganglia may be of great functional significance (18).

PATHOPHYSIOLOGY OF PARKINSONISM

Parkinson's disease is an idiopathic neurodegenerative condition characterized by akinesia/bradykinesia, rigidity, and tremor, the principal causative pathology being loss of dopaminergic neurons from the substantia nigra pars compacta. Much of the research in recent years that has led to greater understanding of the pathophysiology of this condition has resulted from the study of primates made parkinsonian by administration of the neurotoxin MPTP and subsequently studied by a wide range of techniques including single unit recording, metabolic mapping, ligand binding, and *in situ* hybridization.

Briefly, dopamine loss in the striatum leads to overactivity of the pathway from the striatum to GPl. This inhibits pallidosubthalamic neurons, causing disinhibition of the subthalamic nucleus. The resulting overactivity of the STN, and consequently of the GPm, inhibits motor thalamus and cerebral motor cortical mechanisms, and possibly the brainstem loco-motor region (including PPN). Furthermore, underactivity of the intrinsic GPl-GPm connection would further increase activity of GPm. This effect via the indirect pathway is thought to be exacerbated by a simultaneous decrease in activity of the direct pathway, causing decreased GABAergic inhibition of the GPm. Based on this conceptual model of parkinsonism, new treatment strategies are currently being evaluated in which medial pallidal output is reduced by stereotactic neurosurgical procedures to lesion or stimulate the globus pallidus and/or subthalamic nucleus, rather than by dopaminergic action in the striatum.

PATHOPHYSIOLOGY OF DYSKINESIAS

Ballism is a violent dyskinesia, associated in humans with lesions of the STN. Using a primate model of ballism produced by pharmacologic inhibition of the STN, the neural mechanisms were elucidated by studying regional brain 2-deoxyglucose (2-DG) uptake. It was shown that dyskinesia is associated with decrease of excitatory STN efferent activity to the pallidum leading to underactivity of GPm neurons projecting to motor thalamus and brainstem. Because pallidal efferents are themselves GABAergic, this causes disinhibition of motor thalamus, which in turn excites motor cortical areas, leading to inappropriate, involuntary movements.

Huntington's disease (chorea) is characterized by abnormal movements and dementia, the striatum and cerebral cortex bearing the brunt of the disease. Early in disease progression, when chorea may be most prominent, there is relatively selective attrition of striatal neurons projecting to the GPl (17). It is possible to model Huntington's chorea in primates by local blockade of the indirect pathway with GABA antagonists. In this model it was shown that dyskinesia is mediated by disinhibition of the GPl, resulting in "physiologic" inhibition of the STN and, thus, the GPm.

Levodopa-induced dyskinesia refers to the abnormal movements that occur as complica-tions of the treatment of Parkinson's disease and their occurrence can severely limit the usefulness of treatment in the long term. The same phenomenon can be induced in parkinsonian primates in response to prolonged levodopa or dopamine agonist therapy. Using 2-DG uptake it has been shown that in this model the indirect pathway becomes underactive (11). This causes overactivity of the pallidosubthalamic pathway from GPl and physiologic inhibition of the STN and GPm. Conversely, the direct pathway is overactive, further exacerbating the underactivity of GPm.

Experimental studies in this spectrum of apparently different forms of dyskinesia provided, for the first time, functional evidence that all choreiform dyskinesias, irrespective of etiology, share a common neural mechanism, the core features of which are abnormal underactivity of the STN and GPm. They also addressed a long-standing issue in clinical neurology, where the separation or unity of chorea, ballism, and other dyskinesias had been a matter of controversy for many years.

PATHOPHYSIOLOGY OF DYSTONIA

Clinical, experimental, and pharmacologic evidence suggests that dystonia shares properties in common with both akinetic and dyskinetic syndromes. Analysis of the neural mechanisms underlying these two extreme forms of movement disorder indicate that akinesia is associated with abnormally increased output from the medial pallidal segment whereas dyskinesia is associated with abnormally decreased output. It is difficult to reconcile these observations and to retain the notion of motor abnormalities being mediated by simple increases or decreases in GPm activity. Although this simple concept does both fit the data and have predictive capacity in parkinsonism and dyskinesia, it is insufficient to explain dystonia. It seems an inescapable conclusion, therefore, that it must be the precise temporal (and possibly spatial) characteristics of GPm activity that dictate the appearance of dystonia. In certain circumstances overall (average) frequency may be abnormally high and, in others, abnormally low, but this is not per se the crucial factor.

COMMON NEURAL MECHANISMS IN DYSTONIA

The paucity of animal models of dystonia prompts the question as to whether some or all of the manifestations of dystonia in basal ganglia dysfunction, although caused by widely different etiologies, may share a common, generic, pathophysiologic mechanism or whether they are separate entities in this respect. This is an important question. We need to know, for example, whether elucidation of the neural mechanisms underlying levodopa- or dopamine-agonist–induced dystonia will be relevant to that condition alone or will have wider significance for those apparently disparate forms of dystonia for which there is no good animal model (e.g., torsion dystonia). There is some reason for optimism that different forms of dystonia may share common neural mechanisms, although concrete evidence to this effect is scant at present. The first reason is by analogy with choreiform dyskinesias. It has been shown, as detailed above, that in experimental primates that model human forms of chorea of widely differing etiologies, common neural mechanisms within the basal ganglia underlie their expression (12). This has been demonstrated for models of hemiballism (15), Huntington's chorea (13), and levodopa-induced chorea (11). The second reason for such optimism is that in a positron emission tomography (PET) study of human idiopathic torsion dystonia using fluorodeoxyglucose (5), similar regional metabolic changes were observed in the basal ganglia and related nuclei as have been found in 2-DG autoradiographic studies in an experimental primate model of levodopa-induced dystonia (14).

Levodopa- or dopamine-agonist–induced dystonia is seen in humans as a long-term complication of the treatment of Parkinson's disease and can be reliably reproduced in experimental primates made parkinsonian with the neurotoxin MPTP (1). This represents the best animal model currently available for studying dystonia in which the underlying pathology, clinical manifestation, and equivalence to human disease have been clearly demonstrated.

Few hard facts are available correlating the activity or neurochemistry of individual basal ganglia pathways specifically to dystonia. Experimental primate studies on levodopa-induced dystonia and human PET studies in torsion dystonia do, however, appear to agree on the fundamental observation of reduced metabolic activity in the motor regions of the thalamus in dystonia. This probably indicates abnormally reduced activity in the thalamic afferents from the basal ganglia, the majority of which originate from the medial segment of the globus pallidus. This conclusion represents something of a paradox for current models of basal ganglia function in which it has been clearly demonstrated that underactivity of the medial globus pallidus is associated with hyperkinetic choreiform dyskinesia and ballism (3).

DISTINCTION BETWEEN DYSTONIA AND CHOREA

We have put forward the premise that multiple manifestations of dystonia, with differing etiologies, may share a common, generic mechanism in terms of basal ganglia output. It follows, therefore, that elucidation of the underlying pathophysiology of one form of dystonia will permit extrapolation to others. Which form of dystonia is most likely to yield to such mechanistic analysis? We would argue that the most promising candidate is levodopa-induced dystonia, simply because it can be reliably produced in experimental animals.

Dystonia is induced in a significant proportion of parkinsonian (MPTP-exposed) primates receiving long-term treatment with levodopa or dopamine agonists. Such treatment also induces choreiform dyskinesia. In general, dystonia is produced most readily in the most severely parkinsonian animals. Animals displaying chorea early in the course of treatment may show evolution of dystonia as the primary motor disorder with prolonged dopaminergic exposure. Furthermore, chorea and dystonia may coexist in an individual animal. Following a single therapeutic dose, they may occur in different body parts simultaneously, or in the same body part at different times in the dose-response profile. If the latter is the case, dystonia typically appears as a peak-dose effect.

What, then, distinguishes the neural mechanisms underlying chorea and dystonia? The possibilities are either that medial pallidal activity is disrupted in a different manner in the two conditions or that the activity of other pathways must additionally be taken into account. It is, at present, difficult to distinguish between these two possibilities but what little evidence there is suggests that both may be true. In 2-DG experiments in primates the two conditions appear to be separated in only a quantitative sense, with the medial pallidum being even less active in dystonia than in chorea (11,14). Experimental surgical studies, however, point in a different direction because thalamotomy is able to alleviate levodopa-induced chorea but not dystonia, suggesting that pathways from the basal ganglia other than the pallidothalamic projection may be important in dystonia. These might include the connections of the pars reticulata of the substantia nigra, the brainstem reticular formation, and the pedunculopontine nucleus, lesion of which has been reported to improve experimental dystonia (16). The human PET study in torsion dystonia may be particularly informative here. These studies showed decreased medial pallidal (and thus pallidothalamic) neuronal activity in patients who demonstrated dystonia, not chorea. It could be concluded, therefore, that if decreased medial pallidal activity is important in the pathophysiology of dystonia it must become manifest through connections other than, or in addition to, the pallidothalamic pathway.

Another angle on the different mechanisms in chorea and dystonia is to examine how basal ganglia output could be differentially controlled in the two conditions. Medial pallidal activity is essentially controlled by converging inhibitory and excitatory afferents, the former being GABAergic and derived from the striatum and lateral pallidal segment, the latter being glutamatergic fibers from the subthalamic nucleus. In 2-DG studies in primates, the metabolic activity (and thus by inference afferent activity) of the medial pallidum is increased in levodopa-induced dystonia, even though the subthalamic nucleus (and thus its terminals in the medial pallidum) are underactive. In order to explain the 2-DG changes, it must be concluded that inhibitory GABAergic afferents to the medial pallidum are additionally overactive in dystonia. This would be consistent with the notion that the medial pallidum is underactive in this condition and more so than in chorea. Perhaps this is why subthalamic nucleus lesions induce chorea and ballism, but never dystonia. Thus, chorea can occur in situations where glutamate transmission alone is abnormally reduced in the medial pallidum, whereas the generation of dystonia may require a reduction in glutamate and simultaneous enhancement of GABA transmission in the medial pallidal segment.

Recent evidence suggests that, within the pallidal complex, the opioid peptides enkephalin and dynorphin, acting at delta and kappa opioid receptors, can modulate the release of glutamate and GABA (9,10). Furthermore, the synthesis of these peptides appears to be enhanced in neurons projecting to the pallidal complex in animal models of Parkinson's disease following treatment with dopamine-replacing agents that also cause dystonic side effects (e.g., L-DOPA and apomorphine). It is thus an intriguing possibility that altered opioid peptide release may be responsible for abnormalities in amino acid transmission in the globus pallidus in dystonia. These ideas suggest the possibility that antagonists of kappa and delta opioid receptors might be useful as adjuncts to dopamine-replacing agents in Parkinson's disease by allowing expression of the anti-Parkinson effects without generating dystonia.

DYNORPHIN MODULATION OF GLUTAMATE TRANSMISSION

We have explored how subthalamopallidal transmission might be reduced other than by blockade of postsynaptic EAA receptors, focusing on the neuropeptide dynorphin that is colocalized with GABA in striatal neurons projecting to GPm. We suspect a key role for dynorphin in movement disorders because (a) in animal models of Parkinson's disease, there is abnormally decreased expression of the gene coding for dynorphin precursor protein in striatal neurons, and (b) following prolonged exposure to dopaminergic agents in parkinsonism, there is, conversely, abnormally increased expression of dynorphin in striatal neurons. This specifically raises the possibility of a role for dynorphin in the pathophysiology of levodopa-induced dyskinesias.

Dynorphin released by striatal terminals in GPm presumably acts on kappa opiate receptors, which are enriched in this location. We hypothesized that dynorphin modulates glutamate release from subthalamopallidal terminals and, therefore, we studied the effects of kappa agonists on EAA release and uptake mechanisms and on the symptoms of parkinsonism. We discovered that kappa activation in the substantia nigra pars reticulata (the homologue of GPm) selectively reduces glutamate release (10). We demonstrated the functional importance of this finding by showing that, in both rat and primate, injection of the kappa opioid agonist enadoline (CI-977) into the GPm alleviates parkinsonism (2,10). This was replicated by systemic administration of enadoline or the agonist U69,593 (8). Marked synergism between kappa agonists and levodopa was noted (8). The possibility of a combined therapy, conferring increased efficacy of dopaminergic drugs, is attractive because treatment-related dyskinesias are highly correlated with the cumulative dose of dopaminergic agents.

MOLECULAR STUDIES OF STRIATAL MECHANISMS MEDIATING LEVODOPA-INDUCED DYSKINESIA AND DYSTONIA

We have shown that, in animals exhibiting dyskinesias or dystonia following prolonged dopaminergic therapy, striatal D1 receptor levels become elevated relative to the parkinsonian state whereas D2 receptors return toward normal (6). These changes are probably crucial in altering the activity of the direct and indirect striatopallidal pathways and the synthesis of their peptide cotransmitters is known to be controlled differentially by D1 and D2 receptors. In view of the evidence, presented above, that these peptides control amino acid transmission, changes in peptide synthesis in the direct and indirect pathways would have a major impact on basal ganglia physiology. We hypothesize that this scenario underlies the development of levodopa-induced dyskinesia and dystonia and we have, therefore, examined the enkephalin and dynorphin precursors, preproenkephalin A and B (PPE-A and PPE-B) in levodopa-induced dyskinesia, using *in situ* and Northern hybridization (4,7).

We have shown that expression of PPE-B is markedly increased by dopaminergic therapy. This may be a crucial finding, because we have shown both that increased dynorphinergic transmission reduces EAA release from subthalamopallidal terminals (8) and that this is the principal mechanism responsible for the production of dyskinesia in a range of primate models of chorea. We have also identified a novel mechanism by which changes in striatal activity, following prolonged dopaminergic therapy, might reduce glutamate release in the GPm and so elicit dyskinesias. We have demonstrated that dopamine agonists increase the synthesis of the enkephalin precursor PPE-A to a level above that seen in untreated parkinsonism (7). Because we have shown that enkephalin acts to decrease GABA release in the GPl, this change would disinhibit the pallido-subthalamic pathway and, thus, reduce the activity of the STN. These two proposed peptidergic influences concur with our predicted mechanism for dyskinesia based on 2-DG uptake studies, and raises the possibility of opioid antagonist therapy for dyskinesia.

REFERENCES

1. Boyce S, Clarke CE, Luquin R, et al. Induction of chorea and dystonia in parkinsonian primates. *Mov Disord* 1990;5:3–7.

2. Brotchie JM, Hughes NR, Maneuf Y, Mitchell IJ, Crossman AR, Woodruff GN. Anti-parkinsonian effects of the kappa opioid receptor agonist CI-977 in primates. *Eur J Neurosci* 1993;6[Suppl]:119.

3. Crossman AR. A hypothesis on the pathophysiological mechanisms that underlie levodopa- or dopamine agonist-induced dyskinesia in Parkinson's disease: implications for future strategies in treatment. *Mov Disord* 1990;5:100–108.

4. Duty S, Rowell J, Henry B, Crossman AR, Brotchie JM. Regional variations in striatal neuropeptide expression following long-term apomorphine treatment in the 6-hydroxydopamine-lesioned rat. *Brain Res Assoc* 1994;11:49 (abst).

5. Eidelberg D, Moeller JR, Ishikawa T, et al. The metabolic topography of idiopathic torsion dystonia. *Brain* 1995;118:1473–1484.

6. Graham WC, Sambrook MA, Crossman AR. Differential effect of chronic dopaminergic treatment on dopamine D1 and D2 receptors in the monkey brain in MPTP-induced parkinsonism. *Brain Res* 1993;602: 290–303.

7. Henry B, Brotchie JM. Potential of opioid antagonists in the treatment of levodopa-induced dyskinesias in Parkinson's disease. *Drugs Aging* 1996;9:149–158.

8. Hughes NR, McKnight A, Woodruff GN, Crossman AR, Brotchie JM. Anti-parkinsonian effects of *K*-opioid receptor agonists in the reserpine-treated rat. *Mov Disord (in press)*.

9. Maneuf YP, Mitchell IJ, Crossman AR, Brotchie JM. On the role of enkephalin co-transmission in the GABA-ergic striatal efferents to the globus pallidus. *Exp Neurol* 1994;125:65–71.

10. Maneuf YP, Mitchell IJ, Crossman AR, Woodruff GN, Brotchie JM. Functional implications of kappa opioid receptor-mediated modulation of glutamate transmission in the output regions of the basal ganglia in rodent and primate models of Parkinson's disease. *Brain Res* 1995;683:102–108.

11. Mitchell IJ, Boyce S, Sambrook MA, Crossman AR. A 2-deoxyglucose study of the effects of dopamine agonists on the parkinsonian primate brain: implications for the neural mechanisms that mediate dopamine agonist-induced dyskinesia. *Brain* 1992;115:809–824.

12. Mitchell IJ, Jackson AJ, Sambrook MA, Crossman AR. Common neural mechanisms in experimental chorea and hemiballismus in the monkey. Evidence from 2-deoxyglucose autoradiography. *Brain Res* 1985;339: 346–350.

13. Mitchell IJ, Jackson AJ, Sambrook MA, Crossman AR. The role of the subthalamic nucleus in experimental chorea. Evidence from 2-deoxyglucose metabolic mapping and horseradish peroxidase tracing studies. *Brain* 1989;112:1533–1548.

14. Mitchell IJ, Luquin R, Boyce S, et al. Neural mechanisms of dystonia: evidence from a 2-deoxyglucose uptake study in a primate model of dopamine agonist-induced dystonia. *Mov Disord* 1990;5:49–54.

15. Mitchell IJ, Sambrook MA, Crossman AR. Subcortical changes in the regional uptake of [^{3}H]-2-deoxyglucose in the brain elicited by injection of a gamma-aminobutyric acid antagonist into the subthalamic nucleus. *Brain* 1985;108:421–438.

16. Page RD, Sambrook MA, Crossman AR. Thalamotomy for the alleviation of levodopa-induced dyskinesia: experimental studies in the 1-methyl-4-phenyl-1,2,3,6-tetrahydropyridine-treated parkinsonian monkey. *Neuroscience* 1993;55:147–165.

17. Sapp E, Ge P, Aizawa H, et al. Evidence for a preferential loss of enkephalin immunoreactivity in the external globus pallidus in low grade Huntington's disease using high resolution image analysis. *Neuroscience* 1985;64:397–404.

18. Smith Y, Bolam JP. The output neurones and the dopaminergic neurones of the substantia nigra receive a GABA input from the globus pallidus in the rat. *J Comp Neurol* 1989;296:47–64.

Dystonia 3: Advances in Neurology, Vol. 78,
edited by S. Fahn, C. D. Marsden, and M. DeLong.
Lippincott–Raven Publishers, Philadelphia © 1998.

4

Thalamic Single Neuron and Electromyographic Activities in Patients with Dystonia

T. A. Zirh*, Stephen G. Reich, V. Perry, and *Frederick A. Lenz

*Department of Neurosurgery, Johns Hopkins Hospital, Baltimore, Maryland 21287; and
Department of Neurology, Johns Hopkins University, School of Medicine,
Baltimore, Maryland 21287.

Abnormal physiologic activity has been reported in the peripheral and central nervous systems of patients with dystonia. The former includes delayed H-reflex recovery curves in patients with dystonia (33,37,39). Central nervous system activity in patients with dystonia has been studied with positron emission tomographic (PET) scans (6,10,21,34,36). To our knowledge the activity of neurons in the central nervous system has not previously been reported in dystonia or in a model of dystonia (7).

Dystonia has been relieved by neurosurgical procedures such as thalamotomy (5), during which the location of the target is first defined by radiologic studies (23). Thereafter physiologic studies, such as microelectrode recordings (24,32), are carried out to confirm the target (23). These physiologic studies provide a unique opportunity to examine thalamic neuronal activity in patients with dystonia. The results of these studies demonstrate that thalamic activity in the ventralis intermedius (Vim) and ventralis oralis posterior (Vop) is often correlated with and leads electromyographic (EMG) activity. Because a lesion of this area relieves dystonia, this thalamic activity may be involved in the mechanism of dystonia.

METHODS

The operative, physiologic, and analytic methods are outlined briefly here, because they have been detailed in previous reports (23–25, 30–32). Briefly, thalamotomy was carried out as a two-stage procedure. During the first stage of the procedure, the stereotactic coordinates of the anterior and posterior commissures were determined by computed tomography. These coordinates were then used to construct a sagittal map of thalamic nuclei in stereotactic coordinates (15). During the second stage of the procedure, a microelectrode was used to explore the thalamus.

The target location was confirmed by the functional properties of thalamic cells as determined by extracellular recordings. First, Vc was identified as the region where the majority of cells were sensory cells that responded to deep or cutaneous sensory stimulation (20,24). After Vc had been identified, the region anterior to it was explored. In particular, the location of cells with activity related to dystonia was determined. The lesion was made among

---

Abbreviations: GPi, globus pallidus internis; RF, receptive field; SMA, supplementary motor area of cortex; Vc, ventralis caudalis; Vim, ventralis intermedius; Vop, ventralis oralis posterior (14,16).

cells with activity related to dystonia anterior to Vc so as to spare both the internal capsule and Vc (29,31).

The somatosensory examination included light touch, tapping of skin, pressure to skin, joint movement, and deep pressure to muscle, ligament, or tendons. Cells that responded to cutaneous stimulation were classified as cuta-neous sensory cells. Cells that responded to joint movement or pressure to deep structures without a response to stimulation of skin de-formed by these stimuli were classified as deep sensory cells. The receptive field of stimula-tion was then mapped using the modality of stimulation to which the cell responded most consistently.

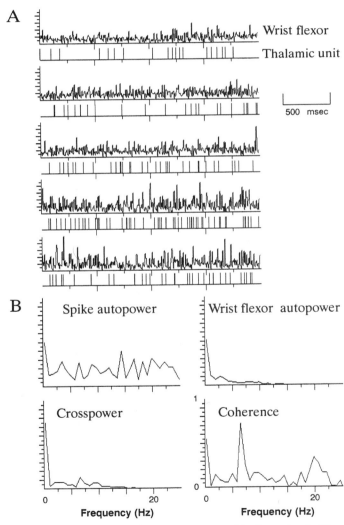

FIG. 1. Thalamic spike train and EMG signals in a patient with dystonia. **A:** The upper panel con-sists of a trace showing the times of occurrence of thalamic action potentials **(upper)** and the en-velope of wrist flexor EMG activity. **B:** The smoothed spike **(upper left)** and EMG autopower spec-tra **(upper right)** and spike × EMG cross-power **(lower left)** and coherence spectra **(lower right)**. See text.

The activity of many cells, particularly those anterior to Vc, was then examined subjectively for dystonia frequency activity during dystonia. EMG activity was monitored from four muscles, including flexors and extensors of the wrist, biceps, and triceps. Thalamic microelectrode and EMG channels were stored on magnetic tape along with a voice channel that recorded cues to movement and details of the somatosensory examination.

Figure 1A shows thalamic and EMG activity during dystonia, and spectral cross-correlation analysis of this activity is shown in Fig. 1B. Initially Fourier transforms were taken of both the EMG signal and the spike train to determine the raw EMG and spike spectra. The raw spectra were then smoothed by frequency averaging of eight contiguous raw spectral estimates. Smoothed spectra are shown in Fig. 1B.

Smoothed cross-power, phase, and coherence spectra were determined by standard calculations (2,12,19,32). The autopower spectrum measures power or intensity of the signal as a function of frequency. Power at dystonia frequency (less than 0.78 Hz, see below) divided by average power for all components in the spike train autopower spectrum was termed autopower signal to noise ratio (SNR). Autopower SNR indicated the extent to which power in the spike train was concentrated at dystonia frequency (2,12,19,32). Smoothed autopower spectra of EMG and thalamic cellular activities for the cell are shown in Fig. 1B.

The cross-spectral function spike × EMG was described in terms of the cross-power, coherence, and phase spectra (2,32). The cross-power spectrum indicated the extent to which power in the two signals occurred at the same frequency with a consistent phase relationship. The coherence was a statistical function used to estimate the probability that two signals were correlated at a given frequency. A coherence of 0 indicated that the two signals were not linearly related, whereas a coherence of 1 indicated that the two signals were identical. As computed in the present study, coherence of greater than 0.42 indicated a significant probability of linear relationship between the two signals ($p < 0.05$; see References 3 and 32).

Spike × wrist flexor EMG cross-spectral function is illustrated in Fig. 1B (lower). The dystonia frequency peak in the cross-power spectrum (left) indicates that the two signals share a large amount of power at dystonia frequency. The coherence at dystonia frequency (right) is greater than 0.42, indicating a significant probability that thalamic and wrist flexor EMG activities are linearly related.

RESULTS

Cellular activity, microstimulation evoked responses, and effects of lesions were studied in the region of thalamus anterior to the cutaneous core of the principal somatosensory nucleus (Vc) of patients undergoing stereotactic thalamotomy for treatment of dystonia. The percentage of cells responding to passive joint movement or to manipulation of subcutaneous structures (deep sensory cells) in the thalamic cerebellar relay nucleus (Vim) was significantly greater in patients with dystonia than in control patients undergoing surgery for treatment of tremor or pain (31).

Lengths of trajectories where all RFs included a single joint were significantly longer in patients with dystonia than in control patients (31). This result suggests that patients with dystonia have reorganized afferent inputs to the thalamic representation of parts of the body undergoing dystonia. The proportion of deep sensory cells responding to movement of more than one joint was significantly higher in patients with dystonia than in control patients indicating a larger representation of the dystonic area in patients with dystonia.

Microstimulation in presumed Vim in patients with dystonia produced simultaneous contraction of multiple forearm muscles, similar to the simultaneous muscle contraction that is characteristic of dystonic movements (25). In some patients a small lesion involving Vim and Vop produced an immediate and dramatic decrease in the dystonic movements. Therefore the results of recordings, microstimulation, and lesions suggest that altered somatosensory activity in Vim and Vop is involved in the mechanism of dystonia.

Crosscorrelation analysis was carried out on EMG activity and thalamic neuronal activity recorded from cells in Vim and Vop in patients with dystonia (25,28). The EMG signals for flexors and extensors of the wrist and elbow exhibited peak EMG power in the lowest frequency band (0 to 0.78 Hz, dystonia frequency) for the majority of epochs studied. Simultaneous contraction (coherence greater than 0.42 and phase angle less than 30 degrees) was often observed for antagonists acting at the wrist and elbow.

The thalamic single unit recordings also reflected dystonia frequency activity. Firing rates were consistently lower in both presumed Vim and Vop of dystonia patients than in control patients. A concentration of spike power at dystonia frequency (SNR greater than 2) was found more frequently for cells in Vim and Vop of dystonia patients than those of control patients. Peak spike power with SNR 2 or greater occurred at dystonia frequency more often for cells in Vop than in Vim. Spike activity in presumed Vim and Vop was often correlated with EMG activity and consistently led EMG activity in all channels. A large number of cells in both presumed Vim and Vop exhibited dystonia frequency activity, which was correlated with and led EMG activity during dystonia. Sensory cells (cells responding to sensory input) were less likely to exhibit peak spike power at dystonia frequency than were nonsensory cells. The coherence and phase of the spike × EMG cross-correlation functions were not significantly different between sensory and nonsensory cells. However, the activity of many sensory cells leads EMG activity when they would be expected to lag because of transmission delays from the periphery to the thalamus.

In normal monkeys and in tremor of Parkinson's disease, motor output from particular thalamic cells is usually directed to the muscles that give rise to afferent input to the same cell (27). In dystonia, thalamic output to a particular muscle was indicated by thalamic activity correlated with and leading EMG activity. In patients with dystonia, thalamic output is more often related to dystonia in muscles other than those giving rise to afferent input (sensory/motor mismatch). This suggests that there is a mismatch of sensory inputs and motor outputs

in dystonia, perhaps related to the reorganization of sensory inputs to Vim/Vop described above. Many sensory cells showed activity leading EMG although the sensory response of these cells predicted that cellular activity should lag EMG. This suggests that sensory activity may drive thalamic activity related to dystonia.

DISCUSSION

The present results indicate that EMG activity in patients with dystonia was concentrated in the lowest frequency range and was characterized by simultaneous contraction of multiple muscles. The activity of cells in Vop but not Vim was dominated by power at dystonia frequency. There was a significant increase in the number of sensory cells in Vim but not Vop. The thalamic representation of afferent inputs from the dystonic part of the body is increased. The activity of cells in Vop and Vim was often correlated with EMG activity and led EMG activity for the majority of spike × EMG pairs. Small lesions in the area of Vim and Vop sometimes dramatically relieved dystonia while stimulation in Vim produced simultaneous contraction of multiple muscles, similar to dystonia (31). These results suggest that activity of cells in both Vop and Vim is involved in the generation of dystonia by different mechanisms.

A greater proportion of sensory cells was found in Vim than in Vop in patients with dystonia. Furthermore, the number of sensory cells in patients with dystonia is significantly greater than control patients in Vim, but not in Vop (31). Stimulation of Vim produced movements characterized by simultaneous contractions of multiple muscles similar to those seen in dystonia. The activity of many sensory cells leads EMG activity where they would be expected to lag because of transmission delays from the periphery to the thalamus. These findings suggest that some sensory cells in Vim may be related to dystonia by motor output of the activity of these cells to the periphery.

The mechanism by which somatosensory processing is altered in dystonia are unclear.

Long loop reflex mechanisms are one type of somatosensory function that is abnormal in hypokinetic disorders (37,39). These reflexes are thought to arise in peripheral movement receptors and be transmitted through dorsal columns, thalamus, cortex, and back to the stretched muscle (8). Long loop reflexes are of increased duration in dystonia (Reference 39; compare Reference 37). A less direct mechanism linking sensory inputs to thalamus with dystonia is sensory modulation of an oscillating network (11,27,38). Alternately, increased sensory inputs to Vim might produce abnormal motor cortex excitability and responses to sensory stimulation, which could drive dystonia (25,31). The sensory/motor mismatch in dystonia patients is reminiscent of the mismatch between RFs (input) and the part of the body where stimulation evokes sensation (projected field, output) in patients with spinal transection (26). These patients have somatotopic reorganization of RF (input) maps but have less complete reorganization of the PF map (output). Failure of the motor (output) map to reorganize in line with changes in the RF map may cause sensory inputs to drive activity in multiple muscles other than the muscle that gives input to the cell.

The present study demonstrates reorganized maps of sensory inputs and sensory/motor mismatches in motor thalamus of patients with dystonia. Reorganization of motor cortical maps has been demonstrated in monkeys trained to perform repetitive tasks (35); reorganization of sensory cortical maps has been demonstrated in monkeys that develop occupational hand cramps as a result of training to repetitive motor behaviors (4,13). Task-specific dystonias, like writer's cramp (22), occur in patients whose occupation includes repetitive motor tasks (see Reference 17). These occupational cramps may be related to motor/sensory mismatch of the type reported in the present review, perhaps secondary to reorganized maps of sensory input. The relationship between spike signals in Vim and dystonia may depend on a sensory mechanism of this type.

A significantly greater proportion of cells in Vop than in Vim are dominated by dystonia frequency activity. Vop has a direct connection to arm motor cortex and to SMA (18), both of which project to the spinal cord (9). SMA influences movement-related activity in motor cortex (1). Thus Vop may influence EMG activity in dystonia by transmission of dystonia-related activity to the spinal cord through SMA or indirectly, through motor cortex. Changes in the somatosensory maps may be related to and contribute to the occurrence of dystonic movements through a sensory/motor mismatch (31), particularly in the case of task-specific dystonias (4,13,35).

Support: Grants to FAL from the MIH (NS2 8598, K08-NS1384, POINS32386-Proj. I and Lily Corp.)

REFERENCES

1. Aizawa H, Tanji J. Corticocortical and thalamocortical responses of neurons in the monkey primary motor cortex and their relation to a trained motor task. *J Neurophysiol* 1994;71:550–560.
2. Bendat JS, Piersol AG. *Random data.* New York: Wiley, 1976.
3. Benignus VA. Estimation of the coherence spectrum and its confidence interval using the FFT. *IEEE Trans Audio Electroacoustic* 1969;17:145–150.
4. Byl NN, Merzenich MM, Jenkins WM. Occupational hand cramps genesis paralleled by degradation of representation in the SI cortex. *Soc Neurosci Abstr* 1995; 21:1757 (abst).
5. Cardoso F, Jankiovic J, Grossman RG, Hamilton W. Outcome after stereotactic thalamotomy for dystonia and hemiballismus. *Neurosurgery* 1995;36:501–508.
6. Ceballos-Baumann AO, Passingham RE, Warner T, Playford ED, Marsden CD, Brooks DJ. Overactive prefrontal and underactive motor cortical areas in idiopathic dystonia. *Ann Neurol* (1995);37:363–372.
7. Crossman AR, Mitchell IJ, Sambrook MA. Neural mechanisms mediating dopamine agonist-induced dystonia in the parkinsonian monkey. *Soc Neurosci Abstr* 1989;15:906.
8. Desmedt JE. *Progress in clinical neurophysiology. Cerebral motor control in man: long loop mechanisms.* Basel: Karger, 1978.
9. Dum RP, Strick PL. The origin of corticospinal projections from the premotor areas in the frontal lobe. *J Neurosci* 1991;11:667–689.
10. Eidelbert D, Moeller JR, Dhawan V, et al. Regional metabolic covariation in idiopathic torsion dystonia: F-fluorodeoxyglucose PET studies. *Mov Disord* 1992;7:436.
11. Elble RJ, Koller W. *Tremor.* Baltimore: Johns Hopkins University Press, 1990.
12. Glaser EM, Ruchkin DS. *Principles of neurobiological signal analysis.* New York: Academic Press, 1976.

13. Hallett M. Is dystonia a sensory disorder? *Ann Neurol* 1995;38:139–140.
14. Hassler R. Anatomy of the thalamus. In: Schaltenbrand G. et al., eds. *Introduction to stereotaxis with an atlas of the human brain.* Stuttgart: Theime Medical Publishers, 1959:230–290.
15. Hawrylyshyn P, Rowe IH, Tasker RR, Organ LW. A computer system for stereotaxic neurosurgery. *Comput Biol Med* 1976;6:87–97.
16. Hirai T, Jones EG. A new parcellation of the human thalamus on the basis of histochemical staining. *Brain Res Rev* 1989;14:1–34.
17. Hochberg FH, Leffert RD, Heller MD, Merriman L. Hand difficulties among musicians. *JAMA* 1983;249:1869–1872.
18. Holsapple JW, Preston JB, Strick PL. The origin of thalamic input to the 'hand' representation in the primary motor cortex. *J Neurosci* 1991;11:2644–2654.
19. Jenkins GW, Watts DG. *Spectral analysis.* San Francisco: Holden-Day, 1968.
20. Jones EG. *The thalamus.* New York: Plenum Publishing, 1985.
21. Karbe H, Holthoff VA, Rudolf J, Herholz K, Heiss WD. Positron emission tomography in dystonia: frontal cortex and basal ganglia hypometabolism. *Mov Disord* 1992;7:437.
22. Lang AE, Weiner WJ. *Movement disorders: a comprehensive survey.* Mount Kisco, NY: Futura Publishing, 1989.
23. Lenz FA, Dostrovsky JO, Kwan HC, Tasker RR, Yamashiro K, Murphy JT. Methods for microstimulation and recording of single neurons and evoked potentials in the human central nervous system. *J Neurosurg* 1988;68:630–634.
24. Lenz FA, Dostrovsky JO, Tasker RR, Yamashiro K, Kwan HC, Murphy JT. Single-unit analysis of the human ventral thalamic nuclear group: somatosensory responses. *J Neurophysiol* 1988;59:299–316.
25. Lenz FA, Jaeger CJ, Seike MS, et al. Cross-correlation analysis of thalamic neuronal and EMG signals in patients with dystonia. *Movement Disorders* 7, Supp. 1:126,1992.
26. Lenz FA, Kwan HC, Martin R, Tasker R, Richardson RT, Dostrovsky JO. Characteristics of somatotopic organization and spontaneous neuronal activity in the region of the thalamic principal sensory nucleus in patients with spinal cord transection. *J Neurophysiol* 1994;72:1570–1587.
27. Lenz FA, Kwan HC, Martin RL, Tasker RR, Dostrovsky JO, Lenz YE. Single neuron analysis of the hu-

man ventral thalamic nuclear group: tremor-related activity in functionally identified cells. *Brain* 1994;117:531–543.
28. Lenz FA, Martin R, Kwan HC, Tasker RR, Dostrovsky JO. Thalamic single-unit activity occurring in patients with hemidystonia. *Stereotact Funct Neurosurg* 1990;54,55:159–162.
29. Lenz FA, Normand SL, Kwan HC, Andrews D, et al. Statistical prediction of the optimal lesion site for thalamotomy in parkinsonian tremor. *Mov Disord* 1995;10:318–328.
30. Lenz FA, Seike M, Lin YC, Baker FH, Richardson RT, Gracely RH. Thermal and pain sensations evoked by microstimulation in the area of the human ventrocaudal nucleus (Vc). *J Neurophysiol* 1993;70:200–212.
31. Lenz FA, Seike MS, Jaeger CJ, et al. Single unit analysis of thalamus in patients with dystonia. *Movement Disorders* 7, Supp. 1:126,1992.
32. Lenz FA, Tasker RR, Kwan HC, et al. Single unit analysis of the human ventral thalamic nuclear group: correlation of thalamic "tremor cells" with the 3-6 Hz component of parkinsonian tremor. *J Neurosci* 1988;8:754–764.
33. Marsden CD, Rothwell JC. The physiology of idiopathic dystonia. *Can J Neurol Sci* 1987;14:521–527.
34. Matsuzaka Y, Aizawa H, Tanji J. A motor area rostral to the supplementary motor area (presupplementary motor area) in the monkey: neuronal activity during a learned motor task. *J Neurophysiol* 1995;68: 653–662.
35. Nudo RJ, Milliken GW, Jenkins WM, Merzenich MM. Use dependent alterations of movement representations in primary motor cortex of adult squirrel monkeys. *J Neurosci* 1996;16:785–807.
36. Playford ED, Passingham RE, Marsden CD, Brooks DJ. Abnormal activation of striatum and supplementary motor area in dystonia: a PET study. *Mov Disord* 1992;7:438.
37. Rothwell JC, Obeso JA, Day BL, Marsden CD. Pathophysiology of dystonias. In: Desmedt JE, ed. *Motor control mechanisms in health and disease,* New York: Raven Press, 1983:851–863.
38. Schnider SM, Kwong RH, Lenz FA, Kwan HC. Detection of feedback in the central nervous system using system identification techniques. *Biol Cybern* 1989;60:203–212.
39. Tatton WG, Bedingham W, Verrier MC, Blair RDG. Characteristic alterations in responses to imposed wrist displacements in parkinsonian rigidity and dystonia musculorum deformans. *Can J Neurol Sci* 1984;11:281–287.

Dystonia 3: Advances in Neurology, Vol. 78,
edited by S. Fahn, C. D. Marsden, and M. DeLong.
Lippincott–Raven Publishers, Philadelphia © 1998.

5

Excitability of Motor Cortex in Patients with Dystonia

Antonio Currà, *A. Berardelli, *Sabine Rona, *S. Fabri, and Mario Manfredi

Department of Neurological Sciences, Instituto Neurologico Mediterraneo Neuromed,Pozzilli, 15, 86077, Italy; and Department of Neurological Sciences, University of Rome "La Sapienza", Viale dell'Università 30, 00185 Rome, Istituto Neuromed Pozzilli (IS) Italy.

Dystonia is characterized by involuntary muscle contractions leading to sustained twisting movements and abnormal postures that occur spontaneously or during specific skilled movements. Observations that patients with symptomatic dystonia often have lesions involving the caudate nucleus, the subthalamus, and thalamus (5,17,18) confirm the role of subcortical structures in the pathophysiology of dystonia. Because the basal ganglia are anatomically connected with the motor cortices their activity influences the function of cortical motor areas (2,30). In dystonia an abnormal basal ganglia output may therefore produce changes at cortical level, resulting in dystonic movements.

Among the various alterations of segmental mechanisms implicated in the regulation of muscle tone are decreased reciprocal inhibition, abnormalities of the H-reflex recovery cycle, and increased excitability of brainstem circuits in patients with cranial dystonia (3,7,9, 19,21,22,23,26,32). Evidence of altered cortical function comes from studies showing that premotor potentials during the preparatory phase of movement have a decreased amplitude in patients with dystonia (10,12,36). Premotor potential studies investigate cortical motor function closely related to movement production but they provide no direct information about the baseline activity of motor cortical areas.

The technique of transcranial magnetic stimulation provides information about corticomotoneuron connections and cortical motor area excitability. Single magnetic pulses delivered to the scalp produce excitatory effects (motor evoked potentials, MEPs) as well as inhibitory effects (silent period, SP) at cortical level. With this technique abnormalities have been detected in patients affected by various movement disorders due to basal ganglia diseases (6,24,25,34).

In patients with dystonia, early studies using electrical cortical stimulation reported normal corticomotoneuron conduction time (11). More recently, Mavroudakis et al. (20) investigated the excitatory and inhibitory effects of low-intensity magnetic stimuli delivered at rest and during facilitation in patients with focal arm dystonia. Although the dystonic group had smaller MEPs elicited at rest than controls, they had a significantly increased amplitude ratio between MEPs measured at rest and during facilitation. In addition, despite having SPs of normal duration, dystonic patients tended to reach their maximal SP duration at lower stimulus intensities than controls. Hence the investigators suggested that the excitatory and the inhibitory cortical circuits explored by transcranial magnetic stimulation are abnormal in patients with dystonia. In normal subjects and in patients with task-specific dystonia, Ikoma et al. (13) studied the MEP changes induced by varying the intensity of magnetic stimulation and the level of background contraction. Magnetic stimulation at increasing intensity elicited greater MEP increases in dystonic patients than in controls. In addition, patients had greater MEP area changes from rest to facilitation on their affected side than controls had on their dominant side. This study also provided interesting findings on the influence of handedness on the duration of SP. Although SPs in the patients' affected side and controls' dominant arm had similar durations, with increasing stimulus intensities the unaffected side of patients showed smaller SP duration increases than did the nondominant arm of controls. This finding confirms previous observations that neurophysiologic abnormalities do not localize exclusively in the affected body parts (9,23).

In normal subjects Kujirai et al. (14) investigated cortical excitability with the "paired magnetic stimulation technique." Magnetic shocks were delivered at varying interstimulus intervals (ISIs) through the (same) stimulating coil in a conditioning-test design. The degree of inhibition varied according to the intensity of the conditioning shock, the length of the ISI, and the muscle condition (rest or contraction). These investigators delivered subthreshold conditioning and suprathreshold test stimuli at ISIs ranging 1 to 15 milliseconds using a focal coil centered on the optimal scalp position to elicit responses in the target muscle at rest. With this paradigm the inhibition produced by the conditioning stimulus on the test response depends exclusively on cortical mechanisms. In normal subjects, the time course of the test response consists of an inhibitory phase (for ISIs 1 to 6 milliseconds) and a facilitatory phase (for ISIs 7 to 15 milliseconds). Using this technique, Ridding et al. (27) studied short-latency intracortical inhibition in normal subjects and in patients with focal, task-specific dystonia. Dystonic patients had a decreased inhibitory phase. In the investigators' opinion this reduction indicates a relative decrease in the excitability of the cortical inhibitory circuits. Hence it suggests one possible pathophysiologic mechanism for the

excessive and inappropriate muscle contraction observed in dystonia.

Paired shocks delivered at longer ISIs (100 to 200) also inhibit the test response in normal subjects and probably do so through cortical mechanisms (16,33). In a recent study of the excitability of cortical motor areas in Parkinson's disease we found that longer ISIs increased inhibition of the test response, whereas shorter ISIs did not (4). Their differential inhibition suggests that the two responses are mediated by different intracortical circuits. Ridding et al. (27) studied patients with dystonia with the subjects at rest. These patients, however, often have difficulty in relaxing their muscle completely. In addition, the amount of short-latency inhibition differs according to whether responses are recorded in muscles at rest or while the subject exerts a background contraction of the target muscle (28). In a study designed to assess corticomotor excitability in a group of patients with upper limb dystonia, to circumvent these problems, we compared responses to paired magnetic stimuli delivered at short and long ISIs, while the subject exerted voluntary contraction. A further reason for studying patients during contraction was that we wanted to compare the behavior of the inhibition induced by paired stimulation with that of the cortical silent period elicited by single shocks, an inhibitory phenomenon obtained only during contraction.

MATERIALS AND METHODS

We studied 11 healthy subjects and ten patients with dystonia of the right upper limb (six women and four men, mean age 36 ± SD 9.7 years). Six patients had task-specific dystonia (writer's cramp), three had segmental dystonia, and one had generalized dystonia (Table 1). All the patients with task-specific dystonia and one of the patients with segmental dystonia stopped taking their medication at least 24 hours before the study. For ethical reasons, the others maintained their therapeutic regimen (trihexyphenidyl). Volunteer controls (three women and eight men, mean age 40 ± SD 11.4 years)

TABLE 1. *Clinical features of patients with dystonia*

Patient	Age	Sex	Type of dystonia	Therapy
1	26	M	Generalized	Trihexyphenidyl
2	27	F	Segmental	—
3	29	F	Writer's cramp	—
4	30	M	Bilateral writer's cramp	—
5	32	F	Writer's cramp	—
6	32	M	Segmental	Trihexyphenidyl
7	36	F	Writer's cramp	—
8	46	F	Segmental	Trihexyphenidyl
9	50	F	Writer's cramp	—
10	52	M	Writer's cramp	—

were all right-handed. Subjects gave their informed consent and the study was approved by the local ethical committee.

Methods for the paired stimulation technique have been described in detail in a previous article (4). In brief, subjects were seated comfortably with their forearms resting on the arms of a chair. Paired magnetic stimuli were delivered through the same round coil (outer diameter 14 cm, maximum magnetic field 2.5 Tesla) by two magnetic stimulators (Novametrix Magstim 200) connected to a Bistim module. To activate predominantly the left hemisphere the coil was held flat over the vertex with the current flowing in a counterclockwise direction when viewed from above. In four subjects with unilateral writer's cramp the stimulating coil was also held with the current flowing in a clockwise direction.

We delivered paired magnetic shocks in a conditioning-test design at short (3, 5, 7, 10, 15, and 20 milliseconds) and long (100, 150, 200, and 250 milliseconds) ISIs. Stimuli were delivered in four blocks of 24 or 32 trials, consisting of eight trials each of three or four conditions: the response to a test shock given alone, and the response of the same shock conditioned by a prior stimulus delivered at different conditioning-test intervals. Within each block, paired shocks at different intervals were randomly intermixed and given every 6 seconds. The test stimulus was given at the fixed intensity of 125% of motor threshold for both types of ISIs. The conditioning stimuli were set at 80% of motor threshold for the short ISI, and at 150% of motor threshold for the long ISI.

Thresholds were determined and paired pulses were tested during a slight voluntary contraction [~20% of maximum voluntary electromyographic (EMG) activity] of the muscle under study.

The methods we used for studying the cortical SP have been detailed in previous papers (24,25). In brief, SPs were elicited by single magnetic shocks delivered at 150% of motor threshold during a maximum voluntary contraction. The duration of the SP was measured from the end of the MEP to the return of continuous EMG activity.

For the paired stimulation technique and the silent period the EMG activity from the FDI muscle contralateral to the side of stimulation was recorded with surface electrodes. Responses were amplified and filtered (Digitimer D160), band-passed (3 Hz to 1 kHz), digitized, and stored on a personal computer through a 1401 CED laboratory interface for the off-line analysis.

All results are expressed as means $\pm$ 1 SEM. Group values (separately for short and long intervals) and differences at single intervals were evaluated with the one-way analysis of variance (ANOVA). The repeated-measures ANOVA was used to compare affected and unaffected sides in patients with unilateral writer's cramp. p values <0.05 were considered significant.

RESULTS

Paired transcranial magnetic shocks elicited responses that had a similar motor threshold in controls and patients (41.1 ± 2.6% and 40.3 ± 1.6%); and in patients with task-specific and non-task-specific dystonia (41.5 ± 2.2%, $n = 6$; 38.5 ± 2.4%, $n = 4$). In patients with writer's cramp the left and the right hemispheres had an identical activation threshold (42.3 ± 1%; $n = 4$ for both hemispheres). In normal subjects and patients conditioning and control responses had a similar mean amplitude (conditioning: 5.2 ± 0.9 mV, control: 2.6 ± 0.7 mV, $n = 11$ normal subjects; conditioning: 3.6 ± 0.6 mV, control: 2.0 ± 0.3 mV, $n = 10$ dystonic patients).

Paired Magnetic Stimuli Delivered at Short Interstimulus Intervals

In controls and patients with dystonia paired magnetic shocks delivered at ISIs of 3 to 7 milliseconds inhibited the test response (controls: 3 milliseconds, 48.7 ± 3.3%; 5 milliseconds, 66 ± 6%; and 7 milliseconds, 87.7 ± 10%; patients: 3 milliseconds, 56.6 ± 10.8%; 5 milliseconds, 61.4 ± 7.1%; and 7 milliseconds, 78 ± 11.7%). ISIs from 10 to 20 milliseconds caused no inhibition of the test response in normal subjects and only mild inhibition in patients (10 milliseconds: 98.7 ± 7.2%; 15 milliseconds: 107.6 ± 15.1%; and 20 milliseconds: 101.7 ± 12.4% in normal subjects; 10 milliseconds: 83.8 ± 11.3%; 15 milliseconds: 83.3 ± 12.8%; and 20 milliseconds: 89.9 ± 11.1% in patients; see Fig. 1). Patients with different types of dystonia showed similar inhibition and no difference emerged between sides in patients with unilateral task-specific dystonia.

Paired Stimuli Delivered at Long Interstimulus Intervals

With long ISIs and suprathreshold conditioning stimuli the time course of the recovery of the test response size differed significantly in patients and normal subjects. In both groups ISIs of 100 and 200 milliseconds elicited a similar response pattern: at 100 milliseconds they markedly suppressed test responses (controls: 16 ± 9.1%, patients: 6.3 ± 3.3%). ISIs of 150 milliseconds only slightly inhibited test responses in normal subjects (79.7 ± 25%), whereas they still markedly reduced the amplitude of the test response in patients (15 ± 6.4%). This difference was statistically significant ($p = 0.017$, ANOVA). At an ISI of 200 milliseconds the test response almost completely recovered (controls: 91.8 ± 25.9%, patients: 81 ± 22.4%; see Fig. 1). An ISI of 250 milliseconds, studied in all dystonic patients and in a subgroup of eight normal subjects, reduced the test response slightly yet not significantly less in patients than in controls (82.6 ± 12.8% vs. 111.2 ± 17.9%).

When patients with task-specific ($n = 6$) and non-task-specific ($n = 4$) dystonia were compared, they showed a similar behavior at intervals of 100 milliseconds (task-specific: 10.5 ± 4.9%; non-task-specific: 0%) and 150 milliseconds (task-specific: 20.6 ± 9.5%; non-task-specific: 6.7 ± 6.7%). At the subsequent intervals, patients with segmental or generalized dystonia were slightly facilitated (200 milliseconds, 107.7 ± 47.4%; 250 milliseconds 110.8 ± 25.3%), whereas patients with task-specific dystonia continued to show inhibition of the test response (200 milliseconds, 63.1 ± 21.1%; 250 milliseconds, 63.9 ± 7.7%). These differences, however, were not statistically significant.

In patients with unilateral writer's cramp ($n = 4$) at all ISIs tested, test responses elicited in the affected and unaffected side had similar mean amplitudes (right hand: 100 milliseconds, 10.8 ± 6.5%; 150 milliseconds, 19.4 ± 11.6%; 200 milliseconds, 37.6 ± 16.8%; 250 milliseconds, 66.7 ± 11.6%; left hand: 100 milliseconds, 20.8 ± 16.9%; 150 milliseconds, 17.4 ± 10.2%; 200 milliseconds, 51.9 ± 19%; 250 milliseconds, 67.8 ± 16.4%).

Cortical Silent Period

A single magnetic shock elicited a slightly shorter silent period in the total group of patients than in controls (110.7 ± 13.9 milliseconds; $n = 10$ vs. 125.8 ± 12.8 milliseconds; $n = 11$). Patients with task-specific focal dystonia had a shorter silent period than in patients with

Paired Magnetic Stimulation at Short ISIs

■ controls   □ patients

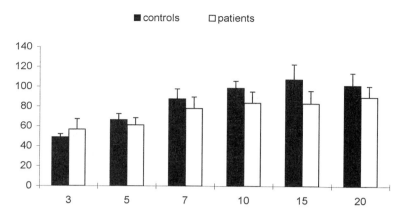

Paired Magnetic Stimulation at Long ISIs

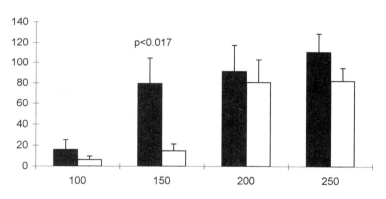

Inter-stimulus Intervals (msec)

FIG. 1. Response to paired magnetic stimuli at short and long ISIs expressed as percentage of an unconditioned control response, in ten patients with dystonia (white columns) and 11 normal subjects (black columns). Each column represents the mean of eight trials per subject; vertical bars are standard errors (SEM). At short ISIs the patients' test response appears slightly more inhibited than in controls, but this difference is not significant. At 150 milliseconds ISI patients' response is significantly more inhibited than that of controls (ANOVA).

segmental or generalized dystonia (90 ± 18.6 milliseconds; $n = 6$ vs. 141.8 ± 6.4 milliseconds; $n = 4$). Owing to the high intersubject variability this last difference was only marginally significant ($p = 0.06$). In patients with task-specific dystonia no significant difference was found between the two sides (right hand: 99.8 ± 25 milliseconds; left hand: 115 ± 30.2 milliseconds, $n = 4$).

DISCUSSION

This study confirms previous findings of normal latency and amplitude of motor responses evoked by transcranial stimulation demonstrating normal corticomotoneuron connection in patients with dystonia.

The motor response threshold similar to those of normal controls suggested that the dystonic patients had normal excitability of cortical motor areas. However, using paired magnetic stimulation we found that long ISIs elicited abnormally inhibited test responses in patients with dystonia. This finding suggests that dystonia increases cortical inhibitory phenomena.

Short Latency Inhibition

With a conditioning-test design, paired pulses given at different interstimulus intervals produce excitatory or inhibitory effects, probably due to activation of different sets of cortical interneurons. Reporting that paired stimuli delivered at 1 to 7 milliseconds ISIs in normal subjects with the muscle at rest produced inhibited test responses, Kujirai et al. (14) and Ridding et al. (27) suggested that they did so by exciting intracortical inhibitory interneurons. In the same test design, short ISIs inhibited test responses in normal subjects also during a voluntary muscle contraction, but in this condition they induced less evident inhibition (28). Although we now confirm test-response inhibition in normal subjects during muscle contraction, the inhibition was less pronounced than that described by others in muscle at rest (28).

In our experiments paired stimuli delivered at short ISIs during a voluntary contraction elicited similar test responses in dystonic patients and normal controls. This contrasts with a report from Ridding et al. (27) noting that test responses recorded in muscles at rest were less inhibited in patients with writer's cramp than in normal subjects. The discrepancy presumably depends on the different state of the muscle during study. Because patients with upper limb dystonia find it difficult to relax their muscles completely, studying these patients during contraction rather than at rest excludes biased responses due to incomplete relaxation.

Long Interstimulus Intervals

Previous studies in normal subjects (4,15, 33) have shown that stimuli delivered at ISIs of 100 and 150 milliseconds elicit inhibited test responses; at longer ISIs test responses progressively recover. We have previously argued that this inhibition arises from activation of cortical inhibitory interneurons.

We have now shown that an ISI of 150 milliseconds elicits a markedly inhibited response in patients with upper limb dystonia. Our findings may help to specify the mechanism responsible for this abnormality. First, we can exclude the possibility that this is due to a difference in the size of the conditioning MEP because patients and normal subjects had MEPs of similar amplitude. Although the intensity of voluntary muscle contraction might have differed in patients and controls we carefully monitored EMG background activity to make sure that it did not. Segmental spinal mechanisms such as refractoriness of spinal motoneurons, after-hyperpolarization potentials, or recurrent inhibition could have intervened. Yet none of these mechanisms produce effects that last longer than 50 to 60 milliseconds (16). Hence we conclude that the difference in the time course of the test response to long ISIs in patients with dystonia and normal subjects depends on cortical mechanisms.

Cortical Silent Period

The cortical SP elicited in response to a single transcranial magnetic stimulus provides a way of investigating inhibitory cortical mechanisms (16,29,37). In this study we found that patients with upper limb dystonia had a slightly shorter SP than normal subjects. Patients with task-specific dystonia had even shorter SPs. One reason why patients with task-specific dystonia had longer SPs could be their anticholinergic medication, a factor reported to lengthen SPs in normal subjects and patients with Parkinson's disease (24). The finding of shorter SPs in our dystonic patients is in line with Mavroudakis's observation (20) that patients with writer's cramp have an abnormally high ratio between SP duration and increased stimulus intensity, thus indicating earlier saturation of cortical inhibitory responses during voluntary activity.

The SP induced by suprathreshold transcranial magnetic stimulus is generated, at least in part, at cortical level and it has been suggested that this inhibition is mediated by the inhibitory neurotransmitter gamma-aminobutyric acid. As in patients with Parkinson's disease, the short-lasting cortical SP in dystonic patients fits in well with the primate model of basal ganglia functioning proposed by DeLong (8). According to this model we have suggested that a reduction in the facilitating effect of the transthalamic motor circuit on the motor cortices would decrease cortical excitation (24).

An important issue is whether the SP and the inhibition elicited by the paired stimulation technique share the same physiologic mechanisms. Although in normal subjects the behavior of these two negative cortical phenomena does overlap, in patients they may behave differently. As in dystonia, also in patients with Parkinson's disease, the two cortical inhibitory phenomena behave differently. In both conditions the cortical SP is shorter whereas the test response with the paired stimulation technique is more inhibited. A short-lasting SP might indicate enhanced cortical excitability, whereas increased inhibition of the test response suggests abnormally reduced cortical excitability in patients. These observations support the notion that distinct cortical interneuronal chains determine these two forms of cortical inhibition.

CONCLUSIONS

The abnormalities described with the paired stimulation technique suggest an increased inhibition of cortical motor areas in dystonia. This agrees with the findings of Féve et al. (12) and Van Der Kamp et al. (36) who reported flattened movement-related cortical potentials in patients with idiopathic and secondary dystonia. The increased inhibition at long ISIs might be related to the slowness of voluntary movement present in patients with dystonia (1,31, 35).

REFERENCES

1. Agostino R, Berardelli A, Formica A, Accornero N, Manfredi M. Sequential arm movements in patients with Parkinson's disease, Huntington's disease and dystonia. *Brain* 1992;115:1481–1495.
2. Alexander GE, Crutcher MD. Functional architecture of basal ganglia circuits: neural substrates of parallel processing. *Trends Neurosci* 1990;13:266–271. Comment in: *Trends Neurosci* 1991;14:55–59.
3. Berardelli A, Rothwell JC, Day BL, Marsden CD. Pathophysiology of blepharospasm and oromandibular dystonia. *Brain* 1985;108:593–608.
4. Berardelli A, Rona S, Inghilleri M, Manfredi M. Cortical inhibition in Parkinson's disease. A study with paired magnetic stimulation. *Brain* 1996;119:71–77.
5. Bhatia KP, Marsden CD. The behavioral and motor consequences of focal lesions of the basal ganglia in man. *Brain* 1994;117:859–876.
6. Cantello R, Gianelli M, Bettucci D, Civardi C. Parkinson's disease rigidity: magnetic motor evoked potentials in a small hand muscle. *Neurology* 1991;41:1449–1456.
7. Cohen LG, Ludlow CL, Warden M, et al. Blink reflex excitability recovery curves in patients with spasmodic dysphonia. *Neurology* 1989;39:572–577.
8. DeLong MR. Primate models of movement disorders of basal ganglia origin. *Trends Neurosci* 1990;13:281–285.
9. Deuschl G, Seifert C, Heinen F, Illert M, Lucking CH. Reciprocal inhibition of forearm flexor muscles in spasmodic torticollis. *J Neurol Sci* 1992;113:85–90.
10. Deuschl G, Toro C, Matsumoto J, Hallett M. The movement related cortical potential is abnormal in patient with writer's cramp. *Ann Neurol* 1995;38:862–868.
11. Thompson PD, Dick JPR, Day BL, et al. Electrophysiology of the corticomotoneurone pathways in patients with movement disorders. *Mov Disord* 1986;1:113–117.
12. Fève A, Bathien N, Rondot P. Abnormal movement related potentials in patients with lesions of the basal ganglia and anterior thalamus. *J Neurol Neurosurg Psychiatry* 1994;57:100–104.
13. Ikoma K, Samii A, Mercuri B, Wassermann EM, Hallett M. Abnormal cortical motor excitability in dystonia. *Neurology* 1996;46:1371–1376.
14. Kujirai T, Caramia MD, Rothwell JC, et al. Corticocortical inhibition in the human motor cortex. *J Physiol (Lond)* 1993;471:501–519.
15. Inghilleri M, Berardelli A, Cruccu G, Priori A, Manfredi M. Motor potentials evoked by paired cortical stimuli. *Electroencephalogr Clin Neurophysiol* 1990;77:382–389.
16. Inghilleri M, Berardelli A, Cruccu G, Manfredi M. Silent period evoked by transcranial stimulation of the human cortex and cervico-medullary junction. *J Physiol (Lond)* 1993;466:521–534.

17. Lee MS, Marsden CD. Movement disorders following lesions of the thalamus or subthalamic region. *Mov Disord* 1994;9:493–507.

18. Marsden CD, Obeso JA, Zarranz JJ, Lang AE. The anatomical basis of symptomatic hemidystonia. *Brain* 1985;108:463–483.

19. Nakashima K, Rothwell JC, Day BL, Thompson PD, Shannon K, Marsden CD. Reciprocal inhibition between forearm muscles in patients with writer's cramp and other occupational cramps, symptomatic hemidystonia and hemiparesis due to stroke. *Brain* 1989;112: 681–697.

20. Mavroudakis N, Caroyer JM, Brunko E, Zegers de Beyl D. Abnormal motor evoked responses to transcranial magnetic stimulation in focal dystonia. *Neurology* 1995;45:1671–1677.

21. Panizza ME, Hallett M, Nilsson J. Reciprocal inhibition in patients with hand cramps. *Neurology* 1989; 39:85–89.

22. Panizza M, Lelli S, Nilsson J, Hallett M. H-reflex recovery curve and reciprocal inhibition of H-reflex in different kinds of dystonia. *Neurology* 1990;40:824–828.

23. Pauletti G, Berardelli A, Cruccu G, Agostino R, Manfredi M. Blink reflex and the masseter inhibitory reflex in patients with dystonia. *Mov Disord* 1993;8: 495–500.

24. Priori A, Berardelli A, Inghilleri M, Accornero N, Manfredi M. Motor cortical inhibition and the dopaminergic system. *Brain* 1994;117:317–323.

25. Priori A, Berardelli A, Inghilleri M, Polidori L, Manfredi M. Electromyographic silent period after transcranial brain stimulation in Huntington's disease. *Mov Disord* 1994;9:178–182.

26. Priori A, Berardelli A, Mercuri B, Manfredi M. Physiological effects produced by botulinum toxin treatment of upper limb dystonia. Changes in reciprocal inhibition between forearm muscles. *Brain* 1995;118: 801–807.

27. Ridding MC, Sheean G, Rothwell JC, Inzelberg R, Kujirai T. Changes in the balance between motor cortical excitation and inhibition in focal, task specific dystonia. *J Neurol Neurosurg Psychiatry* 1995;59:493–498.

28. Ridding MC, Taylor JL, Rothwell JC. The effect of voluntary contraction on corticocortical inhibition in human motor cortex. *J Physiol (Lond)* 1995;487.2: 541–548.

29. Roick H, von Giesen HJ, Benecke R. On the origin of the post-excitatory inhibition seen after transcranial magnetic brain stimulation in awake human subjects. *Exp Brain Res* 1993;94:489–498.

30. Schell GR, Strick PL. The origin of thalamus inputs to the arcuate premotor and supplementary motor areas. *J Neurosci* 1984;4:539–560.

31. Thompson PD, Berardelli A, Rothwell JC, et al. The coexistence of bradykinesia and chorea in Huntington's disease and its implications for theories of basal ganglia control of movement. *Brain* 1988;111:223–244.

32. Tolosa E, Montserrat L, Bayes A. Blink reflex studies in focal dystonias: enhanced excitability of brainstem interneurons in cranial dystonia and spasmodic torticollis. *Mov Disord* 1988;3:61–69.

33. Valls-Solé J, Pascual-Leone A, Wassermann EM, Hallett M. Human motor evoked responses to paired transcranial magnetic stimuli. *Electroencephalogr Clin Neurophysiol* 1992;85:355–364.

34. Valls-Solé J, Pascual-Leone A, Brasil-Neto JP, Cammarota A, McShane L, Hallett M. Abnormal facilitation of the response to transcranial magnetic stimulation in patients with Parkinson's disease. *Neurology* 1994;44:735–741.

35. Van Der Kamp W, Berardelli A, Rothwell JC, Thompson PD, Day BL, Marsden CD. Rapid elbow movements in patients with torsion dystonia. *J Neurol Neurosurg Psychiatry* 1989;52:1043–1049.

36. Van Der Kamp W, Rothwell JC, Thompson PD, Day BL, Marsden CD. The movement-related cortical potential is abnormal in patients with idiopathic torsion dystonia. *Mov Disord* 1995;10:630–633.

37. Wilson SA, Lockwood RJ, Thickbroom GW, Mastaglia FL. The muscle silent period following transcranial magnetic cortical stimulation. *J Neurol Sci* 1993;114:216–222.

Dystonia 3: Advances in Neurology, Vol. 78,
edited by S. Fahn, C. D. Marsden, and M. DeLong.
Lippincott–Raven Publishers, Philadelphia © 1998.

6

Opioid Peptide Precursor Expression in Animal Models of Dystonia Secondary to Dopamine-Replacement Therapy in Parkinson's Disease

Jonathan M. Brotchie, Brian Henry, Christopher J. Hille, and Alan R. Crossman

Division of Neuroscience, School of Biological Sciences, University of Manchester, Manchester, M13 9PT United Kingdom.

Dyskinesias characterized by dystonia and chorea are an almost unavoidable side effect of current dopaminergic treatments for Parkinson's disease. Indeed, dystonia secondary to dopamine-replacement therapy in Parkinson's disease is one of the most commonly encountered forms of dystonia. We believe that the neural mechanisms underlying L-dopa-induced dyskinesia are characterized by decreased GABAergic inhibition of the lateral segment of the globus pallidus (GPl) and decreased glutamatergic excitation of the medial segment of the globus pallidus (GPm). Changes in firing rates of GABAergic and glutamatergic afferents to these regions do not appear to fully account for these changes. We have begun to focus our attention on the possible role of abnormalities in the mechanisms that modulate GABA and glutamate transmission in the basal ganglia in the generation of L-dopa-induced dyskinesia. Opioid peptide transmitters appear to be likely candidates for such a mechanism given that, in the basal ganglia, their synthesis is tightly regulated by dopamine receptor stimulation and that they modulate GABA and glutamate transmission in GPl and GPm.

We have studied opioid peptide precursor expression in animal models of L-dopa-induced dyskinesia. Within the striatum, the expression of pre-proenkephalin-A (PPE-A) and pre-proenkephalin-B (PPE-B) are increased in distinct, topographically organized patterns. We present a model by which enhanced opioid peptide transmission might lead to the appearance of dyskinetic symptoms. These studies open the possibility that subtype-selective antagonists of opioid receptors might prove useful in the treatment of L-dopa-induced dyskinesia and, perhaps, other diseases characterized by dystonic symptoms.

BACKGROUND

Despite tremendous advances over the last decade, dystonia remains one of the greatest challenges facing those interested in understanding the mechanisms underlying movement disorders. Dystonia represents a broad range of movement disorders, each presenting with qualitatively similar symptoms (i.e., sustained muscle contractions) that can affect the musculature in a generalized, segmental, or focal manner. Although similar in symptomatology, the etiology of different disorders characterized by dystonia is very different. However, it is likely that the neural mechanisms underlying dystonia with diverse etiologies show many similarities (see Chapter 3).

The incidence of primary dystonia (i.e., where dystonia is the sole symptom), is probably much greater than previously supposed. It has recently been reported that primary dystonia affects 14 per 100,000 in the North of England (10). In contrast, the incidence of Parkinson's disease is probably in the order of 1 per 1,000. With prolonged dopamine-replacement therapy, parkinsonian patients develop dyskinetic side effects characterized by a mixture of dystonia and chorea (24,29). Dystonia can be seen when the patient is off treatment, at the beginning of a therapeutic effect of a treatment, at peak effect, and/or at the end of treatment. In contrast, chorea usually occurs when the patient is experiencing the peak therapeutic effect of the antiparkinsonian agent. In the long term, it appears that dyskinesias are a virtually unavoidable consequence of dopamine-replacement therapy in Parkinson's disease. For instance, it has been reported that, in young-onset Parkinson's disease, over 80% of patients show L-dopa-induced dyskinesias within 4 years of beginning dopamine-replacement therapy (29). Thus, the dystonic symptoms seen following treatment in Parkinson's disease are probably the most commonly encountered form of dystonia in contemporary neurology. (Throughout this chapter, the term L-dopa-induced dyskinesia will be used to describe dystonia and chorea induced by prolonged treatment of parkinsonian symptoms with L-dopa or other dopamine-replacing agents.)

NEURAL MECHANISMS UNDERLYING DYSTONIA SECONDARY TO DOPAMINE-REPLACEMENT THERAPY IN PARKINSON'S DISEASE

Dyskinesia, indistinguishable from that observed in human parkinsonian patients, is seen in parkinsonian subhuman primates following prolonged L-dopa or dopamine agonist therapy (3,5). We have used the 2-deoxyglucose metabolic mapping approach to study neural activity in primates with L-dopa-induced dyskinesia to determine the neural mechanism underlying the generation of dystonia and chorea (25,27).

These studies are discussed in detail elsewhere (see Chapter 3 of this volume; also Reference 8) but, in essence, have led to the realization that the generation of L-dopa-induced dyskinesia is characterized by decreased GABA-ergic inhibition of the GPl, and decreased glutamatergic excitation of the output regions of the basal ganglia, the GPm, and substantia nigra pars reticulata (SNr).

This general pattern of changes in neural function appears very similar in animals with dyskinesia characterized by dystonia and those where the dyskinesia is predominantly choreic (25) indicating a close functional relationship between chorea and dystonia, and providing the first insight into the possible subcortical mechanisms of dystonia in man. This was an exciting development because it is realistic to expect that advances made in understanding levodopa-induced dystonia will be applicable to other forms of dystonia (e.g., torsion dystonia) for which there is not only no effective treatment, but also no animal model.

However, 2-deoxyglucose studies suggest that the changes in GABAergic and glutamatergic transmission might not be solely due to changes in the firing rate of pallidal and nigral afferents. In recent years, we have become increasingly aware of the powerful role played by opioid peptides utilized by striatal output neurons projecting to GPl, GPm, and SNr, in controlling amino acid transmission and the impact that abnormalities in peptidergic function could have on basal ganglia function.

OPIOID PRECURSOR PEPTIDES

PPE-A and PPE-B are the precursors for a range of opioid peptides used as neurotransmitters within the basal ganglia. PPE-A is a precursor for several enkephalins. A single PPE-A molecule can be processed to produce up to six molecules of Met-enkephalin, a molecule of Leu-enkephalin, and/or the extended enkephalins Met-enkephalin-Arg-Phe and Met-enkephalin-Arg-Phe-Glu-Leu (15). All these PPE-A-derived opioids are relatively selective agonists for δ opioid receptors. PPE-B is often termed prodynorphin, and although this is not, strictly speaking, a misnomer (it is the precursor of all dynorphin synthesized in the brain), it can be confusing, as PPE-B can produce opioid peptides with quite distinct pharmacologic and pharmacokinetic characteristics. Initial stages in the processing of the precursor involve trimming and modification of the C-terminus by enzymes such as carboxypeptidase E. Further processing by enzymes such as the subtilisin-like proteases, termed *proprotein convertases,* then releases the active neuropeptides from PPE-B. At least six proprotein convertases (PC1, 2, 4, 5, furin, and PACE-4) are involved in the production of active opioid peptides in mammalian cells (see, e.g., Reference 11). PPE-B can, depending upon which peptidases were present, give rise to a variety of opioid peptides including a range of dynorphins, Leu-enkephalin, and α-neoendorphin. These opioids are the endogenous ligands for κ, δ, and μ receptors, respectively (20).

OPIOID PEPTIDE PRECURSOR EXPRESSION IN ANIMAL MODELS OF L-DOPA-INDUCED DYSKINESIA

In order to determine whether changes in opioid peptide function might be the "molecular switch" that converts a parkinsonian basal ganglia from one in which L-dopa alleviates symptoms to one in which L-dopa induces dystonia and chorea, we have examined the expression of the high-molecular-weight precursors for opioid peptide transmitters in the striatum of the *N*-methyl-4-phenyl-1,2,3,6-tetrahydropyridine (MPTP)-treated primate model of Parkinson's disease. Two groups of animals were used; one had received acute treatment with apomorphine at a dose sufficient to alleviate parkinsonism. In these animals no dyskinesia was seen. A second group

of animals received similar doses of apomorphine but for a longer period of time. Although apomorphine alleviated parkinsonian symptoms in these animals it also elicited dyskinesia characterized by a mixture of dystonia and chorea.

We and others have previously reported that PPE-A expression is elevated in primate and rodent models of Parkinson's disease (1,13,18, 19,28,33). In the MPTP-treated primate we have found that PPE-A expression is higher in dyskinetic animals than in animals in which treatment reverses symptoms without eliciting dyskinesia. This rise is most marked in sensorimotor and associative regions of the rostral striatum (Fig. 1A). However, other studies in MPTP-treated marmosets and macaques have not been able to detect these elevations in PPE-A expression in dyskinetic animals (19,20). The reason behind this is unclear, but may lie in the details of the methodology. For instance, in those regions of the striatum where we detect our largest changes in expression of PPE-A (i.e., rostrally), previous studies have not taken into account the functional organization of striatum into sensorimotor, associative, and limbic regions. We have found that changes in PPE-A expression do vary between these regions. Another major difference in our study is the use of a control gene, G3PDH, the expression of which acts as a reference for the expression of the gene of interest. We believe that the incorporation of such a control gene reduces the interanimal variability and provides many advantages in the delineation of small changes in gene expression. For instance reference to the control gene will exclude any changes in nonspecific degradation of mRNA. This is a potential problem where it takes several months to prepare all the tissue used in the study, so that some tissues are stored for longer than others. Use of a control gene also reduces any variability due to nonspecific changes in transcription prior to death. Such changes may occur in animals with different ages, different length of disease duration, and different levels of disability. The power of using G3PDH as a control gene is shown by the fact that in our ro-

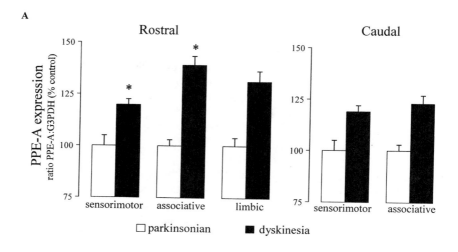

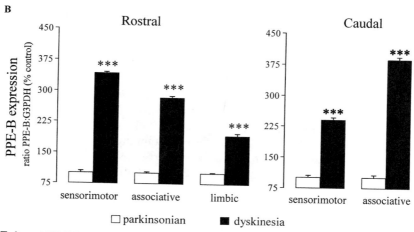

FIG. 1. PPE-A and PPE-B (**A,B**) expression in the MPTP-treated primate with and without L-dopa-induced dyskinesia. Expression of PPE-A and PPE-B was assessed in MPTP-treated primates with and without L-dopa-induced dyskinesia. All animals received apomorphine, at a dose sufficient to alleviate parkinsonian symptoms 45 minutes prior to death. The levels of mRNA were assessed using *in situ* hybridization with 45mer ^{32}S-ATP-3′end-labelled oligoprobes analyzed by optical density measurement of film autoradiographs. Expression of PPE-A and B is expressed relative to the expression of G3PDH. Data represent mean ± SEM ($n = 4$).

dent studies the unlesioned side of 6-OHDA-lesioned rats do not show any significant changes in expression of PPE-A or PPE-B when compared with G3PDH over a range of anti-parkinsonian treatments.

In addition to the changes in PPE-A expression, we have shown, for the first time, that expression of PPE-B is markedly increased in sensorimotor, associative, and limbic regions

of the striatum in L-dopa-induced dyskinesia (Fig. 1B). Increased PPE-B expression shows a marked heterogeneity. Using calbindin immunocytochemistry and acetylcholinesterase histochemistry to define striosome and matrix compartments we have shown that the patches of high PPE-B expression correspond to striosomes. However, it should be noted that the regions of high expression do not completely occupy the striosomal compartment and that, while highest in the striosomes, PPE-B expression is also significantly elevated in the matrix compartment.

Studies in rodents are beginning to prove useful in extending our understanding of the role of changes of expression in opioid precur-

sors in L-dopa-induced dyskinesia. It is well known that dopaminergic agents elicit contraversive rotation in unilateral 6-hydroxydopamine (6-OHDA)-lesioned rats. We and others have discovered that this response shows plasticity, such that repeated administration of L-dopa or apomorphine leads to a marked en-

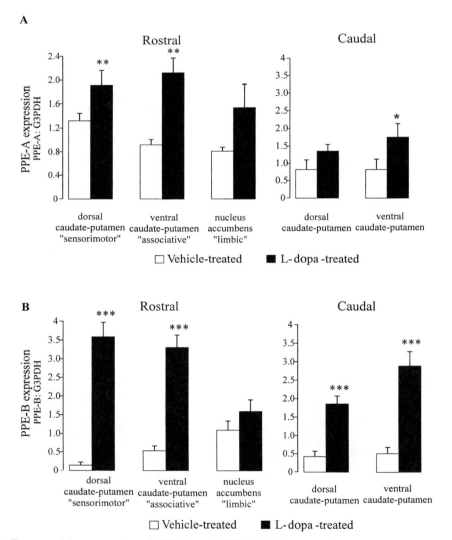

FIG. 2. Topographic expression of PPE-A and PPE-B (**A,B**) expression in the 6-hydroxydopamine-lesioned striatum following repeated L-dopa treatment. Expression of PPE-A and PPE-B was assessed in 6-OHDA-lesioned rats following repeated L-dopa (6.5 mg/kg, twice daily) or vehicle treatment. The levels of mRNA were assessed using *in situ* hybridization with 45mer ^{32}S-ATP-3'end-labeled oligoprobes analyzed by optical density measurement of film autoradiographs. Expression of PPE-A and B in the lesioned striatum is expressed relative to the expression of G3PDH. Data represent mean ± SEM (*n* = 6).

hancement of the rotational response (2,4,17). This phenomenon is quite distinct from the regular, well-characterized, contraversive circling behavior that is often ascribed to receptor "supersensitivity" in this model. Whereas the physical manifestation of this behavioral change is obviously distinct from levodopa-induced dyskinesia (rats do not appear to exhibit dyskinesia under these circumstances), the precipitating factor is the same. As is discussed elsewhere in this volume (Chapter 7) the underlying pathophysiology and pharmacology share many similarities. For example, treatment-induced sensitization is not seen in rats with agents that do not cause dyskinesia in humans when given *de novo* (e.g., bromocriptine) and is attenuated by agents that modulate dyskinesia in the clinic or in MPTP monkeys (14). As in the MPTP-treated primate, drugs that elicit dyskinesia when given *de novo* elevate PPE-A and PPE-B, as in the monkey. The topography of these changes is very similar to those seen in the primate; elevations are seen in both striosome and matrix compartments. The elevations in PPE-A are greatest rostrally whereas PPE-B expression is elevated throughout the striatum (Fig. 2). Agents that do not elicit dyskinesia *de novo* (e.g., bromocriptine and lisuride) do not cause elevations in PPE-A or PPE-B (8).

SPECULATIONS ON THE ROLE OF OPIOID PEPTIDES IN THE NEURAL MECHANISMS UNDERLYING LEVODOPA DYSKINESIA

Given the findings presented above, we hypothesize that the products of PPE-A and PPE-B synthesis might be responsible for the generation of dyskinetic side effects following long-term treatment of parkinsonism.

The major products of PPE-A and PPE-B are generally held to be enkephalins and dynorphin, respectively. From studies in the rat, it has been suggested that enkephalinergic striatal outputs innervate the GPl whereas dynorphinergic striatal efferents are targeted at the output regions of the basal ganglia. We have previously shown that dynorphin, acting at κ opioid receptors, reduces excitatory amino acid (EAA) release in the output regions of the basal ganglia (25) while enkephalin, acting at δ opioid receptors, can reduce GABA release in the GPl (22; see Fig. 3).

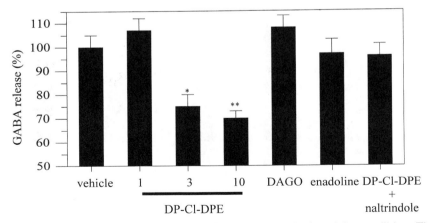

FIG. 3. Delta opioid receptor agonists reduce GABA release in the globus pallidus. The depolarization-evoked release of preloaded [³H]-GABA from slices of rat globus pallidus was measured essentially as described previously (21). The δ opioid agonist DP-Cl-DPE reduced GABA release in a manner that was antagonized by the selective δ opioid antagonist naltrindole. The μ and κ agonists DAGO and enadoline did not reduce GABA release. Data represent evoked GABA release as a percentage of that seen with appropriate vehicle ± SEM (n = 5–7).

We suggest that, following long-term dopaminergic therapy, dopamine receptor stimulation would not only correct the abnormalities in GABA transmission in striatal outputs to GPl, GPm, and SNr, but would also cause excessive release of dynorphin and enkephalin. Enhanced dynorphin levels in the GPm/SNr would reduce glutamate release from subthalamic nucleus efferents and diminish excitation of basal ganglia outputs by the subthalamic nucleus to below normal levels. Thus, GPm/ SNr would become underactive in a manner similar to that observed in other dyskinesias (7,9, 26,30). In addition, enhanced enkephalinergic transmission in GPl would reduce GABA release, perhaps leading to disinhibition of GPl. As a result, the outputs of GPl would be rendered overactive leading to inhibition of the subthalamic nucleus by the GABAergic pallidosubthalamic pathway. Thus, enhanced enkephalin transmission might represent another mechanism, in addition to dynorphinergic reduction of glutamate release, by which increased opioidergic transmission could reduce the excitatory subthalamic drive to the output neurons of the basal ganglia.

This proposed mechanism is appealing because it offers several potential avenues for therapeutic intervention in L-dopa dyskinesia. However, many issues remain to be resolved and caution should be taken in extrapolating elevations in PPE-A and PPE-B levels to enhanced opioidergic transmission in GPl, GPm, and/or SNR. For instance, the processing of PPE-B is complex, and can employ different combinations of proprotein convertases, the expressions of which are regulated by a host of intracellular signaling mechanisms including cAMP, $Ins_{3,4,5} P_3$. Thus, the enhanced PPE-B expression seen in dyskinesia could lead to the formation of several analogues of dynorphin (e.g., $dynorphin_{1-8}$, $dynorphin_{1-17}$). Although most dynorphin analogues are high-affinity agonists at κ opioid receptors (6), shorter analogues tend to be short acting and slightly less selective for κ over δ receptors. Longer analogues are more potent, more selective for the κ receptor, and have longer-lasting actions (6). However, potentially of greater importance is

the fact that PPE-B can also produce Leu-enkephalin (34), which would act preferentially at δ opioid receptors (20), and α-neoendorphin, which would activate μ opioid receptors (20) the functions of which are unknown in the pallidonigral system. It is, thus, apparent that increased PPE-B synthesis might mediate multiple effects by interaction of its peptide products with κ, δ, and possibly μ receptors.

The situation with PPE-A is simpler because all the major products of PPE-A synthesis are enkephalins and have actions mediated primarily through δ opioid receptors. However, we still do not know whether increased PPE-A mRNA levels are translated into protein. Furthermore, we do not know whether such protein, if produced, is transported to terminals, where such terminals might be (i.e., GPl, GPm, SNr, or striatum), or whether it is released. The simple dichotomy between enkephalinergic projections to GPl and dynorphinergic projections to GPm/SNr is also oversimplistic and probably does not hold true in the primate (16). Such problems also apply to interpreting the rise in PPE-B. Indeed as we will discuss below we have been able to demonstrate that activation of κ opioid receptors can reduce glutamate release in the primate, but not rodent, GPl.

Further studies are obviously necessary to characterize the relationship between opioid receptor stimulation and L-dopa-induced dyskinesia. However, we have recently obtained data to suggest that enhanced opioid peptide transmission might indeed be responsible for L-DOPA-induced dyskinesia. Thus, the enhanced locomotor response to L-dopa seen in 6-OHDA-lesioned rats that have received repeated L-dopa treatment is significantly reduced if L-dopa is administered with opioid receptor antagonists (see Chapter 7). Furthermore, in the rodent model, the development, over time, of the hyperkinetic response to dopaminergic agents is correlated with the rise in PPE-B synthesis in sensorimotor and associative (but not limbic) striatum (12). PPE-A synthesis is only significantly elevated after the behavior supersensitivity is well-established and is, therefore, unlikely to contribute to the development of the phenomenon.

Although not proving cause or effect, these findings further support the association between rises in PPE-B expression and L-dopa-induced dyskinesia. The elevation of PPE-A mRNA does not become significant until after the enhanced behavioral response has become established (12). The role of products of PPE-A in the generation of dyskinetic symptoms is thus not clear. We cannot, however, discount the possibility that opioid peptides derived from PPE-A are important in the maintenance of dyskinesia or, that given the topography of changes in expression (i.e., highest in limbic and associative regions of striatum), are responsible for nonmotor side effects of repeated L-dopa treatment in parkinsonism.

THE DIFFERENCE BETWEEN THE NEURAL MECHANISMS UNDERLYING LEVODOPA-INDUCED CHOREA AND DYSTONIA

The model outlined above provides, for the first time, a testable description of how repeated dopamine-receptor stimulation in parkinsonism might lead to the generation of side effects such as dystonia and chorea. However, to date, the model is unable to differentiate between the mechanisms responsible for producing these two quite distinct movement disorders. Thus, although we are well along the road toward understanding the many similarities, the differences between L-dopa-induced chorea and dystonia remain a major challenge to our understanding of movement disorder pathophysiology. Dystonia rather than chorea may result from a combination of one or more of the following:

- Quantitative, topographically organized differences in the levels of abnormalities in peptidergic and classic neurotransmission;
- Differences in the detail of the temporal organization of the changes (i.e., patterning) in space and time, of neuronal firing;
- Additional neural mechanisms.

Quantitative differences between chorea and dystonia were suggested by our previous studies employing 2-deoxyglucose utilization to study nerve terminal activity in L-dopa-induced chorea and dystonia (25). We showed that in L-dopa-induced dyskinesia generally terminal activity in the subthalamic nucleus is significantly increased. This enhanced terminal activity is thought to indicate overactivity of inhibitory pallidosubthalamic terminals projecting from GPl. As described above, we propose that a key mechanism underlying this enhanced pallidosubthalamic activity is increased enkephalinergic inhibition of GABA release in GPl. In this study, we also suggested that 2-deoxyglucose uptake in the subthalamic nucleus as a whole is greater in dystonia than chorea (28; See Fig. 4), perhaps suggesting that there was a simple quantitative difference between the two conditions.

However, recently, more detailed topographic analysis has demonstrated that the enhanced 2-deoxyglucose uptake is actually due to a qualitative difference in the topographic organization of terminal activity in the dystonic compared to the choreic subthalamic nucleus. Thus, nerve terminal activity in the ventral (limbic/associative) subthalamic nucleus is the same in both chorea and dystonia (Fig. 4). However, a marked increase in nerve terminal activity is seen in the dorsal tip of the subthalamic nucleus in dystonic, but not choreic animals (Fig. 4). This finding suggests that the abnormalities in enkephalinergic transmission in the motor loop through the GPl-subthalamic nucleus-GPm/SNr may be important in the generation of dystonia but not chorea. To date it is not known whether the topographic organization of changes in peptide expression might underlie such changes.

An action of dynorphin in GPm/SNr would change basal ganglia output consistent with other forms of dyskinesia. The question arises as to whether additional dynorphinergic mechanisms might be at play in the primate that induce dystonia rather than chorea. A possible lead is suggested by the anatomic distribution of peptidergic projections in the primate. Whereas, in the rat, there is a well-recognized dichotomy between the GABA/enkephalin striatal output to GPl and the GABA/dynorphin/substance P projection to GPm/SNr, in the

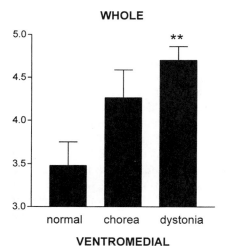

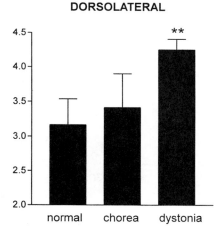

FIG. 4. 2-Deoxyglucose uptake in the subthalamic nucleus in the MPTP-treated primate following dopamine-replacement therapy. Effect of chorea and dystonia. All animals were killed 45 minutes following treatment with apomorphine or L-dopa at a dose that reversed parkinsonian symptoms. Three groups of animals were identified: treated and clinically normal, treatment-induced chorea, treatment-induced dystonia. [3H]-2-deoxyglucose autoradiography was performed as described previously (25). Data represent the ratio of 2-deoxyglucose uptake relative to corpus callosum, mean $\pm$ SEM ($n = 3$ in each group).

monkey and human there is a dynorphin innervation of GPl and an enkephalin innervation of GPm/SNr (17). The dynorphin innervation of GPl in primates appears to be functionally important because we have shown that activation of κ opioid receptors in marmoset GPl reduces glutamate release in a manner similar to that seen in GPm/SNr (Fig. 5). Furthermore, we have also shown that κ receptor activation is enhanced in the GPl of Parkinson's disease patients with treatment-related dyskinesias. We have previously shown, in intracerebral injection studies in primates, that attenuation of glutamate transmission in GPm by the nonselective antagonist kynurenate causes chorea, whereas in GPl it induces dystonia (30). We therefore hypothesize that, following prolonged dopaminergic therapy in Parkinson's disease, choreiform side effects are seen when enhanced dynorphin reduces glutamate input from the subthalamic nucleus to the GPm alone. However, in dystonia we speculate that this effect might be combined with a dynorphin-induced reduction in GPl glutamate release. This would

lead to a reduction in GABAergic inhibition of the GPm/SNr by the direct projection from GPl (32). In this sense, the neural mechanisms within GPm that underlie dystonia would have elements of parkinsonism (underactive GABA) and elements of chorea (underactive glutamate). Such a mechanism is also consistent with the known clinicopathophysiology of Huntington's disease, where in the later stages of the disease (when the GABAergic input to the GPm/SNr degenerates) a shift from chorea to dystonia is seen (31).

Changes in the spatiotemporal patterning of signaling within the dystonic brain may also result from abnormalities in peptidergic function. The fact that peptide transmitters allow communication between neurons over greater distances and times than classic transmitters makes them particularly useful in implementing processes related to lateral inhibition and receptive field size. Enkephalins and dynorphins of different lengths exert actions over different distances and times. Therefore changes in the processing of opioid peptide precursors

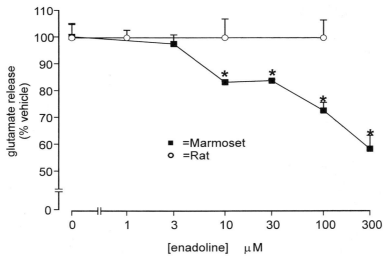

FIG. 5. κ Opioid receptor agonists reduce glutamate release in the primate GPl. Depolarization-evoked release of preloaded [³H]-glutamate was measured from slices of marmoset GPl and the rat homologue globus pallidus. In the marmoset, but not the rat, the κ agonist enadoline reduced glutamate release in a concentration-dependent manner. In the primate study data are the mean of three experiments, in the rodent study data are the mean of six experiments. This reduction in release was antagonized by the selective κ opioid receptors antagonist nor-BNI (10 μM) (data not shown).

could dramatically alter the properties of the neurotransmission, such that the temporal characteristics of peptide-mediated modulation of amino acid transmission could be dramatically altered. To date the properties of peptides in altering the temporal patterning of neuronal activity in animal models of dystonia have not been investigated.

Further studies on peptidergic function in chorea compared to dystonia are required to address the hypotheses resulting from these speculations. However, for the first time we are now in a position where we can begin to develop, and test, specific hypotheses regarding the generation of dystonic symptoms. The understanding of the neural mechanisms responsible for generating dystonic symptoms, and thus a rational therapy, has become an achievable goal.

CONCLUSIONS

There is a strong correlation between enhanced expression of opioid peptide precursor peptides and the appearance of L-dopa-induced dyskinesia. Elucidation of whether the potential products of these precursors are also enhanced and in which regions of the basal ganglia will allow us to test specific hypotheses regarding the generation of dystonic symptoms and allow us to approach the possibility of defining a novel treatment for dystonia seen in L-dopa-induced dyskinesia, perhaps based on selective blockade of opioid receptor subtypes. Similar changes in peptidergic transmission may also underlie other forms of dystonia of basal ganglia origin.

ACKNOWLEDGMENTS

This work was supported by the Dystonia Medical Research Foundation, the Medical Research Council (UK) and the BBSRC.

REFERENCES

1. Augood SJ, Emson PC, Mitchell IJ, Boyce S, Clarke CE, Crossman AR. Cellular localisation of enkephalin gene expression in MPTP-treated cynomolgus monkeys. *Mol Brain Res* 1989;6:85–92.

2. Bevan P. Repeated apomorphine treatment causes behavioural supersensitivity and dopamine D2 receptor hyposensitivity. *Neurosci Lett* 1983;35:185–189.

3. Boyce S, Clarke CE, Luquin R, et al. Induction of chorea and dystonia in parkinsonian primates. *Mov Disord* 1990;5:3–7.

4. Carey RJ. Chronic L-DOPA treatment in the unilateral 6-OHDA rat: evidence for behavioural sensitization and biochemical tolerance. *Brain Res* 1991;568: 205–214.

5. Clarke CE, Boyce S, Robertson RG, Sambrook MA, Crossman AR. Drug-induced dyskinesia in primates rendered hemi-parkinsonian by intracarotid administration of 1-methyl-4-phenyl-1,2,3,6-tetrahydropyridine (MPTP). *J Neurol Sci* 1989;90:307–314.

6. Corbett AD, Paterson SJ, McKnight AT, Magnan J, Kosterlitz HW. Dynorphin1-8 and dynorphin1-9 are ligands for the kappa-subtype of opiate receptor. *Nature* 1982;299:79–81.

7. Crossman AR. Primate models of dyskinesia: the experimental approach to the study of basal ganglia-related involuntary movement disorders. *Neuroscience* 1987;21:1–40.

8. Crossman AR. A hypothesis on the pathophysiological mechanisms that underlie levodopa or dopamine agonist-induced dyskinesia in Parkinson's disease: implications for future strategies in treatment. *Mov Disord* 1990;5:100–108.

9. Crossman AR, Mitchell IJ, Sambrook MA, Jackson A. Chorea and myoclonus in the monkey induced by gamma-aminobutyric acid antagonism in the lentiform complex. The site of drug action and a hypothesis for the neural mechanisms of chorea. *Brain* 1988; 111:1211–1233.

10. Duffy P, Butler AG, Barnes M. The epidemiology of the primary dystonias in the North of England. *Proceedings of the Third International Dystonia Symposium* 1996;22.

11. Dupuy A, Lindberg I, Zhou Y, et al. Processing of prodynorphin by the prohormone convertase PC1 results in high molecular weight intermediate forms. Cleavage at single arginine residues. *FEBS Lett* 1994;337:60–65.

12. Duty S, Brotchie JM. Enhancement of the behavioural response to apomorphine administration following repeated treatment in the 6-hydroxydopamine-lesioned rat is temporally-correlated with a rise in striatal preproenkephalin-B, but not pre-proenkephalin-A, gene expression. *Experimental Neurology* 1997; 144:423–432.

13. Gerfen CR, Mcginty JF, Young III WS. Dopamine differentially regulates dynorphin, substance P and enkephalin expression in striatal neurons; in situ hybridisation histochemical analysis. *J Neurosci* 1991; 11:1016–1031.

14. Gomez-Mancilla B, Bedard PJ. Effect of nondopaminergic drugs on L-DOPA-induced dyskinesias in MPTP-treated monkeys. *Clin Neuropharmacol* 1993;16:418–427.

15. Gubler U, Seeburg P, Hoffman BJ, Gage LP, Udenfriend S. Molecular cloning establishes proenkephalin as precursor of enkephalin-containing peptides. *Nature* 1982;295:206–208.

16. Haber SN, Watson SJ. The comparative distribution of enkephalin, dynorphin and substance P in the human globus pallidus and basal forebrain. *Neuroscience* 1985;14:1011–1024.

17. Henry B, Brotchie JM. Potential of opioid antagonists in the treatment of levodopa-induced dyskinesias in Parkinson's disease. *Drugs Aging* 1996;9:149–158.

18. Herrero M-T, Augood SJ, Hirsch EC, et al. Effects of L-Dopa on preproenkephalin and preprotachykinin gene expression in the MPTP-treated monkey striatum. *Neuroscience* 1995;86:1189–1198.

19. Jolkkonen J, Jenner P, Marsden CD. L-DOPA reverses altered gene expression of substance P but not enkephalin in the caudate-putamen of common marmosets treated with MPTP. *Mol Brain Res* 1995;32: 297–307.

20. Kieffer BL. Recent advances in molecular recognition and signal transduction of active peptides: receptors for opioid peptides. *Cell Mol Neurobiol* 1995;15:615–635.

21. Maneuf YP, Duty S, Hille CJ, Crossman AR, Brotchie JM. Modulation of GABA transmission by diazoxide and cromakalim in the globus pallidus: implications for the treatment of Parkinson's disease. *Expt Neurol* 1996;139:12–16.

22. Maneuf YP, Mitchell IJ, Crossman AR, Brotchie JM. On the role of enkephalin co-transmission in the GABAergic striatal efferents to the globus pallidus. *Expt Neurol* 1994;125:65–71.

23. Maneuf YP, Mitchell IJ, Crossman AR, Woodruff GN, Brotchie JM. Functional implications of kappa opioid receptor-mediated modulation of glutamate transmission in the output regions of the basal ganglia in rodent and primate models of Parkinson's disease. *Brain Res* 1995;683:102–108.

24. Marsden CD, Parkes JD, Quinn N. Fluctuations of disability in Parkinson's disease—clinical aspects. In: Marsden C, Fahn S, eds. *Movement disorders*. London: Butterworth Scientific, 1982:96–122.

25. Mitchell IJ, Boyce S, Sambrook MA, Crossman AR. A 2-deoxyglucose study of the effects of dopamine agonists on the parkinsonian primate brain: implications for the neural mechanisms that mediate dopamine agonist-induced dyskinesia. *Brain* 1992;115:809–824.

26. Mitchell IJ, Jackson A, Sambrook MA, Crossman AR. Common neural mechanisms in experimental chorea and hemiballismus in the monkey. Evidence from 2-deoxyglucose autoradiography. *Brain Res* 1985;339: 346–350.

27. Mitchell IJ, Luquin R, Boyce S, et al. Neural mechanisms of dystonia: evidence from a 2-deoxyglucose uptake study in a primate model of dopamine agonist-induced dystonia. *Mov Disord* 1990;5:49–54.

28. Parent A, Asselin M-C, Cote PY. Dopaminergic regulation of peptide gene expression in the striatum of normal and parkinsonian monkeys. *Adv Neurol* 1996; 69:73–77.

29. Quinn N, Critchley P, Marsden CD. Young onset Parkinson's disease. *Mov Disord* 1987;2:73–91.

30. Robertson RG, Farmery SM, Sambrook MA, Crossman AR. Dyskinesia in the primate following injection of an excitatory amino acid antagonist into the medial segment of the globus pallidus. *Brain Res* 1989;476: 317–322.

31. Sapp E, Ge P, Aizawa H, et al. Evidence for a preferential loss of enkephalin immunoreactivity in the external globus pallidus in low grade Huntington's disease using high resolution image analysis. *Neuroscience* 1995;64:397–404.

32. Smith Y, Bolam JP. The output neurones and the dopaminergic neurones of the substantia nigra receive a GABA input from the globus pallidus in the rat. *J Comp Neurol* 1989;296:47–64.

33. Voorn P, Poest G, Groenwegen HJ. Increase of enkephalin and decrease of substance P immunoreactivity in the dorsal and ventral striatum of the rat after midbrain 6-hydroxydopamine lesions. *Brain Res* 1987;412: 391–396.

34. Zamir N, Palkovits M, Weber E, Mezey E, Brownstein MJ. A dynorphinergic pathway of Leu-enkephalin production in rat substantia nigra. *Nature* 1984;307: 643–645.

Dystonia 3: Advances in Neurology, Vol. 78,
edited by S. Fahn, C. D. Marsden, and M. DeLong.
Lippincott–Raven Publishers, Philadelphia © 1998.

7

Characterization of a Rodent Model in Which to Investigate the Molecular and Cellular Mechanisms Underlying the Pathophysiology of L-dopa-Induced Dyskinesia

Brian Henry, Alan R. Crossman, and Jonathan M. Brotchie

Division of Neuroscience, School of Biological Sciences, University of Manchester, Manchester, M13 9PT United Kingdom.

The most effective and most commonly prescribed treatment for Parkinson's disease is the dopamine precursor L-3,4-dihydroxyphenylalanine (L-dopa) (1,11,24,35). This treatment is highly successful in reversing the hypokinetic symptoms seen in Parkinson's disease in the initial years of treatment (1,3). However, following treatment over an extended period of time many complications are seen. These include "on-off" fluctuations, freezing episodes, nonresponsiveness, or "wearing-off" (2,23,31) and most commonly of all, the abnormal involuntary movements of L-dopa-induced dyskinesia (3). These dyskinesias are dystonic and/or choreiform in nature and can become as debilitating as the Parkinson's disease itself (25,28,32). Following 5 years of L-dopa treatment in Parkinson's disease, up to 80% of patients develop some symptoms of L-dopa-induced dyskinesia (3). It is thus apparent that L-dopa-induced dyskinesia is probably the most common condition in which dystonia is a major symptom.

Conversely, *de novo* administration of bromocriptine or lisuride to both patients and *N*-methyl-4-phenyl-1,2,3,6-tetrahydropyridine (MPTP)-treated macaques does not lead to the development of dyskinesia (4,8,21,30). Unfortunately,

only about 30% of patients respond to the antiparkinsonian effects of bromocriptine (20). Patients who receive bromocriptine monotherapy may also experience psychiatric adverse effects, including confusion, visual hallucinations, and paranoia (7,17) and, therefore, require either bromocriptine plus L-dopa or L-dopa monotherapy. Both of these latter regimens eventually result in dyskinesia (19, 22,26,29).

To understand the neural mechanisms underlying L-dopa-induced dyskinesia, investigate and develop effective adjunct therapies for L-dopa-induced dyskinesia, and screen for novel antiparkinsonian drugs that do not cause dyskinesia, the most valuable asset is an effective animal model that replicates the molecular, cellular, biochemical, and symptomatic changes seen in parkinsonian patients displaying L-dopa-induced dyskinesia. To date, the only animal model that replicates the molecular, cellular, biochemical, and symptomatic changes of L-dopa-induced dystonia has been the MPTP-treated macaque following repeated L-dopa or dopamine-agonist administration (4,6,12). This is an excellent model in almost all respects and will remain the "gold standard" for the investigation of L-dopa-induced dyskinesias. Recently, it has been suggested that MPTP-treated marmosets may also be capable of exhibiting L-dopa-induced dystonia and chorea (27). However, ethical and logistical considerations must lead us to consider nonprimate models that might permit useful advances toward understanding the neural mechanisms underlying L-dopa-induced dystonia. Therefore, a rodent model that replicates the biochemical, molecular, and neural mechanisms underlying L-dopa-induced dyskinesia would be a great advantage. Such a model would not only further understanding of the neural mechanisms underlying L-dopa-induced dyskinesia, but also permit investigation of new antiparkinsonian drugs for their prodyskinetic properties and screening for novel antidyskinetic compounds. Additionally, a rodent model would be less expensive, allow several compounds to be tested *de novo* in a short period of time, and allow subsequent molecular, biochemical, or receptor changes to be investigated following these treatments. No rodent model of L-dopa-induced dyskinesia has been described to date. However, several authors have described a behavioral enhancement of the effects of L-dopa or apomorphine in the unilateral 6-OHDA-lesioned rat model of Parkinson's disease (5,9). Thus, it appears that unilateral 6-OHDA-lesioned rats, when treated repeatedly, show an enhanced level of rotational behavior with increasing length of treatment.

In this chapter, repeated L-dopa treatment of the well-characterized unilateral 6-OHDA-lesioned rat model of Parkinson's disease (33) is used to investigate the possible development of a rodent model of L-dopa-induced dyskinesia. To investigate this possibility, studies were performed to:

- Characterize the behavioral response to repeated L-dopa administration;
- Investigate the modification of this behavioral response by drugs known to reduce L-dopa-induced dyskinesia when coadministered with L-dopa in both patients and MPTP-treated nonhuman primates (10,13,15);

- Investigate the response to *de novo* administration of drugs known not to cause dystonia in patients and MPTP-treated nonhuman primates;
- Investigate alterations in opioid neuropeptide precursors in both rodent and primate models of L-dopa-induced dyskinesia.

EFFECT OF DOPAMINERGIC DRUGS ON ROTATIONAL LOCOMOTION IN THE 6-OHDA-LESIONED RAT MODEL OF PARKINSON'S DISEASE

The effects of various dopaminergic drugs on rotational locomotion of the 6-OHDA-lesioned rat model of Parkinson's disease were investigated. In all 6-OHDA-lesioned rats, stress induced by injection of 1 mL/kg sterile water produced spontaneous rotation ipsiversive to the 6-OHDA lesion immediately following injection (day 0, Fig. 1). Following a single injection of L-dopa (100 mg/kg) and benserazide (25 mg/kg), rotation contraversive to the 6-OHDA-lesion was observed. This response is the well-characterized contraversive rotation that has been much investigated since first described in the early 1970s (33,34). This response is generally held to reflect antiparkinsonian actions. However, this rotational response to L-dopa administration showed a marked plasticity following subsequent injections, rising rapidly and reaching a plateau by approximately day 7. By the end of the 10-day treatment period a 500% increase in the rotational response to the same dose of L-dopa/benserazide was observed (Fig. 1). Following repeated vehicle administration no behavioral alterations were observed, with a low level of rotation ipsiversive to the 6-OHDA lesion observed throughout the test period.

Twice-daily injection of the lower dose of L-dopa (6.5 mg/kg) and benserazide (1.5 mg/kg) showed a more gradual potentiation in response to treatment (Fig. 1). A robust rotational response, contraversive to the 6-OHDA lesion, was not seen until day 7. However, following 7 days of treatment, a rapid increase was ob-

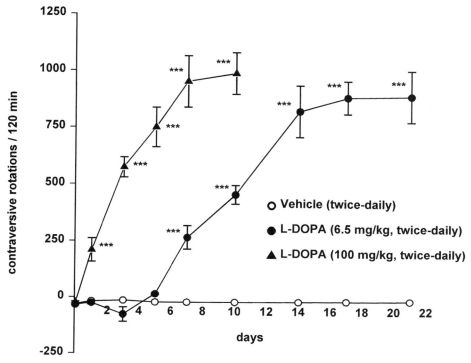

FIG. 1. Behavioral hyperkinesia following repeated L-dopa administration in the 6-OHDA-lesioned rat model of Parkinson's disease. Net 360 degree rotations contraversive to the 6-OHDA lesion were measured following twice-daily (9 a.m. and 5 p.m.) injections of L-dopa (100 mg/kg) and benserazide [25 mg/kg, for 10 days (▲)] L-dopa (6.5 mg/kg) and benserazide [1.5 mg/kg for 21 days (●)], or vehicle (○) in the 6-OHDA-lesioned rat model of Parkinson's disease. Locomotion was assessed for 2 hours following the 9 a.m. injection on days 0, 1, 3, 5, 7, and 10 for the high-dose L-dopa and on days 0, 1, 3, 5, 7, 10, 14, 17, and 21 for the low-dose L-dopa and vehicle. Data are expressed as mean ($\pm$SEM) net rotations contraversive to the 6-OHDA-lesion ($n = 8$). Effect of drug $p < 0.001$, MANOVA; effect of drug over time $p < 0.001$, MANOVA; ***$p < 0.001$ compared with the vehicle group; one-way analysis of variance, Student-Newman-Keuls post hoc analysis.

served following subsequent injections. This potentiated behavioral response reached a plateau by day 14, and by the end of the 21-day treatment period approximately a 500% increase in the rotational response is observed (Fig. 1). Following 21 days vehicle administration, no alteration in behavioral response is observed with only a low level of rotations ipsiversive to the 6-OHDA lesion observed (Fig. 1). Therefore, the rate of onset of this behavioral change is, like dyskinetic symptoms clinically, related to the dose and duration of treatment.

Repeated dopamine-replacement therapy in the 6-OHDA lesioned rat models the precipitating factors for the production of L-dopa-induced dyskinesia in parkinsonian patients (i.e., dopamine depletion of the striatum and subsequent reintroduction in a pulsatile manner). Although rats do not show dystonia and chorea, they do show a novel behavior whereby the rotational response to L-dopa is markedly enhanced with repeated treatment. In the remainder of this chapter, the question of whether the mechanism underlying this behavior is similar to those seen in L-dopa-induced dyskinesia in both patients and MPTP-treated nonhuman primates, and thus whether this model will prove useful in understanding the neural mechanisms underlying symptom generation in patients, will be addressed.

Twenty-one-day *de novo* administration of bromocriptine (5 mg/kg, twice daily) produced a rotational locomotion contraversive to the 6-OHDA-lesion (Fig. 2). However, unlike the response to L-dopa this behavior was not potentiated following subsequent injections. A similar pattern in rotational response was also seen following 21-day *de novo* administration of lisuride (0.1 mg/kg, twice daily, Fig. 2). Inter-

estingly, following a single "priming" dose of L-dopa (100 mg/kg) and benserazide (25 mg/kg) the response to repeated administration (21-day, twice daily) of bromocriptine was potentiated, showing a 300% potentiation in rotational response when compared with "unprimed" (Fig. 3).

Therefore, in the 6-OHDA-lesioned rat *de novo* administration of drugs that do not cause dyskinesia in both patients and MPTP-treated nonhuman primates (i.e., bromocriptine and lisuride) does not lead to an enhancement in response to repeated treatment. However, a behavioral potentiation is observed following re-

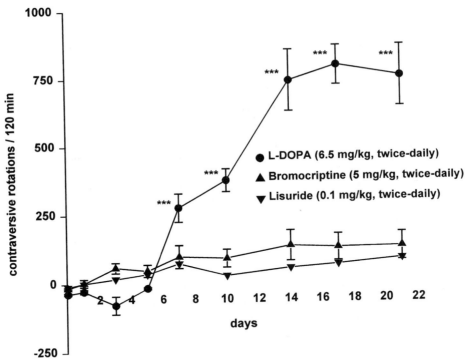

FIG. 2. Behavioral hyperkinesia following repeated L-dopa, bromocriptine, or lisuride administration in the 6-OHDA-lesioned rat model of Parkinson's disease. Net 360 degree rotations contraversive to the 6-OHDA-lesion were measured following twice-daily (9 a.m. and 5 p.m.) injections of L-dopa (100 mg/kg) and benserazide [1.5 mg/kg (●), bromocriptine [5 mg/kg (▲)], or lisuride [0.1 mg/kg (▼)] in the 6-OHDA-lesioned rat model of Parkinson's disease. Locomotion was assessed for 2 hours following the 9 a.m. injection on days 0, 1, 3, 5, 7, 10, 14, 17, and 21. Data are expressed as mean (±SEM) net rotations contraversive to the 6-OHDA-lesion ($n = 8$). Effect of drug $p < 0.001$, MANOVA; effect of drug over time $p < 0.001$, MANOVA; ***$p < 0.001$ compared with the vehicle group; one-way analysis of variance, Student-Newman-Keuls post hoc analysis.

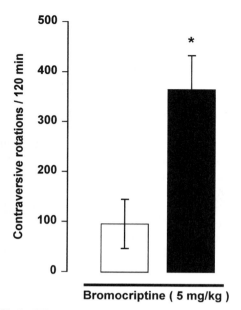

Bromocriptine (5 mg/kg)

FIG. 3. Effects of L-dopa "priming" on rotational locomotion following repeated bromocriptine administration in the 6-OHDA-lesioned rat model of Parkinson's disease. Three weeks post-6-OHDA-lesioned rats were "primed" by a single injection of L-dopa (100 mg/kg) and benserazide (25 mg/kg) or vehicle. Starting on the following day bromocriptine (5 mg/kg) was administered twice daily for 21 days. Net 360 degree rotations contraversive to the 6-OHDA-lesion are shown following 21 days bromocriptine treatment in "L-dopa-primed" (■) or "vehicle-primed" (□) rats. Locomotion was assessed for 2 hours following the 9 a.m. injection on day 21. Data are expressed as mean (±SEM) net rotations contraversive to the 6-OHDA lesion (n = 8). *p <0.05 compared with the "vehicle-primed" group; unpaired, Student's t test.

peated bromocriptine treatment after a single "priming" injection of L-dopa (Fig. 3). In contrast, drugs that elicit dyskinesia in both patients and MPTP-treated primates, or drugs not associated with dyskinesia following *de novo* administration (e.g., bromocriptine or lisuride) following L-dopa-priming, produce a potentiated behavioral response following repeated administration. The fact that a single dose of L-dopa can markedly affect the subsequent response to dopaminergic drugs has major impli-

cations for the design of both clinical trials and experiments where drugs such as apomorphine or L-dopa might be employed either as a diagnostic tool or to assess extent of a dopaminergic lesion.

EFFECT OF COADMINISTRATION OF NONDOPAMINERGIC DRUGS ON L-dopa-INDUCED ROTATIONAL LOCOMOTION IN THE 6-OHDA-LESIONED RAT FOLLOWING REPEATED L-dopa ADMINISTRATION

Previous studies in MPTP-treated primates have shown that several nondopaminergic agents, when coadministered with L-dopa, can reduce L-dopa-induced dyskinesia (15). Coadministration of these compounds with L-dopa was performed in the 6-OHDA-lesioned rat following repeated low-dose L-dopa treatment. Three-weeks postlesion, 6-hydroxydopamine-lesioned rats were treated with L-dopa (6.5 mg/kg) and benserazide (1.5 mg/kg) for 14 days (twice daily, 9 a.m. and 5 p.m.). L-dopa treatment was continued for days 14 to 21. However, nondopaminergic agents (or vehicle) were administered in concert with the a.m. injection of L-dopa. An index of the effect of the nondopaminergic agent on the L-dopa-induced hyperkinesia was attained by expressing the rotational response to L-dopa and drug as a percentage of L-dopa and appropriate vehicle on the following day (i.e., percentage hyperkinesia). Rotational locomotion was assessed for 15 minutes, between 45 minutes to 60 minutes following L-dopa injection.

Coadministration of the α_2-adrenoreceptor antagonist yohimbine (10 mg/kg), the α_2-adrenoreceptor agonist clonidine (1 mg/kg), or the 5-hydroxytryptamine (5-HT) uptake inhibitor 5-MDOT (2 mg/kg), completely abolished the L-dopa-induced hyperkinesia (Fig. 4). Propranolol, the β-adrenoreceptor antagonist, produced a 35% reduction in L-dopa-induced hyperkinesia, whereas low-dose administration of the nonselective opioid receptor antagonist naloxone (0.01 mg/kg) had no effect on the L-dopa-induced hyperkinesia seen following repeated L-dopa administration in the 6-OHDA-lesioned rat (Fig. 4).

To test that reductions in hyperkinesia seen following repeated L-dopa administration in the 6-OHDA-lesioned rat were not due to non-specific reductions in spontaneous locomotion, all drugs used were administered to clinically normal rats and spontaneous locomotion assessed. Naloxone, propranolol, and 5-MDOT had no effect on spontaneous locomotion. Yohimbine increased spontaneous locomotion, whereas it was significantly decreased by clonidine (data not shown). Therefore, in agreement with an MPTP-treated macaque study (15), clonidine acts to reduce L-dopa-induced hyper-

kinesia through a nonspecific mechanism, whereas yohimbine, 5-MDOT, and propranolol caused a specific reduction in L-dopa-induced hyperkinesia. This suggests that the pharmacologic profile of the potentiated response is identical in both the 6-OHDA-lesioned rat model of Parkinson's disease following repeated L-dopa administration, and the MPTP-treated nonhuman primate model of Parkinson's disease, displaying dopamine-agonist-induced dyskinesias. These studies also suggest that further studies on the role of α_2-adrenoreceptors and 5-HT receptors in the neural mechanisms underlying L-dopa-induced dyskinesia might be of great interest.

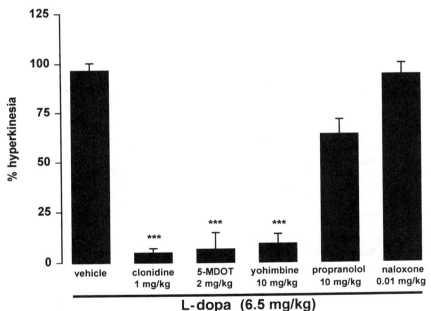

FIG. 4. Effects of coadministration of nondopaminergic drugs on L-dopa-induced rotational loco-motion in the 6-OHDA-lesioned rat following repeated L-dopa administration. Following 14 days, twice-daily, L-dopa administration in the 6-OHDA-lesioned rat, a behavioral hyperkinesia is observed. On days 14 to 21 rats were injected with L-dopa (6.5 mg/kg) and benserazide (1.5 mg/kg). Net 360 degree rotations contraversive to the 6-OHDA lesion were measured following L-dopa (6.5 mg/kg) and benserazide (1.5 mg/kg) plus nondopaminergic drug or L-dopa and benserazide plus vehicle and are expressed as a percentage of the next-day vehicle. All drugs were administered to give maximal effect at 45 minutes following L-dopa administration, the period previously determined as being the peak effect of L-dopa. Locomotion was assessed for 15 minutes (45 to 60 minutes following L-dopa administration). Data are expressed as mean (±SEM) percentage hyperkinesia ($n = 8$). ***$p < 0.001$ compared with the vehicle group; one-way analysis of variance, Student-Newman-Keuls post hoc analysis.

EFFECT OF REPEATED DOPAMINE-REPLACEMENT THERAPY ON EXPRESSION OF STRIATAL OPIOID PEPTIDE PRECURSORS IN BOTH THE 6-OHDA-LESIONED RAT AND THE MPTP-TREATED NONHUMAN PRIMATE MODEL OF PARKINSON'S DISEASE

Several studies have demonstrated that alterations in opioid peptide precursors occur following both dopamine depletion and repeated dopamine-replacement therapy in animal models of Parkinson's disease (14,16,18,36). Utilizing *in situ* hybridization with ^{35}S-labeled oligonucleotide probes targeted to mRNA transcripts encoding the large-molecular-weight opioid peptide precursors, pre-proenkephalin-A and pre-proenkephalin-B, alterations were investigated in striatal tissue from both 6-OHDA-lesioned rats following repeated L-dopa (6.5 mg/kg, twice a day) administration

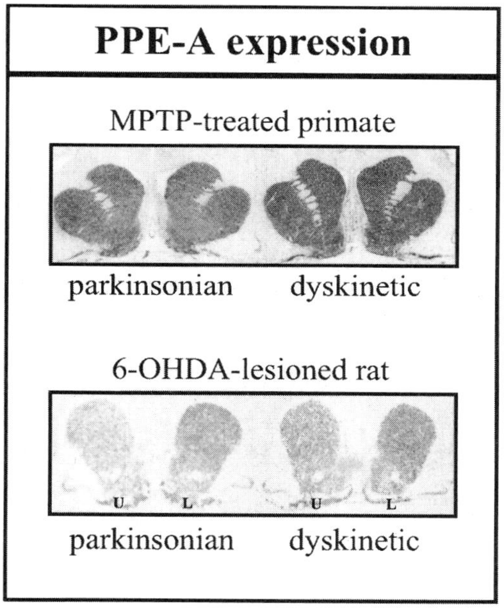

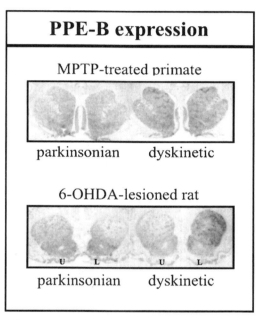

FIG. 5. Striatal expression of the enkephalin precursor pre-proenkephalin-A in the 6-OHDA-lesioned rat following repeated L-dopa administration and MPTP-treated macaque displaying dopamine-agonist-induced dyskinesia. Autoradiographs of *in situ* hybridization utilizing an oligonucleotide probe targeted against the enkephalin precursor, pre-proenkephalin-A, in striatal sections from the 6-OHDA-lesioned rat model of Parkinson's disease [lesioned *(L)* or unlesioned *(U)* striatum] following repeated vehicle or L-dopa (6.5 mg/kg) and benserazide (1.5 mg/kg) administration (twice daily, 21 days) and the MPTP-treated macaque following either dopamine-agonist reversal of parkinsonian symptoms (without dyskinesia) or displaying dopamine-agonist-induced dyskinesia.

FIG. 6. Striatal expression of the dynorphin precursor pre-proenkephalin-B in the 6-OHDA-lesioned rat following repeated L-dopa administration and MPTP-treated macaque displaying dopamine-agonist-induced dyskinesia. Autoradiographs of *in situ* hybridization utilizing an oligonucleotide probe targeted against the dynorphin precursor, pre-proenkephalin-B, in striatal sections from the 6-OHDA-lesioned rat model of Parkinson's disease [lesioned *(L)* or unlesioned *(U)* striatum] following repeated vehicle or L-dopa (6.5 mg/kg) and benserazide (1.5 mg/kg) administration (twice daily, 21 days) and the MPTP-treated macaque following either dopamine-agonist reversal of parkinsonian symptoms (without dyskinesia) or displaying dopamine-agonist-induced dyskinesia.

or MPTP-treated macaques displaying dopamine-agonist-induced dyskinesia. Three weeks post-6-OHDA-lesion, with subsequent vehicle administration (twice daily, 21 days), an increase in pre-proenkephalin-A and decrease in pre-proenkephalin-B is observed in the lesioned striatum when compared with the unlesioned (Figs. 5 and 6). Following 21-day low-dose L-dopa (6.5 mg/kg, twice daily) administration in the 6-OHDA-lesioned rat model of Parkinson's disease, a marked increase in pre-proenkephalin-B and a further increase in pre-proenkephalin-A is observed (Figs. 5 and 6). In MPTP-treated macaques displaying dopamine-agonist-induced dyskinesias, an increase in striatal pre-proenkephalin-A and pre-proenkephalin-B expression was observed when compared with MPTP-treated macaques following dopamine-agonist reversal of parkinsonian symptoms (Figs. 5 and 6).

Thus, in both rodent and primate models of dopamine-agonist-induced dyskinesia, alterations in mRNA expression of the opioid peptide precursors, pre-proenkephalin-A and pre-proenkephalin-B, are qualitatively very similar. Although minor regional differences in pre-proenkephalin-B expression are observed in the rat and primate model of L-dopa-induced dyskinesia, the rodent model may be useful in investigating the mechanisms underlying the regulation of neuropeptide synthesis following dopamine-replacement therapy in Parkinson's disease. In fact, as discussed elsewhere in this volume, (chapters 3 and 6) recent evidence suggests that increased opioid peptide transmission in striatal efferents may not only provide a marker of neuronal activity, but may underlie the genesis of dyskinetic symptoms.

CONCLUSION

Repeated L-dopa treatment of the 6-OHDA-lesioned rat induces an enhanced rotational response with a pharmacologic profile identical to that of L-dopa-induced dyskinesia in primates. Following repeated L-dopa or dopamine-agonist administration in both the 6-OHDA-lesioned rat and the MPTP-treated macaque, identical alterations in the striatal

opioid peptide precursors, pre-proenkephalin-A and pre-proenkephalin-B, are observed.

The MPTP-treated macaque model will no doubt remain the "gold-standard" animal model for investigating L-dopa-induced dyskinesia. However, this novel rodent model of L-dopa-induced dyskinesia may provide a useful addition to investigate possible novel antiparkinsonian compounds for their dyskinetic producing properties. It will also aid our understanding of the molecular and neural mechanisms underlying L-dopa-induced dyskinesia and help in developing adjuncts to dopamine agonists that may reduce the symptoms of L-dopa-induced dyskinesia seen following long-term L-dopa therapy in Parkinson's disease.

ACKNOWLEDGMENTS

The authors acknowledge the financial support of the Dystonia Medical Research Foundation and the Medical Research Council (UK).

REFERENCES

1. Barbeau A. L-dopa therapy in Parkinson's disease—a critical review of nine years experience. *Can Med Assoc J* 1969;101:59–68.
2. Barbeau A. The clinical physiology of side effects in long-term L-dopa therapy. *Adv Neurol* 1974;5:347–365.
3. Barbeau A. High-level levodopa therapy in severely akinetic parkinsonism patients: twelve years later. In: Rinne VK, Klinger M, Stamm G, eds. *Parkinson's disease: current progress, problems and management.* Amsterdam: Elsevier, 1980:229–239.
4. Bedard PJ, Di Paolo T, Falardeau P, Boucher R. Chronic treatment with L-dopa, but not bromocriptine induces dyskinesia in MPTP-parkinsonian monkeys. Correlation with [^{3}H]Spiperone binding. *Brain Res* 1986;379:294–299.
5. Bevan P. Repeated apomorphine treatment causes behavioural supersensitivity and dopamine D2 receptor hyposensitivity. *Neurosci Lett* 1983;25:185–189.
6. Burns RS, Chiueh CC, Markey SP, Ebert MH, Jacobowitz DM, Kopin IJ. A primate model of parkinsonism: selective destruction of dopaminergic neurons in the pars compacta of the substantia nigra by N-methyl-4-phenyl-1,2,3,6-tetrahydropyridine. *Proc Natl Acad Sci USA* 1983;80:4546–4550.
7. Calne DB, Plotkin C, Williams AC, Nutt JG, Neophytides A, Teychenne PF. Long-term treatment of parkinsonism with bromocriptine. *Lancet* 1978;8 (Apr):735–738.

8. Calne DB, Teychenne PF, Claveria LE, Eastman R, Greenacre JK, Petrie A. Bromocriptine in parkinsonism. *BMJ* 1974;4:442–444.

9. Carey RJ. Naloxone reverses L-dopa induced overstimulation effects in a Parkinson's disease animal model analogue. *Life Sci* 1991;48:1303–1308.

10. Carpentier AF, Bonnet AM, Vadailhet M, Agid Y. Improvement of levodopa-induced dyskinesia by propranolol in Parkinson's disease. *Neurology* 1996;56: 1548–1551.

11. Cotzias GC, Papavasiliou PS, Gellene R. Modification of parkinsonism: chronic treatment with L-dopa. *N Engl J Med* 1969;280:337–345.

12. Crossman AR, Clarke CE, Boyce S, Robertson RG, Sambrook MA. MPTP-induced parkinsonism in the monkey: neurochemical pathology, complications of treatment and pathophysiological mechanisms. *Can J Neurol Sci* 1987;14:428–435.

13. Durif F, Vadailhet M, Bonnet AM, Blin J, Agid Y. Levodopa-induced dyskinesias are improved by fluoxetine. *Neurology* 1995;45:1855–1858.

14. Frayne S, Mitchell IJ, Sharpe PT, Crossman AR. Distribution of enkephalin gene expression in the striatum of the parkinsonian primate: implications for dopamine-induced dystonia. *Mol Neuropharmacol* 1991; 1:53–58.

15. Gomez-Mancilla B, Bedard PJ. Effect of nondopaminergic drugs on L-dopa-induced dyskinesias in MPTP-treated monkeys. *Clin Neuropharmacol* 1993; 16:418–427.

16. Herrero MT, Augood SJ, Hirsch EC, et al. Effects of L-dopa on preproenkephalin and preprotachykinin gene expression in the MPTP-treated monkey striatum. *Neuroscience* 1995;68:1189–1198.

17. Hoehn MM. Result of chronic levodopa therapy and its modification by bromocriptine in Parkinson's disease. *Acta Neurol Scand* 1985;71:97–106.

18. Jolkkonen J, Jenner P, Marsden CD. L-dopa reverses altered gene expression of substance P but not enkephalin in the caudate-putamen of common marmosets treated with MPTP. *Brain Res Mol Brain Res* 1995;32:297–307.

19. Kartzinel R, Teychenne P, Gillespie MM, et al. Bromocriptine and levodopa (with or without carbidopa) in parkinsonism. *Lancet* 1976;7 (Aug): 272–275.

20. Lees AJ. Comparison of therapeutic effects of levodopa, levodopa and selegiline, and bromocriptine in patients with early, mild Parkinson's disease: three year interim report. *BMJ* 1993;307:469–472.

21. Lees AJ, Stern GM. Sustained bromocriptine therapy in previously untreated patients with Parkinson's disease. *J Neurol Neurosurg Psychiatry* 1981;44:1020–1023.

22. Lieberman A, Kupersmith M, Estey E, Goldstein M. Treatment of Parkinson's disease with bromocriptine. *N Engl J Med* 1976;295:1400–1404.

23. Marsden CD, Parkes JD. 'On-off' effects in patients with Parkinson's disease on chronic levodopa therapy. *Lancet* 1976;1:292–296.

24. Marsden CD, Parkes JD, Quinn N. Fluctuations of disability in Parkinson's disease—clinical aspects. In: Marsden C, Fahn S, eds. *Movement disorders.* London:Butterworth Scientific, 1982:96–122.

25. Nutt JG. Levodopa-induced dyskinesia. *Neurology* 1990;40:340–345.

26. Parkes JD, Debono AG, Marsden CD. Bromocriptine in parkinsonism: long-term treatment dose response, and comparison with levodopa. *J Neurol Neurosurg Psychiatry* 1976;39:1101–1108.

27. Pearce RKB, Jackson M, Smith L, Jenner P, Marsden CD. Chronic L-dopa administration induces dyskinesias in the 1-methyl-4-phenyl-1,2,3,6-tetrahydropyridine-treated common marmoset *(Callithrix Jacchus).* *Mov Disord* 1995;10:731–740.

28. Poewe WH, Lees AJ, Stern GM. Dystonia in Parkinson's disease: clinical and pharmacological features. *Ann Neurol* 1988;23:73–79.

29. Rinne UK. Early combination of bromocriptine and levodopa in the treatment of Parkinson's disease: A 5-year follow-up. *Neurology* 1987;37:826–828.

30. Rinne UK. Lisuride, a dopamine agonist in the treatment of early Parkinson's disease. *Neurology* 1989; 39:336–339.

31. Shaw KM, Lees AJ, Stern GM. The impact of treatment with levodopa in Parkinson's disease. *Q J Med* 1980;49:283–293.

32. Tolosa ES, Martin WE, Cohen HP. Dyskinesias during levodopa therapy. *Lancet* 1975;21 (June):1381–1382.

33. Ungerstedt U. 6-hydroxy-dopamine induced degeneration of central monoamine neurons. *Eur J Pharmacol* 1968;5:107–110.

34. Ungerstedt U, Arbuthnott GW. Quantitative recording of rotational behaviour in rats after 6-hydroxy-dopamine lesions of the nigrostriatal dopamine system. *Brain Res* 1970;24:485–493.

35. Yahr MD, Duvosin RC, Schear MJ, Barrett RE, Hoehn MM. Treatment of parkinsonism with levodopa. *Arch Neurol* 1969;21:343–354.

36. Zeng BY, Jolkkonen J, Jenner P, Marsden CD. Chronic L-dopa treatment differentially regulates gene expression of glutamate decarboxylase, preproenkephalin and preprotachykinin in the striatum of 6-hydroxy-dopamine-lesioned rat. *Neuroscience* 1995;66:19–28.

Dystonia 3: Advances in Neurology, Vol. 78,
edited by S. Fahn, C. D. Marsden, and M. DeLong.
Lippincott–Raven Publishers, Philadelphia © 1998.

8

Abnormal Cerebellar Output in the Genetically Dystonic Rat

*Mark S. LeDoux and †Joan F. Lorden

*Department of Neurology, University of Tennessee College of Medicine, Memphis, Tennessee 38163; and †University of Alabama at Birmingham, Birmingham, Alabama 35294.

Spontaneous mutations are natural experiments that provide opportunities to test novel hypotheses about mechanisms underlying pathologic phenomena. The dystonic (Jfl:SD-dt) rat is a spontaneous mutant discovered in the Sprague-Dawley strain (52). The dt rat exhibits a severe, generalized, progressive, dystonic motor syndrome after a period of normal development. The dt rat may provide a vehicle for understanding the biochemical and physiologic defects in human dystonia. Beginning at approximately postnatal day 12, locomotion is seriously impaired by twisting movements and postures that involve the muscles of the neck, trunk, and limbs (52). The motor syndrome is characterized by twisting of the axial musculature, clasping of the paws, and frequent falls. The movements are reduced or absent when the animals are at rest. The gross morphology of the brain is normal and there is no evidence of lesions or degeneration in the central or peripheral nervous systems in Golgi or Nissl-stained material (52). Because anatomic examination of the brains from dt rats was unrevealing, biochemical, pharmacologic, and neurophysiologic studies were undertaken.

Twisting movements and postures similar to those of the dt rat are generally attributed to dysfunction of the basal ganglia (13). Neuro-chemical studies on the GABAergic, cholinergic, and dopaminergic systems of the basal ganglia of the dt rat have been uninformative (6,54,60,62). Both biochemical and physiologic evidence, however, point to the olivo-cerebellar system as the site of a functional defect.

In normal rats, harmaline causes a generalized tremor by inducing rhythmic activity in inferior olivary (IO) neurons, which in turn evoke complex spike discharges in Purkinje cells in cerebellar cortex (74). Dystonic rats do not exhibit a tremor in response to harmaline, although other tremorogenic agents with different mechanisms of action are effective in the mutants (53). Single-unit recording in dt rats demonstrates that IO neurons show a normal increase in the rate and rhythmicity of firing in response to harmaline, although Purkinje cells do not (73,74). Because harmaline is thought to influence the firing of Purkinje cells indirectly through action on IO neurons, this suggests a defect in the transmission of information from the IO to Purkinje cells in the dt rat.

The IO receives a dense GABAergic innervation in rats and other species (19–22,63). IO afferents arise from multiple areas including the spinal cord, brainstem, deep cerebellar nuclei (DCN), and frontal cortex (77). GABAergic input from the DCN to the IO is thought to be important in the regulation of IO activity and particularly in governing electrotonic coupling between IO cells (19–21,70). In addition to the somata and dendrites of IO neurons, the axon hillock and initial segment also receive GABAergic input (22). These synapses may serve a different function than those on the soma and dendrites. GABAergic projections to cell bodies and dendrites of IO neurons may arise from a variety of cerebellar and noncerebellar sites. The projection to the axon hillock and initial segment is, however, thought to be exclusively cerebellar in origin (19,22). Therefore, GABAergic IO afferents may regulate both the electronic coupling of cells and the subsequent transmission of impulses. These observations suggest at least two possible causes for the failure of transmission of action potentials from IO neurons to Purkinje cells: a defect specific to IO neurons, or increased IO afferent GABAergic activity in the region of the axon hillock and initial segment.

The DCN are a site of major abnormalities in the dt rat. In comparison to normal rats, glucose utilization is significantly elevated in the DCN of the dt rat, suggesting increased activity at this site (9). The DCN receive dense GABAergic input from Purkinje cells. The synthetic enzyme for GABA, glutamic acid decarboxylase (GAD), is readily detected in the DCN where it is located primarily in the terminals of Purkinje cells. In comparison with normal rats, dt rats show increases in GAD activity (64) and decreases in ^{3}H-muscimol binding (6) that are specific to the DCN.

Although biochemical and electrophysiologic studies established the olivocerebellar network as clearly abnormal in the dt rat, they did not prove that pathologic output signals from this network were required for the expression of the dt rat's dystonic motor syndrome. The first goal of the studies presented here was to determine if cerebellar output is critical to the generation of the dt rat motor syndrome. The second goal was to identify the electrophysiologic features of cerebellar output in the awake dt rat.

IS CEREBELLAR OUTPUT CRITICAL TO THE EXPRESSION OF THE DT RAT MOTOR SYNDROME?

Damage to the cerebellum in adult or developing animals is known to produce severe postural and locomotor deficits (35,55). Experimental evidence shows, however, that the cerebellum is not essential to the generation of locomotor rhythms. Animals lacking a cerebellum instead provide evidence that the cerebellum plays a role in the coordination and calibration of movements and in the adaptive plasticity of motor systems (35,78). Optican and Robinson (65) reported that ablations of the cerebellum altered only the metrics of saccadic eye movements and the ability of animals to adaptively repair saccades made hypometric by weakening an eye muscle. Similarly, CBX has been shown to prevent adaptation of the vestibuloocular reflex, but not to block the reflex itself (67). The presence of an erroneous signal from an adaptive or error-correcting mechanism could mask the functional integrity of other mechanisms essential to posture and locomotion.

In order to test the hypothesis that cerebellar output is essential to the expression of the rat disease, normal and dt rats were subjected to cerebellectomy (CBX) (44,47). Although ablation studies are generally used to disrupt normal behavior, there is evidence that the removal of an erroneous signal may in some cases restore function. One example is the Sprague effect in which transection of the commissure of the superior colliculus or lesions of the substantia nigra reinstate visual orienting behavior in hemianopic cats (83). In addition, weaver mice, mutants with a clear morphologic abnormality of the cerebellum, benefit from CBX (30). In these mice, lesions of the vermis are as effective as complete CBX.

To assess the effects of CBX on the mutant rats, a series of age-appropriate behavioral tests was selected (1,44,47). These included righting on a surface, climbing a wire-mesh incline, and homing (traversing a passageway to return to a home cage). In normal rat pups, the ability to perform these tasks is acquired early in development, prior to the behavioral deterioration of the dt rats (1,44,47,52). The mutant rats were observed to determine how the progression of the disease affected previously established motor function. The effects of CBX were then evaluated by observing changes in the frequency of occurrence of motor signs of the rat disease as well as changes in task performance.

Normal and dt rats bred in the laboratory were tested prior to surgery on either postnatal day 15 or 20. In dt rats, the severity of the motor syndrome was assessed by counting the occurrence of twisting movements of the neck and trunk, paw clasps, falls, and pivoting over a 5-minute observation period (44,47,52). Both normal and dt rats were examined for overall levels of activity and tested on righting reflex time, climbing, and homing (1,44,47).

Separate groups of normal and dt rats underwent CBX by subpial suction at either 15 or 20 days of age. CBX included the dorsal half of the lateral vestibular nucleus (dLV). An additional group of 15-day-old dt rats received bilateral kainic acid injections into the entopeduncular nuclei (ENTO) as a control for nonspecific lesion effects. This nucleus was chosen because, along with the substantia nigra pars reticulata, it serves as a main output nucleus of the basal ganglia (32). All rats were ambulatory upon recovery from anesthesia. Behavioral testing was repeated 3 days after surgery. Groups of 18- or 23-day-old dt and normal rats were also tested as age-matched unoperated controls.

In order to provide a background against which the behavioral effects of CBX can be judged, the performance of groups of untreated normal and dt rats on behavioral tasks on postnatal days 15, 18, 20, and 23 is presented in Fig. 1 (44,47). The data for the day 15 and 20 groups are the preoperative performance of the CBX rats. Over the period from 15 to 23 days of age, normal rats showed little variation on the behavioral measures (Fig. 1). However, in dt rats, the frequency of occurrence of clinical signs increased with increasing postnatal age (Fig. 1A). Overall levels of activity did not

change significantly in either normal or dt rats (Fig. 1B). On three measures of motor performance (Fig. 1C–F), the dt rats showed consistent and significant deterioration.

In both the 15- and 20-day-old dt groups, CBX produced substantial reductions in all of the characteristic movements of the dt rats (Fig. 2). Significant postoperative reductions in motor signs were observed in both CBX dt lesion groups in comparison with their preoperative conditions. Comparisons between CBX and ENTO lesion groups and the age-matched unoperated controls (18C) at day 18 indicated that reliable differences were present between the CBX group and both the ENTO and 18C groups. At day 23, the CBX group also showed significantly fewer motor signs than the unoperated group (23C). In contrast to the effects of CBX, ENTO lesions increased the frequency of clinical signs in the mutant. The findings in the ENTO group suggest that the dt rat movement disorder cannot be attributed to a nonspecific lesion effect.

The results of behavioral evaluations of CBX and ENTO rats are presented in Fig. 3 (44,47). The effects of CBX and ENTO lesions on the clinical signs of dt rats are summarized in Fig. 3A. Figure 3B shows that postoperative activity levels were similar to preoperative levels. Thus, the reductions in motor signs that followed CBX were not due to a general decrease in activity levels. As seen in Fig. 3C, an improvement in righting time was seen after surgery. Other comparisons between preoperative and postoperative performance for this group were not statistically significant (Fig. 3D–F). Thus, in the young dt CBX group that underwent surgery on day 15, the lesion generally prevented deterioration in motor performance.

In the older dt CBX group that received surgery on day 20, significant improvement in comparison with preoperative performance was evident (Fig. 3). The reduction in clinical signs seen in older CBX dt rats (Fig. 3A) was paralleled by significant decreases in righting time (Fig. 3C), and improvement in climbing (Fig. 3D) and homing (Fig. 3E–F). All effects were significant in comparison with preopera-

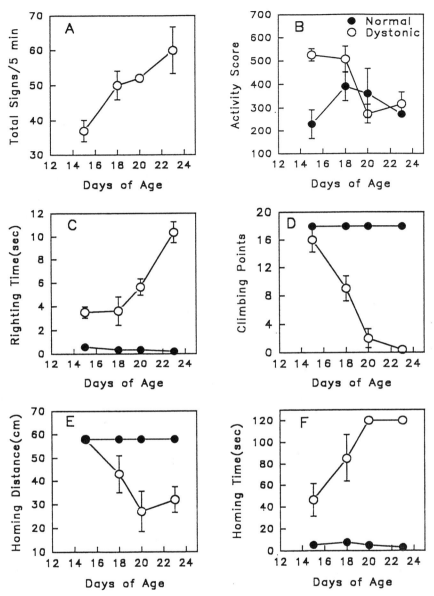

FIG. 1. The natural history of the rat disease was followed from postnatal days 15 to 23. All values are means ± SEM. **A:** The total number of clinical signs over a 5-minute period. **B:** Activity scores for a 15-minute period, following 2 minutes of acclimation. **C:** Righting reflex times, each point is an average of five trials. **D:** Scores for climbing a wire mesh incline set at 30, 45, or 70 degrees from horizontal. Scores are total points earned in three trials at each angle. **E:** Homing task, the longest distance covered in three trials was recorded. **F:** Time to complete the homing task. (From ref. 47, with permission.)

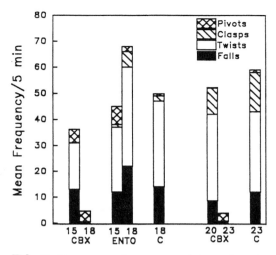

FIG. 2. The mean frequency of four discrete motor signs characteristic of the dt rat counted before (day 15 or 20) and after (day 18 or 23) CBX or ENTO lesions. Unoperated dt controls *(C)* 18 or 23 days of age are also included for comparison. (From ref. 47, with permission.)

tive values, except for homing distance. Comparisons of the older CBX group at day 23 with age-matched unoperated dt rats and CBX normal rats, indicated that the dt CBX group did not differ from normal rats on any measure but showed significant improvement in comparison with the unoperated 23-day-old dt rats on all measures, except homing distance. When the postoperative performance of young and old dt CBX rats was compared directly, they differed only on the performance of the climbing task. Thus, the age at which dt rats underwent CBX had little effect on their final level of performance on the behaviors studied.

The data presented in Fig. 3 document the finding that CBX eliminates the signs of the rat disease, prevents the progressive deterioration of motor performance in young dt rats, and improves performance on several tasks in older dt rats. The long-term consequences of the lesion were examined in a separate group of six dt rats that underwent CBX on postnatal day 15. These animals survived into adulthood without further treatment. As adults, they showed gait ataxia. However, they used all limbs in locomotion and

were able to raise the head, shoulders, and ventral surface of the trunk off the ground. This argues against a simple loss of muscle tone as an explanation for the decrease in clinical signs. The dramatic reduction in signs of the movement disorder seen 3 days postlesion persisted, even in animals followed for over 6 months. All rats continued to grow, reaching normal adult weights. At no time was it necessary to provide hand feeding or other types of support. Both males and females were able to mate successfully and females were able to rear their offspring. CBX is now routinely employed to obtain homozygote breeders.

CBX eliminated the signs of the movement disorder in the dt rat and produced a significant and permanent improvement in motor performance. The decrease in clinical signs observed in the CBX rats cannot be attributed to a nonspecific effect such as akinesia. There was no evidence of hypoactivity in the CBX rats. General observation revealed that the positive effects of CBX were present immediately upon recovery from anesthesia. Specific tests of motor performance revealed improvement in function within 3 days of the lesion and long-term observations confirmed the enduring nature of the effect. The CBX dt rats did show some of the impairments seen following CBX in normal animals. Mostly notably, all of the CBX dt rats exhibited an ataxic gait. In the dt rat, however, the presence of a malfunctioning cerebellum is more debilitating than the complete absence of a cerebellum. In the central nervous system, an abnormal signal may be worse than no signal at all.

It is not possible to rule out the presence of abnormalities elsewhere in the brain of the dt rat. It is possible that the cerebellum is required for the behavioral expression of dysfunction at another site within the nervous system such as the basal ganglia. The long-term improvement induced by CBX in the behavioral capacity of the mutant indicates, however, that other defects are not sufficient to produce the movement disorder. In addition, the poor survival of untreated dt rats (52) cannot be attributed to an unidentified defect.

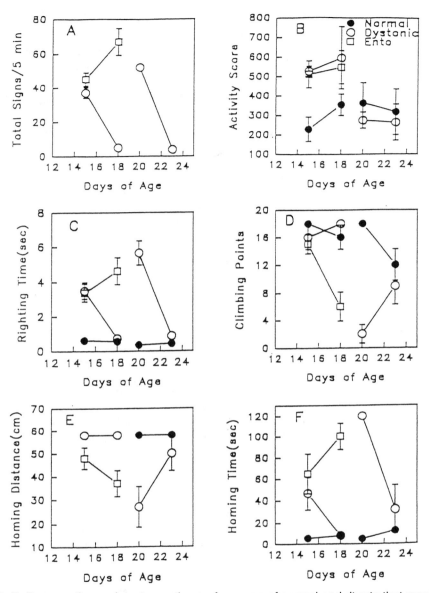

FIG. 3. A–F: Preoperative and postoperative performance of normal and dt rats that received CBX at day 15 or 20 and dt rats that received ENTO lesions at day 15. All values are means ±SEM. Behavioral tasks are the same as those in Fig. 1. The results for normal rats are not included in **A** because they did not exhibit abnormal motor signs. In addition, the results for normal rats at 15 and 18 days are excluded from **E** because of overlap with the dt CBX group. (From ref. 47, with permission.)

DO ALL CEREBELLAR NUCLEI AND DORSAL PORTIONS OF THE LATERAL VESTIBULAR NUCLEI CONTRIBUTE TO THE DT RAT MOTOR SYNDROME?

Because CBX included all DCN and the dLV, it was not possible to determine the relative importance of specific nuclei in the generation of the dt rat motor syndrome. In a follow-up study, the motor function of 15-day-old dt rats was tested before and after the creation of bilateral electrolytic or excitatory amino acid (EAA) lesions of specific cerebellar nuclei (44,48). Bilateral lesions of the medial cerebellar nucleus (MCN), nucleus interpositus (INT), lateral cerebellar nucleus (LCN), and dLV were made in separate groups of dt rats. Rats were tested again on postnatal day 20. Unoperated dt rats of the same age served as controls.

The frequency of four motor signs (falls, twists, clasps, pivots) was determined for each rat. In addition, rats were tested on several standard measures of neonatal motor performance (1,44,47,48). The tests of homing, climbing, hanging, and righting provide, for the dt rat, practical, age-appropriate measures of motor function. These tests were not intended, however, to specifically test the function of individual cerebellar nuclei.

Electrolytic lesions were made with parylene-coated stainless steel electrodes. Fiber-sparing EAA lesions were made with either kainic acid or N-methyl-DL-aspartic (NMDA) acid diluted in sterile normal saline. A blind analysis of the histologic material (150 cases) allowed for inclusion of only those cases with appropriately placed lesions. After histologic analysis, a total of 78 cases remained in seven groups: CTRL (control, $N = 12$), MCN ($N = 11$), INT ($N = 11$), LCN ($N = 10$), dLV ($N = 12$), EAA-MCN ($N = 11$), and EAA-dLV ($N = 11$). The NMDA and kainic acid cases did not significantly differ on any measure for either the EAA-MCN or EAA-dLVN group. Therefore, NMDA and kainic acid cases were pooled.

All lesion groups were compared with the control group. Selected lesion effects were contrasted to assess the relative importance of individual nuclei to the dt rat motor syndrome. The effects of MCN and dLV lesions were compared because both regions play important roles in the control of axial musculature, posture, and balance (34,57,71,72). In contrast, the LCN plays an important role in the control of voluntary movements and coordination of the distal extremities (36,39). Therefore, the effects of MCN and LCN lesions were compared because of their relationships to different aspects of movement. In addition, electrolytic and EAA lesion groups were contrasted to assess the contribution of fiber damage to the effects of electrolytic lesions.

The mean weight of all groups increased over postnatal days 15 to 20. However, using day 15 weight as a covariate, the day 20 weight of the control group ($M = 41.6$ g) was significantly greater than that of the dLV ($M = 36.4$ g) and MCN ($M = 34.7$ g) EAA lesion groups. There were no significant differences between the electrolytic lesion groups and the control group. Although there was a tendency for the control group to be less active than the lesion groups, there were no differences in activity levels among the lesion groups.

As in the case of CBX, all DCN lesions produced a reduction in the total number of abnormal motor signs on day 20 in comparison with the control group (Fig. 4). The largest effect was produced by electrolytic dLV lesions. This group differed significantly from the MCN lesion group. There were no other significant group differences. When components of the motor syndrome were analyzed separately, there were lesion effects on falls, clasps, and twisting, but not pivoting.

Figure 5 shows the effects of DCN lesions on homing time, homing distance, righting time, and climbing points. The performance of unoperated dystonic control rats deteriorated on homing time, homing distance, righting, and climbing from day 15 to 20. All lesions prevented deterioration on one or more measures of motor performance during this time. Overall, however, the electrolytic and EAA-dLV lesions had the largest and most widespread positive effects on motor performance. All lesions reduced day 20 righting time in

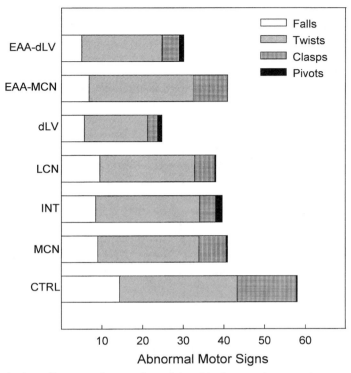

FIG. 4. Selective lesion effects on the number of day 20 abnormal motor signs counted during a 5-minute observation period. Four discrete motor signs were observed: falls, twists, clasps, pivots. (From ref. 48, with permission.)

comparison with the control group. The largest effect on righting time was produced by electrolytic dLV lesions. All rats showed some loss in climbing ability between days 15 and 20. The rats in the MCN, electrolytic dLV, and EAA-dLV groups had the smallest decline in climbing scores between days 15 and 20 in comparison with unlesioned control rats. The largest effect on climbing scores was seen in rats with electrolytic dLV lesions. Homing time increased and homing distance decreased for the dystonic control group from day 15 to 20 (Fig. 5C and D). Only the electrolytic dLV group demonstrated a statistically significant improvement in homing time and homing distance in comparison with the control group. However, there was a tendency for electrolytic MCN lesions to prevent deterioration in both homing time and homing distance. Hanging time for the controls increased by a mean of

36.0 seconds from day 15 to 20. There was no significant lesion effects on hanging time.

From postnatal days 15 to 20, untreated dt rats show a progressive increase in the frequency of abnormal motor signs and progressive decrease on several measures of motor function including righting, climbing, and homing. Electrolytic and EAA lesions of the cerebellar nuclei and dLV improved motor performance and decreased the severity of the dt rat motor syndrome without impairing general activity. The performance of the dystonic rats on the hanging test suggests that the reductions in clinical signs and improvements in motor function demonstrated by the lesion groups were not the result of weakness or hypotonia. In addition, the activity measure excluded a simple hypokinetic effect.

No single lesion used in this study had effects as large as those obtained with CBX

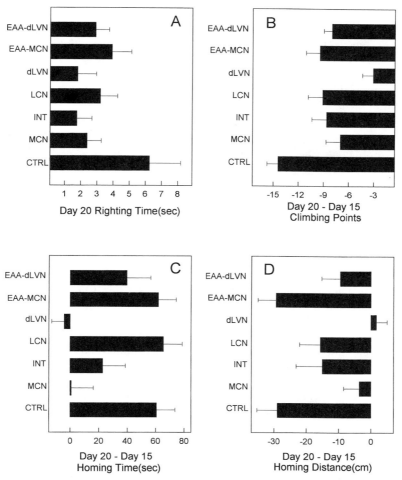

FIG. 5. A–D: Selective lesion effects on four measures of motor performance. (From ref. 48, with permission.)

(44,47,48). Rats subjected to a total CBX showed a 90% reduction in abnormal motor signs with complete elimination of twisting and clasps. In the dt rat, CBX on day 15 prevented deterioration in climbing, homing, and righting. Normal and dt rats that received CBX on day 15 could not be distinguished on day 20 righting or homing times. In this experiment, the largest effect on abnormal motor signs was the approximately 60% fewer signs in the electrolytic dLV lesion group in comparison to unoperated controls. Although selective lesions did not produce the profound effects of CBX, all selective lesions had a positive effect on the

dt rat motor syndrome and reduced the deterioration in motor performance that occurs in unoperated dt rats. The positive effect of the DCN and dLV lesions supports the hypothesis that the expression of the dt rat motor syndrome depends on abnormal cerebellar output, although no single region of the cerebellum appears to account for the entire motor syndrome.

Most functional descriptions of the cerebellum are based on dividing it into three longitudinal zones with the flocculonodular lobe treated separately (10–12,82). These three divisions each include cerebellar cortex, underlying white matter, and associated nuclei: a medial zone projecting to the MCN and dLV; an intermediate zone projecting to the INT; and a lateral zone projecting to the LCN. The cerebellar nuclei or dLV provide the final output from each longitudinal zone.

The DCN demonstrate both divergence and convergence of projections (5,66). The MCN projects to multiple mesencephalic sites and has bilateral, but mainly crossed, projections to the reticular and vestibular nuclei and spinal cord (24,25,31,82). Fiber-sparing kainic acid lesions show that the MCN exerts a crossed inhibitory and an ipsilateral excitatory influence on extensor postural tone (34). The INT projects to the red nucleus, thalamus, pontine reticular tegmental nucleus, pretectal nuclei, zona incerta, medullary reticular formation, and superior colliculus (17,24,25,31,82). The LCN also projects to the red nucleus, thalamus, and medullary reticular formation (24,25,31, 82). The lateral vestibulospinal tract originates mainly from the dLV and terminates in the anterior horn of the spinal cord (61). In the rat, dLV projections to lumbosacral segments of the spinal cord predominate (69). The lateral vestibulospinal tract plays a critical role in the maintenance of tone in antigravity muscles so that balance can be preserved during various movements (57). Unilateral lesions of the lateral vestibular nucleus (LVN) can cause scoliosis in rats thereby emphasizing the critical role of the LVN in the control of axial musculature (2). In view of the widespread projections from the DCN and dLV to important motor and premotor structures, an abnormal signal from these nuclei could have marked effects at many levels of the motor system.

In the present study, the dLV lesions were most effective in reducing clinical signs and improving motor performance. This suggests that the dLV, like the DCN, plays an important role in the expression of the dt rat motor syndrome. The EAA-dLV lesions were, however, less effective than electrolytic lesions. Because of the central location of the dLV, electrolytic lesions of this nucleus invariably and unavoidably damaged a larger portion of the output from adjacent nuclei than lesions of the DCN. Thus, the dLV lesions were probably more similar to CBX than DCN lesions in terms of ex-

tent. Although less effective than the electrolytic lesions, the EAA-dLV lesions were still more effective than the INT and LCN lesions. The particular effectiveness of electrolytic and EAA dLV lesions may be a consequence of the role that this structure plays in the maintenance of posture. Improvement in balance and posture would have a substantial impact on all the tests of motor performance used in this study.

On several measures, the MCN lesions were as effective or nearly as effective as the dLV lesions. This may be attributed to two factors. First, lesions of the MCN are likely to damage fibers of passage from the vermis to the dLV. It is possible that elimination of an abnormal signal from Purkinje cells is functionally better than leaving this connection intact. Second, the MCN plays an important role in the maintenance of posture (34,71,72). Lesions that improve the postural stability of the dt rats will produce a greater enhancement of their general performance on tests such as climbing, homing, and righting than lesions with effects that might be seen mainly in the distal extremities.

The individual DCN and dLV operate in parallel so that spatially and temporally correct movements can occur (78). The inability of behavioral and motor testing to clearly differentiate lesion groups may be explained by the parallel processing of different movement components by individual nuclei. Because the motor tasks used in this study were functionally complex, it is likely that more than one nucleus was involved in each task. Lesions of individual nuclei were associated with modest generalized improvements in motor function and decreases in abnormal motor signs rather than specific changes on a particular test or a decrease of one abnormal motor sign.

WHAT ARE THE DISTINGUISHING FEATURES OF THE ABNORMAL SIGNAL FROM THE CEREBELLAR NUCLEI IN THE AWAKE dt RAT?

Although lesion studies established the DCN as critical to the dt rat motor syndrome, they did not reveal the mechanisms by which cerebellar output distorts normal motor function. A characterization of neuronal signals in the DCN of the awake dt rat will serve as a first step in delineating the effects of abnormal cerebellar output on the motor system (44,45). In addition, awake recordings from the DCN may help to clarify the conflicting results of biochemical and electrophysiologic studies of the olivocerebellar loop in the dt rat. When compared with normal rats, DCN GAD activity is increased (64), DCN muscimol binding is decreased (6), DCN glucose utilization is increased (9), Purkinje cell firing rates are decreased (74), and MCN firing rates are increased (51) in the dt rat. In the absence of electrophysiologic information, the biochemical data might suggest that Purkinje cell firing rates are high and DCN firing rates are low in the dt rat.

Under urethane anesthesia, the firing rate of MCN cells in dt rats was nearly twice the rate seen in normals (51). In addition, the firing pattern of both MCN and INT neurons was more regular in dt than in normal rats. It is not known how these findings under urethane anesthesia relate to DCN neuronal activity in awake dt rats. It is possible that the differences in MCN neuronal activity between normal and dt rats are caused by differential sensitivity to urethane. In addition, it is not known if these physiologic abnormalities involve cells in the LCN or if this pathophysiology observes a medial to lateral gradient across the DCN.

Single-unit activity was obtained from the MCN, INT, and LCN in awake normal and dt rats between and including postnatal days 12 and 26 (44,45). All pups were housed with their dams until sacrifice and removed from their cages only for surgery and recording from the DCN.

Rats were anesthetized for surgery with intraperitoneal injections of ketamine and xylazine. After scalp reflection, an indifferent lead was screwed into parietal skull and the underlying dura into posterior parietal cortex. Small burr holes were made in the frontal and caudal occipital bones and U-shaped skull posts were tunneled extradurally between the pairs of burr holes in each bone. A burr hole was made over the cerebellum for access to the DCN. A plastic dam was placed around the cerebellar access site to prevent acrylic from occluding the burr hole. A flat-head, machine screw was placed, head down, on the midline, midparietal region and the entire assembly was secured to the skull with dental acrylic.

Single-unit recordings were obtained at least 4 hours after full recovery from anesthesia or on the day following surgery. Rats were placed in a soft foam-lined container that left the face fully exposed and the head bolt was secured to a restraining device. Potentials were recorded extracellularly with parylene-coated tungsten microelectrodes. Small electrolytic marking lesions were created at each recording site with a direct current lesion maker. Between 2,000 and 8,200 spikes were obtained for each cell. There were no significant differences between normal and dt rats in the number of spikes recorded.

The distinctiveness of the activity recorded from DCN cells in dt rats is apparent in Figure 6. For descriptive purposes, a burst can be defined as a group of two or more spikes both preceded and followed by relatively long interspike intervals (ISIs). The spike trains from normal rats exhibited occasional bursts of variable duration. In contrast, the number of spikes per burst varied over a narrow range for DCN cells from dt rats. Most bursts in dt rats had less than five spikes.

Spike trains from normal rats showed ISI histograms with mild positive skew and non-rhythmic autocorrelations. In contrast, spike trains from dt rats showed bursting firing patterns, rhythmic autocorrelations, and strongly skewed or bimodal ISI histograms. Bimodality and the rhythmicity of autocorrelations increased with increasing postnatal age in the dt rats. The average firing rate ($\pm$ SD) for DCN cells was 36.6 ± 18.3 Hz in normal rats and 41.2 ± 18.4 Hz in dt rats.

The effects of urethane on DCN neuronal firing rates are striking when compared with the results from awake recordings. Under urethane anesthesia (51), MCN firing rates were significantly higher in dt ($M = 23.7$) than in normal rats ($M = 12.8$). In contrast to the re-

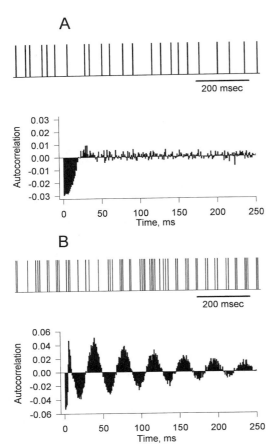

FIG. 6. Representative portions of spike trains and autocorrelations for the cell's entire spike train. **A:** Spike train from a DCN cell of a normal rat. **B:** Spike train from a DCN cell of a dt rat.

sults obtained under general anesthesia, DCN firing rates were much higher in both normal and dt rats in the awake preparation. Although the difference in DCN neuronal firing rates between normal and dt rats was not statistically significant, there was a trend toward higher firing rates in dt rats. In addition, the pattern of firing was markedly different between normal and dt rats. DCN cells from dt rats showed frequent short bursts of activity that usually consisted of only two to five spikes and, in this regard, appear to be different from bursts of activity by DCN neurons that occur during normal motor activity (59).

Single-unit recordings from the MCN, INT, and LCN support the conclusions of lesion studies by showing that the cerebellar output signal from each of the DCN is abnormal. The dt rat's disordered olivocerebellar physiology did not appear to spare any of the cerebellar output nuclei. In addition, no single nucleus stood out as being much more abnormal than its neighbors.

An analysis of *in vitro* recordings from the DCN (37), the *in vivo* response of DCN neurons in the climbing fiber deafferented rat to iontophoretically applied GABA (7), the long-term consequences of climbing fiber deafferentation in the DCN and LVN (8,40), and DCN GABAergic activity in the dt rat suggest that pathologic hyperpolarization of the DCN neuronal membrane is responsible for the highly distinctive DCN spike train characteristics seen in the dt rat. A review of previous electrophysiologic studies of the olivocerebellar network can provide considerable insight into the pathophysiology of the dt rat motor syndrome.

The neurotoxin 3-acetylpyridine (3-AP) destroys IO neurons (18) and eliminates the climbing fiber projection to Purkinje cells. The 3-AP-treated rat develops a movement disorder with features similar to the dt rat motor syndrome (52,76). However, whereas the dt rat motor syndrome gets progressively worse with increasing postnatal age, the 3-AP-treated rat typically shows some degree of motor recovery and a change in the clinical appearance of its motor syndrome during the weeks and months following IO lesioning.

The initial effects of climbing fiber destruction are an elimination of Purkinje cell complex spikes (14,68), an increase in Purkinje cell simple-spike rate (14,68), increased glucose utilization in the DCN (3), and decreased neuronal firing rates in the DCN and LVN (4). The long-term consequences of climbing fiber deafferentation are much different: the Purkinje cell simple-spike firing rate is similar to that demonstrated by intact animals, and the firing rate of DCN neurons is increased and exhibits a bursting pattern (8).

When GABA was applied to rat DCN neurons several months after 3-AP IO destruction, the sensitivity of DCN neurons to GABA was markedly reduced. Nearly all neuronal firing was depressed by GABA in a dose-dependent manner in control rats that did not receive 3-AP (7). Bicuculline increased DCN neuronal firing rates in control rats, but had little or no effect on DCN neurons from the 3-AP treated rats. These findings suggest that a long-term consequence of climbing fiber deafferentation is decreased postsynaptic sensitivity of DCN neurons to the inhibitory transmitter GABA. Intracellular recordings of synaptic potentials in the LVN of long-term 3-AP treated rats (40) support the iontophoretic studies in the DCN. One month after climbing fiber deafferentation, inhibitory postsynaptic potentials recorded from LVN neurons after stimulation of Purkinje cell axons were relatively small in size and increased in latency (40).

In the dt rat, GABA receptor density is decreased in the DCN (6). This presumed downregulation of GABA receptors in the dt rat may be the consequence of increased GABAergic transmission at Purkinje cell terminals. The average Purkinje cell firing rate is slightly higher in awake dt than in normal rats (46). Decreased activity in climbing fiber collaterals to the DCN could also contribute to decrease the ratio of excitatory to inhibitory inputs to the DCN in the dt rat (80). The complex spike firing rate is significantly lower in dt than in normal rats (46). Decreased excitatory drive to the DCN could result in membrane hyperpolarization.

Jahnsen (37) has shown that in DCN neurons there is a rebound train of spikes in response to injection of hyperpolarizing current. The rebound burst is both voltage and time dependent. With small hyperpolarizing pulses, the rebound does not reach the spike threshold. The number of spikes produced by hyperpolarizing pulses that cause the rebound to reach threshold is correlated with the size of the hyperpolarizing pulse. In addition, longer hyperpolarizations increase the number and frequency of rebound spikes.

Llinás and Mühlethaler (50) extended Jahnsen's work by showing that a depolarizing current step delivered at the resting membrane potential elicits tonic firing in DCN neurons whereas the same current step delivered from a hyperpolarized level elicits all-or-none burst responses. More important with regard to the intrinsic excitability of DCN neurons was the demonstration of a low-threshold inactivating calcium-dependent conductance that generates rebound excitation following transient membrane hyperpolarization. The bursting shown by DCN neurons in the dt rat may be the manifestation of the intrinsic excitability of DCN neurons superimposed on a hyperpolarized resting membrane potential.

CONCLUSIONS

The positive results of eliminating the DCN in the dt rat suggest that abnormal cerebellar output can have significant deleterious effects at multiple sites within the motor system. However, the electrophysiologic consequences of the dt rat's DCN output signal at recipient nuclei have not been determined. In addition, the precise mechanisms by which this signal produces a dystonic motor syndrome are not known. The dt rat is a unique vehicle for understanding the pathophysiologic basis of a movement disorder not associated with gross or microscopic structural abnormalities of the brain or peripheral nervous system (23,38,58). Continued study of the dt rat may provide critical insights into the functional organization of motor systems and pathophysiology of movement disorders in general.

Lesion studies in the dt rat along with several lines of clinical evidence suggest that the olivocerebellar network and associated vestibular pathways should be considered as potential contributors to the pathophysiology of both generalized and focal human dystonia and that the basal ganglia are unlikely to be the sole site of abnormality in the primary dystonias. In addition to the basal ganglia (13), secondary dystonia has been associated with lesions of a wide variety of neural structures including the midbrain (27,39,42), pons (29,56), and cerebellum (26,41,43,79). Recordings from the thalamus in humans with generalized dystonia have shown that abnormal neuronal activity is present in both pallidal and cerebellar receiving zones (49). Not only pallidal (33,81), but also cerebellar lesions have been associated with significant improvements in the signs of generalized dystonia (15,16,28,84). Finally, movement disorders with known genetic defects such as Huntington's disease are characterized by expression of the abnormal gene product throughout the neuraxis (75); the same might be expected in DYT1 and other primary dystonias.

ACKNOWLEDGMENTS

This work was supported by grants from NIH (NS 01593-01) and the Dystonia Medical Research Foundation.

REFERENCES

1. Altman J, Sudarshan K. Postnatal development of locomotion in the laboratory rat. *Anim Behav* 1975;23: 896–920.
2. Barrios C, Arrotegui JI. Experimental kyphoscoliosis induced in rats by selective brain stem damage. *Int Orthop* 1992;16:146–151.
3. Batini C, Benedetti F, Buisseret-Delmas C, Montarolo PG, Strata P. Metabolic activity of intracerebellar nuclei in the rat: effects of inferior olive inactivation. *Exp Brain Res* 1984;54:259–265.
4. Batini C, Billard JM. Release of cerebellar inhibition by climbing fiber deafferentation. *Exp Brain Res* 1985;57:370–380.
5. Bava A, Cicirata F, Giuffrida R, Licciardello S, Panto M. Electrophysiologic properties and nature of ventrolateral thalamic nucleus neurons reactive to converging inputs of paleo- and neocerebellar origin. *Exp Neurol* 1986;91:1–12.
6. Beales M, Lorden JF, Walz E, Oltmans GA. Quantitative autoradiography reveals selective changes in cerebellar GABA receptors of the rat mutant dystonic. *J Neurosci* 1990;10:1874–1885.
7. Billard JM, Batini C. Decreased sensitivity of cerebellar nuclei neurons to GABA and taurine: effects of long-term inferior olive destruction in the rat. *Neurosci Res* 1991;9:246–256.
8. Billard JM, Daniel H. Persistent reduction of Purkinje cell inhibition on neurones of the cerebellar nuclei after climbing fibre deafferentation. *Neurosci Lett* 1988;88:21–26.
9. Brown LL, Lorden JF. Local cerebral glucose utilization reveals widespread abnormalities in the motor system of the rat mutant dystonic. *J Neurosci* 1989;9: 4033–4041.
10. Buisseret-Delmas C. Sagittal organisation of the olivocerebellonuclear pathway in the rat. I. Connections with the nucleus fastigii and the nucleus vestibularis lateralis. *Neurosci Res* 1988;5:475–493.
11. Buisseret-Delmas C. Sagittal organisation of the olivocerebellonuclear pathway in the rat. II. Connections with nucleus interpositus. *Neurosci Res* 1988;5: 494–512.
12. Buisseret-Delmas C. Sagittal organisation of the olivocerebellonuclear pathway in the rat. III. Connections with the nucleus dentatus. *Neurosci Res* 1988;7: 131–143.
13. Calne DB, Lang AE. Secondary dystonia. In: Fahn S, Marsden CD, Calne DB, eds. *Advances in neurology: dystonia 2.* New York: Raven Press, 1988:9–33.
14. Colin F, Manil J, Desclin JC. The olivocerebellar system. I. Delayed and slow inhibitory effects: an overlooked salient feature of cerebellar climbing fibers. *Brain Res* 1980;187:3–27.
15. Cooper IS. Dystonia. In: Schaltenbrand G, Walker AE, eds. *Stereotaxy of the human brain.* New York: Georg Thieme Verlag, 1982:544–561.
16. Crosby EC, Schneider RC, DeJonge BR, Szonyi P. The alterations of tonus and movements through the interplay between the cerebral hemispheres and the cerebellum. *J Comp Neurol* 1966;127:1–91.
17. Daniel H, Billard JM, Anguat P, Batini C. The interposito-rubral system. Anatomical tracing of a motor control pathway in the rat. *Neurosci Res* 1988; 5:87–112.
18. Desclin JC, Escubi J. Effects of 3-acetylpyridine in the central nervous system of the rat, as demonstrated by silver methods. *Brain Res* 1974;77:349–364.
19. de Zeeuw CI, Holstege JC, Ruigrok TJH, Voogd J. Ultrastructural study of the GABAergic, cerebellar and mesodiencephalic innervation of the cat medial accessory olive: anterograde tracing combined with immunocytochemistry. *J Comp Neurol* 1989;284:12–35.
20. de Zeeuw CI, Holstege JC, Ruigrok TJH, Voogd J. Mesodiencephalic and cerebellar terminals terminate upon the same dendritic spines in the glomeruli of the cat and rat inferior olive: an ultrastructural study using a combination of [³H]leucine and wheat germ agglutinin coupled horseradish peroxidase anterograde tracing. *Neuroscience* 1990;34:645–655.
21. de Zeeuw CI, Ruigrok TJH, Holstege JC, Jansen HG, Voogd J. Intracellular labeling of neurons in the medial accessory olive of the cat: II. Ultrastructure of dendtritic spines and their GABAergic innervation. *J Comp Neurol* 1990;300:478–494.
22. de Zeeuw CI, Ruigrok TJH, Holstege JC, Schalekamp MPA, Voogd J. Intracellular labeling of neurons in the medial accessory olive of the cat: III. Ultrastructure of axon hillock and initial segment and their GABAergic innervation. *J Comp Neurol* 1990;300:495–510.
23. Fahn S. Dystonia: where next? In: Quinn NP, Jenner PG, eds. *Disorders of movement: clinical, pharmacological and physiological aspects.* San Diego: Academic Press, 1989:349–357.
24. Faull RLM. The cerebellofugal projections in the brachium conjunctivum of the rat. II. The ipsilateral and contralateral descending pathways. *J Comp Neurol* 1978;178:519–536.

25. Faull RLM, Carman JB. The cerebellofugal projections in the brachium conjunctivum of the rat. I. The contralateral ascending pathway. *J Comp Neurol* 1978; 178:495–518.

26. Fletcher NA, Stell R, Harding AE, Marsden CD. Degenerative cerebellar ataxia and focal dystonia. *Mov Disord* 1988;4:336–342.

27. Foltz EL, Knopp LM, Ward AA Jr. Experimental spasmodic torticollis. *J Neurosurg* 1959;16:55–72.

28. Fraioli B, Guidetti B, la Torre E. The stereotaxic dentatotomy in the treatment of spasticity and dyskinetic disorders. *J Neurosurg Sci* 1973;17:49–52.

29. Gibb WRG, Lees AJ, Marsden CD. Pathological report of four patients presenting with cranial dystonias. *Mov Disord* 1988;3:211–221.

30. Grüsser-Cornehls U. Compensatory mechanisms at the level of the vestibular nuclei following post-natal degeneration of specific cerebellar cell classes and ablation of the cerebellum in mutant mice. In: Flohr H, ed. *Post-lesion neural plasticity.* Berlin: Springer-Verlag, 1988:431–442.

31. Haroian AJ, Massopust LC, Young PA. Cerebellothalamic projections in the rat: an autoradiographic and degeneration study. *J Comp Neurol* 1981;197:217–236.

32. Heimer L, Alheid GF, Zaborszky L. Basal ganglia. In: Paxinos G, ed. *The rat nervous system. Vol 1. Forebrain and midbrain.* Sydney:Academic Press, 1985: 347–353.

33. Iacono RP, Kuniyoshi SM, Lonser RR, Maeda G, Inae AM, Ashwal S. Simultaneous bilateral pallidoansotomy for idiopathic dystonia musculorum deformans. *Pediatr Neurol* 1996;14:145–148.

34. Imperato A, Nicoletti F, Diana M, Scapagnini U, DiChiara G. Fastigial influences on postural tonus as studied by kainate lesions and by local infusion of GABAergic drugs in the rat. *Brain Res* 1984;295: 51–63.

35. Ito M. *The cerebellum and neural control.* New York: Raven Press, 1984.

36. Ivry RB, Keele SW, Diener HC. Dissociation of the lateral and medial cerebellum in movement timing and movement execution. *Exp Brain Res* 1988;73:167–180.

37. Jahnsen H. Electrophysiological characteristics of neurones in the guinea-pig deep cerebellar nuclei *in vitro. J Physiol* 1986;372:129–147.

38. Jankovic J, Fahn S. Dystonic disorders. In: Jankovic J, Tolosa E, eds. *Parkinson's disease and movement disorders.* Baltimore: Williams & Wilkins, 1993;337–374.

39. Jankovic J, Patel SC. Blepharospasm associated with brainstem lesions. *Neurology* 1983;33:1237–1240.

40. Karachot L, Ito M, Kanai Y. Long-term effects of 3-acetylpyridine-induced destruction of cerebellar climbing fibers on Purkinje cell inhibition of vestibulospinal tract cells of the rat. *Exp Brain Res* 1987; 66:229–246.

41. Khara JS, Calabrese VP. Cerebellar degeneration and Meige's syndrome. *South Med J* 1991;84:387–388.

42. Krauss JK, Mohadjer M, Braus DF, Wakhloo AK, Nobbe F, Mundinger F. Dystonia following head trauma: a report of nine patients and review of the literature. *Mov Disord* 1992;3:263–272.

43. Lauterbach EC, Price ST, Wilson AN, Kavali CM, Jackson JG, Kirsh AD. Dystonia after subcortical lesions: clinical and pathophysiologic implications. *Mov Disord* 1994;9:43A.

44. LeDoux MS. *A functional and neurophysiological examination of cerebellar output in the mutant rat dystonic (dt).* Ann Arbor, MI: University Microfilm, 1995.

45. LeDoux MS, Hurst DC, Lorden JF. Single-unit activity of cerebellar nuclear cells in the awake genetically dystonic rat. *Neurosci Abstr* 1995;21:271.

46. LeDoux MS, Lorden JF. Single-unit activity of cerebellar Purkinje cells in the awake genetically dystonic rat. *Neurosci Abstr* 1996;22:1629.

47. LeDoux MS, Lorden JF, Ervin JM. Cerebellectomy eliminates the motor syndrome of the genetically dystonic rat. *Exp Neurol* 1993;120:302–310.

48. LeDoux MS, Lorden JF, Meinzen-Derr J. Selective elimination of cerebellar output in the awake genetically dystonic rat. *Brain Res* 1995;696:91–103.

49. Lenz FA, Seike MS, Jaeger CJ, et al. Single unit analysis of thalamus in patients with dystonia. *Mov Disord* 1997;12:9A.

50. Llinás R, Mühlethaler M. Electrophysiology of guinea-pig cerebellar nuclear cells in the *in vitro* brain stem-cerebellar preparation. *J Physiol* 1988;404:241–258.

51. Lorden JF, Lutes J, Michela VL, Ervin J. Abnormal cerebellar output in rats with an inherited movement disorder. *Exp Neurol* 1992;118:95–104.

52. Lorden JF, McKeon TW, Baker HJ, Cox N, Walkley SU. Characterization of the rat mutant dystonic (dt): a new animal model of dystonia musculorum deformans. *J Neurosci* 1984;4:1925–1932.

53. Lorden JF, Oltmans GA, McKeon TW, Lutes J, Beales M. Decreased cerebellar 3′,5′-cyclic guanosine monophosphate levels and insensitivity to harmaline in the genetically dystonic rat (dt). *J Neurosci* 1985; 5:2618–2625.

54. Lorden JF, Oltmans GA, Stratton SE, Mays LE. Neuropharmacological correlates of the motor syndrome of the genetically dystonic rat (dt). In: Fahn S, Marsden CD, Calne DB, eds. *Advances in neurology: dystonia 2.* New York: Raven Press, 1988:277–298.

55. Manni E, Dow RS. Some observations on the effects of cerebellectomy in the rat. *J Comp Neurol* 1963;121:189–194.

56. Maraganore DM, Folger WN, Swanson JW, Ahlskog JE. Movement disorders as sequelae of central pontine myelinolysis: report of three cases. *Mov Disord* 1992;7:142–148.

57. Marlinsky VV. Activity of lateral vestibular nucleus neurons during locomotion in the decerebrate guinea pig. *Exp Brain Res* 1992;90:583–588.

58. McGeer EG, McGeer PL. The dystonias. *Can J Neurol Sci* 1988;15:447–483.

59. McKay WA. Unit activity in the cerebellar nuclei related to arm reaching movements. *Brain Res* 1988; 442:240–254.

60. McKeon TW, Lorden JF, Oltmans GA, Beales M, Walkley SU. Decreased catalepsy response to haloperidol in the genetically dystonic (dt) rat. *Brain Res* 1984;308:89–96.

61. Mehler WR, Rubertone JA. Anatomy of the vestibular nucleus complex. In: Paxinos G, ed. *The rat nervous system, vol. 2, hindbrain and spinal cord.* Sydney: Academic Press, 1985:185–219.

62. Naudon L, Clavel N, Delfs JM, Lorden JF, Chesselet MF. Differential expression of glutamic acid decarboxylase mRNA in cerebellar Purkinje cells and deep cerebellar nuclei of the genetically dystonic rat. *Neurosci Abst* 1996;22:1649.

63. Nelson BJ, Adams JC, Barmack NH, Mugnaini E. Comparative study of glutamate decarboxylase immunoreactive boutons in the mammalian inferior olive. *J Comp Neurol* 1989;286:514–539.

64. Oltmans GA, Beales M, Lorden JF. Glutamic acid decarboxylase activity in micropunches of the deep cerebellar nuclei of the genetically dystonic (dt) rat. *Brain Res* 1986;385:148–151.

65. Optican LM, Robinson DA. Cerebellar-dependent adaptive control of primate saccadic system. *J Neurophysiol* 1980;44:1058–1076.

66. Rispal-Padel L, Troiani D, Harnois C. Converging cerebellofugal inputs to the thalamus. *Exp Brain Res* 1987;68:59–72.

67. Robinson DA. Adaptive gain control of the vestibulo-ocular reflex by the cerebellum. *J Neurophysiol* 1976; 39:954–969.

68. Savio T, Tempia F. On Purkinje cell activity increase induced by suppression of inferior olive activity. *Exp Brain Res* 1985;57:456–463.

69. Shamboul KM. Lumbosacral predominance of vestibulospinal fiber projections in the rat. *J Comp Neurol* 1980;192:519–530.

70. Sotelo C, Gotow T, Wassef M. Localization of glutamic-acid-decarboxylase-immunoreactive axon terminals in the inferior olive of the rat, with special emphasis on anatomical relations between GABAergic synapses and dendrodendtritic gap junctions. *J Comp Neurol* 1986;252:32–50.

71. Sprague JM, Chambers WW. Regulation of posture in intact and decerebrate cat. I. Cerebellum, reticular formation, vestibular nuclei. *J Neurophysiol* 1953;16: 451–463.

72. Sprague JM, Chambers WW. Control of posture by reticular formation and cerebellum in the intact, anesthetized and unanesthetized and in the decerebrate cat. *Am J Physiol* 1954;176:52–64.

73. Stratton SE, Lorden JF. Effect of harmaline on cells of the inferior olive in the absence of tremor: differential response of genetically dystonic and harmaline-tolerant rats. *Neuroscience* 1991;41:543–549.

74. Stratton SE, Lorden JF, Mays LE, Oltmans GA. Spontaneous and harmaline-stimulated Purkinje cell activity in rats with a genetic movement disorder. *J Neurosci* 1988;8:3327–3336.

75. Strong TV, Tagle DA, Valdes JM, et al. Widespread expression of the human and rat Huntington's disease gene in brain and nonneural tissues. *Nat Genet* 1993; 5:259–265.

76. Sukin D, Skedros DG, Beales M, Stratton SE, Lorden JF, Oltmans GA. Temporal sequence of motor disturbances and increased glutamic acid decarboxylase activity following 3-acetylpyridine lesions in adult rats. *Brain Res* 1992;426:82–92.

77. Swenson RS, Castro AJ. The afferent connections of the inferior olivary complex in rats. An anterograde study using autoradiographic and axonal degeneration techniques. *Neuroscience* 1983;8:259–275.

78. Thach WT, Goodkin HP, Keating JG. The cerebellum and the adaptive coordination of movement. *Ann Rev Neurosci* 1992;15:403–442.

79. Tranchant C, Maquet J, Eber AM, Dietemann JL, Franck P, Warter JM. Cerebellar cavernous angioma, cervical dystonia and crossed cortical diaschisis. *Rev Neurol (Paris)* 1991;147:599–602.

80. van der Want JJL, Wiklund L, Guegan M, Ruigrok T, Voogd J. Anterograde tracing of the rat olivocerebellar system with Phaseolus vulgaris leucoagglutinin(PHA-L). Demonstration of climbing fiber collateral innervation of the cerebellar nuclei. *J Comp Neurol* 1989; 288:1–18.

81. Vitek JL, Evatt M, Zhang J, et al. Pallidotomy is an effective treatment for patients with medically intractable dystonia. *Mov Disord* 1997;12:31A.

82. Voogd J, Gerritts NM, Marani E. Cerebellum. In: Paxinos G, ed. *The rat nervous system. Vol. 2. Hindbrain and spinal cord.* New York: Academic Press, 1985: 251–291.

83. Wallace SF, Rosenquist AC, Sprague JM. Ibotenic acid lesions of the lateral substantia nigra restore visual orientation behavior in the hemianopic cat. *J Comp Neurol* 1990;296:222–252.

84. Zervas NT. Long-term review of dentatectomy in dystonia musculorum deformans and cerebral palsy. *Acta Neurochir* 1977;24[Suppl]:49–51.

Dystonia 3: Advances in Neurology, Vol. 78,
edited by S. Fahn, C. D. Marsden, and M. DeLong.
Lippincott–Raven Publishers, Philadelphia © 1998.

9

Clinical-Genetic Spectrum of Primary Dystonia

*Susan B. Bressman, *Deborah de Leon, *Deborah Raymond, †Laurie J. Ozelius, †Xandra O. Breakefield, *Torbjoern G. Nygaard, ‡Laura Almasy, §Neil J. Risch, and ‖Patricia L. Kramer

Department of Neurology, College of Physicians and Surgeons of Columbia University and the Presbyterian Hospital, New York, New York 10032; †The Molecular Neurogenetics Unit, Neurology, Massachusetts General Hospital and Harvard Medical School, Boston, Massachusetts 02114; ‡Department of Genetics, Southwest Foundation for Biomedical Research, San Antonio, Texas 78227; §Department of Genetics, Stanford University, Stanford, California 94305; and the ‖Department of Neurology, Oregon Health Sciences University, Portland, Oregon 97201.

Dystonia is classified into two major etiologic subtypes: primary or idiopathic and secondary or symptomatic (see Table 1). Although the term *idiopathic* is firmly entrenched in the literature, the time has probably arrived to drop this adjective. As responsible loci are mapped and genes are cloned, "idiopathic" no longer distinguishes the primary dystonias from other inherited conditions that may produce dystonic movements such as Hallervordan-Spatz, Huntington's disease, dopa-responsive dystonia, or X-linked dystonia-parkinsonism. The term *primary dystonia* is preferable because it does not denote a lack of knowledge about pathogenesis but rather relies on clinical characterization only. Under this clinical definition of primary dystonia, the criteria are (a) dystonia is the *only* neurologic sign except for tremor and (b) historical data and laboratory workup do not reveal an exogenous (e.g., neuroleptic exposure, perinatal asphyxia) or other inherited or degenerative cause for dystonia.

Based on the bimodal age at onset distribution and clustering of clinical features, primary dystonia is divided into two main clinical subtypes: (a) early onset (younger than 28 years,

with a median onset of 9 years), which usually starts in a leg or arm and then progresses to involve other limbs and the trunk, and (b) late-onset (older than 28 years, with a median onset of 45 years), which usually starts in cervical, cranial, or brachial muscles and tends to remain localized in distribution (16,28). In addition, a third rarer clinical subtype has been described in several families in which there is both early and late-onset of symptoms; dystonia may begin in either a limb or cervical-cranial muscles and spread to several body regions may occur (5,9,21).

EARLY-ONSET PRIMARY DYSTONIA (OR DYSTONIA MUSCULORUM DEFORMANS)

Inheritance Pattern

The first reports of early-onset (younger than 28 years) primary dystonia, almost 90 years ago, described two important features of this disease that were not fully appreciated for decades: the disease is familial (37), and it is more common in Jews of Eastern European an-

TABLE 1. *Etiologic classification of dystonia[a]*

Primary dystonia (dystonia is the only sign and history/lab unrevealing)
  Childhood and adolescent limb-onset
    Autosomal dominant, penetrance 30%
    Often spreads to other limbs; infrequent cranial involvement
    Vast majority due to DYT1 (chr 9q)
      In Ashkenazim: Single DYT1 founder mutation accounts for >90% of cases
      In non-Jewish families: Many different mutation "events" (may be same mutation)
  Mixed phenotype: onset in childhood or adult, may begin in limb, neck, or cranial muscles
    Autosomal dominant, incomplete penetrance
    Cranial involvement with dysarthria/dysphonia common; limb involvement produces tonic posturing but
      gait brisk
    Mapped to chr 8-DYT6 in Mennonite/Amish families
  Adult cervical, cranial, or brachial-onset
    Autosomal dominant with very reduced penetrance; some families higher penetrance
    Dystonia usually remains localized; in rare families there is spread
    Not DYT1 or DYT6
    Mapped to chr 18p (DYT7) in one German torticollis family
Secondary dystonia
  Associated with hereditary neurologic syndromes
    Dopa-responsive dystonia (DRD or DYT5)
    Myoclonic dystonia
    Lubag (X-linked parkinsonism-dystonia or DYT3)
    Rapid-onset dystonia-parkinsonism
    Wilson's disease
    Gangliosidoses
    Metachromatic leukodystrophy
    Lesch-Nyhan syndrome
    Homocystinuria
    Hartnup disease
    Glutaric acidemia
    Leigh's disease
    Familial basal ganglia calcifications
    Hallervorden-Spatz disease
    Dystonic lipidosis (sea-blue histiocytosis)
    Ceroid-lipofuscinosis
    Ataxia-telangiectasia
    Neuroacanthocytosis
    Intraneuronal inclusion disease
    Huntington's disease
    Neuroacanthocytosis
    Machado-Joseph's disease/SCA3
    Mitochondrial encephalomyopathies/Leber's disease
  Due to known environmental cause
    Perinatal cerebral injury
    Encephalitis, infectious and postinfectious
    Head trauma
    Pontine myelinolysis
    Primary antiphospholipid syndrome
    Stroke
    Tumor
    Multiple sclerosis
    Cervical cord injury or lesion
    Peripheral injury
    Drugs
    Toxins
  Dystonia as part of parkinsonism
  Psychogenic dystonia

[a]DYT2, autosomal recessive in Gypsies/not mapped; DYT3, X-linked dystonia parkinsonism (Lubag); DYT4, autosomal dominant whispering dysphonia in Australian family/not mapped; DYT5, dopa-responsive dystonia/14q-GTPCH gene.

cestry (42). In 1970, Eldridge (15) proposed that early-onset primary dystonia is inherited as an autosomal-recessive trait in Jews and an autosomal-dominant trait in non-Jews. For close to 20 years this view was widely accepted. More recent studies from Israel (43) and the United States (6,33), as well as reanalysis of Eldridge's original data (32), indicate that the disorder is *not* autosomal recessive in Jews; it is transmitted in an autosomal-dominant fashion, with reduced (30%) penetrance. The age-adjusted risk for all first-degree relatives is about 15.5% and for all second-degree relatives it is 6.5%, with no significant sex differences. Parent, offspring, and sibling risks are *not* significantly different. Further, there is no evidence for sporadic cases or new mutations; that is, all cases are inherited (6,33). The study of Bressman and colleagues found that the range of clinical features in the relatives of early-onset Ashkenazi probands is limited. Although the disease in relatives compared to probands is milder, more localized, and has a slightly later age at onset, most share a similar phenotype of early limb-onset dystonia; symptom onset after age 40 and onset in cranial muscles are rare (6). With the subsequent discovery of a founder mutation in this population (see below), the above family study findings have been both confirmed and explained; that is, a single founder mutation underlies almost all early-onset primary dystonia in Ashkenazim and this mutation is limited (early limb-onset) in its expression (7).

Early-onset dystonia in the non-Jewish Caucasian population is also inherited as an autosomal-dominant trait with markedly reduced penetrance (17,24,32,42). A systematic analysis (17) of 96 non-Jewish British probands with generalized, multifocal, and segmental dystonia (the majority had early onset) concluded that approximately 85% of cases are inherited as an autosomal-dominant trait with reduced penetrance of 40%; the remaining 15% are likely to be nongenetic phenocopies. Increased paternal age of singleton cases was found and about 14% of genetic cases are thought to be new mutations. As in the study of Ashkenazi

families, there was variable and often milder expression in affected relatives although, unlike that population, a larger proportion (10% to 15%) of non-Jewish affected family members had late onset (older than 44 years). One proposed explanation for the genetic and clinical differences between these populations is that the disorder among Jews is genetically homogenous, whereas among non-Jews greater genetic heterogeneity of dystonia is likely (33). That is, the most plausible reason for the higher frequency of early-onset dystonia, a dominant disorder, in Jews is the presence of a single founder mutation and genetic drift (33); thus most cases would be due to the same mutation event and clinical homogeneity would be expected. In non-Jews, a heterogeneous population with a lower incidence of disease, the disorder is likely to result from mutation/selection balance so that multiple mutations, including new mutations, would be expected. This greater etiologic heterogeneity among non-Jews might then also explain the greater clinical heterogeneity observed in this population.

DYT1/Genetic Linkage Studies

Ozelius et al. (30) mapped the first primary dystonia locus (named DYT1) in 1989. They studied a large North American non-Jewish family of French-Canadian ancestry, first reported by Johnson et al. (22), and localized the gene to the 9q32-34 region. Subsequently, Kramer and colleagues (23) found linkage of dystonia with markers in the same region in 12 Ashkenazi families. Clinical features were similar in the non-Jewish and 12 Jewish families; onset was early in both (average, 14.4 ± 3 and 13.2 ± 1 years, respectively) and symptoms began in a limb (86% and 90%, respectively) in almost all. In the study of Kramer et al. tightest linkage was found with the gene encoding arginosuccinate synthetase (ASS); subsequent multipoint analysis with markers in the 9q region revealed a similar location for the disease genes in both the Jewish and non-Jewish groups (25) and the same gene is thought to cause dystonia in both. Because the locus for dopamine beta hydroxylase (DBH) maps to the DYT1 9q region and because this enzyme was implicated in several studies of primary dystonia, this candidate locus was evaluated and excluded soon after DYT1 was localized (36).

Since the initial linkage findings, studies of European (41), non-Jewish North American (24), and Ashkenazi (7,31) families confirm that DYT1 is a common cause of early-onset primary dystonia, although it is not responsible for dystonia in all early-onset families (41). In a European study of 27 small families (three Jewish and 24 non-Jewish) there was evidence for linkage to the chromosomal region containing DYT1, with a combined lod score of 3.4 at ASS calculated for 24 families. However, tight linkage to ASS was excluded in 3 non-Jewish families (41). One of the excluded families was thought to have dopa-responsive dystonia; otherwise clinical differences between "DYT1" and "non-DYT1" families were not noted.

Evidence implicating DYT1 was also provided in a study of six non-Jewish North American families of European descent (24). The clinical features of affected members in these six families were similar to each other, and also similar to the non-Jewish and Jewish families first linked to 9q34 (i.e., early limb onset with spread to other limbs and the trunk, also see Table 2). Penetrance, using 9q-linked markers, was 40%. Analyses of haplotypes (a haplotype is a group of alleles from closely linked loci inherited as a unit from one parent) in these non-Jewish families did not suggest linkage disequilibrium (see below for discussion of this term); however, two French-Canadian families shared the same haplotype, suggesting a common ancestor. It is presumed that most early-onset primary dystonia in the non-Jewish population results from different mutation events in the DYT1 gene.

Linkage Disequilibrium of DYT1 with 9q Markers in Ashkenazi Jews

Soon after finding linkage of early-onset primary dystonia with 9q markers in Ashkenazi families, it became apparent that these families share a common 9q haplotype. This sharing of

TABLE 2. *DYT1 phenotype*

	Non-Jewish (Kramer et al. [24][a])	Ashkenazi Jewish (Bressman et al. [7])
No. families	4	52
No. affected	36	90
M:F	1.7:1	1.1:1
Age onset (yr)		
Mean	13.6	12.5
Median	11	9
Range	4–43	4–44
Disease duration (yr)		
Mean	24	23
Range	0.5–61	0.5–66
Site onset		
Limb	33 (92%)	85 (94%)
Leg	21	42
Arm	12	43
Cervical/cranial	3 (8%)	5 (6%)
Neck	1	3
Larynx	1	2
Other cranial	1	0
Site last exam		
Limb	35 (97%)	88 (98%)
Neck	10 (28%)	28 (31%)
Cranial	7 (19%)	7 (8%)
Larynx	4 (11%)	3 (3%)
Other cranial	4 (11%)	5 (6%)
Distribution last exam		
Generalized	25 (69%)	54 (60%)
Multifocal	3 (8%)	10 (11%)
Segmental	2 (6%)	10 (11%)
Focal	6 (17%)	16 (18%)

[a]The four families chosen from seven reported had individual family lod scores >2.0 at 9q34 marker loci; the three not included each had lod scores <1.0.

a *particular* haplotype of alleles more frequently than would be expected by chance is called *linkage disequilibrium*. For markers that are tightly linked to the disease gene, such an association of linked alleles and the disease gene implies the disease is due largely to a single mutation event or founder mutation. Very strong linkage disequilibrium between the DYT1 gene and a haplotype at the 9q marker loci ABL and ASS was found first (31). This was then extended to include four additional polymorphic markers, D9S62a, D9S62b, D9S63, and D9S64 (35). The presence of very strong linkage disequilibrium at the relatively large genetic distance of at least a few centiMorgans also suggests that the mutation is recent; Risch et al. (35) have calculated that the mutation was introduced into the Ashkenazi population about 350 years ago and probably originated in Lithuania or Byelorussia. They also argue that the high current prevalence of the disease in Ashkenazim (estimated to be about 1:3,000 to 1:9,000 with a gene frequency of about 1:2,000 to 1:6,000) is due to the tremendous growth of that population in the eighteenth and nineteenth centuries from a small reproducing founder population (34,35). A founder mutation and genetic drift (changes in gene frequency due to chance events such as migrations, population expansions) rather than a heterozygote advantage (i.e., nonpenetrant DYT1 carriers have some advantage that leads to carriers being more prevalent), is probably responsible for the high frequency of DYT1 dystonia in Ashkenazim. This same mechanism, they argue, also accounts for the high frequency of other genetic diseases (e.g., familial dysautonomia, Bloom's syndrome, BRCA1 - breast/ovarian cancer) in Ashkenazim.

Clinical Expression of the DYT1 Founder Mutation in Ashkenazim

The clinical spectrum of the Ashkenazi DYT1 founder mutation (as defined by the associated haplotype of alleles at the 9q marker loci D9S62b, D9S63, and ASS) was assessed in a study of 174 affected Ashkenazi individuals with both early- and late-onset primary dystonia (7). Over 90% of *both familial and isolated* early limb-onset primary dystonia cases carried the associated haplotype of 9q alleles (Figs. 1 and 2) and the clinical features of (a) first symptoms in a limb, (b) involvement of a leg in the course of disease, and (c) early-onset discriminated between those who had and those who did not have the associated haplotype with about 90% accuracy. The mean age at onset in carriers was 12.5 years. Dystonia began in a limb (arm or leg equally) in 94%, and over 70% of carriers had progression to a generalized or multifocal distribution. Rarely, carriers of the associated haplotype had onset in the neck (3.3%) or larynx (2.2%) and there were no carriers with onset in the facial muscles. Spread to the larynx or other cranial muscles was also uncommon (3.3% and 5.5%, respectively).

Haplotype noncarriers on the other hand, constituted the great majority of late-onset and cervical/cranial-onset cases. The mean age at onset of noncarriers was 36.5 years and all patients with onset after age 44 were noncarriers; 79% of noncarriers had onset in the neck, larynx, or cranial muscles, and dystonia remained

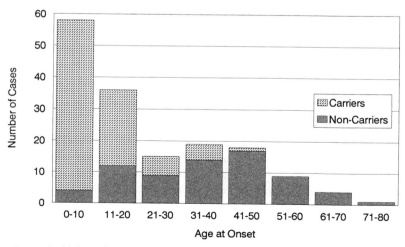

FIG. 1. Age at onset of idiopathic torsion dystonia in Ashkenazi Jewish carriers and noncarriers of the haplotype associated with the DYT1 mutation.

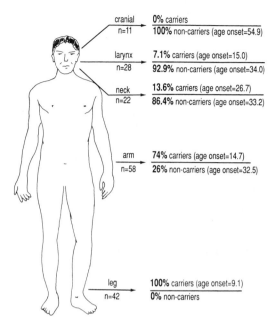

cranial
n=11
0% carriers
100% non-carriers (age onset=54.9)

larynx
n=28
7.1% carriers (age onset=15.0)
92.9% non-carriers (age onset=34.0)

neck
n=22
13.6% carriers (age onset=26.7)
86.4% non-carriers (age onset=33.2)

arm
n=58
74% carriers (age onset=14.7)
26% non-carriers (age onset=32.5)

leg
n=42
100% carriers (age onset=9.1)
0% non-carriers

FIG. 2. The proportion of haplotype carriers and noncarriers for the various sites of onset of idiopathic torsion dystonia.

localized as focal or segmental in almost all (97%) the noncarriers. If divided by site at onset, there was only one group that contained a significant proportion of both carriers and noncarriers, namely those with onset in an arm, and even within this group differences were found between haplotype carriers and noncarriers. Carriers were younger at onset and were more likely to have spread of dystonia to another limb compared with noncarriers, who were older at onset and tended to spread up to the neck and cranial muscles.

In summary, a single founder mutation accounts for over 90% of early limb-onset primary dystonia among Ashkenazim but this mutation event is generally not responsible for late-onset or cervical/cranial-onset dystonia. The clinical-genetic differences observed between haplotype carriers and noncarriers suggest dystonia in noncarriers results from non-genetic factors, other DYT1 mutations, and/or other dystonia genes. Recent linkage studies suggest that at least a proportion of late-onset

and cervical/cranial-onset is due to other dystonia genes (see below).

DYT1 and Causes for Reduced Penetrance and Variable Expression

Although most affected DYT1 gene carriers have early limb-onset dystonia (Table 2), there is still a wide range of disease severity and 70% of gene carriers never express the gene. The cause(s) of low penetrance and variable expression is unknown; possible mechanisms include genomic imprinting, anticipation, modifying genes, and environmental factors. Only a few studies have assessed families for these factors. LaBuda et al. (26) analyzed the pedigrees of four previously published series of early-onset or generalized and segmental families for evidence of genomic imprinting or anticipation. They found that the gender of the transmitting parent did not influence site of onset, age at onset, or distribution of dystonia, except that there was maternal transmission in almost all later-onset cases. The data were also consistent with anticipation, however sampling bias could not be ruled out. A similar trend toward later onset of maternally transmitted dystonia was noted by de Leon et al. (14) in affected Ashkenazi DYT1 gene carriers, but this did not reach statistical significance. This same group found no evidence for anticipation in Ashkenazi and non-Jewish families with dystonia due to DYT1 (2).

Intrafamilial correlations of clinical features, such as age at onset and severity, have also been assessed for evidence of genetic heterogeneity (different genes or alleles producing different phenotypes that "breed true"). A very low correlation for age at onset among 23 first-degree relative pairs was found in one British study of generalized and segmental probands. The authors concluded that there is no evidence of genetic heterogeneity; they suggested that primary dystonia is due to a single gene and that expression may be influenced by environmental factors (18). The influence of environmental factors in precipitating dystonia in DYT1 carriers was suggested in a study by the same group, which found that 16.4% of generalized and segmental primary dystonia cases have a history of peripheral trauma exacerbating or precipitating dystonia (19); the dystonic movements either worsened or began in the same region of the body that was injured. On the other hand, a study of 40 Ashkenazi patients with secondary dystonia (8) found no evidence that the DYT1 gene contributes to secondary dystonia, even in cases that mimic the DYT1 phenotype (i.e., patients with neuroleptic exposure or perinatal asphyxia and early limb-onset dystonia). This study suggests that the DYT1 gene is not commonly precipitated by environmental factors that are known to cause dystonia, such as birth injury or dopamine-blocking agents; however, the role of other modifiers such as peripheral trauma could not be excluded.

LATE-ONSET PRIMARY DYSTONIA

Genetic Epidemiology and Inheritance Patterns

Unlike early-onset dystonia, the genetic contribution to late-onset primary dystonia is not yet clearly established. There have been several systematic family studies of patients with late-onset (11), focal (38,40), or cervical-cranial dystonia (13). The criteria for inclusion in these studies differed; for example the Defazio study excluded writer's cramp whereas the Waddy study included probands with all focal dystonias. Nevertheless, the overall population of patients was similar (primarily late-onset cervical and cranial dystonia). The rates of dystonia in examined parents and siblings (most offspring were not yet past the age at-risk) ranged from 5% (11,13) to 9% (38,40); affected relatives within families usually also had late-onset focal dystonia and in some studies there was a correlation within families of the specific body region affected (13,40). None of the studies found a significant difference between the rates in parents and siblings. The rates of dystonia observed in first-degree relatives in these studies are much higher than the

reported population prevalence (3/10,000) (29) and also significantly higher than control group frequencies (0/142 in the study of Defazio and 1/86 in the study of Stojanovic). The conclusion in all these studies is that the pattern of inheritance of late-onset primary dystonia is consistent with autosomal-dominant transmission with very reduced penetrance, or autosomal dominant with higher penetrance in a subset (and the remainder sporadic/nongenetic).

An alternative approach to help discern whether there is evidence for a genetic basis for late-onset primary dystonia is to assess whether there is phenotypic variation among ethnic groups. That is, as described above, early-onset dystonia was suspected to be genetic in Ashkenazim, and due to a founder mutation, because this form of dystonia is increased in the Ashkenazi population. A similar question can be posed for late-onset dystonia; that is, is adult-onset, or cervical or cranial-onset dystonia more common in any particular ethnic group? Unfortunately, there are few valid epidemiologic data to support differences in disease prevalence among different ethnic groups. Because the disorder is relatively rare in all ethnic groups and because it is often either not detected or misdiagnosed, a true estimate of disease frequency would require a door-to-door study canvassing a very large population. Alternatively, comparisons can be made between ethnic groups attending a clinical center. Such an analysis is not dependent on the actual rate at which members of different ethnic groups seek treatment; however, it is based on the assumption that people attend the clinic because of the severity of symptoms and treatment available, independent of ethnicity. For example, such an analysis assumes that the probability that an Italian-American will attend a clinic for treatment of torticollis versus blepharospasm is not different from that of an Ashkenazi Jew or African-American. Given this caveat, Almasy and colleagues (4) analyzed the clinical features of 786 patients with primary dystonia attending Columbia University's movement disorders clinic. As expected, Ashkenazi Jews had a lower age-at-onset distribution compared with non-Jews. Further, in the early-onset group, Jews were less likely to have onset in the neck and more likely to have onset in a limb. A novel finding was that among late-onset cases, Jews had less cervical and more cranial onset than Caucasian non-Jews. Also, African-Americans showed suggestive differences in both age at onset and site at onset compared with both Jewish and non-Jewish Caucasians, with an intermediate age at onset, a deficit of leg onset, and an excess of cranial and larynx onset. These ethnic variations in age and site at onset suggest there are population differences in disease-causing gene loci or alleles, although environmental differences cannot be excluded.

Linkage Studies Excluding DYT1

Although the relationship between early- and late-onset primary dystonia remains to be fully elucidated, there is mounting evidence that these clinical subtypes are causally distinct, with at least a proportion of late-onset primary dystonia being due to genes other than DYT1. It had been argued that one gene underlies all primary dystonia because all dystonia, regardless of ultimate progression, begins as a focal phenomenon, and also because focal dystonia (particularly writer's cramp) is seen in the relatives of early-onset generalized patients (20,40). Current evidence suggests that genetic differences underlie the clustering of clinical features. As described above, the DYT1 phenotype, as assessed by linkage studies and also the associated DYT1 haplotype in Ashkenazim, is generally one of early onset with first symptoms in a leg or arm; late onset and cervical or cranial onset are uncommon expressions of the DYT1 Ashkenazi founder mutation. The restricted nature of the DYT1 phenotype also has been confirmed by linkage studies excluding DYT1 in families with late onset of symptoms or prominent cervical/cranial involvement.

As described above, for the general population of late-onset or cervical/cranial-onset patients the risk of dystonia in first-degree relatives is low, only 5% to 9%. However, rare large non-Jewish families with more highly penetrant autosomal-dominant late-onset or cervical-cranial predominant dystonia are described; linkage studies in *all* these families have excluded the DYT1 region (1,5,12,21). The DYT1 locus was excluded in four North American families of German ancestry, including one Mennonite family (9,10,12), an Italian family (5), an Australian family (1), and a Swedish family (21). The overall phenotype in these families differs from DYT1 phenotype: the average age at onset is later, and/or onset is commonly in the neck or cranial muscles or there is spread to the cervical or cranial muscles, usually with severe disability. Despite these differences, in each of these families, except for the torticollis families of Bressman et al. (12), there is at least one family member whose phenotype overlaps with the "typical" DYT1 (see Table 3). For example, in one of the North American non-DYT1 families (9), symptom onset was later (average, 28.4 ±14.8 years) and most affected family members had first symptoms in the neck with progression to involvement of both cervical and cranial muscles in all. Yet one affected in this family had onset in a leg in childhood and that individual went on to have generalized dystonia. The clinical features of segmental cervical and cranial dystonia in this family are similar to those of the Italian family described by Bentivoglio et al. (5).

The Mennonite family described by Bressman et al. (10), the Australian family of Ahmad et al. (1), and the Swedish family of Holmgren et al. (21) display an even more varied or mixed clinical picture (Table 3). In all three families there is a wide range in the age at onset with symptoms beginning in either the limbs, neck, larynx, and other cranial muscles; further, dysphonia or dysarthria was prominent in both the Mennonite and Australian families.

Finally, DYT1 was excluded in two families with a phenotype consisting primarily of pure torticollis (12). Unlike the other excluded phenotypes, however, dystonia in these families is similar to that observed commonly in the general population; that is, onset in the neck occurring during adulthood and remaining localized.

TABLE 3. *Clinical features of non-DYT1 families (all non-Jewish)*

	Bressman et al. (9)	Bressman et al. (8,10)	Bressman et al./ Uitti et al. (12,39)	Holmgren et al. (21)	Bentivoglio et al. (5)	Ahmad et al. (1)
No. families	1	2	2	1	1	1
Origin	German-American	Mennonite/Amish German-American	German-American	Swedish	Italian	English Australian
No. affected	7	15 (9 and 6)	7 and 5	7	8	10 (2 with Wilson's)
M:F	3:4	4:11	2:5 and 4:1	4:3	4:4	5:5
Age onset (yr)						
Mean	28.4	18.7	30.9 and 35.2	27	16	ns
Range	7–50	5–38	15–62 and 18–49	17–50	<28 in 7; 1 was 40	13–37
Disease duration (yr)						
Mean	28	23.7	15 and ns	14	ns	ns
Range	10–50	2–69	1–44 and 7–38	0–47	32–71	ns
Site onset						
Limb	1/7	8/15	1/12	2/6	3/7 (1 with neck)	1/10
Leg	1	1	0	0	0	1
Arm	0	7	1	2	3	0
Cervical/cranial	6/7	7/15	11/12	4/6	5/7 (1 with arm)	9/10
Neck	6	3	11	0	5	2
Larynx	1 (with neck)	1	0	1	0	7
Other cranial	0	3	0	3	5	0
Sites at last exam						
Limb	2/7	13/15	2/12	6/7	ns	ns
Leg	1	8	0	4		
Arm	2	13	2	6		
Neck	7/7	7/15	11/12	?		
Cranial	7/7	11/15	0	at least 4/6	ns	ns
Larynx	3	7	0	at least 3		
Other cranial	7	8	0	at least 4		
Distribution last exam						
Generalized	1/7	4/15	0	3/7	2/8	8/10
Multifocal	0	4/15	0	3/7	0	0
Segmental	6/7	6/15	1 (arm and neck)	0	5/8	2/10
Focal	0	1/15	11/12	1/7	1/8	0
Atypical features	Attention/learning disorder					Wilson's disease, progressive dementia

Mapping of Genes for Late-Onset and Cervical/Cranial Dystonia

The most recent development in our understanding of the genetics of primary dystonia is the mapping of two additional gene loci for dystonia. One gene has been localized to chromosome 8 (DYT6) in two Mennonite families (one of these was previously excluded from DYT1, as described above) and another locus (DYT7) has been mapped in a German family with torticollis. The numbering of primary dystonia loci, skipping from DYT1 to DYT6, is confusing but historically based on the inclusion of dystonic disorders that are either not considered primary (i.e., X-linked dystonia-parkinsonism assigned DYT3 and dopa-responsive dystonia assigned DYT5) or clinically described but as yet unmapped (autosomal-recessive dystonia in the Gypsy population assigned DYT2 and dystonia with whispering dysphonia assigned DYT4).

The DYT6 gene was mapped in two families of German-American Mennonite and Amish origin not known to be related but phenotypically similar to each other (4). There were nine affected individuals in one family and six in the other. The average age at onset was 18.7 years (range, 5 to 38 years), with about one-half having onset in childhood and the remainder having onset in adulthood. The disease duration averaged 23 years (range, 2 to 69 years). The spectrum of dystonic symptoms and signs was very broad. Dystonia began in an arm in seven of 15 affected and a leg in one; the remaining members had onset in the neck ($n = 3$), larynx ($n = 1$), tongue ($n = 2$), and facial muscles ($n = 1$). There was spread of disease beyond the site of onset in almost all affected family members (one had only writer's cramp); in most, dystonia affected both the cranial-cervical and limb muscles. The greatest disability stemmed from involvement of cranial-cervical muscles in ten of 15 family members, and from brachial muscles in the remainder. A genome-wide search in the larger family led to the finding of linkage with markers on chromosome 8, with maximum lod score of 3.69 at the anonymous locus D8S1797. Linkage to the same region was then confirmed in the second family

with a maximum lod score of 2.11 at several loci including D8S1797. In these two clinically and ethnically similar families an identical haplotype spanning approximately 40 cM of chromosome 8 cosegregated with the disease. This large shared candidate region suggests these families share a founder mutation from the recent past. The study of other unrelated affected Mennonite individuals for this haplotype may help narrow the candidate region as many linkage studies of families with a mixed phenotype of early and late limb and cervical-cranial dystonia.

DYT7 was mapped in a German torticollis family consisting of seven definitely affected and six possibly affected individuals (27). The pedigree structure was consistent with autosomal-dominant inheritance with reduced penetrance of about 50%. Six of the seven with definite dystonia had torticollis; one of these affected individuals also had mild facial/mandibular involvement (Meige) and one had writer's cramp. The seventh definitely affected person had spasmodic dysphonia. Of those with possible dystonia, five had mild signs of torticollis (muscle hypertrophy or shoulder elevation without head rotation) and one had only postural hand tremor. Hand tremor was also noted in three definitely affected and three others with possible dystonia. The age at onset ranged from 28 to 70 years (mean = 43), and after an average disease duration of 9 years, the dystonia did not progress beyond the sites involved. A genome-wide linkage search was performed and linkage to the region telomeric of D18S1153 on chromosome 18p was found, with a maximum lod score of 3.17. All the affecteds, eight of 16 unaffecteds, and five of the six possibly affected individuals carried the disease haplotype, confirming both the reduced penetrance and variable expression of dystonia in this family. Also, one of the possibly affected individuals, who had tremor only, did not carry the haplotype; this finding underscores the importance of conservative diagnosis, particularly when attributing a relatively common abnormality, such as postural hand tremor, to a relatively rare disease, such as dystonia. The region containing this torticollis gene (DYT7), like DYT6, is large, 30 cM. The strategy to further localize this gene is similar to that planned for DYT6: Other clinically similar families need to be studied, including sporadic cases and small families from the same geographic region who might show linkage disequilibrium. Also, several candidates genes in the linked region are to be assessed.

SUMMARY

Early-Onset Primary Dystonia

Linkage and association studies indicate that mutations in the gene mapped to chromosome 9q34 (DYT1) produce a specific range of clinical features. Primary dystonia due to DYT1 is transmitted as an autosomal-dominant trait with reduced penetrance of 30% to 40%, and mutations in this gene account for most early-onset (younger than 28 years) cases. In over 90% of our Ashkenazi patients with early limb-onset primary dystonia, the disease is due to a single founder mutation in the DYT1 gene, as determined by very strong linkage disequilibrium with a haplotype of 9q alleles at surrounding marker loci. On the other hand, this mutation is rarely responsible for late-onset (older than 28 years) primary dystonia and has not yet been found in any Ashkenazi patients with onset older than 44 years or onset in the facial muscles. The role of other DYT1 mutations in the Ashkenazi population is not clear. Large informative Ashkenazi families with late-onset dystonia have not been identified for linkage studies that might implicate or exclude the DYT1 region; however, among smaller late-onset families and simplex cases, there is no strong evidence to date of another DYT1-associated haplotype (P. L. Kramer, personal communication). The diagnosis of dystonia due to the Ashkenazi founder mutation can be confirmed by testing for the associated haplotype of alleles at the 9q loci D9S62, D9S63, and ASS. In most, but not all, non-Jewish families with early limb-onset primary dystonia, the disease also is due to the DYT1 gene, but multiple mutation events appear to be responsible. That is, there is no evidence for linkage dise-

quilibrium in studies of non-Jewish families (although two French-Canadian families were found to share the same haplotype of 9q34 alleles). Until the gene at DYT1 is identified, testing for DYT1 mutations in non-Jewish early-onset patients remains restricted to those with large multiplex families suitable for linkage analysis. Once the gene is identified, direct mutation screening may be available for Jewish and non-Jewish populations.

Late-Onset Primary Dystonia

Unlike early-onset dystonia, the genetic contribution to late-onset primary dystonia is not established. Several family studies have concluded that there is evidence for autosomal-dominant inheritance with reduced penetrance; in most studies, however, the rates of dystonia in first-degree relatives of late-onset probands are significantly lower (about 5%) than the rates in first-degree relatives of early-onset probands (15%).

The relationship between early- and late-onset primary dystonia remains to be fully elucidated. It has been argued that the same gene underlies both early- and late-onset primary dystonia based on the fact that all dystonia, regardless of ultimate progression, begins as a focal phenomenon, and also because later-onset focal dystonia (particularly writer's cramp) is occasionally seen in the relatives of early-onset generalized patients. There is mounting evidence, however, that etiologic differences underlie the clustering of clinical features and that different genes are responsible for early- and late-onset primary dystonia.

Rare large non-Jewish families with highly penetrant autosomal-dominant late-onset or cervical-cranial predominant dystonia are described, and linkage studies of seven such families have been reported; the DYT1 locus was excluded in all seven families. Mapping of genes in these "non-DYT1" families is underway and to date two loci (DYT6 and DYT7) have been identified. The DYT6 locus on chromosome 8 was mapped in two North American Mennonite families with a "mixed phenotype" of both childhood and adult-onset dystonia beginning in both limb and cervical-cranial muscles. Most affecteds in these families had progression of signs to involve multiple body regions and cervical and cranial dystonia (e.g., dysphonia, dysarthria, blepharospasm, torticollis) produced the greatest disability in most. The DYT7 locus was mapped in a German family primarily affected with adult-onset torticollis. The role of these two loci in the general population of late-onset primary dystonia needs to be assessed. Because most cases of adult-onset primary dystonia are sporadic, this question may remain unanswered until after identification of these genes and their gene products.

REFERENCES

1. Ahmad F, Davis MB, Waddy HM, Oley CA, Marsden CD, Harding AE. Evidence for locus heterogeneity in autosomal dominant torsion dystonia. *Genomics* 1993; 15:9–12.
2. Almasy L, Bressman SB, deLeon D, Risch N. No evidence for anticipation in 9q34-linked idiopathic torsion dystonia. *Genet Epidemiol* 1995;12:326.
3. Almasy L, Bressman SB, deLeon D, Risch NJ. Ethnic variation in clinical expression of idiopathic torsion dystonia. *Mov Disord* 1997;12:715–721.
4. Almasy L, Bressman SB, Kramer PL, et al. Idiopathic torsion dystonia linked to chromosome 8 in two Mennonite families. *Ann Neurol* (*in press*).
5. Bentivoglio AR, Albanese A, Del Grosso, et al. A large Italian family affected by idiopathic torsion dystonia with complete penetrance not linked to DYT1. *Neurology* 1996;46[Suppl]:A385 (abst).
6. Bressman SB, deLeon D, Brin MF, et al. Idiopathic dystonia among Ashkenazi Jews: evidence for autosomal dominant inheritance. *Ann Neurol* 1989;26:612– 620.
7. Bressman SB, deLeon D, Kramer PL, et al. Dystonia in Ashkenazi Jews: clinical characterization of a founder mutation. *Ann Neurol* 1994;36:771–777.
8. Bressman SB, deLeon D, Raymond D, et al. The role of the DYT1 gene in secondary dystonia. *Neurology* (*in press*).
9. Bressman SB, Heiman GA, Nygaard TG, et al. A study of idiopathic torsion dystonia in a non-Jewish family: evidence for genetic heterogeneity. *Neurology* 1994; 44:283–287.
10. Bressman SB, Hunt AL, Heiman GA, et al. Exclusion of the DYT1 locus in a non-Jewish family with early onset dystonia. *Mov Disord* 1994;9:626–632.
11. Bressman SB, Rassnick H, Almasy L, et al. Inheritance of late-onset idiopathic torsion dystonia. *Neurology* 1995;45[Suppl 4]:A457 (abst).
12. Bressman SB, Warner TT, Almasy L, et al. Exclusion of the DYT1 locus in familial torticollis. *Ann Neurol* 1996;40:681–684.
13. Defazio G, Livrea P, Guanti G, et al. Genetic contribution to idiopathic adult-onset blepharospasm and cranial-cervical dystonia. *Eur Neurol* 1993;33: 345– 350.
14. deLeon D, Bressman SB, Brin MF, Risch NJ, Fahn S. Torsion dystonia in Ashkenazi Jews: is there evidence for an imprinted gene? *Mov Disord* 1992;7:292.
15. Eldridge R. The torsion dystonias: literature review and genetic and clinical studies. *Neurology* 1970;20 [Suppl]:1–78.
16. Fahn S, Marsden CD, Calne DB. Classification and investigation of dystonia. In: Marsden CD, Fahn S, eds. *Movement disorders 2*. London: Buttersworth, 1987: 332–358.
17. Fletcher NA, Harding AE, Marsden CD. A genetic study of idiopathic torsion dystonia in the United Kingdom. *Brain* 1990;113:379–396.
18. Fletcher NA, Harding AE, Marsden CD. Intrafamilial correlation in idiopathic torsion dystonia. *Mov Disord* 1991;6:310–314.
19. Fletcher NA, Harding AE, Marsden CP. The relationship between trauma and idiopathic torsion dystonia. *J Neurol Neurosurg Psychiatry* 1991;54:713–717.
20. Harding AE. Movement disorders: genetic aspects. In: Marsden CD, Fahn S, eds. *Movement disorders 3*. London: Butterworths, 1994:46–64.
21. Holmgren G, Ozelius L, Forsgren L, et al. Adult-onset idiopathic torsion dystonia is excluded from the DYT1 region (9q34) in a Swedish family. *J Neurol Neurosurg Psychiatry* 1995;59:178–181.
22. Johnson W, Schwartz G, Barbeau A. Studies on dystonia musculorum deformans. *Arch Neurol* 1962;7:301–313.
23. Kramer LP, Ozelius L, deLeon D, et al. Dystonia gene in Ashkenazi Jewish population located on chromosome 9q32-34. *Ann Neurol* 1990;27:114–120.
24. Kramer PL, Heiman GA, Bressman SB, et al. The DYT1 gene on 9q34 is responsible for most cases of early limb-onset idiopathic torsion dystonia in non-Jews. *Am J Hum Genet* 1994;55:468–475.
25. Kwiatkowski OJ, Ozelius L, Kramer PL, et al. Torsion dystonia genes in two populations confined to a small region on chromosome 9q32-34. *Am J Hum Genet* 1991;49:366–371.
26. LaBuda MC, Fletcher NA, Korczyn AD, et al. Genomic imprinting and anticipation in idiopathic torsion dystonia. *Neurology* 1993;43:2040–2043.
27. Leube B, Doda R, Ratzlaff T, Kessler K, Benecke R, Auberger G. Idiopathic torsion dystonia: assignment of a gene to chromosome 18p in a German family with adult onset, autosomal inheritance and purely focal distribution. *Hum Mol Genet* 1996;5:1673–1677.
28. Marsden CD, Harrison MSG. Idiopathic torsion dystonia (dystonia musculorum deformans): a review of forty-two patients. *Brain* 1974;97:793–810.
29. Nutt JG, Muenter MD, Aronson A, Kurland LT, Melton LJ III. Epidemiology of focal and generalized dysto-nia in Rochester, Minnesota. *Mov Disord* 1988; 3: 188–194.
30. Ozelius L, Kramer PL, Moskowitz CB, et al. Human gene for torsion dystonia located on chromosome 9q32-34. *Neuron* 1989;2:1427–1434.
31. Ozelius LJ, Kramer PL, deLeon D, et al. Strong allelic association between the torsion dystonia gene (DYT1) and loci on chromosome 9q34 in Ashkenazi Jews. *Am*

J Hum Genet 1992;50:619–628.

32. Pauls DL, Korczyn AD. Complex segregation analysis of dystonia pedigrees suggests autosomal dominant inheritance. *Neurology* 1990;40:1107–1110.

33. Risch NJ, Bressman SB, deLeon D, et al. Segregation analysis of idiopathic torsion dystonia in Ashkenazi Jews suggests autosomal dominant inheritance. *Am J Hum Genet* 1990;46:533–538.

34. Risch NJ, deLeon D, Fahn S, et al. ITD in Ashkenazi Jews-genetic drift or selection?-reply. *Nature Genet* 1995;11:14–15.

35. Risch NJ, deLeon D, Ozelius LJ, et al. Genetic analysis of idiopathic torsion dystonia in Ashkenazi Jews and their recent descent from a small founder population. *Nature Genet* 1995;9:152–159.

36. Schuback D, Kramer P, Ozelius L, et al. Dopamine beta-hydroxylase gene excluded in four types of hereditary dystonia. *Hum Genet* 1991;87:311–316.

37. Schwalbe W. Eine eigentumliche tonische Krampfform

38. Stojanovic M, Cvetkovic D, Kostic VS. A genetic study of idiopathic focal dystonias. *J Neurol* 1995;242:508–511.

39. Uitti RJ, Maraganore DM. Adult-onset familial cervical dystonia: report of a family including monozygotic twins. *Mov Disord* 1993;8:489–494.

40. Waddy HM, Fletcher NA, Harding AE, Marsden CD. A genetic study of idiopathic focal dystonias. *Ann Neurol* 1991;29:320–324.

41. Warner TT, Fletcher NA, Davis MB, et al. Linkage analysis in British and French families with idiopathic torsion dystonia. *Brain* 1993;116:739–744.

42. Zeman W, Dyken P. Dystonia musculorum deformans; clinical, genetic and pathoanatomical studies. *Psychiatr Neurol Neurochir* 1967;70:77–121.

43. Zilber N, Korcyn AD, Kahana E, et al. Inheritance of idiopathic torsion dystonia among Jews. *J Med Genet* 1984;21:13–26.

mit hysterischen Symptomen, Thesis, Berlin, 1908.

Dystonia 3: Advances in Neurology, Vol. 78,
edited by S. Fahn, C. D. Marsden, and M. DeLong.
Lippincott–Raven Publishers, Philadelphia © 1998.

10

The Gene (DYT1) for Early-Onset Torsion Dystonia Encodes a Novel Protein Related to the Clp Protease/Heat Shock Family

*Laurie J. Ozelius, *Jeffrey W. Hewett, *Curtis E. Page, †Susan B. Bressman, ‡Patricia L. Kramer, *Christo Shalish, †Deborah de Leon, §Mitchell F. Brin, †Deborah Raymond, *David Jacoby, *John Penney, ‖Neil J. Risch, †Stanley Fahn, *James F. Gusella, and *Xandra O. Breakefield

*Molecular Neurogenetics Unit, Massachusetts General Hospital, Charlestown, Massachusetts 02129 and Departments of Neurology and Genetics and Neuroscience Program, Harvard Medical School, Boston, Massachusetts 02114; †Dystonia Clinical Research Center, Department of Neurology, Columbia Presbyterian Medical Center, New York, New York 10032; ‡Department of Neurology, Oregon Health Sciences University, Portland, Oregon 97201; §Movement Disorders Center, Mount Sinai Hospital, New York, New York 10029; and ‖Department of Genetics, Stanford University, Stanford, California 94305.

Early-onset, generalized torsion dystonia is the most severe form of hereditary dystonia (see Chapter 9). The syndrome follows an autosomal-dominant mode of inheritance with reduced penetrance, such that 60% to 70% of gene carriers do not express any symptoms. This disease has highest prevalence in the Ashkenazi Jewish population, due to a founder mutation, with an estimated gene carrier frequency of up to 1/2,000 (41). The mutant gene is about tenfold less frequent in other ethnic populations (32,49). The gene responsible for early-onset dystonia, termed DYT1, was initially mapped to human chromosome 9q34 (38). This positional information was refined (36) and used to identify the DYT1 gene (37), as reviewed here.

The clinical spectrum of early-onset dystonia is similar across all ethnic populations (4). Symptoms usually begin as a twisting in of the foot/leg or hand/arm between 9 and 13 years of age, and spread to involve twisting contractions of other limbs within 5 years (4,18).

There have been few clues as to the etiology of this disease. Based on cases of secondary dystonia, the alteration in function is believed to reside in the midbrain or striatum (3,6), but there is no obvious neuropathology in hereditary cases of dystonias (22,23,49). Although this distinctive lack of neuropathology has made it difficult to determine exactly which neuronal pathways are disrupted in dystonia, genetic studies of another dystonic syndrome, dopa-responsive dystonia, have implicated insufficiency of dopaminergic input to the striatum in childhood-onset dystonia (11,15,44). In contrast to dopa-responsive dystonia, early-onset dystonia does not respond well to drug treatment, although high-dose anticholinergic medication has proven effective in some individuals (12). In the converse situation, drug-induced dystonias are almost always caused by disruption of dopaminergic neurotransmission. Neuroleptic drugs that act by blocking dopamine D2 receptors can cause acute dystonic reactions (30). Also brief periods of dystonia can be produced at the beginning and end of L-dopa treatment of Parkinson patients (30). Positional cloning of the dystonia gene was undertaken as a means to identify the primary defect in early-onset dystonia, as well as to elucidate eventually the neurons and neurotransmitter circuitry in the disease.

POSITIONAL CLONING OF THE DYT1 GENE

The initial strategy was to map the location of the dystonia gene by linkage analysis in a large kindred with multiple members affected with typical early-onset dystonia and to use rigorous diagnostic criteria for affected members, to avoid phenocopies. A genomic search located the responsible gene to a 30-centiMorgan (cM) region on chromosome 9q34 in a non-Jewish family from upstate New York (38)

(Fig. 1), which had been described initially by Dr. Andre Barbeau and colleagues (24). In subsequent studies a collection of Ashkenazi Jewish families with a similar syndrome was used to confirm linkage to the same chromosomal region, assuming that the high incidence of early-onset dystonia in this population resulted from a founder mutation (27). The position of the DYT1 gene was further refined to 5 cM [approximately 5,000 kilobases (kb) of DNA] by recombination events in these families (27). Genetic studies in other non-Jewish and Jewish families were consistent with localization of the DYT1 gene to this region in all families with typical early-onset dystonia of sufficient size for linkage analysis (26,28).

The next goal was to reduce the size of the chromosomal region known to contain the DYT1 gene to one compatible with cloning of the genomic region and searching for genes

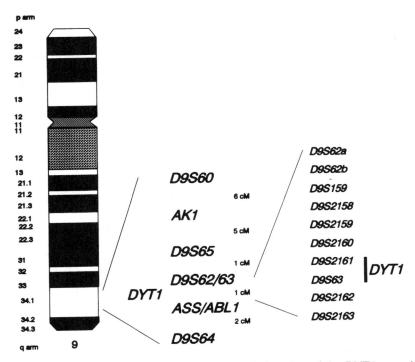

FIG. 1. Chromosomal location of DYT1 gene. The genetic location of the DYT1 gene is shown on a Giemsa-metaphase banded human chromosome 9 *(left column)* with flanking genetic markers. Middle column, genetic map (39); right column, physical order of polymorphic markers flanking DYT1 (36).

within it. This effort was facilitated by the Ashkenazic Jewish founder mutation, which is responsible for essentially all cases of early-onset torsion dystonia in this population (4). The presence of this founder mutation was deduced by analysis of DNA for a particular set of polymorphic variations in sequence (markers) around the DYT1 gene (41). This defining haplotype occurs in the heterozygous condition (since the mutation is autosomal dominant) and defines the presence of the predisposing mutation in both affected individuals and unaffected gene carriers. Analysis of this haplotype in combination with the heritage of affected Ashkenazi Jewish kindreds revealed that the founder mutation was introduced about 350 years ago (20 generations) in the geographic region of Lithuania and Byelorussia (41). These affected kindreds then represent an extensive interrelated pedigree derived from the same ancestral parents. Such a large pedigree allows for many meiotic transmissions of the disease gene, with each meiotic event having the potential for exchanges of DNA sequence (recombinations) around the DYT1 gene. Fine localization of the DYT1 gene was achieved by identification of 13 polymorphic variations in the critical region and typing of 64 Ashkenazi individuals with typical early-onset dystonia for these variations (36). Variations in the flanking ends of the haplotype (due to historic recombinations) served to localize the DYT1 gene to an interval of less than 1 cM (less than 1,000 kb). The cloned markers circumscribing the gene were used to screen a library of human genomic DNA cloned in large capacity (300 to 500 kb) vectors, termed *yeast artificial chromosomes* (YACs). YAC clones were isolated in an overlapping array. In this way a set of contiguous genomic clones (a contig) spanning 600 kb was generated across ten of the 13 markers flanking the DYT1 gene. A critical region of 150 kb, as defined by the closest markers coinheriting with the disease gene, was considered the region most likely to contain the dystonia gene (36).

The next step of the search was to identify genes within the 150-kb critical region. This genomic region was first subcloned into smaller capacity (30 to 40 kb) cosmid vectors to facilitate identification of genes (37). A set of 11 cosmids with overlapping sequences, which spanned the 150-kb region, was aligned by virtue of common sequences and restriction enzyme sites. These cosmids were then digested with different restriction enzymes and cloned into vectors designed to elucidate the exon portion of genes. These "exon amplification" vectors allow identification of exons by virtue of the splice sites flanking them, which are used in processing of RNA transcripts to remove intronic sequences between exons in generating messenger RNA (5,7). Twenty-eight unique exons were identified and cloned, and used to screen cDNA libraries from human tissues, including fetal brain and several regions of adult brain, cortex and substantia nigra. In this way five cDNAs were identified that were encoded in this critical region (Fig. 2). These cDNAs were extended by overlapping of cDNA clones with shared sequences and by polymerase chain reaction (PCR) extension from 5' and 3' ends (14). When these cDNAs were aligned across the genomic cosmid contig they appeared to cover most of the 150 kb and thus may account for all the genes in this region.

cDNAs were screened for mutations initially using a method termed *single-strand conformational polymorphism* (SSCP) analysis, which allows resolution of sequence differences by altered migration of renatured DNA under conditions of gel electrophoresis (21,35). First-strand cDNA was synthesized from messenger RNA isolated from patient and control lymphoblast cultures and amplified as 100- to 300-bp fragments using PCR. Fortunately all five messages were expressed at sufficient levels in lymphoblasts to generate cDNA fragments for analysis. Sequencing of fragments with altered migration revealed a number of polymorphic variations in coding and noncoding regions of all five genes, which were found in both affected and control individuals (Fig. 2). One alteration, a deletion of three base pairs (GAG), corresponding to a triplet codon for glutamic acid, was uniquely found in patients with early-onset dystonia.

cDNA DQ1

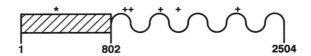

Polymorphisms: C/T @ 343, proline/proline   **Transcript size:**   2.7 kb

cDNA DQ2

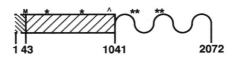

Polymorphisms: C/T @ 288,alanine/alanine   **Transcript size:**   2.2 kb, 1.4 kb
                      G/C @ 688, aspartic acid/histidine
                      G/T @ 1232
                      C/G @ 1255
                      del/T @ 1464
                      T/A @ 1495

Mutation: del/GAG @ 946, del/glutamic acid

cDNA DQ3

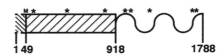

Polymorphisms: A/G @ 156, glutamic acid/glutamic acid   **Transcript size:**   1.8 kb
                      A/G @ 420, lysine/lysine
                      T/C @ 801, glycine/glycine
                      AC/CT @ 1005
                      G/A @ 1063
                      (T)n @1273
                      T/A @ 1724
                      A/G @ 1751

cDNA DQ4

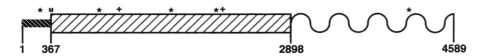

Polymorphisms: G/A @ 225
                      C/T @ 840, alanine/alanine
                      G/A @ 1696, valine/isoleucine   **Transcript size:**   4.5 kb
                      C/T @ 2172, histidine/histidine
                      G/A @ 4225

TABLE 1. *Genotype of GAG deletion in candidate cDNA in affected individuals and controls*

Categories	Families	Genotype in individuals		
		+/+[a]	+/−	−/−
Controls				
Ashkenazi Jewish (AJ)	130	130	0	0
Non-Jewish (NJ)	137	137	0	0
Affected and obligate carriers[b] in 9-linked families				
AJ founder haplotype	64	0	173	0
NJ	4	0	88	0
Affecteds of unknown linkage[c]				
Typical	19	5	36[d]	0
Uncertain	38	34	4	0
Atypical	76	76	0	0

[a]+, GAGGAG; −, GAG (del).
[b]Lod score > +2 for 9q34 markers (Ref. 26).
[c]Families too small for linkage analysis.
[d]From 14 families.

Extended genetic studies confirmed that the GAG deletion was present in the heterozygous state in most individuals affected with early-onset dystonia, as well as in obligate carriers of this disease gene (Table 1). For these studies, screening of the mutation was simplified by using PCR amplification of the target region from genomic DNA isolated from blood samples, followed by digestion with the restriction enzyme BseRI, which cuts the control fragment, but not the mutant fragment (Fig. 3). The deletion was shown to coinherit with the disease in four non-Jewish families with early-onset dystonia, which were large enough to establish likely linkage to chromosome 9q34, and to be present in all carriers of the Ashkenazi Jewish founder mutation (173 cases in 64 families); it was never found in controls (27). The screen was then extended to include other individuals with symptoms encompassing the broad classification of primary, early-onset dystonia. These individuals were subdivided into three categories depending on the confidence with which they were diagnosed to have typical early-onset dystonia (by S.B. prior to knowledge of mutational status). The typical group (74% of whom carried the GAG deletion) consisted of individuals with classic symptoms of early-onset dystonia, in which onset occurred in a limb prior to 28 years of age and spread to involve at least one other limb, but not cranial muscles. The uncertain group (10% with GAG deletion) included individuals for which diagnosis was not clear-cut, in that onset of limb dystonia commenced after the age of 45 years; onset occurred before 28 years but in cervical or cranial muscles; symptoms spread from limbs to cranial muscles; or patients had other neurologic problems. The four cases out of 38 with uncertain dystonia that carried the GAG deletion in DYT1 fell into two types: two individuals had early onset

◄——————————

FIG. 2. Sequence variations in cDNAs in DYT1 region. Diagrams are scaled representations of each of the four cDNA transcripts in the critical region. The striped black box indicates 5′untranslated sequence; the striped white box indicates deduced open reading frame; and the wavy line indicates 3′untranslated sequences. The dashed lines at the 5′end of the open reading frame of cDNAs DQ2 and DQ3 indicate that no stop codon 5′to the first predicted methionine (M) has been found. The numbers flanking the open reading frame box indicate the beginning and end of the cDNAs and the nucleotide position of the predicted start and stop codons. Regions generating SSCP shifts are indicated above the transcript diagram: + marks those for which nucleotide changes have not yet been determined; * marks the location of known nucleotide changes corresponding to SSCP shifts; ^ marks the GAG-deletion in cDNA DQ2. (From reference 37, with permission.)

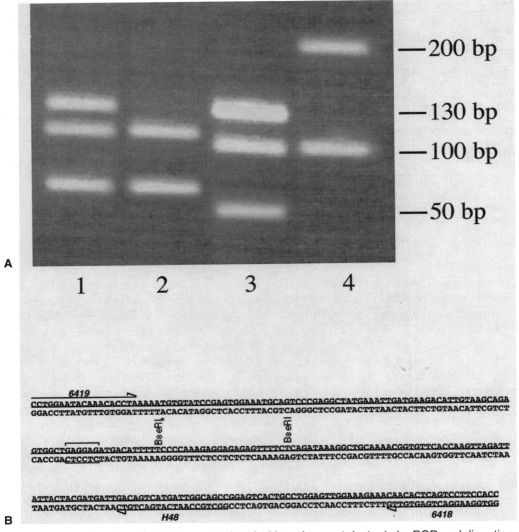

FIG. 3. Resolution of GAG deletion associated with early-onset dystonia by PCR and digestion. **A:** Digestion of PCR fragment with BseRI. PCR products were generated from genomic DNA with primers 6419 and H48 and the 200 bp product was digested with BseRI. Bands of 120 bp and 70 bp were generated from control DNA *(lane 2)*, whereas a novel band of 130 bp was generated from affected individuals with the GAG-deletion *(lane 1)*, because of the loss of a BseRI site. Lane 3 and 4 are markers: 3 = PCR products of specific sizes (50, 100, and 130 bp) and 4 = 100 bp ladder (Pharmacia). **B:** Sequence surrounding GAG-deletion. Normal genomic/cDNA sequence of torsinA showing position of primers *(arrows)*; the GAGGAG sequence *(bracketed)* in which the GAG deletion occurs; and BseRI sites (*, site lost as a result of the deletion). (From reference 37, with permission.)

in a limb, but with subsequent spread to the head or neck; the two others had typical early-onset dystonia complicated by other neurologic conditions, polio, and concurrent head trauma. The most distinguishing features of DYT1

GAG-deletion dystonia therefore are onset before 28 years in a limb with spread to at least one other limb, and, usually, with no involvement of cervical or cranial muscles. The atypical group comprised individuals whose symptoms were not typical of early-onset dystonia, for example, having focal or segmental cervical-cranial dystonia or only writer's cramp; none of these 76 individuals had a GAG deletion.

The identification of a single mutation (GAG deletion) responsible for almost all typical cases of early-onset dystonia representing a number of different ethnic groups is remarkable. There are a few examples of other diseases in which a recurrent type of discrete mutational change underlies a specific syndrome, including achondroplasia (2), hypokalemic periodic paralysis (13,20), and hypertrophic cardiomyopathy (47). There are two possible explanations for the recurrence of the same disease-related mutation across ethnic groups: (a) all cases are ancestrally related and actually bear the identical mutation, or (b) the same mutation has arisen independently, but is the only change (or perhaps one of a few) that causes that particular disease phenotype. For the GAG deletion in early-onset dystonia the latter explanation appears to be valid, as analysis of polymorphisms in the immediate vicinity (5 kb) of the DYT1 gene revealed two different flanking haplotypes in association with the deletion. It is assumed then that other mutations in the DYT1 may account for the 16% of typical cases that lack the GAG deletion. It remains possible that distinct types of mutations in DYT1 may underlie other forms of dystonia or other neurologic diseases.

CHARACTERISTICS OF THE DYT1 GENE

The DYT1 gene is estimated to be about 8 kb and encodes two mRNAs, estimated from northern blots as 1.8 and 2.2 kb, which have a fairly ubiquitous tissue distribution (37). The cloned cDNA (DQ2) is 2 kb and contains a predicted open reading frame of 998 base pairs (bp) with two poly A addition sites at the 3'end. It is not clear at this time whether the full 5'end is cloned, as the open reading frame continues 5'to the predicted translational start site (ATG). The deduced protein, termed *torsinA,* is 332 amino acids in length with a calculated molecular weight of 37,813 Daltons and pI 6.8. This gene and the deduced protein have about 70% homology at the nucleotide and amino acid level with an adjacent gene in the genome, termed *DQ1,* encoding a related protein, termed *torsinB.* These two genes are in opposite orientations in the genome (with 3'ends nearest to each other) and are assumed to have arisen from a tandem duplication of an evolutionary precursor gene. The DQ1 gene product also has a relatively ubiquitous tissue distribution by northern blot analysis, but its message is distinguished from that of DYT1 (DQ2 cDNA) by being 2.8 kb.

A search of genomic and cDNA databases reveals that DYT1 represents a unique member of a larger gene family that spans a broad range of species. A protein closely related to torsinA has been deduced from DNA sequence of the worm, *Caenorhabiditis elegans.* Homologous sequences (approximately 50% identity) were also found in the expressed sequence tag site (ESTS) database corresponding to human, mouse, and rat torsinA and torsinB, as well as to two other torsin-related proteins, termed *torp1* and *torp2.* Figure 4 shows an amino acid sequence alignment of these predicted proteins. They share a single hydrophobic domain near the N-terminal, which could be involved in intracellular trafficking into or across a membrane; six cysteine residues, presumably important in secondary protein structure; several possible phosphorylation sites, indicating possible differences in activation states; and an ATP-binding site (see below). The pair of glutamic acids (one of which is deleted in dystonia) is conserved in human torsinA and torsinB, and flanked by cysteine residues, suggesting it is part of a functional domain.

Certain discrete elements in torsinA suggest a distant relationship to two other protein families, which share some similar functions: the family of heat shock proteins and proteases [HSP 100/Clp family (40)] which occurs primarily in prokaryotes, but has also been described in some eukaryotes; and the primarily eukaryotic family of ATPases associated with a variety of cellular activities [AAA family (8)]. Both families bind ATP and/or have ATPase activity, function as oligomeric complexes with other proteins, and mediate a range of related

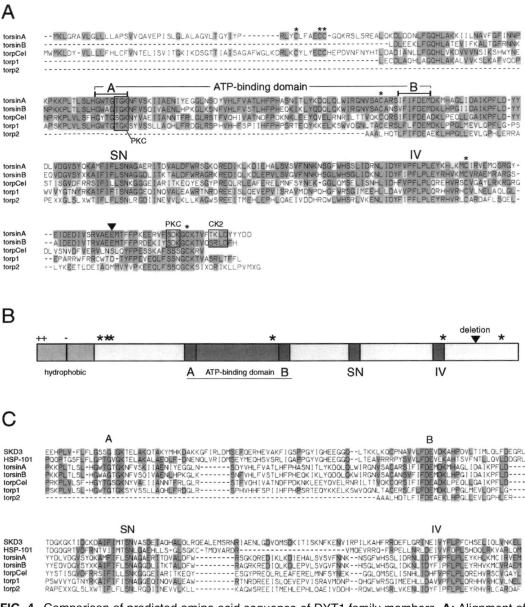

FIG. 4. Comparison of predicted amino acid sequence of DYT1 family members. **A:** Alignment of torsins and torps. TorsinA and torsinB are encoded by cDNAs DQ2 and DQ1, respectively. TorpCel is the predicted amino acid sequence from a *C. elegans* genomic sequence. Torp-1 and torp-2 correspond to overlapping expressed sequence tag cDNAs from human and mouse, respectively. The solid triangle represents the site of the GAG (E) deletion in torsinA. Conserved cysteine residues are represented by *. Darkly shaded residues are identical to a consensus sequence; highly shaded residues are similar. Conserved possible phosphorylation sites for protein kinase C (PKC) and casein kinase 2 (CK2) are boxed. **B:** Schematic representation of torsinA domains. The N-terminal region *(left)* contains about 40 hydrophobic amino acids, preceded by two basic residues *(K, R)* and bisected by a polar and an acidic residue *(Q, E)*. The ATP-binding domain is indicated along with its conserved A and B motifs. Two additional motifs conserved with the HSP100 family (SN and IV) are shaded. **C:** Comparison of torsins and torps with two representative members of the HSP100 family. SKD3, from mouse is an HSP100 family member of class 2M; HSP101 from soybean is a heat shock protein of class 1B (43). Shaded residues are identical to a consensus sequence. The conserved motifs (A, B, SN, and IV) occur in all seven proteins. (Reprinted in part from reference 37, with permission.)

functions. Members of these gene families typically function in folding or unfolding of other proteins and in guidance to correct cellular locations; regulation of dynamic cellular processes, such as signaling and gene transcription; and recovery or protection from stress by renaturation of degraded proteins. Figure 4C compares the torsin family to two representative members of the HSP100 protein family: HSP101, a heat shock protein from soybeans in the HSP100 subfamily 1B; and SKD3, a ubiquitous mouse protein in the subfamily 2M (40,43). The most robust feature is a conserved NTP-binding sequence comprising two motifs: the nucleotide-binding site "A" followed approximately 60 amino acids later by the Mg^{2+}-binding site "B" (46). In a conserved stretch of 140 amino acids that include the nucleotide binding domain, torsin family members are 25% to 30% identical to HSP100 family proteins. Key residues of the HSP100 consensus site IV (43) and another site (SN; Fig. 4C) are also conserved, but consensus site V is absent in the torsins.

Typically proteins in these two families form doughnut-like rings of identical subunits with ATP mediating binding of these subunits (e.g., Reference 42). This ring then stacks with one or more other rings composed of a set of different subunits. Stacking is typically mediated by the carboxy terminus of the primary ring. Thus a mutation in the carboxy portion of the HS1U protein complex (HSP/Clp family) blocks association with the HS1V protein complex, and thereby inhibits proteolytic activity in a dominant manner (31). Similarly a number of mutations in the carboxy terminal of the FtSH protein (filamentation temperature-sensitive member of the AAA family) block protein translocation in *Escherichia coli* (1). By analogy, the GAG deletion in the carboxy region of torsinA could prevent function of a complex formed with another set of proteins, even if only a few members of the heteromeric torsinA structure bore the mutation. In this model the mutant torsinA would act in a dominant-negative fashion to suppress function of normal torsinA.

IMPLICATIONS FOR DYSTONIA

This is the first demonstration, to our knowledge, of a role for any members of the HSP100/Clp protease or AAA families in a human disease, and suggests the possibility of a new type of genetic disease state that confers a susceptibility to a "second hit." This is particularly intriguing in the context of early-onset dystonia where only 30% or so of gene carriers manifest the disease state, and where there has been some suggestion that physical trauma may precipitate symptoms (16). Although the broad range of functions of these protein families does not point to a specific function for torsinA, common features of the family suggest two biochemical handles for torsinA: ATPase activity and binding to another protein.

An understanding of early-onset dystonia should also provide insight into developmental plasticity in the basal ganglia. Early-onset dystonia has several clinical features that suggest developmental disruption of temporal and spatial patterning in this region of the brain. Detailed clinical analysis of many patients with the Ashkenazi Jewish founder mutation has shown that when symptoms have an early onset (mean age 9 years) they occur most frequently in a foot and tend to generalize to many other body parts (88% of cases; Reference 4). When symptoms begin somewhat later (mean age 15 years), they usually start in the arm and have a decreased tendency to generalize (36%). (These two categories account for 95% of affected cases with this founder mutation.) Individuals with the founder mutation who pass the age of 28 years without symptoms (60% to 70% of gene carriers) usually remain symptom-free for life. Thus the earlier the onset of symptoms, the more likely they are to occur in a lower body part and to involve more body parts, although usually not the head and neck (Fig. 5). These observations are consistent with a dorsal-ventral pattern of development affecting dopaminergic input to the basal ganglia, which continues to undergo synaptic restructuring during the postnatal period (17,45). This developmental gradient overlies a somatotopic

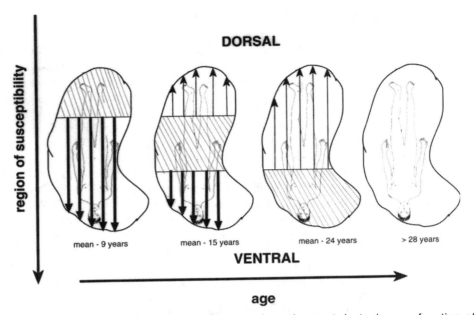

FIG 5. Hypothetical model of neuronal involvement in early-onset dystonia as a function of age. Dystonic symptoms are believed to arise through neuronal dysfunction in the basal ganglia. Neurons in this region of the brain have an anatomic patterning corresponding to the movements they subserve in the body, which can be represented roughly as an inverted homunculus. In early-onset dystonia the physical site of onset of symptoms and tendency to generalize as a function of age can be represented as a zone of susceptibility (cross-hatched area) moving ventrally in the basal ganglia with age. Clinical analysis of carriers of the Ashkenazi Jewish founder mutation (4) reveals that the earlier the onset of symptoms, the more likely they are to commence in lower limbs and the greater the tendency *(thick black arrows)* to generalize and involve upper parts of the body. With increasing age onset, symptoms tend to involve progressively higher body parts, and still tend to progress upward. By 28 years of age or older, carriers of the early-onset gene have passed the age of susceptibility and have only a small remaining chance of manifesting any symptoms. Still, as gene carriers, these "escapees" are at equal risk as affected gene carriers for having affected children.

distribution of neuronal connections in the basal ganglia subserving movements of different body parts (inverted homunculus) (9). This model of neuronal involvement provides a platform for evaluating subtle neuromorphologic and physiologic changes in dystonia, and the changes that occur in dystonia may provide insight into components of pattern formation.

Dystonia has for long been the most poorly understood, but common, member of a group of movement disorders, including Huntington's disease and Parkinson's disease. Hereditary dystonia differs importantly from these other two neurodegenerative syndromes in that there is no apparent neuronal degenera-

tion. Still there is an interrelatedness in these syndromes in that dystonic symptoms can be seen in early-onset cases of Parkinson's disease and in Huntington's disease (48), and parkinsonian symptoms appear in two hereditary forms of dystonia, including rapid onset in later years and untreated dopa-responsive dystonia (10,34). Possibly the biggest clue as to the pathogenesis of early-onset dystonia comes from investigation of individuals suffering from dopa-responsive dystonia, which, in contrast to early-onset dystonia, can be virtually cured by administration of L-dopa (33,44). Positional cloning of the genes responsible for this condition has revealed two enzymes necessary for L-dopa synthesis, GTP cyclohydrolase I (15) and tyrosine hydroxylase (25,29). Thus childhood-onset dopa-responsive dystonia is caused by an insufficiency of dopaminergic input into the striatum. In this model, deficits of dopaminergic innervation to the striatum would appear as dystonia in early life and as parkinsonism in later life. The lack of response to L-dopa in early-onset DYT1 patients, in the presence of no apparent loss of dopaminergic neurons, suggests a possible deficiency in storage, release, reuptake, or reception of dopamine in the striatum.

Identification of the DYT1 gene should pave the way for better diagnosis and understanding of functional alterations in early-onset dystonia. The elucidation of a common mutation in about 75% of affected individuals from a wide range of ethnic backgrounds will greatly simplify DNA diagnosis. Heretofore DNA diagnosis for this form of dystonia has only been possible for individuals of Ashkenazi-Jewish descent and a panel of DNA polymorphisms was needed to define the founder haplotype. Now the common mutation can be revealed in individuals of different ethnic backgrounds by a single PCR and gel assay. DNA diagnosis will be useful not only for genetic counseling in families with affected members, but also for differential diagnosis in individuals having dystonia of unknown etiology. Further, given the observation that the best response to anticholinergic therapy tends to be in patients treated early in the course of the disease (19), it may prove useful to identify gene carriers prior to onset of symptoms in order to reduce the time between onset of symptoms and treatment. The identification of the DYT1 gene also provides a means to localize the neurons in the brain involved in dystonia by virtue of *in situ* hybridization to the corresponding mRNA and immunocytochemical detection of the protein, torsinA. Further, knowledge of the gene sequence and structure will allow creation of genetically authentic transgenic animals to pursue the molecular etiology of this disease, and potentially to serve as experimental models for therapy.

ACKNOWLEDGMENTS

We thank all the families who participated in these studies for providing samples and inspiration. We thank K. Sims, A. Buckler, D. Schuback, H. McFarlane, P. Crawford, M. Anderson, T. Gasser, E. Smith, S. Teitz, J. Yount, N. Smith, V. Ramesh, and M. Rutter for help and advice with experimental protocols; M. McDonald for access to cDNA libraries; and S. McDavitt for skilled preparation of this manuscript. This work was supported by the Dystonia Medical Research Foundation (P.K., S.B., M.B., S.F., J.G., L.O., X.O.B.); the Histadrut Foundation, which provided the sequencer used in these studies (L.O., X.O.B.); the Jack Fasciana Fund for the Support of Dystonia Research (X.O.B., L.O.); and NIH grants NS28384 (X.O.B.), NS26656 (S.F., S.B.), NS24279 (X.O.B., J.G.), HG00169 (J.G.), and HG00348 (N.R.).

REFERENCES

1. Akiyama Y, Shirai Y, Ito K. Involvement of FtsH in protein assembly into and through the membrane. *J Biol Chem* 1994;269:5225–5229.
2. Bellus GA, Hefferon TW, Ortiz de Luna TI, et al. Achondroplasia is defined by recurrent G380R mutations of FGFR3. *Am J Hum Genet* 1995;56:368–373.
3. Bhatia KP, Marsden CD. The behavioural and motor consequences of focal lesions of the basal ganglia in man. *Brain* 1994;117:859–876.
4. Bressman SB, de Leon MS, Kramer PL, et al. Dystonia in Ashkenazi Jews: clinical characterization of a founder mutation. *Ann Neurol* 1994;36:771–777.
5. Buckler AJ, Chang DD, Graw SL, Brook JD, Haber DA, Sharp PA. Exon amplification: a strategy to isolate mammalian genes based on RNA splicing. *Proc Natl Acad Sci USA* 1991;88:4005–4009.
6. Calne DB, Lang AE. Secondary dystonia. *Adv Neurol* 1988;50:9–33.
7. Church DM, Stotler CJ, Rutter JL, Murrell JR, Trofatter JA, Buckler AJ. Isolation of genes from complex sources of mammalian genomic DNA using exon amplification. *Nat Genet* 1994;6:98–105.
8. Confalonieri F, Duguet M. A 200-amino acid ATPase module in search of a basic function. *Bioessays* 1995;17:639–650.
9. Crutcher MD, DeLong MR. Single cell studies of the primate putamen. *Exp Brain Res* 1984;53:233–243.
10. Dobyns WB, Ozelius LJ, Kramer PL, et al. Rapid-onset dystonia-parkinsonism. *Neurology* 1993;43:2596–2602.
11. Endo K, Tanaka H, Saito M, et al. The gene for hereditary progressive dystonia with marked diurnal fluctuation maps to chromosome 14q. In: Segawa M, Nomura

Y, eds. *Monographs in neural sciences age-related do-pamine-dependent disorders.* New York: Karger, 1995:120–125.

12. Fahn S, Marsden CD. The treatment of dystonia. In: Marsden CD, Fahn S (eds). *Movement disorders 2.* London: Butterworths, 1987:359–382.

13. Fontaine E, Bale-Santos J, Jurkat-Rott K, et al. Mapping of the hypokalaemic periodic paralysis (HypoPP) locus to chromosome 1q31-32 in three European families. *Nat Genet* 1994;6:267–272.

14. Frohman MA, Dush MK, Martin GR. Rapid production of full-length cDNAs from rare transcripts: amplification using a single gene-specific oligonucleotide primer. *Proc Natl Acad Sci USA* 1988;85:8998–9002.

15. Furukawa Y, Mizuno Y, Narabayashi H. Early-onset parkinsonism with dystonia. Clinical and biochemical differences from hereditary progressive dystonia or DOPA-responsive dystonia. *Adv Neurol* 1996;69: 327–337.

16. Gasser T, Bove CM, Ozelius LJ, et al. Haplotype analysis at the DYT1 locus in Ashkenazi Jewish patients with occupational hand dystonia. *Mov Disord* 1996;11:163–166.

17. Graybiel AM. Correspondence between the dopamine islands and striosomes of the mammalian striatum. *Neuroscience* 1984;13:1157–1187.

18. Greene P, Kang UJ, Fahn S. Spread of symptoms in idiopathic torsion dystonia. *Mov Disord* 1995;10:143– 152.

19. Greene P, Shale H, Fahn S. Analysis of open-labeled trial in torsion dystonia using high dosages of anticholinergics and other drugs. *Mov Disord* 1988;2:237– 254.

20. Grosson CL, Esteban J, McKenna-Yasek D, Gusella JF, Brown RH. Hypokalemic periodic paralysis mutations: confirmation of mutation and analysis of founder effect. *Neuromuscul Disord* 1995;6:27–31.

21. Hayashi K, Yandell DW. How sensitive is PCR-SSCP? *Hum Mutat* 1993;2:388–346.

22. Hedreen JC, Zweig RM, DeLong MR, Whitehouse PJ, Price DL. Primary dystonias: A review of the pathology and suggestions for new directions of study. *Adv Neurol* 1988;50:123–132.

23. Hornykiewicz O, Kish SJ, Becker LE, Farley I, Shannak K. Biochemical evidence for brain neurotransmitter changes in idiopathic torsion dystonia (dystonia musculorum deformans). In: Fahn S, Marsden CD, Calne DB (eds). *Advances in neurology, vol. 50.* New York: Raven Press, 1988:157–165.

24. Johnson W, Schwartz G, Barbeau A. Studies on dystonia musculorum deformans. *Arch Neurol* 1962;7:301– 313.

25. Knappskog PM, Glatmark T, Mallet J, Ludecke B, Bartholome K. Recessively inherited L-DOPA-responsive dystonia caused by a point mutation (Q381K) in the tyrosine hydroxylase gene. *Hum Mol Genet* 1995;4: 1209–1212.

26. Kramer P, Heiman G, Gasser T, et al. The DYT1 gene on 9q34 is responsible for most cases of early-onset idiopathic torsion dystonia (ITD) in non-Jews. *Am J Hum Genet* 1994;55:468–475.

27. Kramer PL, de Leon D, Ozelius L, et al. Dystonia gene in Ashkenazi Jewish population is located on chromosome 9q32-q34. *Ann Neurol* 1990;27:114–120.

28. Kwiatkowski DJ, Ozelius L, Kramer PL, et al. Torsion dystonia genes in two populations confined to a small region on chromosome 9q32-34. *Am J Hum Genet* 1991;49:366–371.

29. Ludecke B, Dworniczak B, Bartholome K. A point mutation in the tyrosine hydroxylase gene associated with Segawa's syndrome. *Hum Genet* 1995;95:123–125.

30. Marsden CD, Obeso JA, Zarranz JJ, Lang AE. The anatomical basis of symptomatic hemidystonia. *Brain* 1985;108:463–483.

31. Missiakas D, Schwager F, Betton J-M, Georgopoulos C, Raina J. Identification and characterization of HS1V HS1U (ClpQ ClpY) proteins involved in overall proteolysis of misfolded proteins in *Escherichia coli.* *EMBO J* 1996;15:6899–6909.

32. Nutt JG, Muenter MD, Aronson A, Kurland LT, Melton LJ. Epidemiology of focal and generalized dystonia in Rochester, Minnesota. *Mov Disord* 1988; 3:188–194.

33. Nygaard TG, Marsden CD, Fahn S. Dopa-responsive dystonia: long-term treatment response and prognosis. *Neurology* 1991;41:174–181.

34. Nygaard T, Wilhelmsen K, Risch N, et al. Linkage mapping of dopa-responsive dystonia (DRD) to chromosome 14q. *Nature Genet* 1993;5:386–391.

35. Orita M, Suzuki Y, Sekiya T, Hayashi K. Rapid and sensitive detection of point mutations and DNA polymorphisms using the polymerase chain reaction. *Genomics* 1989;5:874–879.

36. Ozelius LJ, Hewett J, Kramer P, et al. Fine localization of the torsion dystonia gene (DYT1) on human chromosome 9q34: YAC map and linkage disequilibrium. *Genome Res* 1997;7:483–494.

37. Ozelius LJ, Hewett JW, Page CE, et al. A strong candidate for the early onset torsion dystonia gene (DYT1) encodes an ATP-binding protein. *Nat Genet.* 1997; 17: 40–48

38. Ozelius L, Kramer PL, Moskowitz CB, et al. Human gene for torsion dystonia located on chromosome 9q32-q34. *Neuron* 1989;2:1427–1434.

39. Ozelius LJ, Kwiatkowski DJ, Schuback DE, et al. A genetic linkage map of human chromosome 9q. *Genomics* 1992;14:715–720.

40. Perier F, Radeke CM, Raab-Graham KF, Vandenberg CA. Expression of a putative ATPase suppresses the growth defect of a yeast potassium transport mutant: identification of a mammalian member of the Clp/HSP104 family. *Gene* 1995;152:157–163.

41. Risch N, de Leon D, Ozelius LJ, et al. Genetic analysis of idiopathic torsion dystonia of Ashkenazim for a small founder population. *Nat Genet* 1995;9:152–159.

42. Rohrwild M, Pfeifer G, Santarius U, et al. The ATP-dependent HslVU protease from *Escherichia coli* is a four-ring structure resembling the proteasome. *Nat Struct Biol* 1997;4:133–136.

43. Schirmer EC, Glover JR, Singer MA, Lindquist S. HSP100/Clp proteins: a common mechanism explains diverse functions. *TIBS* 1996;21:289–296.

44. Segawa M. Introduction. In: Segawa M, Normura Y (eds). Age-related dopamine-dependent disorders, Vol. 14. *Monogr Neural Sci.* Basel: Karger, pp 1–8.

45. Szele FG, Dowling JJ, Gonzales C, Theveniau M, Rougon G, Chesselet M-F. Pattern of expression of highly polysialylated neural cell adhesion molecules in the developing and adult rat striatum. *Neuroscience* 1994;60:133–144.

46. Walker JE, Sarasti M, Runswick MS, Gay NS. Distantly related sequences in the alpha- and beta-subunits of ATP synthase, myosin, kinases and other ATP-

requiring enzymes and a common nucleotide binding fold. *EMBO J* 1982;1:945–950.

47. Watkins H, Thierfelder L, Auan R, et al. Independent origin of identical beta cardiac myosin heavy-chain mutations in hypertrophic cardiomyopathy. *Am J Hum Genet* 1993;53:1180–1185.

48. Young AB, Shoulson I, Penney JB, et al. Huntington's disease in Venezuela: neurologic features and functional decline. *Neurology* 1986;36:244–249.

49. Zeman W, Dyken P. Dystonia musculorum deformans: clinical, genetic and pathoanatomical studies. *Psychiatr Neurol Neurochir* 1967;10:77–121.

Dystonia 3: Advances in Neurology, Vol. 78,
edited by S. Fahn, C. D. Marsden, and M. DeLong
Lippincott–Raven Publishers, Philadelphia © 1998

11

The Role of the DYT1 Gene in Secondary Dystonia

*Susan B. Bressman, *Deborah de Leon, *Deborah Raymond,
*Paul E. Greene, †Mitchell F. Brin, *Stanley Fahn, ‡Laurie J. Ozelius,
‡Xandra O. Breakefield, §Patricia L. Kramer, and ‖Neil J. Risch

*Department of Neurology, Columbia-Presbyterian Medical Center, New York, New York 10032;
†Department of Neurology, Mount Sinai Medical Center, New York, New York 10029; ‡Molecular
Neurogenetics Unit, Neurology, Massachusetts General Hospital, Charlestown, Massachusetts 02129,
and Harvard Medical School, Boston, Massachusetts 02114; §Department of Neurology, Oregon
Health Sciences University, Portland, Oregon 97201; and ‖Department of Genetics, Stanford
University, Stanford, California 94305.*

Until recently, the diagnosis of primary (or idiopathic) dystonia rested solely on clinical criteria aimed at excluding secondary causes of dystonia such as perinatal asphyxia, exposure to dopamine-receptor blockers, trauma, and neurologic disorders such as Wilson's disease and dopa-responsive dystonia (9). Although the classification of dystonia as either primary or secondary appears straightforward, the diagnosis is frequently uncertain in practice. Many of the ascribed causes of secondary dystonia are based on historical information or subtle clinical findings, and have no diagnostic radiologic, serologic, or other pathologic marker. Another confounding issue in the diagnosis of secondary dystonia is the debated causal relationship between some environmental factors (specifically, neuroleptic exposure, perinatal asphyxia, and head and peripheral trauma) and dystonia; it is unclear whether these common insults alone are sufficient to cause dystonia or, as proposed in several studies, whether they precipitate or exacerbate symptoms in genetically predisposed individuals (8,13). Even more critically, some have questioned if certain of these factors play any role at all, particularly in patients with a phenotype of primary dystonia (12,14).

The recent finding of linkage disequilibrium of primary dystonia and a haplotype of 9q34 alleles in Ashkenazi Jews now allows for the laboratory confirmation of one genetic subtype of primary dystonia (22,23). The presence of the associated haplotype of 9q34 alleles in an affected individual indicates that dystonia is due to a founder mutation in the DYT1 gene. This mutation accounts for at least 90% of early (younger than 28 years of age) limb and cervical-onset primary dystonia in Ashkenazim (23); it is an infrequent cause of late-onset primary dystonia, and was not present in any cases beginning in facial muscles or starting after age 44 years (3). Using this information on the phenotypic range of the Ashkenazi founder mutation, we studied Ashkenazi patients with a variety of clinical subtypes of secondary dystonia. We were particularly interested in studying patients we considered phenotypically similar to patients with the DYT1 founder mutation (i.e., phenocopies). Our intention was to determine whether our clinical classification of secondary dystonia was appropriate or whether there is evidence to support the contention that environmental factors precipitate dystonia in those with an inherited susceptibility.

MATERIALS AND METHODS

Clinical Features

We ascertained patients from a computerized database of patients diagnosed with dystonia and treated before January 1, 1995 by members of the Movement Disorders Group at Columbia Presbyterian Medical Center. In our previously published studies of primary dystonia in Ashkenazi Jews, our diagnostic criteria were normal neurologic examination except for dystonia, normal laboratory evaluation including computerized tomography (CT) or magnetic resonance imaging (MRI) and serum ceruloplasmin, no marked improvement of dystonia with a levodopa trial, and a history that excluded environmental causes of dystonia; specifically, perinatal asphyxia and exposure to dopamine-receptor blocking agents were systematically assessed in all patients (2,3,20,22, 23). Any patient who did not fully meet these criteria was excluded, even if primary dystonia was considered as a second possible diagnosis. It was from this group (n = 118) of Ashkenazi patients with diagnoses of possible secondary dystonia, and possible primary dystonia, that we recruited subjects for study. We targeted the group of patients with symptom onset before age 28 years (n = 51), as this is the group most likely to contain patients harboring the founder mutation (3,23). The etiologic categories of secondary dystonia we included were (a) perinatal asphyxia; (b) exposure to dopamine-receptor blocking agents (tardive); (c) head trauma; (d) peripheral trauma; (e) suspected but unconfirmed heredodegenerative disorder; (f) structural abnormality; (g) psychogenic dystonia; and (h) infection. Patients with secondary dystonia due to identified inherited disorders (e.g., Wilson's disease or dopa-responsive dystonia) were not included.

We did not use a family history of dystonia as a criterion to exclude cases as possibly secondary. Also, because we were interested in studying patients in whom we entertained diagnoses of both possible secondary and possible primary dystonia, previously published criteria for secondary etiologies (6,10,19,24) were not fulfilled in all cases. We identified patients as Ashkenazi Jews as described (2). Participating patients and their family members gave informed consent.

Outpatient office charts were reviewed to determine pertinent historical data such as birth and neonatal events; type, dosage, and duration of treatment with dopamine-receptor blocking agent and temporal relation to dystonia; type and extent of peripheral or head trauma and temporal relation to dystonia; and history of infectious or psychiatric illness. We also reviewed charts to determine clinical features including age and site of onset of dystonia, distribution of dystonia at most recent examination, any other neurologic abnormalities, and the results of imaging or other laboratory studies. Clinical confirmation of the diagnosis of possible secondary dystonia was performed after chart review by one investigator (S.B.B.) blinded to the genetic data.

DNA Methods, Probes, and Polymorphism Analysis

Blood was obtained by venipuncture from consenting affected individuals and family members as necessary for phasing. DNA was extracted from lymphoblastoid lines or whole blood as described (1). Analyses of dinucleotide repeat polymorphisms for the loci D9S62a (32/37), D9S62b (1290/1301), D9S63, and ASS were carried out on genomic DNA as described (16,21).

Statistical Analyses

Based on previous studies (3,23), we considered individuals likely to carry the DYT1 Ashkenazi haplotype if they carried on the same chromosome the "2", "8", and "16" alleles at D9S62a, b, and D9S63, respectively, or the "16" and "12" alleles at D9S63 and ASS, respectively, or the full haplotype of alleles, "2", "8", "16", and "12". Linkage phase was determined in all potential haplotype carriers, (i.e., individuals who had two or more of the associated alleles). The carrier frequency of this haplotype was compared between the current group of subjects and the primary dystonia patients we previously reported (3,23).

RESULTS

Forty patients were available and agreed to participate in this study; 25 patients (13 females and 12 males) were less than age 28 years (early onset) when symptoms began (Table 1). Among the 25 with early onset, ten had a diagnosis of perinatal asphyxia or static encephalopathy. Medical and birth records documented at least two of the following markers of perinatal asphyxia in five of the ten: Apgar score less than 3, need for more than 5 minutes of resuscitation, cyanosis, fetal decelerations, meconium staining, or neonatal seizures. Written documentation of perinatal asphyxia was lacking for the remaining five, and the diagnoses were based on historical information of cyanosis, need for resuscitation, or delayed milestones. The remainder of the early-onset group consisted of 15 patients with dystonia attributed to a variety of etiologies: tardive dystonia due to dopamine-receptor blocking agents ($n = 5$), peripheral trauma ($n = 4$), another suspected inherited disorder ($n = 2$), structural abnormality ($n = 2$), psychogenic dystonia ($n = 1$), and measles infection ($n = 1$). In cases thought to be due to dopamine blockers, trauma, or infection, the exposure or insult occurred within 6 months of the onset of dystonia except for two individuals (No. 11 and No. 16). One of these was a 14-year-old boy who developed right arm and then right leg dystonia within weeks after minor right arm trauma; CT scanning showed mild ventricular asymmetry with enlargement on the left suggesting a longstanding occult left hemisphere injury; the contributions of both the immediate peripheral injury and a remote central injury were considered in this individual. The other patient first complained of right arm cramping at age 8; however no posturing or other involuntary movements were noted in physician records. Subsequently, at age 18 years, he developed

generalized dystonia after 4 years of treatment with neuroleptic medications; whether this patient had dystonia prior to neuroleptic exposure has never been clarified. Three patients (Table 1, No. 9 with perinatal asphyxia, No. 12 with tardive dystonia, and No. 21 with another suspected inherited disorder) had a family history of dystonia. For the patient with perinatal asphyxia, the family member was examined and a diagnosis of primary dystonia was confirmed; testing indicated that this relative had the haplotype of 9q alleles characteristic of the founder mutation.

Of the 25 patients with early onset, 11 had normal examinations except for dystonia and normal radiologic studies. Of these 11, nine had onset in a limb or the neck: three patients with perinatal asphyxia; four patients with tardive dystonia; one man who developed torticollis 4 days after peripheral injury; and one woman whose dystonia began in the setting of measles infection.

There were 15 patients (four men and 11 women) with onset of dystonia after age 28 years (Table 2); in 12 patients dystonia was thought to be due to dopamine-blocking agents, two were psychogenic and one began after head and neck trauma. One (No. 8) had a family history of dystonia.

Of the 40 patients tested, 39 did not have the haplotype of associated alleles. Only one individual (Table 1, No. 24) carried the associated haplotype; she had clinical features typical of carriers (i.e., childhood onset in a limb with spread to other limbs and no other neurologic or laboratory abnormalities). Her symptoms emerged during a mild nonencephalopathic exanthematous illness diagnosed as measles infection; although a causal relationship to measles was questioned, a possible infectious or immune mechanism was postulated by the examining physician.

Using the clinical criteria for secondary dystonia of (a) examination abnormalities in addition to dystonia, and/or (b) abnormal laboratory findings, and/or (c) history of an established cause for dystonia such as perinatal asphyxia, or exposure to dopamine blocker or

TABLE 1. *Clinical features in 25 patients with secondary dystonia with onset age 28 years or younger*

Age at onset (yr)	Site of onset	Age last exam (yr)	Dystonia distribution at last exam	Etiology	Other findings and abnormal laboratory
1) 2	Legs	27	Legs, trunk, arms, tongue	Birth asphyxia, not documented	Dysarthria, spasticity
2) 3.5	Arms	25	Arms	Birth asphyxia, documented	Delayed milestones, mild ataxia and dysarthria, arm tremor
3) 4	Arm	31	Neck, arms, trunk, legs, tongue, jaw	Birth asphyxia, documented	
4) 4	Larynx	6	Larynx	Birth asphyxia, documented	
5) 6	Arm	27	Arms, jaw, face	Birth asphyxia, not documented	Delayed milestones, mild cognitive impairment, seizures, mild dysmetria and tremor
6) 7	Leg	29	Face, jaw, tongue, pharynx, larynx, neck, trunk, arms, legs	Birth asphyxia, not documented	Delayed milestones, dysarthria, slow fine motor movements
7) 8	Neck, trunk, arm	57	Neck, trunk, arm	Birth asphyxia, not documented	
8) 9	Face and hand	12	Face, arms, legs	Birth asphyxia, documented	Chorea, mild dysarthria, clumsy fine motor movements
9) 10	Face and tongue	55	Face, tongue, jaw, neck, arms	Birth asphyxia, not documented	Mild hemiparesis
10) 16	Neck and arm	27	Neck, trunk, arms	Birth asphyxia, documented	
11) 18	Legs	38	Neck, arms, legs	Cramping of right arm at age 9 yr; frank dystonia after treatment with neuroleptics	
12) 18	Neck	19	Neck	Tardive	
13) 22	Legs	38	Face, tongue, jaw, neck, trunk, arms, legs	Tardive	
14) 23	Face and jaw	27	Face, jaw, tongue, neck, arms	Tardive	
15) 26	Neck and arms	26	Neck and arms	Tardive	

16) 12	Arm	22	Right arm and leg	Peripheral trauma (soft tissue injury to right arm) weeks before onset, and remote central trauma suspected	MRI left ventricular enlargement
17) 14	Arm	17	Right arm and leg	Peripheral trauma (soft tissue injury to right arm) days before onset	Mild muscle atrophy and reflex asymmetry; myoclonic jerks
18) 19	Leg	20	Leg	Peripheral trauma (surgery of affected leg) 6 months before onset	Myoclonic jerks
19) 23	Neck	23	Neck	Peripheral trauma (fractured clavicle) days before onset	
20) 8	Arm	34	Right arm and leg	Suspected left thalamic tumor by pneumoencephalography and angiography—irradiated	Hemiparesis and hemisensory loss after radiation; CT nl, MRI after radiation left basal ganglia lesion
21) 13	Arms and leg	19	Arms and leg	Paroxysmal dystonia in addition to interictal dystonia	Paroxysms resolved with carbamazepine
22) 15	Arm	23	Right arm	Suspected developmental abnormality	Tics, parkinsonism, clumsy right motor movements, right hyperreflexia, nystagmus; MRI left cerebellar and cerebral hemisphere atrophy
23) 19	Arm	38	Face, tongue, pharynx, arms, legs	Suspected inherited disorder (consanguinity)	Parkinsonism, dysarthria, ophthalmoparesis
24) 8	Leg	21	Arms, legs, neck, and trunk	Measles infection days before onset	
25) 23	Neck	33	Neck, arms, trunk, legs	Psychogenic	Tremor, paralysis

TABLE 2. *Clinical features in 15 patients with secondary dystonia with onset older than age 28 years*

Age at onset (yr)	Site of onset	Age last exam	Dystonia distribution last exam	Etiology	Other findings and abnormal laboratory
1) 29	Leg	44	Face, tongue, neck, arms, trunk, legs	Tardive	
2) 34	Leg	37	Leg	Tardive	Mild limb chorea; CT agenesis of corpus callosum
3) 34	Thumb	82	Face, jaw, tongue, larynx, neck, arms, trunk	Tardive	
4) 36	Leg	38	Arms and leg	Tardive	
5) 37	Face	38	Face, jaw, tongue, larynx, neck	Tardive	
6) 39	Neck	41	Face, jaw, neck	Tardive	
7) 44	Face and tongue	45	Face, tongue, neck, arms, trunk	Tardive	
8) 44	Face	55	Face	Tardive	
9) 52	Face	67	Face, larynx, neck, trunk	Tardive	
10) 60	Neck	64	Neck, left arm, and leg	Tardive	
11) 60	Face	64	Face, tongue, neck	Tardive	
12) 72	Tongue	79	Jaw, tongue, pharynx	Tardive	
13) 40	Neck	70	Face, neck, trunk	Peripheral trauma	
14) 31	Neck	32	Neck	Psychogenic	
15) 32	Leg	33	Legs	Psychogenic	Head tremor

trauma, there were no misdiagnoses of primary dystonia due to the common DYT1 mutation.

DISCUSSION

This study confirms the accuracy of clinical criteria in diagnosing individuals with secondary versus primary dystonia. Genetic cases due to the DYT1 founder mutation are very rarely clinically misclassified as secondary dystonia, even among patients with secondary dystonia and neurologic features typical of the DYT1 phenotype. Previous studies of primary dystonia used different methods to exclude patients or families thought to have other causes for dystonia (2,8,11,17,26,27,28); most concur that the examination should be normal except for dystonia (although many studies also allowed for tremor beyond that considered normal or physiologic), that the CT or MRI should be normal, and that Wilson's disease, dopa-responsive dystonia, and other inherited disorders should be ruled out. This definition of primary dystonia, particularly with regard to genetic studies that exclude individuals with subtle neurologic or radiologic abnormalities, has not been validated because no test was available to detect genetic cases. The present findings support prior descriptive studies, including seminal descriptions of early-onset primary dystonia (17,27), that stressed the need to distinguish primary dystonia based on the clinical examination. This study also confirms that exclusionary historical criteria (i.e., exposure to dopamine-blocking agents and perinatal asphyxia) be included as diagnostic criteria of primary dystonia due to DYT1. Indeed, it is in the group with perinatal asphyxia and tardive dystonia that we found seven of the nine patients who mimic the typical DYT1 phenotype; that is, individuals with normal examinations except for dystonia, unremarkable radiologic studies, and early onset of symptoms in limb or cervical muscles. Based on these clinical features, we would have expected 90% to be haplotype carriers (3,23), whereas we found no carriers in this group in the present study ($p \ll 0.001$).

Our findings indicate that perinatal asphyxia and neuroleptics may produce a dystonic syndrome in the absence of a genetic susceptibility, verifying the category of secondary or symptomatic dystonia. A significant proportion of our tardive cases, however, had late or cranial-onset of symptoms (i.e., 12 of 17 tardive cases were over 28 years of age at onset of symptoms, and seven had first symptoms in cranial muscles). These are clinical features rarely observed in carriers of the DYT1 founder mutation (3). Thus, that these individuals tested as non-DYT1 carriers is not surprising. Similarly, a study of ten Ashkenazi patients with late onset of occupational dystonia also found that none carried the associated haplotype (15). The genetic basis of late-onset and cranial-onset dystonia is not yet known, although a proportion may be inherited as autosomal-dominant traits (7,25,26). Further, linkage studies have excluded the DYT1 gene in several large families with apparent autosomal-dominant inheritance of late-onset or cranial-predominant dystonia (4,5,18), suggesting the presence of other non-DYT1 susceptibility genes. Neuroleptic exposure (or other environmental factors) possibly may modify expression of these other mutations.

We did not use a family history of dystonia to distinguish primary and secondary dystonia, and our findings suggest that it should not be included as a diagnostic feature. There were four patients with a family history of dystonia and none of them had the DYT1-associated haplotype. We did not personally examine the relatives of three of the patients, two first-degree relatives with writer's cramp and one second-degree relative with blepharospasm, so that findings could not be confirmed. However, one patient, with early cranial-onset dystonia and a mild left hemiparesis due to perinatal asphyxia, had a cousin with early limb-onset dystonia who carried the DYT1-associated haplotype. The lack of the associated haplotype in this patient from a family known to carry the DYT1 haplotype provides a strong argument for stringent diagnostic criteria for primary dystonia in genetic linkage and association studies.

Although we found no evidence to implicate either perinatal asphyxia or neuroleptic exposure as precipitants of dystonia due to the DYT1 Ashkenazi founder mutation, the role of other environmental and genetic factors remains unknown. Previous study suggests that peripheral trauma may precipitate or exacerbate primary dystonia (13). We had four patients with onset of symptoms before age 28 years and peripheral trauma as a cause of dystonia. However, among these there was only one phenocopy of the DYT1 Ashkenazi founder mutation. One possible explanation for the paucity of patients with trauma-induced secondary dystonia is that some patients with trauma preceding dystonia may have been included in our group with primary dystonia. Unlike exposure to neuroleptic medication and birth asphyxia, which are exhaustively investigated and always considered causative in the evaluation of dystonia patients, minor trauma either may have been missed in the initial evaluation or may not have been considered causal by the examining physician.

We estimated the lifetime penetrance of the DYT1 mutation to be 30% (2); even among the definitely affected, the range of clinical features is broad (3). There is no explanation for this markedly reduced penetrance or variable expression. Future study comparing variably affected and unaffected DYT1 gene carriers may help sort out the contribution of trauma and other environmental and genetic factors in DYT1 gene expression.

ACKNOWLEDGMENTS

This work was supported by grants NS26656 and NS28384 from the National Institutes of Health and a Dystonia Clinical Research Center grant and individual grants from the Dystonia Medical Research Foundation.

REFERENCES

1. Breakefield XO, Bressman SB, Kramer PL, et al. Linkage analysis in a family with dominantly inherited torsion dystonia: exclusion of the pro-opiomelanocortin and glutamic acid decarboxylase genes and other chromosomal regions using DNA polymorphisms. *J Neurogenet* 1986;3:159–175.
2. Bressman SB, de Leon D, Brin MF, et al. Idiopathic dystonia among Ashkenazi Jews: evidence for autosomal dominant inheritance. *Ann Neurol* 1989;26:612–620.
3. Bressman SB, de Leon D, Kramer PL, et al. Dystonia in Ashkenazi Jews: Clinical characterization of a founder mutation. *Ann Neurol* 1994;36:771–777.
4. Bressman SB, Heiman GA, Nygaard TG, et al. A study of idiopathic torsion dystonia in a non-Jewish family: evidence for genetic heterogeneity. *Neurology* 1994; 44:283–287.
5. Bressman SB, Hunt AL, Heiman GA, et al. Exclusion of the DYT1 locus in a non-Jewish family with early-onset dystonia. *Mov Disord* 1994;9:626–632.
6. Burke RE, Fahn S, Gold AP. Delayed onset dystonia in patients with "static encephalopathy". *J Neurol Neurosurg Psychiatry* 1980;43:789–797.
7. Defazio G, Livrea P, Guanti G, et al. Genetic contribution to idiopathic adult-onset blepharospasm and cranial-cervical dystonia. *Eur Neurol* 1993;33:345–350.
8. Eldridge R. The torsion dystonias: literature review and genetic and clinical studies. *Neurology* 1970;20: (part 2):1–79.
9. Fahn S, Marsden CD, Calne DB. Classification and investigation of dystonia. In: Marsden CD, Fahn S, eds. *Movement disorders.* Boston: Butterworth, 1987:33–358.
10. Fahn S, Williams DT. Psychogenic dystonia. *Adv Neurol* 1988;50:431–455.
11. Fletcher NA, Harding AE, Marsden CD. A genetic study of idiopathic torsion dystonia in the United Kingdom. *Brain* 1990;113:379–395.
12. Fletcher NA, Harding AE, Marsden CD. A case-control study of idiopathic torsion dystonia. *Mov Disord* 1991;6:304–309.
13. Fletcher NA, Harding AE, Marsden CD. The relationship between trauma and idiopathic torsion dystonia. *J Neurol Neurosurg Psychiatry* 1991;54:713–717.
14. Fletcher NA, Harding AE, Marsden CD. Idiopathic torsion dystonia—reply [letter]. *Mov Disord* 1992;7: 388.
15. Gasser T, Bove CM, Ozelius LJ, et al. Haplotype analysis at the DYT1 locus in Ashkenazi Jewish patients with occupational hand dystonia. *Mov Disord* 1996;11:163–166.
16. Henske EP, Ozelius LJ, Gusella JF, et al. A high resolution linkage map of chromosome 9q34. *Genomics* 1993;17:587–591.
17. Herz E. Dystonia, part 2 (clinical classification). *Arch Neurol Psychiatr* 1944;51:319–355.
18. Holmgren G, Ozelius L, Forsgren L, et al. Adult onset idiopathic torsion dystonia is excluded from the DYT1 region (9q34) in a Swedish family. *J Neurol Neurosurg Psychiatry* 1995;59:178–181.
19. Kang UJ, Burke RE, Fahn S. Natural history and treatment of tardive dystonia. *Mov Disord* 1986;1:193–208.
20. Kramer PL, de Leon D, Ozelius L, et al. Dystonia gene in Ashkenazi Jewish population is located on chromosome 9q32-34. *Ann Neurol* 1990;27:114–120.
21. Kwiatkowski DJ, Henske EP, Weimer K, et al. Construction of a GT polymorphism map of human 9q. *Genomics* 1992;12:229–240.
22. Ozelius LJ, Kramer PL, de Leon D, et al. Strong allelic association between the torsion dystonia gene (DYT1) and loci on chromosome 9q34 in Ashkenazi Jews. *Am J Hum Genet* 1992;50:619–628.
23. Risch NJ, de Leon D, Ozelius L, et al. Genetic analysis

of idiopathic torsion dystonia in Ashkenazi Jews and their recent descent from a small founder population. *Nat Genet* 1995;9:152–159.

24. Saint Hilaire MH, Burke RE, Bressman SB, et al. Delayed-onset dystonia due to perinatal or early childhood asphyxia. *Neurology* 1991;41:216–222.

25. Stojanovic M, Cvetkovic D, Kostic VS. A genetic study of idiopathic focal dystonias. *J Neurol* 1995; 242:502–511.9.

26. Waddy HM, Fletcher NA, Harding AE, et al. A genetic study of idiopathic focal dystonias. *Ann Neurol* 1991; 29:320–324.

27. Zeman W, Dyken P. Dystonia musculorum deformans; clinical, genetic and pathoanatomical studies. *Psychiatr Neurol Neurochir* 1967;70:77–121.

28. Zilber N, Korczyn AD, Kahana E, et al. Inheritance of idiopathic torsion dystonia among Jews. *J Med Genet* 1984;21:13–20.

Dystonia 3:Advances in Neurology, Vol. 78,
edited by S. Fahn, C. D. Marsden, and M. DeLong
Lippincott–Raven Publishers, Philadelphia © 1998

12

Familial Cervical Dystonia, Head Tremor, and Scoliosis: A Case Report

Drake D. Duane

Arizona Dystonia Institute/Arizona State University, Scottsdale, Arizona 85258.

Familial generalized dystonia has been linked to a specific gene locus, q34 on chromosome 9, and has been labeled DYT1 (9). Although both tremor and dystonia not uncommonly occur in dystonic individuals as well as their family members, essential tremor (ET) does not link with the DYT1 chromosome 9 locus (1,4). Because individuals with generalized dystonia may have relatives with focal dystonia, it is possible that the DYT1 gene locus also may be responsible for some forms of focal dystonia.

Likewise, patients with focal dystonia themselves or their relatives may exhibit tremor. In some cases, this tremor is a slower, less rhythmic or "dystonic" tremor; in others, it shares characteristics observed in what is otherwise called "essential" tremor (8). Tremor distribution in patients with focal dystonia most commonly affects the head, followed by head and hands, followed by hands only, and least commonly affects voice alone (3). A description of tremor in relatives of those with cervical dystonia (CD) increases the probability of tremor occurring in affected patients, as well as increasing the probability that there will be dystonic manifestations beyond the neck region (3).

The first published report of multiple family members in the same generation affected with CD was in 1896 by Thompson, in which two brothers and two sisters were described. As there were allegedly no other family members demonstrating dystonic symptoms or signs, the conclusion was drawn that the genetic mecha-

nism was likely autosomal recessive (12). The family was of Caucasian English Christian ancestry.

Focal dystonia has been previously described in multiple family members whether by history or by direct examination (5,7,11,14), including twins (6,13). It is unclear in such families what genetic mechanism underlies these associations, but autosomal dominance appears likely. A recent report from Germany in one family with multiple affected members with CD suggests linkage with chromosome 18p (10).

CURRENT CASE REPORT

This report is of a German Christian ancestry family residing in Nebraska without history of consanguinity in which three male members of generation II have adult-onset CD. The index case (II, 4) has been in remission for nine years. A female sibling in this generation had adolescent-onset scoliosis. The deceased father of this nine-member generation was said to have had long-standing, adult-onset head "shaking" but without recorded head rotation or tilt.

The two female offspring of the index case demonstrate in one (III, 11) adolescent-onset scoliosis and in the other (III, 10) a history of onset of CD at age 33 in which there have been two periods of exacerbation with no period of remission. Their brother is said to be asymptomatic but has not been examined. A granddaughter of an unaffected sister from the index generation (II, 2) has late-childhood-onset scoliosis. The abbreviated family tree is presented in Fig. 1.

Six of the nine members of the second generation have been examined, and one additional sib submitted blood samples. The scoliotic daughter of the index case (III, 11) was both examined and supplied a blood sample. Her sister (III, 10) affected with fluctuating CD has been examined and has provided blood samples for analysis. Blood samples were sent to the National Hospital Queen Square, London, England, for DNA analysis.

The oldest affected brother (II, 3) with torticollis also exhibits a vertical head and mild postural hand tremor. The father of this generation is described as having a chronic horizontal head shaking. Neither of the other two brothers has tremor nor do any of the relatives in this generation or in generation III that have been examined nor are any others described as having tremor. The onset of his CD was in 1982 at the age of 53 years. The characteristics of the CD are a phasic retrocollis with slight right rotation and dystonic vertical head and bilateral postural hand tremor with secondary vocal

tremor, as well as mild lower cranial dystonia. The patient was examined by the author in September of 1992 in his home state of Nebraska, at the same time and place as the other family members in this report.

Patient II, 4, the index case, had onset of CD in 1977 at the age of 47. The character then was tonic, right rotation without tremor. Placed on oral anticholinergic therapy in 1985, this patient went into remission within a few weeks of the introduction of this medication. He had first been examined in 1985, was subsequently reexamined in 1987, and like his older brother, was examined again in September of 1992. Although subjectively feeling as though at times the neck muscles are tight, there is no evidence of distorted nuchal posture and range of motion of the cervical spine is completely free.

Patient III, 6, had onset of CD in 1965 at the age of 31. The CD is a tonic right rotation with slight right lateral tilt but no evidence of cranial or other site of dystonia or tremor. None of these three men have been aware of scoliosis and spine films done on the index case in 1985 failed to reveal evidence of scoliosis.

In none of the affected or unaffected family members was there a history of perinatal stress,

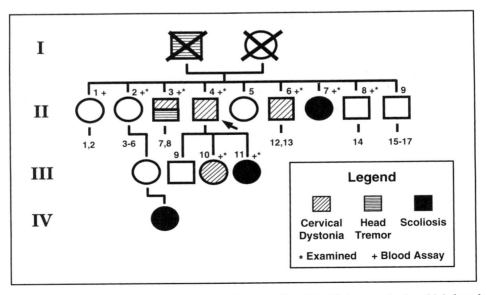

FIG. 1. Abbreviated family tree of family "A" of German/Scottish-Irish ancestry in which four family members have cervical dystonia, two have head tremor, and three have scoliosis.

painful injury antecedent to the onset of symptoms, or evidence of autoimmune disorder by history. In none was there elevated titers of antinuclear antibody or rheumatoid factor, nor was there evidence of abnormalities of copper or ceruloplasmin levels. The index case II, 4, has a slightly elevated creatine kinase level whereas all the others studied do not. The youngest examined sib (II, 8) has slightly elevated levels of thyroglobulin antibody, whereas none of the others have this or elevated levels of thyroid microsomal antibody. All three affected brothers are right-handed as are all of their sibs except for one unaffected sister (II, 2) who is left-handed. Only two of the sibship are blue-eyed (II, 6 and II, 7). Both affected daughters (III, 10 and III, 11) are brown-eyed. The sister with scoliosis (III, 11) holds a writing instrument in a tightened hand posture but not one construed to represent dystonia. None of the three affected brothers gave a history of transitory symptoms of dystonia or tremor antecedent to the date of CD onset.

DISCUSSION

Whether by direct examination or by history, patients with CD have increased frequency of relatives with tremor most commonly described as affecting the head. Next most frequent is the recalled occurrence of scoliosis in first-degree relatives (2). The true occurrence of familial CD is unclear but by history, in one study, was reported at 6% with the same investigation describing facial dystonia in 5% of relatives and spasmodic dystonia in 1%. Family history of parkinsonism was similar in frequency to that of a control group of spine pain patients (2). Demonstrations to all patients were given to distinguish rest tremor with bradykinesia from postural tremor aiding in the distinction between parkinsonism and non-parkinsonian tremor.

One other family in the author's personal experience demonstrated multiple family members with CD; in that instance, three family members were known to have CD, two of whom were examined. The sister of one of those affected with CD exhibited adductor spasmodic dysphonia and head tremor. Tremor

also occurred in three other family members, head in two and hands in one. One of the CD patients in that family, a woman with onset of her symptoms in her early 40s, succumbed suddenly without identified cause in her mid-50s. That patient's brain has been placed in the brain bank at McLean Hospital, Belmont, Massachusetts. Although genetic blood studies were drawn from several of those family members the results of none of these, unfortunately, have been reported to the author.

Personal communication with the late Professor Anita Harding in 1995 and reconfirmed in 1996 with Dr. Nicholas Wood of the National Hospital Queen Square indicates no linkages to the DYT1 gene locus in this family "A." In light of the recent report of a similar family with multiple affected with CD from Germany being linked to chromosome 18p, our colleagues in England are currently investigating whether that site may be linked in this family. A conundrum for the genetic research is whether to include evidence of scoliosis of adolescent or later onset as an *affected* family member or in future studies whether to include as affected family members those with scoliosis as well as those with only tremor.

Personal observations with over 1,500 patients seen in the last 25 years with CD suggest that up to 25% of patients with CD are aware of scoliosis or have X-ray evidence of scoliosis antecedent to or concurrent with the onset of their cervical symptomatology. This raises the possibility that among the manifestations of dystonia may be scoliosis in isolation. The extent to which, however, the general population of scoliotics represents dystonia is unclear, but would seem to be low given the 4% in females and 2% in males frequency of scoliosis.

The association of CD with tremor in this family and in general is interesting because ET does not link to the DYT1 gene locus. But whether other gene loci may produce both dystonic head tremor and CD is not clear because direct observation of affected family members is uncommon, further complicating the already difficult decision making as to whether the described family member has a dystonic or essential-type tremor. The association, however, between rhythmic oscillation of the head and dystonically induced distorted posture is robust and improbably related to chance.

Efforts are now under way to examine additional members of this family and to draw serum samples from them for DNA analysis.

CONCLUSIONS

The observations in this family argue for clinical investigators to continue to study family history in depth and recurrently, as serial inquiry often increases the yield. Whenever possible, one should actually examine the allegedly affected as well as unaffected family members. This case report reinforces the probability that a strong factor in the etiology of focal dystonic movement disorders and tremor is genetic, although the relationship between these two clinical phenomena is obscure. Whether the heterogeneity in clinical manifestation is solely under genetic control is not clear; therefore, continued efforts at investigating potential mitigating epigenetic factors when patients are evaluated is appropriate. The eventual determination of the genetic marker in this family may clarify etiology and pathogenesis of focal dystonia and assist in determining whether there is a relationship, genetic or otherwise, between CD, head and/or hand tremor, and scoliosis.

ACKNOWLEDGMENTS

This work was supported in part by funds provided by the Foundation for Clinical Neuroscience.

REFERENCES

1. Conway D, Bain PG, Warner TT, et al. Linkage analysis with chromosome 9 markers in hereditary essential tremor. *Mov Disord* 1993;8:374–376.
2. Duane DD, Case JL, LaPointe LL. Thyroid/immune dysfunction and familial movement disorder in cervical dystonia. *Neurology* 1991; 41 [Suppl 1]:292.
3. Duane DD, Clark M, Gottlob L, et al. The influence of family history of tremor on cervical dystonia. *Mov Disord* 1993;8:313–314 (abst).
4. Dürr A, Stevanin BS, Jedynak CP, et al. Familial essential tremor and idiopathic torsion dystonia are different genetic entities. *Neurology* 1993;43: 2212–2214.
5. Eldridge R. The torsion dystonias: literature review and genetic and clinical studies. *Neurology* 1970; 20[Suppl]:1–78.
6. Elite R, Ince SE, Chernow B, et al. Dystonia in 61-year-old identical twins: observations over 45 years. *Ann Neurol* 1984;16:356–358.
7. Gilbert GJ. Familial spasmodic torticollis. *Neurology* 1977;27:11–13.
8. Jedynak CP, Bonnet AM, Agid Y. Tremor and idiopathic dystonia. *Mov Disord* 1991;6:230–236.
9. Kramer PL, deLeon D, Ozelius L, et al. Dystonia gene in Ashkenazi Jewish population is located on chromosome 9q32-34. *Ann Neurol* 1990;27: 114–120.
10. Leube B, Rudnicki D, Ratzlaff T, et al. Idiopathic torsion dystonia: assignment of a gene to chromosome 18p in a German family with adult onset, autosomal dominant inheritance and purely focal distribution. *Hum Mol Genet* 1996;5:1673–1678.
11. Stojanovic M, Cvetkovic D, Kostic VS. A genetic study of idiopathic focal dystonias. *J Neurol* 1995; 242:508–511.
12. Thompson JH. A wry-necked family. *Lancet* 1896; 2:24.
13. Uitti RJ, Manganese DM. Adult onset familial cervical dystonia; report of a family including monozygotic twins. *Mov Disord* 1993;8:489–494.
14. Waddy HM, Fletcher NA, Harding AE, Marsden CD. A genetic study of idiopathic focal dystonias. *Ann Neurol* 1991;29:320–324.

Dystonia 3: Advances in Neurology, Vol. 78,
edited by S. Fahn, C. D. Marsden, and M. DeLong
Lippincott–Raven Publishers, Philadelphia © 1998

13

The Epidemiology of the Primary Dystonias in the North of England

*Philip O.F. Duffey, *†Anthony G. Butler, ‡Maurice R. Hawthorne, and *†Michael P. Barnes

School of Clinical Neurosciences, The Medical School, University of Newcastle upon Tyne, NE2 4NR, United Kingdom; †Hunters Moor Regional Rehabilitation Centre, Newcastle upon Tyne, NE2 4NR, United Kingdom; and ‡The North Riding Infirmary, Middlesbrough, Cleveland, TS1 5JE, United Kingdom.

Epidemiologic studies of dystonia are few in number and there are no published data giving the prevalence of the primary dystonias in the United Kingdom. This paucity of information has been acknowledged by a number of authors (16,22) and recently Hewer (11) stated that there were insufficient data to allow estimation of clinical need. The comprehensive review of neuroepidemiology in the United Kingdom by Cockerell et al. (4) also omits dystonia from the table of conditions whose prevalence is given. Although indigenous information is lacking, studies from Israel, China, Japan, Egypt, and the United States do exist. The findings of these studies and others are summarized in Table 1.

The seminal paper of Schwalbe (20) described dystonia in three Jewish siblings and subsequently many have recognized the prevalence of primary torsion dystonia to be comparatively high in Jewish populations (3,5,8,24). Using information housed in the National Registry of Neurological Diseases in Israel, Alter et al. (1) were able to show dystonia to be most common in Jews of Eastern European ancestry. Data from this survey have been expanded and reviewed on two further occasions (14,25), the last being in 1984 when Zilber et al. calculated a prevalence ratio for primary torsion dystonia in Ashkenazi Jews of 4.3 per

100,000 (the prevalence ratio rose to 6.8 per 100,000 when the analysis was restricted to those cases whose fathers were born in Russia, Poland, or Romania). Despite the nature of primary torsion dystonia as observed in Ashkenazim, particularly the tendency of the dystonia to become generalized (2), and the detailed demographic information available to the authors of these papers, it is apparent that the calculated prevalence of dystonia in the population studied increased at each assessment and clearly case ascertainment has been incomplete. Risch et al. (19) make the same assertion in their critique of these studies. In the same paper, data held in the Dystonia Medical Research Centre at the Columbia Presbyterian Medical Centre in New York are used by Risch and colleagues to generate a crude point prevalence rate. Then, citing the work of Bressman et al. (2) in which it was shown that 50% of cases in this geographic area had not had a prior diagnosis of primary torsion dystonia and adjusting for that portion of the sample too young to have yet manifest their dystonia, they estimate the true prevalence of primary torsion dystonia among the Ashkenazim to be 11.06 per 100,000. This figure is significantly greater than any previously given.

The epidemiologic survey of dystonia performed by Nutt et al. (18), which incorporates

TABLE 1. *Studies reporting the prevalence of primary dystonia*

Authors	Year of publication	Population	Location	Dystonia prevalence[a]	
				Generalized	Focal
Eldridge (5)	1970	Unselected	USA	0.29	—
Eldridge (5)	1970	Jewish	USA	2.5	—
Korczyn et al. (14)	1980	Jewish	Israel	0.96	—
Korczyn et al. (14)	1980	Non-Jewish	Israel	0.17	—
Zilber et al. (25)	1984	Ashkenazim	Israel	4.3	—
Li et al. (15)	1985	Unselected	Republic of China	5.0	3[b]
Nutt et al. (18)	1988	Unselected	Rochester, USA	3.4	29.5
Giménez-Roldán et al. (10)	1988	Gypsy	Spain	2.0	—
Kandil et al. (12)	1994	Unselected	Assuit, Egypt	None identified	10[b]
Risch et al. (19)	1995	Ashkenazim	New York, USA	11	—
Nakashima et al. (17)	1995	Unselected	Tottori, Japan	0.2	6.12

[a] Crude rates expressed per 100,000 population.
[b] Cervical dystonia alone was identified.

the work of Duane and colleagues, is one of the most detailed of its kind and is the source of much of the information given in standard neurology texts (13), reviews, and educational literature (7,16,23). In this study cases were acquired by review of hospital records and consultation notes made between 1950 and 1982 from clinics throughout Rochester, Minnesota. Records from these institutions are widely regarded as being extremely accurate and it is likely that few, if any, of the cases of dystonia recognized by the medical staff in the region were omitted from the survey. The number of cases on which the prevalence figures were calculated is small: 31 patients with primary focal dystonia and three with primary generalized dystonia. The study therefore generated very wide confidence limits, 17.2 to 47.9 per 100,000 and 0.41 to 12.4 per 100,000 for focal and generalized dystonia, respectively, at the 95% interval. This shortcoming is acknowledged by the authors but seldom disclosed when the findings are cited. In addition, Nutt and colleagues comment on difficulties experienced while differentiating between cases of primary and secondary dystonia. They describe two patients with oromandibular dystonia who also had extensive cerebrovascular disease, which in one case was found at postmortem to have caused infarction within the brainstem, diencephalon, and cerebral hemispheres, and another patient with oromandibular dystonia plus ataxia and a peripheral neuropathy. It is conceivable that each of these

patients may have had a secondary dystonia. Given the small total number of cases the final estimation of prevalence of primary dystonia would be reduced significantly if these cases were omitted from the Rochester study.

The population studies undertaken in China (15) and Egypt (12) were mammoth; 63,195 individuals were sampled in the former study and 42,000 in the latter. The reported prevalence of primary focal dystonia in each study was 3 and 10 per 100,000 respectively. It is interesting to note, however, that neither study reported cases of primary focal dystonia other than torticollis and that Kandil et al. (12) identified no cases of generalized dystonia. It seems unlikely that the primary dystonias are truly so limited in these populations and one must suspect that case ascertainment was incomplete. This suspicion is reinforced by the observation that the tendency of torticollis to be more common in females reported in Rochester (18) and reproduced in the United Kingdom (21) was reversed in Egypt.

The most recent epidemiologic survey of dystonia is that of Nakashima et al. performed in the Tottori prefecture in Japan (17). The methodology of this survey is not dissimilar to that of Nutt et al. in being records based. The calculation of prevalence excludes two patients with primary writing tremor. Whether this condition is a focal dystonia or a variant of essential tremor has been the subject of some debate. However, even if the prevalence figure is recalculated using these patients, the prevalence of focal dystonias in Western Japan remains significantly less than in Rochester. The authors suspect genetic factors to be responsible for this difference.

In summary it is evident that the body of work concerning the epidemiology of primary dystonia is not large. With the exception of the figure postulated by Risch et al. (19) the prevalence rates calculated for the United States, Israel, and Japan were derived from diagnosed cases and each is likely to underestimate the true disease prevalence. The presence of a significant number of undiagnosed cases of dystonia within the community has been the experience of a number of authors (2,9). The surveys undertaken in Egypt and China ought to have provided superior results; however, in each case this is in doubt given the nature of the cases identified. A need for further studies is therefore established.

METHODS

The catchment area for this study comprises the counties of Northumberland, Tyne and Wear, Durham, and Cleveland in the northeast of England. The region contains both rural and urban areas with major conurbations existing around the cities of Newcastle, Middlesborough, and Sunderland. The sample population is calculated to be 2,605,100 (United Kingdom Office for National Statistics, Estimated Residential Population Mid-1995). There are certain advantages to performing an epidemiologic survey of dystonia in this area. It is relatively insular and served by only 12 neurologists operating from three centers. In addition the manner in which treatment is funded has meant that the administration of botulinum toxin is largely restricted to two clinics in the region through which all patients, bar a small number with blepharospasm, are funnelled. As a consequence one of these clinics has become the second largest in the United Kingdom when ranked by quantity of botulinum toxin used (Speywood Pharmaceuticals Ltd., personal communication). This centralization has facilitated the collection of data and assessment of patients.

The survey may be divided into three phases that have run from 1993 onward. In the first phase the records of neurologists, and otolaryngeal and ophthalmic surgeons in the region were reviewed. The examination of case notes was not restricted to those coded for dystonia; it also included case notes coded for any unspecified disorder of movement or gait not attributed to a specific disease. Added to this list of patients were those known to the Dystonia Society, a charitable organization representing individuals with dystonia and campaigning for increased awareness of the condition.

In the second phase of the study measures were taken to heighten the awareness of dystonia in the region; articles describing dystonia were placed in local newspapers, a series of radio discussions on the subject were given, and on two occasions a short video sequence illustrating the more common forms of dystonia was screened on the regions' independent television channel. In all cases information was given to enable interested individuals to contact the researchers. In addition, seminars for family physicians and other medical practitioners on the subjects of dystonia and the use of botulinum toxin were organized, in conjunction with the Dystonia Society, in 1993, 1994, and 1996.

Finally, a postal survey was undertaken in a well-defined area within the region already exposed to phases one and two of the study. A brochure containing pictorial representations of the various focal dystonias and information regarding the concept of dystonia was delivered to 45,383 households containing 101,766 individuals. The targeted addresses were contained within three postal codes; most were within a single town boundary, its suburbs, and neighboring villages. The demographic characteristics of this community were considered to be representative of the region as a whole. The aim of the postal survey was to gauge, albeit crudely, whether a significant number of individuals with dystonia remained to be identified after the first two stages of the study.

Patients identified by these means in whom a diagnosis of dystonia was thought possible were interviewed and examined. Demographic and medical details were obtained and if appropriate the dystonia was classified according to anatomic distribution. Individuals fulfilling the diagnostic criteria for primary dystonia as defined by the Ad Hoc Committee of the Dystonia Medical Research Foundation (6) and known to be both exhibiting their condition and resident in the catchment area on the designated prevalence date of January 1, 1996 were included in the study. A history of exposure to neuroleptic drugs or other agents known to be capable of producing dystonia were cause for exclusion.

RESULTS

A total of 372 individuals who fulfill the inclusion criteria of this study have been identified. The characteristics of these patients are shown in Table 2. These figures can be used to generate crude point prevalence ratios of 14.28 per 100,000 (95% confidence interval 12.8 to 15.76) for primary dystonia, 1.42 per 100,000 for generalized dystonia (95% confidence interval 0.95 to 1.89), and 12.86 per 100,000 for focal dystonia (95% confidence interval 11.45 to 14.25). It is interesting to note that approximately 10% of these cases were not previously known to any medical practitioner. The postal survey performed within part of the region generated 41 positive replies, which when investigated added a further three cases of primary dystonia to the 16 known previously within the specified area: two cases of writer's cramp and

one case of spasmodic dysphonia. It might be anticipated that a postal survey applied to the entire region would increase the known number of cases by a similar proportion.

The relative frequencies of the various types of focal dystonia are also shown in Table 2. It is noted that in this population-based survey only cervical dystonia is encountered more frequently than isolated blepharospasm while writer's cramp and spasmodic dysphonia each account for a similar and relatively small proportion of the total cases. This finding differs from the experience of Soland and colleagues based on referrals to clinics in London (21). In their review of the sex prevalence of the focal dystonias, Soland et al. divide their patient population into the following proportions: spasmodic torticollis 44%, cranial dystonia 19%, writer's cramp 19%, blepharospasm 11%, spasmodic dysphonia 4%, oromandibular dystonia 3%. Referral bias may account for this discrepancy. Previous studies have found a female preponderance for focal dystonia in the craniocervical region and a tendency for writer's cramp to be more common in males (21). The findings of this survey tend to support such a notion although statistical significance was reached for cases of cervical dystonia and blepharospasm only. Analysis of the group as a whole, without regard for anatomic location of the dystonia, shows that females have a relative risk of 2.1 (95% confidence interval 1.65 to 2.56) in comparison to males.

TABLE 2. *The epidemiology of the primary dystonias in the North of England*

Type of dystonia	Number of cases	%	Mean age of onset	Male:female ratio	p value (chi^2)
Generalized	37	9.9	16.7	1:1.3	ns[a]
Cervical	159	42.7	40.7	1:2.2	<0.0001
Blepharospasm	78	21.0	58.8	1:3.6	<0.0001
Segmental-cranial	24	6.5	49.6	1:3	ns
Spasmodic dysphonia	22	5.9	53.0	1:4.5	ns
Writer's cramp	19	5.1	37.9	1.4:1	ns
Segmental-axial/limb	15	4.0	28.9	1:4	ns
Focal-limb	13	3.5	26.8	2.3:1	ns
Oromandibular	3	0.8	47.6	Female	ns
Multifocal	2	0.5	45.5	Female	ns

[a]ns, not statistically significant.

DISCUSSION

This study is the first to document the prevalence of primary dystonia in the United Kingdom. The findings confirm that primary dystonia is considerably more prevalent than a number of better known neurologic conditions, such as myotonic dystrophy, myasthenia gravis, and motor neuron disease (4). The work has implications with regards to medical education and service provision, particularly the finance of botulinum toxin clinics. The discrepancy between the true disease prevalence and that reported here is difficult to estimate. It is acknowledged that the mechanisms established to conduct this survey continue to generate eligible cases and it may be necessary to revise the estimate of prevalence upward in the years to come.

ACKNOWLEDGMENTS

The authors gratefully acknowledge the statistical advice of Joyce French. This study has been supported by financial contributions from Allergan Ltd., Speywood Pharmaceuticals (UK) Ltd., Northern and Yorkshire Regional Health Authority, and The Dystonia Society of the United Kingdom (North-east division).

REFERENCES

1. Alter M, Kahana E, Feldman S. Differences in torsion dystonia among Israeli Ethnic Groups. *Adv Neurol* 1976;14:115–120.
2. Bressman SB, de Leon D, Brin M, et al. Idiopathic torsion dystonia among Ashkenazi Jews: evidence for autosomal dominant inheritance. *Ann Neurol* 1989;26: 612–620.
3. Cooper IS, Cullinan T, Riklan M. The natural history of dystonia. *Adv Neurol* 1976;14:157–169.
4. Cockerell OC, Sander JWAS, Shorvon SD. Neuroepidemiology in the United Kingdom. *J Neurol Neurosurg Psychiatry* 1993;56:735–738.
5. Eldridge R. The torsion dystonias: clinical, genetic, pathological, biochemical and therapeutic aspects. *Neurology* 1970;20:1–78.
6. Fahn S. Concept and classification of dystonia. *Adv Neurol* 1988;50:1–8.
7. Fahn S. Dystonia: phenomenology, classification, etiology, genetics, biochemistry and pathology. In: Fahn S, Marsden CD, Jankovic J, eds. *A comprehensive review of movement disorders for the clinical practitioner.* New York: Columbia University College of Physicians and Surgeons, 1996:341–376.
8. Flateau E, Sterling W. Progressiver Torsionspasms bie Kindern, *Z Gesamte Neurol Psychiatr* 1911;7:586–612.
9. Fletcher NA, Harding AE, Marsden CD. A genetic study of idiopathic torsion dystonia in the United Kingdom. *Brain* 1990;113:379–395.
10. Giménez-Roldán S, Delgado G, Marín M, Villanueva JA, Mateo D. Hereditary torsion dystonia in Gypsies. *Adv Neurol* 1988;50:73–81.
11. Hewer RL. The epidemiology of disabling neurological disorders. In: Greenwood R, Barnes MP, McMillan TM, Ward CD, eds. *Neurological rehabilitation.* London:Churchill Livingstone, 1993:4.
12. Kandil MRA, Tohamy SA, Fattah HA, Ahmed HN, Farwiez HM. Prevalence of chorea, dystonia and athetosis in Assiut, Egypt: a clinical and epidemiological study. *Neuroepidemiology* 1994;13:202–210.
13. Kurtzke JF. Neuroepidemiology. In: Bradley WG, Daroff RB, Fenichel GM, Marsden C, eds. *Neurology in clinical practice.* 3rd ed. Boston: Butterworth-Heinemann, 1991:545–560.
14. Korczyn AD, Kahana E, Zilber N, Streifler M, Carasso R, Alter M. Torsion dystonia in Israel. *Ann Neurol* 1980;8:387–391.
15. Li S, Schoenberg BS, Wang C, et al. A prevalence study of Parkinson's disease and other movement disorders in the Peoples Republic of China. *Arch Neurol* 1985;42:655–657.
16. Marsden CD, Quinn NP. The dystonias. *BMJ* 1990; 300:139–144.
17. Nakashima K, Kusumi M, Inoue Y, Takahashi K. Prevalence of focal dystonias in the western area of Tottori Prefecture in Japan. *Mov Disord* 1995;10: 440–443.
18. Nutt JG, Muenter MD, Aronson A, Kurland LT, Melton LJ. Epidemiology of focal and generalised dystonia in Rochester, Minnesota. *Mov Disord* 1983; 3:188–194.
19. Risch N, de Leon D, Ozelius L, et al. Genetic analysis of idiopathic torsion dystonia in Ashkenazi Jews and their recent descent from a small founder population. *Nat Genet* 1995;9:152–159.
20. Schwalbe W. Eine eigentumliche tonische Krampfform mit hysterischen Symptomen. *Medicin und Chirurgie.* Berlin:Universitats-Buchdruckerei von Gustav Schade, 1980.
21. Soland VL, Bhatia KP, Marsden CD. Sex prevalence of focal dystonias. *J Neurol Neurosurg Psychiatry* 1996;60:204–205.
22. Spinella GM, Sheridan PH. Research opportunities in dystonia: National Institute of Neurological Disorders and Stroke workshop summary. *Neurology* 1994;44: 1177–1179.
23. Tanner CM, Goldman SM. Epidemiology of movement disorders. *Curr Opin Neurol* 1994;7:343–345.
24. Zador J. Le spasme torsion: parallele des tableaux cliniques entre la race juive et les autres races. *Rev Neurol* 1936;72:365.
25. Zilber N, Korczyn AD, Kahana E, Kalman F, Alter M. Inheritance of idiopathic torsion dystonia among Jews. *J Med Genet* 1984;21:13–20.

Dystonia 3:Advances in Neurology, Vol. 78,
edited by S. Fahn, C. D. Marsden, and M. DeLong
Lippincott–Raven Publishers, Philadelphia © 1998

14

Abnormal Brain Networks in DYT1 Dystonia

David Eidelberg

*Movement Disorders Center and Functional Brain Imaging Laboratory, North Shore University
Hospital, Manhasset, New York 11030.*

INTRODUCTION

Brain Circuitry in Dystonia: Animal Models

The brain metabolic abnormalities underlying idiopathic torsion dystonia (ITD) are currently unknown. Nonetheless, several experimental models have been proposed to explain the functional mechanisms underlying the hyperkinetic movement disorders including ITD. For example, Crossman (4) proposed that levodopa induced dyskinesias that may occur through a selective deactivation of the subthalamic nucleus (STN) mediated through the indirect striatopallidal pathway. This results in a reduction in the functional activity of the internal pallidum (GPi), which is the major inhibitor of ventral thalamic outflow to the motor cortex. An alternative mechanism for the production of hyperkinesia invokes the direct striatopallidal pathway. This pathway is inhibitory and serves to suppress GPi directly without concomitant deactivation of STN. In their experimental model of dystonia, Mitchell et al. (16) suggested that the direct pathway may be pathologically overactive leading to GPi suppression and to consequent functional accentuation of thalamic inputs to cortical motor areas. Thus, whether through underaction of the indirect pathway or through overaction of the direct pathway, or both, reductions in inhibitory pallidothalamic outflow appear to underlie the manifestations of hyperkinesia in experimental animal models.

In spite of the utility of animal models in the understanding of the pathophysiology of movement disorders, direct parallels to human disease are not always justified. Nonetheless, functional brain imaging has provided the possibility of investigating hypotheses concerning mechanisms of disease in living human patients. In particular, positron emission tomography (PET) imaging with ^{18}F-fluorodeoxyglucose (FDG) has provided a useful means of assessing neuronal function through the measurement of local glucose utilization. Additionally, metabolic interactions between brain regions can be quantified utilizing network analytical strategies for the identification of unique neuronal circuits associated with different neurodegenerative processes. We have developed a network analytical approach known as the Scaled Subprofile Model (SSM; 1,7,18). This mathematical model is based on principal-components analysis (PCA) and allows for the extraction of specific patterns of regional metabolic covariation. By computing subject scores for these patterns, we can quantify the expression of disease-related neural networks in individual patients and in normal control subjects. We have utilized this approach extensively in the study of Parkinson's disease (PD) and other movement disorders.

This work was supported by a generous grant from the Dystonia Medical Research Foundation and by NIH NS RO1-35069.

Abnormal Brain Networks in Parkinsonism and Normal Aging

In our early studies, we identified a specific pattern of regional metabolic covariation associated with PD (6,7). This pattern was characterized by relative hypermetabolism of the lentiform nucleus and thalamus covarying with metabolic decreases in the primary and association motor cortices. Subject scores for this pattern, representing its expression in the brains of individual patients, were found to correlate significantly with independent measures of clinical disability as measured by the Unified Parkinson's Disease Rating Scale (UPDRS; 13). Additionally, we found that these subject scores also correlated with presynaptic nigrostriatal dopaminergic function as measured by striatal uptake of [18F]fluorodopa (FDOPA) (6,8). We have subsequently demonstrated that this metabolic covariation pattern was identified in four independent cohorts of PD patients scanned on different tomographs of varying resolution (7). These findings led us to conclude that this regional metabolic covariation pattern is a reliable and reproducible network marker of the parkinsonian disease process. In subsequent studies, we developed a technique of computing the expression of this network in individual subjects. We referred to this algorithm as topographic profile rating (TPR; 8,9). We used this approach to compute subject scores for the original PD-associated pattern on a prospective case-by-case basis (7,9). We found these measures of network expression to be highly predictive of independent measures of clinical disability (9). In parallel studies, we found that a related pattern of regional metabolic *asymmetries* could differentiate early-Stage PD from normals with an accuracy comparable to FDOPA/PET (8). Moreover, using the TPR algorithm, we found that this metabolic covariance pattern reliably distinguished drug-responsive from drug-resistant parkinsonians even at the earliest stages of clinical disability (Hoehn and Yahr Stage I) (8). This finding contrasts with FDOPA/PET in which such a differentiation could not be achieved in the same patients. These findings

lend credence to our notion that regional metabolic covariance patterns can serve as reliable network markers of disease processes in prospective clinical studies.

Recently, we expanded the application of network imaging to the study of human neurophysiology *in vivo*. We scanned 42 PD patients with FDG/PET in an awake unmedicated state prior to unilateral ventral pallidotomy. Subsequently, we obtained intraoperative measurements of GPi single-unit activity in the same patients in an identical awake, unmedicated state. We found that GPi firing rates were highly correlated with the expression of a pattern characterized by covarying metabolism in the pallidum, ventral thalamus, and pons—a topographic distribution compatible with the anatomic projection fields of the pallidum (20). This result demonstrates that functional connectivity may be obtained utilizing SSM network analysis and that the expression of the PD network marker was associated with measurable abnormalities in pallidal neuronal activity. Moreover, in our PET study of alterations in brain metabolism subsequent to pallidotomy (11), we noted that operative changes in the expression of this pattern were highly correlated with clinical outcome following surgery. These findings indicate that regional metabolic covariance patterns identified with SSM can indeed be construed as spatially distributed neural networks.

SSM network analysis can also be applied to model specific neurodegenerative processes. In a separate series of investigations, we identified regional metabolic covariance patterns associated with the normal aging process (17). In that study we found that an age-related pattern identified in a cohort of 20 patients accurately predicted chronologic age in a separate cohort of 130 other normatives scanned at another PET center. Moreover, subject scores for this pattern were also found to be highly reproducible within subjects. Having demonstrated the presence of a quantifiable aging-related marker in normals, we utilized this network approach to examine the relationship between normal aging and parkinsonism. In a recent study we used TPR to calculate the expression of the age-related pattern in 37 PD patients (12). By quantifying subject scores for the aging pattern in these patients, we obtained an estimate of metabolic age in the patients (i.e., the age predicted solely on the basis of FDG/PET). We then calculated the difference between this estimate of metabolic age and actual chronologic age. For normal aging, it was expected that the metabolic age and real age should be similar, and that the difference would be near zero. In a case of accelerating aging as has been proposed for PD (2), computed metabolic age might overestimate true age. On the other hand, in a situation where a pathologic process supplants normal aging and disrupts the normal age-metabolism relationship, computed metabolic age may consistently underestimate true chronologic age. In our investigation we noted a significant underestimation of real age by FDG/PET in PD patients, suggesting that aging and parkinsonism are independent and dissociated neurodegenerative processes. We also used linear extrapolation to determine the duration of the parkinsonian preclinical period. We estimated this interval to be approximately 5 years, a finding consistent with estimates derived through longitudinal FDOPA/PET measurements in single patients (19). Thus, network imaging with SSM allows for the development of comprehensive models of disease progression that may be useful in understanding the natural history of neurodegenerative processes.

Abnormal Brain Networks in Idiopathic Torsion Dystonia

The results of network analysis in ITD contrast with those described above in parkinsonism. In our original study of ITD, we scanned 11 ITD patients with predominantly right-sided symptomatology (10). We found that ITD was characterized by a significant regional metabolic covariation pattern characterized by lentiform hypermetabolism that was dissociated from metabolic activity in the thalamus. Importantly, these changes were associated with covariate metabolic *increases* in primary motor and premotor areas including supple-

mentary motor areas (SMAs). These findings in ITD contrast with PD in that the metabolic activity of the lentiform nucleus (including the pallidum) do not covary with thalamic metabolism, and that the cortical motor regions are functionally overactive, even at rest. Additionally, we found that subject scores for the ITD pattern correlated significantly with independent Fahn-Marsden dystonia ratings.

We interpreted these results as evidence of overactivity of neural networks involving associative motor regions. Moreover, the dissociation between lentiform and thalamic metabolism in ITD suggested the possibility of a functional inhibition of GPi, as has been postulated as a mechanism for hyperkinesia (14). We interpreted this metabolic dissociation as indicating an overactivity of direct inhibitory projections from the putamen to GPi releasing the ventral tier thalamic nuclei from their normal pallidofugal inhibition (7). (The relative lentiform hypermetabolism noted by us may relate to the increase in GPi afferents through the direct pathway.) Once the ventral thalamus has been unyoked from the GPi, its projections to motor cortices appear to be increased, thereby accentuating glucose metabolism in these cortical regions. These findings are compatible with the results of motor activation studies of ITD (3), as well as being consistent with experimental animal models of dystonia (4,16) as described above.

ABNORMAL BRAIN NETWORKS IN DYT1 DYSTONIA

Although most of the ITD patients in the above study had action-only dystonia, and therefore were not moving during the time of PET imaging, the possibility of contamination by concurrent motor activity could not be discounted. Moreover, the patients were selected from a variety of genotypes with significant clinical variability by restricting the SSM analysis to nonmanifesting carriers of the DYT1 gene. To address the problem of concurrent movement during PET, as well as the genotypic and phenotypic variability inherent in our first study, we developed a new methodology for data analysis by restricting SSM analysis to nonmanifesting carriers of the DYT1 gene and normal controls.

We scanned a group of seven nonmanifesting DYT1 gene carriers and ten age-matched normal control subjects with FDG/PET using an Advance tomograph (General Electric Medical Systems, Milwaukee, WI). The performance characteristics of this instrument have been described elsewhere (5). This 18-ring bismuth germanate whole-body tomograph produces 35 slices with an axial field of view of 15 cm and a resolution of 4.2 mm [full width at half maximum (FWHM)] in all directions. In each PET study subjects were positioned in the scanner using a Laitinen stereoadapter (Sandstrom Trade and Technology, Inc., Welland, ON) (15) with three-dimensional laser alignment with reference to the orbitomeatal (OM) line. All studies were performed with the subject's eyes open in a dimly lit room and minimal auditory stimulation. The time course of ^{18}F radioactivity was determined by sampling

radial arterial blood. We calculated global and regional cerebral metabolic rates for glucose (GMR and rCMRGlc, respectively) in all FDG/PET studies on a pixel by pixel basis employing the autoradiographic method as described by us previously (7,21,22).

SSM analysis was performed on the combined group of DYT1 carriers and normal volunteers blind to gene status as described elsewhere (7–9). We identified a significant covariance pattern (first principal component) that accounted for 32% of subject × region variance. This network was characterized by bilateral lentiform hypermetabolism and thalamo-lentiform dissociation associated with covarying resting state increases in SMA metabolism (Fig. 1). Subject scores from this pattern were abnormally elevated in the nonmanifesting DYT1 carriers (Fig. 2, left), indicating a genotype-related increase in brain network expression in these clinically normal individuals.

We subsequently used TPR to calculate the expression of this pattern in five *affected* ITD

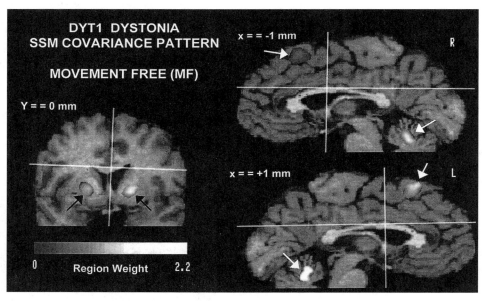

FIG. 1. Display of the regional covariance pattern associated with DYT1 dystonia identified using the Scaled Subprofile Model (SSM) in a combined group of nonmanifesting DYT1 carriers and age-matched normal volunteers. Region weights have been mapped on standardized Talairach MRI sections. This pattern was characterized by relatively increased metabolism in the lentiform nucleus, supplementary motor areas, and cerebellar hemispheres.

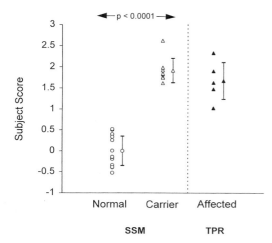

FIG. 2. Scatter diagram of the individual subject scores for the brain network depicted in Fig. 1 measured in normals *(open circles)*, nonmanifesting gene carriers *(open triangles)*, and affected DYT1 dystonia patients *(filled triangles)*. Mean subject scores for the DYT1 network were abnormally elevated in both nonmanifesting DYT1 carriers and dystonia patients (*p* <0.001).

patients with the DYT1 genotype scanned with FDG as described above. We noted an abnormal increase in the expression of this network in the symptomatic cohort analogous to that found in the nonmanifesting carriers (Fig. 2, right). These findings demonstrated that the metabolic network abnormalities associated with the DYT1 genotype were present and reproducible in independent gene-bearing cohorts with and without clinical manifestations of dystonia.

These results indicate that our previous findings of relative lentiform and SMA hypermetabolism and lentiform-thalamic dissociation in ITD (10) are essential features of this disorder and not artifacts of movement. The two covariance topographies are compared in Fig. 3. Both patterns are characterized by significant network-related metabolic increases (region weight 1 or greater, reflecting values 2 or more standard deviations from the neutral value of 0; 7,10) in the lentiform nucleus and SMA. Similarly, the ratio of region weights for the thalamus and the lentiform nucleus are approxi-

mately 0.2, indicating considerable metabolic dissociation (as compared with the corresponding region weight ratio of 0.9 in the PD network; 7–9). As expected in a network identified in *affected* dystonia patients, the ITD pattern was characterized by considerably higher region weights in both SMA and lateral premotor region as compared with the movement-free pattern identified in the nonmanifesting DYT1 carriers. The DYT1 pattern also included a major cerebellar contribution that was not evident in the earlier pattern. The reason for this disparity may relate to the limited cerebellar sampling of the tomograph utilized in the original study. Nonetheless, the cause for network-related cerebellar hypermetabolism in DYT1 dystonia remains unclear, and may suggest a potential role for this structure in the pathophysiology of this disorder.

It is also important to note that the mean expression of the DYT1 pattern did not differ in nonmanifesting gene carriers and affected dystonia patients. This suggests that while this metabolic brain network may be linked to the DYT1 genotype, its abnormal expression in individual subjects may be a necessary but not sufficient criterion for the development of symptoms. Indeed, it is likely that other brain networks are expressed in symptomatic individuals that relate directly to the clinical manifestations of disease. The identification of these patterns may be valuable in understanding the specific mechanisms of dystonia. Moreover, it is also conceivable that such movement-related patterns may be expressed abnormally, but to a lesser degree, in nonmanifesting carriers. Should this be the case, the mathematical relationship between subject scores for the movement-free and the movement-related patterns may be a critical determinant of the functional threshold needed to be reached for the development of symptoms. These metabolic networks, either individually or in combination, may serve as useful metabolic markers for studying the natural history of ITD and for quantitatively assessing the utility of potential therapeutic strategies.

The actual role of these networks in mediating abnormal motor function in ITD is still

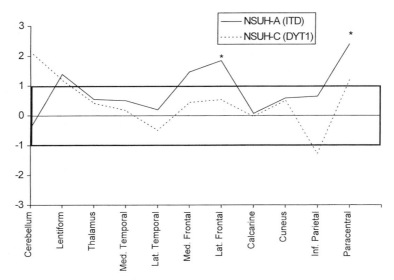

FIG. 3. Comparison of the DYT1 network with that previously identified in a previous study of ITD patients (10). (NSUH-A and NSUH-C refer to the different tomographs used in the identification of each of these patterns; see text.) Lentiform hypermetabolism with thalamic metabolic dissociation was a common feature of both patterns. Region weights for lateral frontal cortex and SMA *(asterisks)* were higher in the ITD-related pattern, as may be expected with the inclusion of affected patients. Cerebellar region weights were higher in the DYT1 pattern, suggesting a functional role for this structure in the pathogenesis of DYT1 dystonia. [Regions with weights of magnitude ≥1 *(outside of box)* account for over 50% of the variance in the normalized metabolic data ($p < 0.001$) and contribute significantly to the abnormal dystonia networks. Regions with weights of magnitude <1 *(in box)* do not contribute significantly to these networks.]

unclear. It would be of great interest to perform motor activation studies in these clinically asymptomatic but metabolically perturbed DYT1 carriers. These experiments may be crucial in delineating the relationship between altered network expression in the resting state and abnormal functional activation of motor circuits during the execution of controlled movement tasks (3). Additionally, an important challenge for the future lies in the understanding of the somatotopic differences in brain metabolism that underlie the different forms of dystonia. The spatial resolution of currently available PET instruments does not allow for the delineation of abnormally functioning groups of neurons underlying the various somatic distributions of dystonia subtypes. Indeed, functional magnetic resonance imaging methods may ultimately permit investigators to identify the specific abnormal neuronal populations responsible for the different clinical forms of dystonia.

ACKNOWLEDGMENT

Special thanks to Ms. Lauren Moran for assistance in manuscript preparation.

REFERENCES

1. Alexander GE, Moeller JR. Application of the scaled subprofile model to functional imaging in neuropsychiatric disorders: a principal component approach to modeling brain function in disease. *Hum Brain Mapping* 1994;2:79–94.
2. Calne DB, Peppard RF. Aging of the nigrostriatal pathway in humans. *Can J Neurol Sci* 1987;14:424–427.
3. Ceballos-Baumann AO, Passingham RE, Warner T, et al. Overactive prefrontal and underactive motor cortical areas in idiopathic dystonia. *Ann Neurol* 1995;37:363–372.

4. Crossman A. A hypothesis on the pathophysiological mechanisms that underlie levodopa or dopamine agonist-induced dyskinesia in Parkinson's disease: implications for future strategies in treatment [Review]. *Mov Disord* 1990;5:100–108.

5. DeGrado TR, Turkington TG, Williams JJ, et al. Performance characteristics of a whole-body PET scanner. *J Nucl Med* 1994;35:1398–1406.

6. Eidelberg D, Moeller JR, Dhawan V, et al. The metabolic anatomy of Parkinson's disease: complementary ^{18}F-fluorodeoxyglucose and ^{18}F-fluorodopa positron emission tomographic studies. *Mov Disord* 1990;5: 203–213.

7. Eidelberg D, Moeller JR, Dhawan V, et al. The metabolic topography of parkinsonism. *J Cereb Blood Flow Metab* 1994;14:783–801.

8. Eidelberg D, Moeller JR, Dhawan V, et al. Early differential diagnosis of Parkinson's disease with ^{18}F-fluorodeoxyglucose and positron emission tomography. *Neurology* 1995;45:1995–2004.

9. Eidelberg D, Moeller JR, Ishikawa T, et al. Assessment of disease severity in parkinsonism with ^{18}F-fluorodeoxyglucose and PET. *J Nucl Med* 1995;36:378–383.

10. Eidelberg D, Moeller JR, Ishikawa T, et al. The metabolic topography of idiopathic torsion dystonia. *Brain* 1995;118:1473–1484.

11. Eidelberg D, Moeller JR, Ishikawa T, et al. Regional metabolic correlates of surgical outcome following unilateral pallidotomy for Parkinson's disease. *Ann Neurol* 1996;39:450–459.

12. Eidelberg D, Moeller JR, Kazumata K, et al. Comparative rates of metabolic degeneration in Parkinson's Disease and normal aging *Mov Disord* 1996;11:3 (abst).

13. Fahn S, Elton RL. UPDRS Development Committee. Unified Parkinson disease rating scale. In: Fahn S, Marsden CD, Calne D, Goldstein M, eds. *Recent developments in Parkinson's disease,* vol. 2. Floral Park, NJ: Macmillan, 1987:293–304.

14. Hallet M. Physiology of basal ganglia disorders: an overview [Review]. *Can J Neurol Sci* 1993;20:177–183.

15. Laitinen LV, Liliequist B, Fagerlund M, Eriksson AT. An adapter for computed tomography-guided stereotaxis. *Surg Neurol* 1985;23:559–566.

16. Mitchell IJ, Luquin R, Boyce S, et al. Neural mechanisms of dystonia: evidence from a 2-deoxyglucose uptake study in a primate model of dopamine agonist-induced dystonia. *Mov Disord* 1990;5:49–54.

17. Moeller JR, Ishikawa T, Dhawan V, et al. The metabolic topography of normal aging. *J Cereb Blood Flow Metab* 1996;16:385–398.

18. Moeller JR, Strother SC. A regional covariance approach to the analysis of functional patterns in positron emission tomographic data. *J Cereb Blood Flow Metab* 1991;11:A121–135.

19. Morrish PK, Sawle GV, Brooks DJ. The rate of progression of Parkinson's disease. A longitudinal [^{18}F] DOPA study. *Adv Neurol* 1996;69:427–431.

20. Parent A, Hazrati LN. Functional anatomy of the basal ganglia. I. The cortico-basal ganglia-thalamo-cortical loop. *Brain Res Brain Res Rev* 1995;20:91–127.

21. Phelps ME, Huang SC, Hoffman EJ, et al. Tomographic measurement of local cerebral glucose metabolic rate in human with ^{18}F-2-fluoro-2-deoxy-D-glucose. Validation of method. *Ann Neurol* 1979;6:371–388.

22. Takikawa S, Dhawan V, Robeson W, et al. Noninvasive quantitative FDG/PET studies using an estimated input function derived from a population arterial blood curve. *Radiology* 1993;188:131–136.

Dystonia 3: Advances in Neurology, Vol. 78,
edited by S. Fahn, C. D. Marsden, and M. DeLong
Lippincott–Raven Publishers, Philadelphia © 1998

15

Activation Positron Emission Tomography Scanning in Dystonia

*†‡Andrés O. Ceballos-Baumann and *†David J. Brooks

*MRC Cyclotron Unit, Hammersmith Hospital, London, United Kingdom, †Institute of Neurology, London, United Kingdom, and ‡Neurologische Klinik der Technischen Universität München, München, D-81675 Germany.

Dystonia is characterized by involuntary muscular co-contractions causing twisting movements and abnormal posturing. A genetic locus has been identified on chromosome 9q34 in some Jewish and non-Jewish families with idiopathic torsion dystonia (ITD) (33), although considerable genetic heterogeneity occurs in ITD (54). Histopathologic studies of ITD generally show no abnormality, although cell loss in the basal ganglia or brainstem nuclei has been reported in occasional cases (24,57).

The pathophysiology of dystonia remains unclear; in most cases of acquired dystonia there are structural basal ganglia or thalamic lesions (3,34,40). Marsden et al. (34) therefore hypothesized that dystonia could arise from abnormal pallidal and/or ventral thalamus output to the premotor areas. Peripheral nerve and central motor conduction is normal in dystonia but there is impaired reflex inhibition of antagonists (45). Secondary dystonia is uncommon where the corticospinal tract is damaged, suggesting that an intact pyramidal pathway may be necessary in order to manifest dystonia. The N30 component of the median nerve somatosensory evoked potential (SEP) shows an enhanced amplitude in some patients with dystonia (43) and this has been postulated to reflect supplementary motor area (SMA) overactivity. In contrast, the late phase of the Bereitschaftspotential is attenuated in patients with writer's cramp (WC) and this, plus an observed decreased amplitude of the N30 component of the SEP in patients with spasmodic torticollis, would be more in favor of the SMA being under- rather than overactive (14,36).

Structural imaging [computed tomography (CT) and magnetic resonance imaging (MRI)] is invariably normal in ITD. Positron emission tomography (PET) provides a means of studying regional cerebral function in humans in vivo under both resting and activating conditions. Studies on resting blood flow and metabolism in dystonia have tended to yield conflicting results. Normal, increased, and decreased resting striatal metabolism have all been reported in dystonia cases and this, in part, may reflect the heterogeneity of the cohorts of patients examined (12,16,25,30,37,49). Familial, sporadic, dopa-responsive, and secondary dystonias have all been grouped together at times and early studies concentrated on hemi- and focal dystonics in order to perform side-to-side comparisons of basal ganglia function. Activation studies with $H_2{}^{15}O$ PET provide a noninvasive method of studying activity of central motor pathways in dystonic patients and are potentially more informative than resting studies.

Tempel and Perlmutter (51) examined the integrity of central sensory connections in a group of 11 patients with idiopathic hemi- or focal dystonia, six of whom had WC. They used vibrotactile stimulation to activate the sensorimotor cortex (SMC), and measured the resultant increase in blood flow. The dystonic subjects had a normal pattern of resting regional cerebral blood flow (rCBF) but showed a significant attenuation of the contralateral SMC blood flow response to tactile stimulation (80% of normal). This was true whether the affected or "normal" hand was stimulated. The authors suggested that this attenuated SMC activation was a consequence of excessive inhibitory output to the cortex from the basal ganglia in dystonia. More recently, the same workers compared the cerebral activation associated with vibrotactile stimulation in six unilateral writer's cramp cases and eight age-matched normal controls (52). Similar findings were obtained, but in this study attenuated activation of caudal SMA was also noted in the dystonia group.

Whereas this PET activation work focused on the sensory system in idiopathic dystonia, the present paper relates to studies with motor activation in patients with idiopathic dystonia (7,8), acquired hemidystonia (AHD) (10), and WC before and after effective botulinum toxin (BOTX) treatment (5,10,11). Four activation paradigms were used: (a) execution of paced joystick movements in freely selected directions in ITD and AHD; (b) imagination of these movements in ITD; (c) paced continuous stereotyped writing in writer's cramp patients; (d) imitation of dystonic writing in healthy controls.

The paradigm involving performance of paced joystick movements in freely selected directions that we employed in the studies on ITD and AHD has been previously used to demonstrate impaired activation of the striatum and mesial frontal cortex in Parkinson's disease (28,41) and frontal cortex in motor neuron disease (31). Based on this previous work we regard this paradigm to be a robust activation task that examines both preparatory and executive aspects of motor function. The paradigms involving imagery and writing served to focus on different aspects of the motor system: Imagination of movements disassociates activity of

the motor decision and executive systems; and an automatic and overlearned task done continuously such as stereotyped writing examines executive motor activity. Imitation of dystonic writing by healthy controls should help to differentiate between primary activation phenomena causing dystonia and secondary phenomena due to muscle spasm. Finally, the writing paradigm in writer's cramp allows one to examine the functional effects of BOTX when clinically effective.

MATERIALS AND METHODS
Patient Selection
Idiopathic Torsion Dystonia (ITD)

Nine patients with ITD (mean age 33 ± 13 years, 4 women and 5 men, range 20 to 55 years, Table 1) and six control subjects (mean age 39 ± 13 years, 6 men, range 20 to 59 years) were recruited. Head movements artifact (patients 6, 7) and noncompliance during the scan (patient 4) led to rejection of the data set of three patients and therefore the sets of six out of the nine ITD patients were analyzed.

Acquired Hemidystonia (AHD)

Five patients (two women and three men) with AHD (mean age 36 ± 14 years, range 20 to 59 years, Tables 2 and 3) and five healthy right-handed control subjects (mean age 39 ± 14 years, range 20 to 59 years) were scanned. All five patients had dystonic posturing at rest and on action in the absence of other system involvement.

Writer's Cramp (WC) Patients

Six right-handed patients (two women and four men, see Table 4) with WC (mean age 53 ± 11 years, range 35 to 66 years) had PET, five of them twice (before and after BOTX) along with six healthy right-handed control subjects (one woman and five men, mean age 47 ± 13 years, range 35 to 69 years). Five of the six WC patients benefited clinically from BOTX injections. Patient 4 declined to come back for the

TABLE 1. Clinical characteristics and genetic information on 9 idiopathic torsion dystonia patients

Pat. no.	Sex	Age at study (yr)	Age at onset (yr)	Distribution of dystonia	Ashkenazi haplotype carrier	Movement score[a]	Disability score[a]	Drug treatment
1	F	47	37	Multifocal	−	8	3	Trihexiphenidyl 15 mg/d; Clonazepam 0.5 mg t.i.d.
2	M	24	9	Focal, dystonic writer's cramp	+	4	2	Nil
3	F	21	5	Generalized	−	31	13	Trihexiphenidyl 100 mg/d; Baclofen 30 mg
5	M	47	11	Multifocal	+	15	6	Nil
8	F	20	6	Generalized	+	12	3	Trihexiphenidyl 40 mg/d
9	M	39	15	Generalized	−	24	8	Nil
4	M	25	5	Generalized	−	17	9	Baclofen 60 mg/d; Trihexiphenidyl 60 mg/d
6	M	22	7	Generalized	−	32	16	Nil
7	F	55	12	Generalized	−	34	14	Tetrabenazine 75 mg/d

The scans of the lower 3 patients were technically not satisfactory and could not be included in the group analysis.

[a]Movement and disability scores according the Fahn-Marsden dystonia scale.

From ref. 8, with permission.

TABLE 2. *Acquired hemidystonia patient details: sex, age, onset, type of dystonia*

Case	Sex	Age at study (yr)	Age at onset (yr)	Onset and handedness before onset	Type and side of hemidystonia contralateral to lesion
1	F	59	Childhood	No hemiplegia, slow progression during childhood, exacerbation after wrist trauma at age 54, handedness not remembered	Fixed at hand, intensified by action in leg and arm, left-sided
2	F	20	10	No hemiplegia, slow progression over 4 years, right-handed	Fixed at hand and foot, intensified by action in leg, arm, and face, right-sided
3	M	23	18	5 months after 5 months of hemiplegia, slow progression over years, left-handed	Mobile, intensified by action, left-sided
4	M	43	28	6 years after 1 year of hemiplegia, slow progression over years, right-handed	Mobile, intensified by action, right-sided
5	M	35	12	2 weeks after 2 weeks of hemiplegia, slow progression right-handed	Mobile, intensified by action, left-sided

postinjection scan due to his disappointment with the effect of BOTX as it resulted in a temporary but significant paresis of the right hand. The remaining five patients had technically satisfactory follow-up scans 2 to 5 weeks after BOTX injections when clinical benefit was apparent.

All subjects gave informed written consent. The studies were approved by the Hammersmith Hospital Ethics Committee, and permission to administer radioactivity was obtained from the Administration of Radioactive Substances Advisory Committee of the Department of Health, UK.

Methods

All subjects had between 8 and 12 sequential rCBF scans with $H_2^{15}O$ over the course of 2 1/2 hours with their eyes closed. The light was dimmed and the background noise consisted of the fans of the electronic equipment. Changes in rCBF compared to the reference state (rest condition) were used as an index of the regional synaptic activity. Four scans were performed for each of the experimental conditions. During the rest condition subjects were asked to relax with the arms and hands in the most comfortable position possible. They were

TABLE 3. *Acquired hemidystonia patient details: etiology of hemidystonia and structural imaging findings*

Case	Etiology	Contralateral lesion site	Additional MRI/CT findings
1	Vascular, perinatal	Lentiform ncl. centered on globus pallidus	—
2	Vascular, presumed perinatal	Lentiform ncl. centered on globus pallidus	Slight hemiatrophy
3	Head trauma	Low R thalamus signal on T1-weighted image	Slight temporal horn dilatation
4	Head trauma	Scattered low density at lentiform nucleus and posterior limb of internal capsule	Slight bilateral ventricular dilatation
5	Head trauma	Posterolateral thalamic infarction	Right occipital and right temporal infarction, mild cerebellar atrophy

From ref. 6, with permission.

TABLE 4. *Writer's cramp patient clinical details*

Case	Sex	Age at study (yr)	Age at onset (yr)	Clinical characteristics of writer's cramp (WC) (all on right side)	Other affected areas	Time period free of BOTX treatment before 1st scan	Target muscles (all on right side) and BOTX dose	Improvement (change in %) in self-rated function[a] before and after BOTX plus whether script improved
1	M	35	25	Simple, II and III finger extension, hand pronation, discomfort on writing	—	12 months	Ext. dig. ind. prop. (40 U Dysport®)	40%, improvement of script
2	F	66	63	Simple WC, tremor, discomfort on writing	Meige's syndrome	No BOTX before	Ext. carpi rad. + uln. (80 U), flex. carpi rad. + uln. (120 U Dysport®)	80%, impressive improvement of script
3	M	56	48	Simple WC, thumb flexion at IPJ, hand supination, pain on writing	—	4 months	Flex. poll. longus (100 U Dysport®)	50%, script appeared normal before and after BOTX
4	M	49	45	Dystonic WC, tremor, discomfort on writing	—	4 months	Ext. carpi rad. (80 U) + uln. (80 U Dysport®)	No improvement
5	M	65	61	Simple WC, finger flexion II and III, tremor, discomfort	Blepharospasm	4 months	Flex. dig. sup. (40 U) + prof. (60 U Dysport®)	50%, improvement of script
6	F	49	32	Dystonic WC, hand supination, curling in of fingers III–V, thumb adduction	—	8 months	Flex. dig. prof. (60 U Dysport®)	40%, improvement of script

[a] Patients were asked to rate their writing function in percent of normal before and after BOTX treatment.
From ref. 11, with permission.

told beforehand that they would be hearing pacing tones like during the activating condition and were instructed not to react.

The activating condition in the ITD and AHD patients consisted of moving a joystick, freely choosing at each pacing tone in which direction to move it. During the free-selection task subjects had to spontaneously select and execute joystick movements, paced every 3 seconds. There were four possible directions of joystick movement: forward, back, left, or right. The subjects moved the joystick after each pacing tone. The mean time from the tone to the completion of the joystick movement was recorded for each subject (response time) as well as the number of errors that occurred when the subject failed to complete the movement because of reduced movement amplitude. AHD patients were also studied while performing the movements with the unaffected hand and ITD patients and their controls while imagining the joystick movements. In order to enhance compliance during the imagination task in the ITD study, subjects were asked after each scan in which direction they had moved the joystick in their mind.

WC patients (two sessions, before and after BOTX) and their controls were scanned while continuously writing the three letter word "dog." The controls had an additional activating condition that consisted of imitating dystonic writing. The subjects were paced by a tone so that they wrote the word "dog" every 4 seconds. Writing the stereotyped word at this rate ensured continuous script. Subjects had a 40×40 cm board with a paper roll suspended above their thorax as they lay supine. The board was angled in the most comfortable position for the subject emulating as far as possible his or her physiologic writing position. Writing was performed with a Papermate fibertip pen. Subjects were instructed to write in the dark with their eyes closed. A plastic surround helped the subject to assess the writing space available in semidarkness. Subjects were allowed to write words on top of each other, although this occurred only exceptionally. In practice, all subjects were able to write fluently in a supine position in the darkness. Subjects had at least two trials of 100 seconds writing positioned while in the scanner, so that they felt confident with the paradigm prior to scanning. They were trained to write continuously and adapt their writing speed to the cueing tones. All subjects wrote in lines (less than four) during the 100 seconds of the task and all writer's cramp patients developed dystonia.

All subjects were closely observed by two light-enhancing video monitors and in the scanning room by one of us (A.O.C-B.). Movements of the hand and arm were recorded by a video camera to assess dystonic posturing.

Data Acquisition

A slow bolus technique was used (46). Fifteen millicuries (mCi) of $H_2^{15}O$ in 3 cc of normal saline was loaded into intravenous tubing (25 gauge) attached to a cannula in an antecubital vein. This was then flushed into the subject over 20 seconds by an automatic pump at a rate of 10 ml/min. Scanning commenced 0 to 5 seconds before onset of rise in head counts (30 to 45 seconds after initiation of the slow bolus) and the time from rise to peak count rate was 30 to 40 seconds, depending on the individual circulation time. Scanning lasted 90 seconds. The pacing tones commenced 10 seconds before scanning for both the resting and activated state. The interval between successive $H_2^{15}O$ administrations was 10 minutes. The measurement of regional brain radioactivity was carried out with PET (953-B, Siemens-CTI, Knoxville, TN) with the interplane septa retracted (47). This scanner utilizes block technology detectors and contains 16 individual rings, each 6.5-mm thick axially, resulting in a total of 31 measured planes (direct and cross) covering an axial field of view of 10.65 cm. In three-dimensional (3-D) mode, the scanner is able to acquire sinograms between any pair of opposing detectors, resulting in a total of 256 sinograms (1).

A 20-minute transmission scan using rotating rods of $^{68}Ge/^{68}Ga$ was performed for attenuation correction with the septa in place. 2-D blank and transmission scans (septa extended) were used to reconstruct a 3-D attenuation map. Oblique lines of coincidence for which the attenuation correction factor had not been measured were obtained by forward projection through the 3-D map (53). After a 30-second delay, emission data were acquired in a 90-second frame, beginning 0 to 5 seconds before the rising phase of the head curve. The head curve recorded the whole brain net true count rate over time. The attenuation-corrected emission data were reconstructed as 31 axial planes by filtered back projection with a Hanning-filter of 0.5 cycles/pixel, giving a reconstructed transaxial resolution of 8.5-mm full width at half maximum. The reconstructed images contained 128×128 pixels, each measuring 2.09 $\times$ 2.09 mm.

Imaging Transformation

All calculations and image manipulations were carried out with Sun SPARC 2 computers (Sun Computers Europe Inc., Surrey, UK) using Analyze version 6.0 image display software (BRU, Mayo Foundation) (44) and PRO MATLAB (MathWorks, Inc., Natick, MA). Statistical maps of significant blood flow change were then derived using SPM software (MRC Cyclotron Unit, London, UK). The 31 contiguous 3.5-mm scan slices were interpolated to 43 planes. To correct for any head movement between scans, all head images were aligned on a voxel by voxel basis using a 3-D automated image registration algorithm (AIR) (56).

To facilitate group analysis, the intercommissural (AC-PC) line was identified (22) and the volume transformed into standard stereotactic space (50). The stereotactically normalized images contained 26 planes of $2 \times 2 \times 4$ mm voxels corresponding to the horizontal sections in the Talairach atlas. Each image was smoothed with a Gaussian filter of $10 \times 10 \times 6$ mm to increase signal to noise.

Statistical Analysis

We used statistical parametric mapping (SPM) for data analysis (19). The effect of variance in global on focal cerebral ^{15}O activity

at rest and on activation was removed following an analysis of covariance (20) and images were scaled to a global mean rCBF of 50 ml/100 ml/min. Normalized mean rCBF (relative rCBF: rrCBF) values and the associated variance of such mean rrCBF values across conditions were determined for each pixel in the 3-D data set.

To determine the volumes of significant activity elicited in the brain by the motor task within groups, the t statistic was applied to the mean rrCBF values obtained for each voxel for the four rest and four motor states. This generated a statistical parametric map (SPM{t}) of significant rrCBF changes associated with the motor task. In such an SPM{t} those voxels whose significance values exceed a defined threshold are displayed in three orthogonal projections. The level of the threshold is set to correct for the effective number of independent tests constituting the SPM, which is less than the actual number of voxels because neighboring voxels are not truly independent due to applied smoothing (21). The stereotactic coordinates of the most significant sites of change were determined and correlated with the stereotactic atlas (50). The voxels showing maximally significant motor task activation were used to estimate the change in normalized rCBF (rrCBF) due to smoothing: Such rrCBF changes corresponded to spherical regions of approximately 15 mm in diameter centered on the chosen coordinates.

We carried out a statistical analysis within and between groups. For the former we calculated SPMs comparing writing with rest, for the latter we calculated SPMs showing regions where rrCBF changes between the resting and the activated state were significantly different in patients compared to controls at a threshold of omnibus $p < 0.001$. Phantom studies suggest that this threshold avoids false positives (1). In this last analysis, the between-group comparison tests for differences in both amplitude and extent of activation for the two cohorts of subjects. It is most sensitive to differences in voxels where little activation occurred in one group and significant activation occurred in the other. This analysis explicitly tests for the interaction term reflecting a group difference in the rrCBF activations (6,8,31,55).

RESULTS

Task Performance

Idiopathic Torsion Dystonia

ITD patients made the same number of joystick movements as controls, but more incomplete movements. Patient 3 was the only one who had significant action dystonia in the performing hand during the task, and this patient displayed more errors than the other patients. However, control subject 4 made a similar percentage of errors and there was no significant difference between the groups. Mild dystonic posturing in the performing hand was recorded in patient 9 and discrete "overflow" into the legs was observed in patients 8 and 9. The mean response times were on average 16% slower in the ITD group ($p < 0.03$, paired t test).

Acquired Hemidystonia

The number of completed joystick movements and errors was similar in both groups although the AHD group were on average 53% slower when moving the dystonic arm and 12% slower when moving the "unaffected" arm compared to controls moving their dominant right hand. All patients displayed dystonic posturing during the task. This was severe in patients 1, 2, and 5. Patient 5 nevertheless was quicker than most controls in moving the joystick with both the dystonic and the "unaffected" arm. All patients displayed minor involuntary associated movements with the unaffected side when moving the dystonic arm. This was most apparent in patients 3, 4, and 5.

Writer's Cramp

Monitoring during the scan and counting the number of written words "dog" on the paper in relation to the number of the pacing tones showed that all WC patients and controls wrote the word "dog" with fewer than 5% omissions. The size of the script and the number of lines used for writing during the 100 seconds of writing (3 to 5) was not different for the two groups. Study of the videotape recordings during writing showed that time spent writing and initial writing posture was also similar in both groups. There was no evidence that normal volunteers spent more time waiting for cues than patients. Patients did not conspicuously raise their arm from the writing surface or interrupt their writing. However, patients 1 and 2 used excessive force to write and in all patients mild dystonic posturing was observed, most conspicuously in patient 5 where curling in of fingers III, IV, and V occurred.

Extent of Positron Emission Tomography Data

The data common to all subjects extended axially from 20 mm below to 68 mm above the intercommissural line. This field of view included both the superior cerebellum and SMA.

Idiopathic Torsion Dystonia

Comparing changes in rCBF associated with performance of the executive motor task with the right hand, the ITD patients showed enhanced activation in the following areas at a threshold of omnibus $p < 0.001$: left lateral premotor cortex (lateral area 6), rostral SMA (rostral medial area 6), mesial area 8, right dorsolateral prefrontal cortex (areas 9, 46), and anterior cingulate cortex (area 32). There was also enhanced activation of the left lentiform nucleus. At a lower threshold omnibus $p < 0.01$, enhanced activation for the patients in ITD was also seen in the right anterior insula, right medial temporal gyrus (area 21), and both lentiform nuclei (right 8 mm, left -8 to $+4$ mm relative to ACPC line) and bilateral lower premotor cortex (area 6) adjacent to insula. At a $p < 0.001$ level of significance, the patients showed impaired activation of caudal SMA (mesial area 6), posterior cingulate (area 31), and mesial parietal cortex (areas 5 and 7). At a lower threshold of $p < 0.01$ impaired activation was seen bilaterally in the shoulder area of SMC in ITD (Fig. 1).

A between-group comparison of activation changes in ITD patients compared to controls

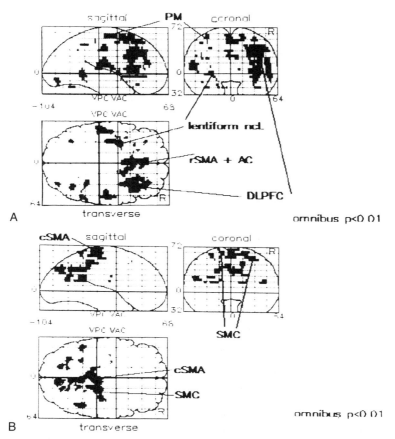

FIG. 1.   A and B: An SPM showing impaired and enhanced rCBF increases compared with controls when patients with ITD perform paced joystick movements in freely selected directions with the right hand. The results have been displayed as statistical maps in three projections: coronal, sagittal, and transverse according to the stereotactic space of the atlas of Talairach and Tournoux. The black areas show all voxels with statistically significant enhanced activation in the AHD group compared with the control group above a threshold of omnibus *p* <0.01. Areas showing no significant change are white. Each pixel in the whole-brain data set is displayed along the line of sight onto each of the three projections. In order to locate the position of a voxel, its position should be compared in each of the three different projections. Striatal, premotor, and prefrontal areas are relatively overactive in ITD **(A)** and motor executive cortex (caudal supplementary area and sensorimotor cortex) is underactive **(B)**. (From ref. 8, with permission.)

while imagining the movements versus rest did not yield any significant differences in patterns of activation between the groups. Both groups showed a similar activation pattern with activation in the following areas: occipital lobe (A18), left lentiform nucleus, left posterior thalamus, bilateral insula, bilateral parietal cortex, bilateral dorsolateral prefrontal cortex (areas 9, 46), rostral SMA, and lateral premotor cortex with sparing of SMC.

Acquired Hemidystonia

AHD patients using their dystonic arm showed enhanced activation compared with control subjects using their right arm in the following areas at a threshold of omnibus *p* <0.001: bilateral SMC, contralateral premotor cortex (lateral area 6), dorsal prefrontal cortex, insula and mesial superior parietal cortex, and ipsilateral cerebellum. At a lower threshold

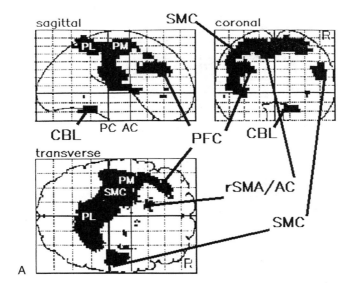

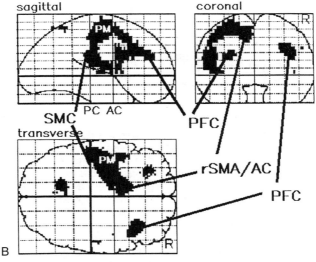

FIG. 2. A: AHD: enhanced activation—dystonic arm. Comparison of differences in levels of activation between five patients with AHD and five age-matched healthy controls during paced joystick movements with the dystonic arm in freely selected directions (omnibus *p* <0.01). **B:** AHD: enhanced activation—"normal" or unaffected arm. Comparison of differences in activation between five patients with AHD and five age-matched normal controls during paced joystick movements with the unaffected arm in freely selected directions (omnibus *p* <0.01). The images have been flipped before to make a comparison with the normal control group possible. PC, posterior commissure; AC, anterior commissure; PM, premotor cortex; rSMA, rostral SMA; AC, anterior cingulate; PFC, prefrontal cortex; SMC, sensorimotor cortex; PL, parietal cortex; CBL, cerebellum. (From ref. 6, with permission.)

Overactivity in patients before Botx versus controls

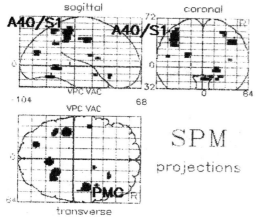

Overactivity in patients after Botx versus controls

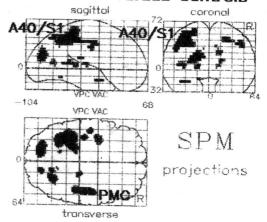

Underactivity in patients before Botx versus controls

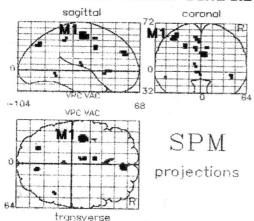

Underactivity in patients after Botx versus controls

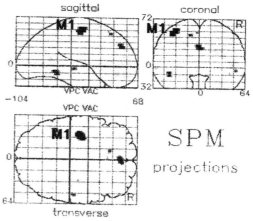

FIG. 3. Writer's cramp. Comparison of differences in levels of activation between six patients with writer's cramp before and five after BOTX versus six normal controls during paced stereotyped writing (omnibus $p < 0.001$). Note the expansion of the parietal cortex overactivity (mainly area 40 / S1) after successful BOTX therapy and the unaltered focus of underactivity in M1. PC, posterior commissure; AC, anterior commissure; A 40/ S1, area 40 / primary sensory cortex; M1, primary motor cortex; PMC, premotor cortex. (From ref. 11, with permission.)

omnibus $p < 0.01$, enhanced activation for the patients in AHD was also seen in the rostral SMA (mesial area 6), contralateral somatosensory area (SI/II), anterior cingulate (area 32), contralateral lower prefrontal, ipsilateral insula, and ipsilateral superior parietal. There was no significantly impaired activation. The AHD patients using the "unaffected" arm showed enhanced activation compared with control subjects in the following areas at a threshold of omnibus $p < 0.001$: contralateral premotor, ipsilateral dorsal prefrontal, and contralateral SMC. At a lower threshold omnibus $p < 0.01$, enhanced activation was also seen in the rostral SMA, anterior cingulate (area 32), contralateral insula/lower premotor and lower prefrontal, mesial parietal, and contralateral somatosensory area (SI/II). There was no significantly impaired activation (Fig. 2). Single subject analysis showed a similar pattern of cortical overactivity in the five AHD patients.

Writer's Cramp

Writing and simulating dystonic writing in controls led to a similar robust activation pattern involving the whole of the motor system. Stereotyped writing activated both dorsal prefrontal areas (right >>left), cingulate cortex, SMA, parietal cortex, the contralateral premotor cortex, sensorimotor cortex, both insulae, thalami, basal ganglia, and vermis. There was only a little ipsilateral premotor activation. In normal controls, writing in a dystonic posture increased the activation of ipsilateral parietal cortex and to a lesser degree orbitofrontal cortex, but not dorsal prefrontal areas or the basal ganglia.

Comparison of Writer's Cramp Patients before Botulinum Toxin with Controls

The WC patients compared with control subjects while writing showed enhanced activation in the following areas: ipsilateral lateral premotor cortex, lower premotor-insular cortex, superior mesial parietal, contralateral parietooccipital and parietal cortex (S1/area 40), and vermis. At a lower threshold of omnibus p <0.01, enhanced activation for the WC patients was also seen in the dorsal prefrontal cortex, contralateral lateral premotor, anterior cingulate, and rostral SMA (mesial area 6).

The WC patients showed impaired activation compared with control subjects of contralateral primary motor cortex, caudal SMA, mesial prefrontal, anterior cingulate, mesial parietal cortex (area 7/5), and thalamus. The primary motor cortex (M1) focus was located over the hand area of the precentral gyrus and extended toward the premotor cortex.

Comparison of Writer's Cramp Patients after Botulinum Toxin with Controls

The treated WC patients showed greater activation compared with control subjects while writing in contralateral insula and inferior premotor cortex, and ipsilateral inferior premotor cortex, bilateral parietal (area 40/S1) and ipsilateral posterior parietal, contralateral parietooccipital cortex and ipsilateral thalamus. At omnibus p <0.01 no increased activation of rostral SMA and dorsolateral prefrontal cortex (DLPFC) was evident.

Impaired activation compared with control subjects was detected in contralateral primary motor cortex, mesial prefrontal, and ipsilateral temporal cortex area 21/37.

Comparison of Writer's Cramp Patients before and after Botulinum Toxin Treatment

After BOTX patients showed enhanced activation compared with before treatment in the following areas: mesial parietal area 7, contralateral parietal S1/area 40, contralateral caudal SMA, and ipsilateral anterior insula and thalamus.

After treatment patients showed reduced activation of anterior cingulate, vermis, and right cerebellar hemisphere (Fig. 3).

DISCUSSION

This study of ITD when activity due to paced joystick movements in freely selected directions was compared with rest produced two main findings. First, rostral premotor areas (lateral area 6 and SMA), the dorsal prefrontal cortex, and lentiform nucleus showed a greater degree of activation than found for control subjects. Second, there was impaired activation of caudal SMA and sensorimotor cortex. A picture is therefore emerging in which dystonic limb movement appears to be associated with inappropriate overactivity of basal ganglia-frontal association area projections but underfunctioning of the primary executive areas (sensorimotor and caudal premotor cortex). The former may explain the involuntary movements and the latter the associated bradykinesia. The cause of this imbalance in cerebral function in ITD remains uncertain; the authors postulate that the pathology of dystonia may directly affect both the basal ganglia and motor executive cortex, disinhibiting function of the former and inhibiting function of the latter.

Is, then, inappropriate overactivity of rostral premotor and dorsal prefrontal cortex secondary to release of basal ganglia inhibition a common feature of all dystonic syndromes? In common with ITD, the acquired dystonia patients showed increased rostral premotor and DLPFC activation in association with arm movement. This was also evident in the hemisphere contralateral to the lesion. In contrast to the ITD patients, however, the secondary dystonia group showed raised rather than reduced primary motor cortex activation when moving the affected arm. We interpreted the common observations in ITD and AHD as being compatible with overactivity of accessory motor areas underlying dystonia, regardless of its etiology. However, in contrast to patients with ITD overactivity, rather than underactivity, of primary motor cortex was observed. This discrepancy may reflect the fact that the AHD patients had isolated structural basal ganglia or thalamic lesions disrupting striato-thalamic-frontal projections whereas in ITD cases the basal ganglia and motor cortex may both be affected by the pathology.

It could be argued that the overactivity of the rostral premotor and the DLPFC in dystonia patients on limb movement reflects the additional physical or mental effort required to overcome involuntary co-contraction. If additional mental effort were the reason for this enhanced activation of frontal areas, we would expect the same frontal areas to be overactive in patients with other disorders who also found the joystick task difficult, such as patients with Parkinson's disease and motor neuron disease. In fact these groups of patients showed underactivity in frontal association areas compared with controls (2,31). In Parkinson's disease patients activation of SMA and DLPFC could only be achieved after administration of dopaminergic agents re-

lieved the akinesia (2). Against increased physical effort being the cause of the frontal overactivity (6) are the results in patients with AHD. When these patients moved their "unaffected" hand, these movements were not associated with any increased effort and were performed with similar velocity and accuracy to controls, but led to overactivity of premotor and prefrontal cortex, possibly due to subcortical convergence of inappropriate commands to the other hemisphere secondary to the discrete basal ganglia or thalamic lesions. Finally, when normal controls simulate dystonic writing requiring increased effort there is also no increase in the level of DLPFC activation (5).

If frontal association area overactivity in dystonia does not reflect increased effort, does it represent inappropriate use of motor planning circuitry? Imagination of movements disassociates activity of the motor decision and executive systems (7). As with controls, imagination of limb movement in ITD led to significant activation of dorsolateral prefrontal and anterior supplementary motor areas, lentiform nucleus, but not sensorimotor cortex. No significant differences in levels of activated rCBF changes were found between the normal and dystonic cohorts suggesting that their ability to plan and prepare movements is preserved and that the main dysfunction in ITD lies within the motor executive system (7). By motor executive system we mean those cortical areas that have been specifically shown to have a level of activity dependent on the force, velocity, and frequency of movement in PET and nonhuman primate electrophysiology studies and which are not primarily associated with motor planning (13,27,35,48). These areas include the primary motor cortex and caudal SMA, but not rostral SMA or prefrontal areas.

Can the abnormality in idiopathic dystonia within the executive system be examined more closely? Moving a joystick in freely selected directions requires motor decision making, preparation, and execution and therefore does not focus on the executive motor system. Stereotyped, continuous writing in contrast is a complex but automatic and overlearned motor task requiring no decision making. During the joystick task, subjects could freely "think" for approximately 2 seconds about which of the four possible directions they would select to move the joystick once they heard the pacing tone (every 3 seconds) and then execute the movement as swiftly as possible. The executive component occupied only approximately 15% of the scanning time. The writer's cramp study focused on the motor executive system by keeping the task automatic and avoiding pauses in motor output.

Stereotyped writing was associated with pronounced activation of the motor system with robust responses in bilateral dorsal prefrontal areas, right more than left, anterior cingulate cortex, premotor cortex and SMA, parietal cortex, the contralateral sensorimotor cortex, both insulae, thalami, basal ganglia, and vermis.

There were three main findings (9) in the WC patients where dystonia was induced by continuous stereotyped writing and then relieved by transiently causing selective muscle weakness with BOTX injections: First, impaired activation of motor executive areas (primary motor cortex and caudal SMA) was found when dystonia is present. Second, comparing the patient group before and after BOTX, this treatment resulted in enhanced activation of parietal cortex and motor accessory areas, but failed to normalize the impaired activation of primary motor cortex. Third, frontal association areas and parietal association areas showed greater activation in writer's cramp patients than normal controls.

The overactivity of prefrontal association areas in WC was less conspicuous than in the studies on ITD using freely selected joystick movements as a paradigm. We assume that the predominantly executive, automatic, and overlearned task that was our writing paradigm attenuated the extent of the premotor and prefrontal overactivity. Because overactivity of DLPFC and rostral SMA was not evident after BOTX it could be argued that this prefrontal overactivity is a secondary rather than a primary phenomenon. The motor effort required in our writing task is far greater than that required for joystick movements; however our findings make it unlikely that the increased prefrontal activation seen during freely chosen joystick movements in ITD is an epiphenomenon.

The more demanding executive character of our writing task led to more obvious impairment of activation in the primary motor cortex M1 when WC as opposed to ITD patients were compared with controls. The underactivity of motor cortex in idiopathic dystonia has now been described in three different studies using different activation paradigms. It was described in two previous studies by Tempel and Perlmutter (51,52) where sensory pathways were activated with vibrotactile stimulation in patients with idiopathic dystonia and subsequently with a subgroup of patients with WC. Moreover, the underactivity in the primary motor cortex in our WC cases was not significantly altered by clinically effective BOTX injections when patients came back for rescanning. Could the reduced level of motor cortex activation in WC represent an epiphenomenon of dystonic posturing? If this were so, as the dystonia was abolished after BOTX, one would expect the reduced SMC activation to normalize, which it did not. Additionally, reduced motor cortex activation (Fig. 4) was not present in acquired dystonia due to basal ganglia lesions (6) or when healthy controls simulated dystonic posturing while writing (5). For these reasons, we regard the attenuated primary motor cortex activation in idiopathic dystonia as representing a primary deficit. Interestingly, caudal SMA activation responded to BOTX and so one possibility is that raised SMA activity may drive the motor improvement following this treatment.

Reduced motor cortex activation in ITD is in accord with electrophysiologic data: Deuschl et al. (14) studying patients with WC found an attenuation of the late phase of the Bereitschaftpotential prior to movement and suggested a deficiency of contralateral motor cortex activation just prior to the initiation of voluntary movements in patients with focal dystonia. The underactivity of motor cortex demonstrated with PET is synaptic and so

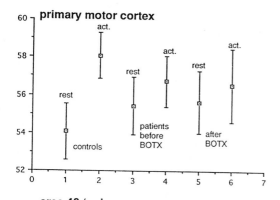

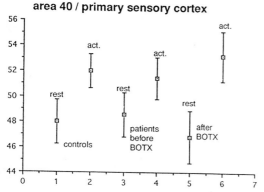

FIG. 4. Graphic representations of mean H₂¹⁵O uptake scaled as rCBF normalized to a global rCBF of 50 ml/100 ml/min with associated standard deviations in resting and activated states. The graphs illustrate the rCBF changes in the control group, and in the writer's cramp patient group before and after BOTX treatment at rest and during stereotyped writing. Areas contralateral to the writing arm *(right arm)* are depicted: primary motor cortex (−40, −12, 48), area 40 /primary sensory cortex (−22, −28, + 48). Note the similar impaired activation effects in M1 before and after BOTX and the enhancement in area 40 / S1 activation after successful BOTX therapy. Rest, resting state; act, activated state. (From ref. 11, with permission.)

could represent either reduced defective excitatory or inhibitory activity of intrinsic interneurons. Alternatively, it could represent decreased excitatory or inhibitory afferent input from SMA. As transcranial magnetic stimulation has suggested increased motor cortex excitability in WC (26) we postulate that the decreased activation we observe represents a

primary loss of interneuron inhibition of efferent projections from the premotor cortex and motor cortex to the spinal cord.

The therapeutic effects of BOTX in dystonia cannot be solely explained in terms of producing local weakness of the overactive muscles. Distant effects of BOTX injections are often observed, such as the improvement of oromandibular dystonia of Meige's syndrome after isolated periorbital injections to treat blepharospasm (4,17). "Diffusion" of the toxin to lower parts of the face may occur but there is no observable weakness of the oromandibular musculature, whereas weakness can be readily detected in the injected orbicularis oculi muscles. Gelb et al. (23) have suggested that central reorganization must take place after BOTX as the pattern of muscle activity changes in patients with cervical dystonia. It is thus likely that changes in afferent input occur and, if this is the case, there may be a neural substrate in the form of reorganization of cortical blood flow.

We found increased activation of premotor areas, primary sensory cortex, and posterior (area 7) and inferior parietal cortex (area 40) in the BOTX-treated group when compared with the same patient group of patients before BOTX. We know that there is reciprocal connectivity between primary sensory cortex and parietal areas 5, 7, and 40 (38). The posterior and inferior parietal areas represent secondary sensory association centers and their overactivity could be the result of reorganizational changes in primary sensory areas that project to these higher association centers. These changes may result from the blockade of the neuromuscular junction of the γ motor neurons, which is thought to lead to a reduction in spindle afferent activity (29). In rat masseter muscles it has been shown that BOTX consistently reduces the spindle afferent discharges (18).

Comparing the activation effects after BOTX treatment with the same group of patients before the injections we found enhanced activation in premotor areas, especially in caudal SMA. Caudal premotor accessory areas all have direct corticospinal projections (15) and could be directly affected by BOTX-induced disconnection with anterior horn cells. We feel, however, that the BOTX-induced overactivity of premotor areas is more likely to be secondary to the observed parietal release as parietal areas project directly to premotor cortex (39). An alternative explanation for the observed premotor and parietal overactivity after BOTX could be that it results from a change in movement strategy. The motor system may use a variety of different strategies to achieve the same final motor output. A change in strategy results from the weakness induced by BOTX requiring a degree of semiautomatic motor tasks such as writing.

A remote possibility is that the cortical flow changes found in our study following BOTX are related to the uptake of the light chain of the neurotoxin into the neuroaxis (42). It seems more likely, however, that the changes are a direct consequence of the BOTX-induced deafferentation of anterior horn cells and this would also be in accord with the cortical reorganization observed after denervation in traumatic upper limb amputees (32).

CONCLUSIONS

ITD, WC, and AHD are all associated with overactivity of premotor cortex. The functional substrate of dystonia appears to lie at the level of the motor executive rather than the motor planning system because imagination of movements is not affected in this disorder. The overactivity of frontal association areas may be the cause of the involuntary movements, represent an adaptive mechanism to aid in inhibiting dystonic movements, or simply be secondary to the excessive striatal output as observed in ITD. Underactivity of motor cortex is associated with idiopathic but not acquired dystonia secondary to discrete lesions in the lentiform nucleus or thalamus. This suggests that in idiopathic dystonia the basal ganglia and motor cortex are both affected by the pathology. The beneficial effects of BOTX in WC patients are associated with further overactivity of parietal association areas, possibly due to a change in movement strategy or more likely to cortical reorganization following deafferentation with anterior horn cells. These cortical changes may

in part be responsible for the symptomatic relief induced by BOTX treatment.

SUPPORT

Dr. Ceballos-Baumann was supported by Forschungsstipendium Ce 33/3-1 of the Deutsche Forschungsgemeinschaft, Bonn, and by Grant 9307059N of the Medical Research Council, London.

REFERENCES

1. Bailey DL, Jones T, Friston KJ, et al. Physical validation of statistical parametric mapping. *J Cereb Blood Flow Metab* 1991;11(Suppl 2):S150(abst).
2. Brooks DJ, Jenkins IH, Passingham RE. Positron emission tomography studies on regional cerebral control of voluntary movement. In: Mano N, Hamada I, De Long MR, eds. *Role of the cerebellum and basal ganglia in voluntary movement*. Amsterdam: Excerpta Medica, 1993:267–274.
3. Burton K, Farrell K, Li D, Calne DB. Lesions of the putamen and dystonia: CT and magnetic resonance imaging. *Neurology* 1984;34:962–965.
4. Ceballos-Baumann AO, Gasser T, Dengler R, Oertel WH. Lokale Injektionsbehandlung mit Botulinum-Toxin A bei Blepharospasmus, Meige Syndrom und Spasmus hemifacialis. Beobachtungen an 106 Patienten. *Nervenarzt* 1990;61:604–610.
5. Ceballos-Baumann AO, Passingham RE, Marsden CD, Brooks DJ. Differential brain activation in idiopathic and simulated writer's cramp: a PET study. *J Neurol* 1995;242[Suppl 2]:S47(abst).
6. Ceballos-Baumann AO, Passingham RE, Marsden CD, Brooks DJ. Motor reorganisation in acquired hemidystonia: a PET activation study. *Ann Neurol* 1995;37:746–757.
7. Ceballos-Baumann AO, Passingham RE, Stephan KM, et al. Cerebral activation with performing and imagining movement in idiopathic torsion dystonia (ITD): a PET study. *Neurology* 1994;44:837S(abst).
8. Ceballos-Baumann AO, Passingham RE, Warner T, et al. Overactivity of prefrontal and underactivity of motor cortical areas in idiopathic dystonia: a PET activation study. *Ann Neurol* 1995;37:363–372.
9. Ceballos-Baumann AO, Sheean G, Passingham RE, et al. Cerebral activation with stereotyped writing in patients with writer's cramp before and after botulinum toxin treatment: a PET study. *Neurology* 1995; 45 (suppl 4):8345(abst).
10. Ceballos-Baumann AO, Sheean G, Passingham RE, et al. Motor reorganisation after botulinum toxin treatment for writer's cramp: a PET study. *Mov Disord* 1995;10:389(abst).
11. Ceballos-Baumann AO, Sheean G, Passingham RE, et al. Botulinum toxin does not reverse the cortical dysfunction associated with writer's cramp: a PET study. *Brain* 1997; 120:571–582.
12. Chase TN, Tamminga CA, Burrows H. Positron emission tomographic studies of regional cerebral glucose

metabolism in idiopathic dystonia. *Adv Neurol* 1988;50:237–241.

13. Dettmers C, Fink GR, Lemon RN, et al. Relation between cerebral activity and force in the motor areas of the human brain. *J Neurophysiol* 1995;74:802–815.

14. Deuschl G, Toro C, Matsumoto J, Hallett M. Movement related cortical potentials in writer's cramp. *Ann Neurol* 1995;38:862–868.

15. Dum RP, Strick PL. The origin of corticospinal projections from the premotor areas in the frontal lobe. *J Neurosci* 1991;11:667–689.

16. Eidelberg D, Moeller JR, Ishikawa S, et al. The metabolic topography in idiopathic torsion dystonia. *Brain* 1995;118:1473–1484.

17. Elston JS. Long-term results of treatment of idiopathic blepharospasm with botulinum toxin injections. *Br J Ophthalmol* 1987;71:664–668.

18. Filippi GM, Errico P, Santarelli R, et al. Botulinum A toxin effects on rat jaw muscle spindles. *Acta Otolaryngol (Stockh)* 1993;113:400–404.

19. Friston KJ, Frackowiak RSJ. Imaging functional anatomy. In: Lassen NA, Ingvar DH, Raichle ME and Friberg L, eds. *Brain work and mental activity*. Copenhagen: Munksgaard, 1991:267–277.

20. Friston KJ, Frith CD, Liddle PF, et al. The relationship between global and local changes in PET scans. *J Cereb Blood Flow Metab* 1990;10:458–466.

21. Friston KJ, Frith CD, Liddle PF, Frackowiak RS. Comparing functional (PET) images: the assessment of significant change. *J Cereb Blood Flow Metab* 1991;11:690–699.

22. Friston KJ, Passingham RE, Nutt JG, et al. Localisation in PET images: direct fitting of the intercommissural (AC-PC) line. *J Cereb Blood Flow Metab* 1989;9:690–695.

23. Gelb DJ, Yoshimura DM, Olney RK, et al. Change in pattern of muscle activity following botulinum toxin injections for torticollis [see comments]. *Ann Neurol* 1991;29:370–376.

24. Gibb WR, Kilford L, Marsden CD. Severe generalised dystonia associated with a mosaic pattern of striatal gliosis. *Mov Disord* 1992;7:217–223.

25. Gilman S, Junck L, Young AB, et al. Cerebral metabolic activity in idiopathic dystonia studied with positron emission tomography. *Adv Neurol* 1988;50:231–236.

26. Ikoma K, Samii A, Mercuri B, et al. Abnormal motor excitability in dystonia. *Neurology* 1996;46:1371–1376.

27. Jenkins HJ, Passingham RE, Frackowiack RSJ, Brooks DJ. The effect of movement rate on cerebral activation: a study with positron emission tomography. *Mov Disord* 1994;9[Suppl 1]:P486.

28. Jenkins IH, Fernandez W, Playford EE, et al. Impaired activation of the supplementary motor area in Parkinson's disease is reversed when akinesia is treated with apomorphine. *Ann Neurol* 1992;32:749–757.

29. Kaji R, Shibasaki H, Kimura J. Writer's cramp: a disorder of motor subroutine [Editorial]. *Ann Neurol* 1995;38:837–838.

30. Karbe H, Holthoff VA, Rudolf J, et al. Positron emission tomography demonstrates frontal cortex and basal ganglia hypometabolism in dystonia. *Neurology* 1992;42:1540–1544.

31. Kew JJ, Leigh PN, Playford ED, et al. Cortical function in amyotrophic lateral sclerosis. A positron emission tomography study. *Brain* 1993;58:655–680.

32. Kew JJM, Ridding MC, Rothwell JC, et al. Reorganisation of cortical blood flow and transcranial magnetic stimulation maps in human subjects after upper limb amputation. *J Neurophysiol* 1994;2517–2524.

33. Kwiatkowski DJ, Ozelius L, Kramer PL, et al. Torsion dystonia genes in two populations confined to a small region on chromosome 9q32-34. *Am J Hum Genet* 1991;49:366–371.

34. Marsden CD, Obeso JA, Zarranz JJ, Lang AE. The anatomical basis of symptomatic hemidystonia. *Brain* 1985;108:463–483.

35. Matsuzaka Y, Aizawa H, Tanji J. A motor area rostral to the supplementary motor area (presupplementary motor area) in the monkey: neuronal activity during a learned motor task. *J Neurophysiol* 1992;68:653–662.

36. Nardone A, Mazzini L, Zaccala M. Changes in EMG response to perturbations and SEP's in a group of patients with idiopathic spasmodic torticollis. *Mov Disord* 1992;7(Suppl 1):125(abst).

37. Otsuka M, Ichiya Y, Shima F, et al. Increased striatal 18F-dopa uptake and normal glucose metabolism in idiopathic dystonia syndrome. *J Neurol Sci* 1992;111:195–199.

38. Pandya DN, Seltzer B. Intrinsic connections and architectonics of posterior parietal cortex in the rhesus monkey. *J Comp Neurol* 1982;204:196–210.

39. Petrides M, Pandya DN. Projections to the frontal lobe from the posterior-parietal region in the rhesus monkey. *J Comp Neurol* 1984;228:105–116.

40. Pettigrew LC, Jankovic J. Hemidystonia: a report of 22 patients and a review of the literature. *J Neurol Neurosurg Psychiatry* 1985;48:650–657.

41. Playford ED, Jenkins IH, Passingham RE, et al. Impaired mesial frontal and putamen activation in Parkinson's disease: a positron emission tomography study. *Ann Neurol* 1992;32:151–161.

42. Poulain B, Tauc L, Maisey EA, et al. Neurotransmitter release is blocked intracellularly by botulinum neurotoxin, and this requires uptake of both toxin polypeptides by a process mediated by the larger chain. *Proc Natl Acad Sci USA* 1988;85:4090–4094.

43. Reilly JA, Hallett M, Cohen LG, et al. The N30 component of somatosensory evoked potentials in patients with dystonia. *Electroencephalogr Clin Neurophysiol* 1992;84:243–247.

44. Robb RA, Hanson DP. A software system for interactive and quantitative visualization of multidimensional biomedical images. *Australas Phys Eng Sci Med* 1991;14:9–30.

45. Rothwell JC, Day BL, Obeso JA, et al. Reciprocal inhibition between muscles of the human forearm in normal subjects and in patients with idiopathic torsion dystonia. *Adv Neurol* 1988;50:133–140.

46. Silbersweig D, Stern E, Frith CD, et al. Detection of thirty-second cognitive activations in single subjects with positron emission tomography: a new low dose H215O regional cerebral blood flow three-dimensional imaging technique. *J Cereb Blood Flow Metab* 1993;13:617–629.

47. Spinks TJ, Jones T, Bailey DL, et al. Physical performance of a positron emission tomograph for brain imaging with retractable septa. *Phys Med Bull* 1992;37:1637–1655.

48. Stephan KM, Fink GR, Passingham RE, et al. Functional anatomy of the mental representation of upper

extremity movements in healthy subjects. *J Neurophysiol* 1995;73:373–386.

49. Stoessl AJ, Martin W, Clark C, et al. PET studies of cerebral glucose metabolism in idiopathic torticollis. *Neurology* 1986;36:653–657.

50. Talairach J, Tournoux P. *Co-planar stereotaxic atlas of the human brain.* Stuttgart, New York: Thieme, 1988.

51. Tempel LW, Perlmutter JS. Abnormal vibration-induced cerebral blood flow responses in idiopathic dystonia. *Brain* 1990;113:691–707.

52. Tempel LW, Perlmutter JS. Abnormal cortical responses in patients with writer's cramp. *Neurology* 1993;43:2252–2257.

53. Townsend DW, Geissbuhler A, Defrise M, et al. Fully three-dimensional reconstruction for a PET camera with retractable septa. *IEEE Trans Med Imaging* 1991; 10:505–512.

54. Warner TT, Fletcher NA, Davis MB, et al. Linkage analysis in British and French families with idiopathic torsion dystonia. *Brain* 1993;58:739–744.

55. Weiller C, Chollet F, Friston KJ, et al. Functional reorganization of the brain in recovery from striato-capsular infarction in man. *Ann Neurol* 1992;31: 463–472.

56. Woods RP, Cherry SR, Mazziotta JC. Rapid automated algorithm for aligning and reslicing PET images. *J Comput Assist Tomogr* 1992;16:620–633.

57. Zweig RM, Hedreen JC, Jankel WR, et al. Pathology in brainstem regions of individuals with primary dystonia. *Neurology* 1988;38:702–706.

Dystonia 3: Advances in Neurology, Vol. 78,
edited by S. Fahn, C. D. Marsden, and M. DeLong
Lippincott–Raven Publishers, Philadelphia © 1998

16

Advanced Neuroimaging Methods in the Study of Movement Disorders: Dystonia and Blepharospasm

*John C. Mazziotta, †Michael Hutchinson, ‡Terry D. Fife, and §Roger Woods

Division of Brain Mapping, Departments of Neurology, Radiological Sciences, and Molecular and Medical Pharmacology, UCLA School of Medicine, Los Angeles, California 90024; †Departments of Neurology and Radiology, New York University Medical Center, New York, New York 10016; ‡Department of Neurology, Barrow Neurological Institute, University of Arizona College of Medicine, Phoenix, Arizona 85013; and §Division of Brain Mapping, Department of Neurology, UCLA School of Medicine, Los Angeles, California 90024.

Movement disorders, in general, and dystonia, in particular, represent a diverse and heterogeneous set of nervous system dysfunctions. With regard to dystonic syndromes, neuroimaging techniques have not, to date, provided consistent results that have added new insights into the cause of these disorders or new directions for their treatment. This is due, in part, to the fact that most methods used to date in the evaluation of patients with dystonic syndromes have had relatively low spatial and temporal resolution and the methods used to study patients among laboratories have varied greatly. This is true both for structural imaging with X-ray computed tomography (CT) and magnetic resonance imaging (MRI) as well as for functional imaging with positron emission tomography (PET) and single photon emission computed tomography (SPECT).

Another reason for the lack of consistent results stems from the heterogeneous nature of the disorders themselves. Both primary idiopathic dystonias as well as secondary forms can present in a wide variety of ways reflecting a diverse and largely unknown set of etiologies (1,19,20,22,24,34,35). Further complicating the picture is the fact that patients can be studied at different stages in their disorders, with varying degrees of severity, and in a wide range of behavioral states. In most cases, subjects have been studied in "resting" conditions where the behavioral state of the patient is largely undefined except for the fact that they were not instructed to perform a specific task. Modern structural and functional neuroimaging techniques employ methods with improved spatial resolution as well as much more well-developed paradigms for selecting homogeneous groups of patients, studying them under well-defined and controlled conditions, and analyzing the resulting data with tools better suited for finding abnormalities in distributed systems that span many neuroanatomic sites (33).

Dystonic syndromes that occur secondary to structural lesions in the brain have been well documented with conventional CT and MRI techniques (29). These would include cerebral hemorrhages, trauma, and infarctions.

Modern neuroimaging approaches to the study of movement disorders and dystonic syndromes should provide greater insight into their causes and allow for the monitoring of experimental therapies developed for their treatment. These techniques will also allow for the exploration and examination of hypotheses that have a role in causing these abnormal involuntary movements. For example, the concept that plastic reorganization in the adult brain may, in part, induce the chronic movement disorders seen in dystonic patients has recently been put forward (3) and can be examined and rigorously studied in humans using functional imaging techniques.

In this chapter, advanced neuroimaging methods of use in the study of dystonic syndromes are discussed with regard to both structure and function. Blepharospasm and Meige's syndrome are used to illustrate a novel behavioral paradigm used to explore these particular movements.

ADVANCED STRUCTURAL AND FUNCTIONAL IMAGING TECHNIQUES

Structure

Methods

Current MRI produces the most detailed, high-resolution images of the human brain *in vivo*. Even with the high spatial resolution and contrast-to-noise ratio available with modern conventional MRI units, the selective differentiation of thalamic subnuclei and subregions of the basal ganglia and brainstem have not yet been possible. Two approaches are being explored to increase both the spatial resolution and contrast-to-noise ratio with MRI imaging. The first involves the use of higher field magnets with dedicated head coils. The second involves signal averaging of repeated imaging sessions of the same subject. This latter technique is analogous to evoked potential averaging of electroencephalographic (EEG) data where the averaging process enhances the true signal as the random noise and unrelated events are diminished in their magnitude.

High-Field MRI Imaging

Conventional MRI devices operate at 1.5 Tesla (T). With such a device excellent images of normal neuroanatomy and detailed imaging of pathologic processes are possible in *in vivo* human studies. The use of higher field magnets with proper radiofrequency head coils and pulse sequences can extend this already excellent performance to an even greater range. Research MRI devices, functioning from 3 to 5 T, have been built and are in experimental use. Experience with a 3-T device in our own laboratory demonstrates the capacity of the instrument to produce images showing substructures of the hippocampus (Fig. 1) as well as details of the thalamus, basal ganglia, and brainstem. High spatial resolution coupled with good contrast-to-noise ratios makes such an approach both feasible and practical. When combined with echo planar imaging capabilities, these image sets can be obtained not only at high quality but also rapidly in time (e.g., as fast as a tenth of a second).

Magnetic Resonance Image Averaging

Signal averaging is a common data processing technique that enhances the sensitivity to detect events embedded in background noise. A common example of this approach in neurologic diagnoses is the EEG evoked potential. In this technique, EEG data acquired during stimulus presentation are averaged, in a time-locked fashion, during many repetitions of the stimulus presentation. The resultant event-related potentials emerge from the EEG data as the random activity in the EEG is minimized by the averaging process. Thus, despite the fact that in a single trial, the event-related signal would be undetectable, a clear electrophysiologic response can be identified relative to the stimulus presentation.

The same approach can be applied to imaging data. Previous attempts to achieve this signal enhancement with MRI data have not proven very fruitful. Capitalizing on the idea that this lack of signal enhancement may be due to physiologic and voluntary motion by the subject during the long MRI acquisition period, Holmes and colleagues (15,16) aligned and registered data sets acquired from the same subject during 16 identical MRI data acquisitions. Resultant MRI averaged images reveal

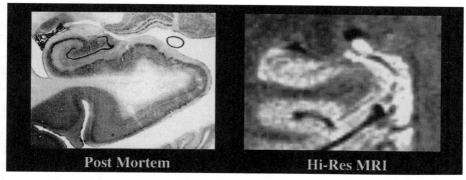

FIG. 1. Hippocampal anatomy. **A:** Normal hippocampus seen in coronal section from a postmortem specimen process with Weil stain. Notice the detailed substructures within the hippocampus. **B:** Coronal image of a normal adult volunteer acquired using MRI at 3 T. Note the detailed anatomy of the hippocampal substructures including white matter and cellular layers. When compared with the postmortem specimen, it is clear that the anatomic resolution of high-field MRI approaches that of histologic analysis. Images courtesy of Mark Cohen, Ph.D., and Susan Bookheimer, Ph.D., of UCLA.

remarkably improved anatomic detail and spatial resolution. They demonstrate clear enhancement over the raw data acquired in any given image set. Thus, such an approach can be used to improve spatial resolution and the image quality of *in vivo* MRI data acquisitions, providing increased anatomic detail in the evaluation of patients with movement disorders and dystonic syndromes. With this technique, substructure of the thalamus and basal ganglia can be identified, bridging gray matter that spans the anterior limb of the internal capsule between the caudate and putamen can be seen, and the separation between putamen, external capsule, claustrum, and extreme capsule can be identified.

The practical disadvantage to this approach is the fact that 16 separate MRI data acquisition periods were required to realize this improved image quality. Given the relatively long image acquisition time required in conventional MRI scanning, such an approach would be generally impractical. Fortunately, the development of echo planar imaging drastically reduces the data acquisition time for MRI. Because echo planar hardware and algorithms are increasingly available on conventional MRI devices, for the purposes of functional MRI, data acquisition times will fall precipitously.

Thus, with short (a few seconds per image set) data acquisition times, averaged MRI data sets should be acquired in the same or less time than a single conventional imaging session. The result is improved spatial resolution acquired in a faster time frame.

Applications

The increased spatial resolution available through the use of either of the above techniques, or both combined, should provide the most detailed anatomic images of structures important in the evaluations of dystonic syndromes in patients during life. Specifically, high-resolution images of the basal ganglia should provide specific information about the size, shape, volume, and orientation of the putamen, globus pallidus, caudate, substantia nigra, and the fiber pathways that surround and connect them. The same is true for the subnuclei of the thalamus, particularly the ventrolateral and ventroanterior nuclei. High-resolution imaging of the brainstem and cerebellum may be able to identify specific nuclear complexes in terms of volume and shape. All of these measurements will be made more sensitive by comparing left/right asymmetries in patients with asymmetric dystonic syndromes.

Functional Imaging

Methods

Current neuroimaging methods of use in the evaluation of movement disorders include functional MRI (fMRI), magnetic resonance spectroscopy (MRS), PET, and SPECT (33). Functional MRI provides semiquantitative estimates of changes in blood flow based on differences in venous oxygen concentrations when brain regions are compared in two different states. Rapid growth of this technique and its increasing availability using conventional MRI devices modified for the method, should make this an attractive means of evaluating patients once appropriate diagnostic criteria are developed. The strategy for its use dictates the requirement for comparing two states. Sample strategies are provided below.

PET and SPECT both employ the administration, either by intravenous injection or inhalation, of radioactive compounds that trace physiologic pathways in the human brain. Both techniques are capable of measuring cerebral perfusion, either in a single state or in the same comparative fashion discussed above for fMRI (10,23). In addition, PET can measure the extraction and metabolism of oxygen and glucose (17), protein synthesis, amino acid uptake, and cerebral pH. Both PET and SPECT can be used with radiolabeled ligands to evaluate presynaptic neurotransmitter integrity (e.g., dopaminergic) (28,32) or postsynaptic receptor function (2,36). An ever-increasing number of both pre- and postsynaptic tracers have been developed for both techniques, thereby increasing the number of neurochemical systems that can be assayed using these functional imaging methods. PET produces data that are quantitative, uniform in resolution across the field of view, and employ positron-emitting isotopes with short half-lives (2 minutes to 2 hours, typically). More expensive than SPECT, access to PET centers is generally limited to larger medical centers and requires the close proximity of a cyclotron capable of producing positron-emitting isotopes.

The spatial resolution of SPECT imaging is somewhat less than that of PET and the technique is less rigorously quantitative. Measurements of oxygen or glucose metabolism have not yet been developed. Nevertheless, SPECT instruments are available in most hospital settings and the single photon emitting radioisotopes are produced commercially and can be purchased on a regional or national basis.

Magnetic resonance spectroscopy allows for the assay of specific chemical compounds in the brain without the requirement for administering ionizing radiation. Most typically, proton spectroscopy is used because of its higher signal and because modifications of conventional MRI devices allow them to make such measurements. Nevertheless, the spatial resolution with this technique is low compared with PET or SPECT. No consistent proton spectroscopy data are currently valuable in patients with dystonic syndromes. Spectroscopic measurement of sodium, phosphorus, and other elements requires specialized hardware and is still in developmental stages but promises to provide an even broader range of *in vivo* chemical assays.

Functional Imaging Strategies

The typical functional imaging strategy to increase the detection sensitivity for brain abnormalities has been to compare two different states in the same subject, thereby utilizing the subject or patient as his or her own control (10,23) (Table 1). This approach has been the mainstay for evaluating normal brain function, in which a reference state is compared to a stimulated state (e.g., eyes closed versus eyes open). Studies of this type have provided insights into the complexities of the distributed motor system, its topographic organization, and the centers in the brain important for initiating, executing, and maintaining voluntary movements (12,13). The same strategy can be used in patients with dystonic syndromes to compare cerebral networks that govern the abnormal movements. Functional imaging observations have been obtained in patients with dystonia in terms of blood flow (4,5,26), glucose metabolism (6,9,11,18,21,31), and neurotransmitter systems (25,30,32).

TABLE 1. *List of behavioral paradigms and states useful in evaluating patients with movement disorders and dystonia when employing functional imaging techniques*

Resting studies in normals
"Activation" tasks in normal subjects
"Activation" tasks in patient groups
Sleep-wake studies in normal subjects and patients
Comparison of involuntary movements vs. normal states in patients with episodic movement disorders
Comparison of topographic sensory and motor representations in normal subjects vs. movement disorder patients

Although the study of voluntary movements in patients with dystonia should prove increasingly insightful, it is also possible to compare different degrees of abnormal involuntary movements in the same patient. One approach is to evaluate the patients in an awake state that minimizes movements compared with a state where movements are maximized. Typical of most movement disorders, involuntary movements are minimized when patients are relaxed, nonstressed, and in specific postures. Imaging under these conditions could provide a reference state with minimal movements. Conversely, a stressful environment, postures that maximize the movements, and other provocations will provide a target state where, for a given patient, involuntary movements are maximized. Comparison of these two states should provide insights into the brain networks that cause or produce the involuntary activity. By studying populations of patients where the differential between the minimal and maximal degree of movements varies, a graded distribution of system involvement can be developed.

A further extrapolation of the minimization-maximization strategy is to compare patients with involuntary movements in the awake state when the movements are occurring versus sleep where involuntary movements typically cease. There are three important prerequisites for the use of this strategy. First, there should be no consistent focal functional changes between wake and sleep conditions in normal subjects. This condition has been satisfied by studies in our own laboratory (18) as well as

others (14). Second, differential changes between the wake and sleep states in movement disorder patients must be focal rather than global because, in the latter case, global normalization of data required for between-state comparisons will dilute or eliminate the opportunity to detect widely distributed changes between the two conditions. Finally, rigorous methods must be available to precisely align and register data sets from the same subject between states. This criterion has been satisfied by the development of such appropriate algorithms (38). An example of the use of the wake-sleep paradigm for evaluating movement disorders is discussed below in the section on Meige's syndrome.

BLEPHAROSPASM AND MEIGE'S SYNDROME

In order to evaluate the sleep-wake strategy, a comparative study between the two states was performed in patients with Meige's syndrome and in normal age-matched controls using PET measurements of cerebral glucose metabolism (18). Six patients had blepharospasm and dystonia of the muscles of the neck or larynx (mean age 69, range 67 to 72 years). None had a prior history of neurologic disorders or neuroleptic exposure prior to the onset of involuntary movements. The duration of their syndrome ranged from 3 to 14 years. All had obtained some degree of relief from botulinum toxin injections and the time from their last treatment ranged from a few days to 14 weeks. Two patients had torticollis to the right, three had spasmodic dysphonia, and three had diminished left arm swing. Three patients were on oral medications [triazolam (Halcion), amitriptyline hydrochloride (Elavil), clonazepam (Klonopin), baclofen] but these medications were discontinued 12 hours prior to imaging. Six normal controls (mean age 66, range 57 to 72 years) were identified. None had a history of neurologic or neuropsychiatric disorders. All had normal general medical and neurologic examinations. Both patients and controls had normal T1-weighted MRI studies.

Three-dimensional PET studies (7,8) were performed with fluorine-18 fluorodeoxyglucose (FDG). During the FDG uptake period subjects were videotaped. The first scan was performed in the wake state and the second scan was performed during sleep, after a night of sleep deprivation. In the sleep study, the stages of sleep were determined by simultaneous EEG monitoring and the injection of FDG occurred after the subject was in stage 2 sleep by EEG criteria.

Sleep studies were registered to the wake studies and the two data sets for each subject were then globally normalized by obtaining an overall value for all data points within an outer cerebral boundary obtained at every tomographic plane. A ratio of global values between the wake-sleep studies was used to normalize the sleep study to be equivalent to that of the wake study. Data sets from the two states were then subtracted to give differential maps of relative hyper- or hypometabolism between the two states. The subtracted images were superimposed on each subject's MRI scan and regions of interest were then drawn for specific cortical and subcortical zones. Because of the limited axial field of view, regions of interest for the cerebellum and brainstem could only be obtained in four of the six subjects. Patient values were compared with results from control subjects using two-tailed t tests. For the cerebellar values in the Meige group, the Mann-Whitney rank-sum test was used for data comparison because these values were not normally distributed.

Sleep-wake subtraction studies in normal subjects did not show any areas of focal change. In both the patients and the controls, the PET findings were remarkably symmetric despite the fact that several patients had asymmetries in their neurologic examination. In the patient group, two structures showed significant deviation from the normal population. Both the thalamus ($p < 0.006$) and the cerebellum ($p < 0.03$) had relative hypometabolism compared with control subjects in the sleep state. Because the cerebellar studies were only available in a subset of the patient group, these results must be considered with caution.

It is important to note that the relative metabolic changes in the thalamus and cerebellum seen in the patient group were not readily apparent in the wake study alone. The use of the wake-sleep subtraction studies allowed these observations to be made and evaluated as significant. It should also be noted that the three criteria for performing valid wake-sleep studies were met in this initial experiment. First, no focal metabolic changes were seen during sleep in normal subjects. Changes were limited to -0.5% and $+1.8\%$, confirming previous findings by Heiss and coworkers (14). Second, focal changes were identified in the patient studies in two brain regions. Third, valid and accurate alignment of registration methods exist for the presubtraction alignment of data (38).

These results indicate the potential of functional imaging, here demonstrated with PET but also possible with SPECT and fMRI, to reveal cerebral circuitry of importance in movement disorders and for suggesting plausible pathophysiologic mechanisms that underlie them. The sleep-wake paradigm can detect small but significant changes that can be of biological importance in understanding the pathophysiology of these complex and heterogeneous movement disorders syndromes.

NEUROPLASTICITY AS A POTENTIAL MECHANISM IN THE PRODUCTION OF DYSTONIA

The wealth of information derived from animal studies [see Byl et al. (3) for review] indicates that normal learning can result in changes in the somatosensory representation of appropriate cortical regions. More recently, it has been proposed that repetitive strain injuries can produce learning-induced dedifferentiation of the representation of primary sensory-motor cortex in adult monkeys (3). These investigators demonstrated that repetitive movements produced in a specific form and in an appropriate behavioral context caused a degradation of sensory-controlling fine motor movements. This resulted in a movement control disorder in monkeys and a reorganization of the primary somatosensory cortical areas. That is, primary somatosensory cortex was dedifferentiated for cortical representations of the skin of the hand manifested by receptive fields that were ten to 20 times larger than normal and the emergence of receptor fields that covered the entire glabrous surface of individual digits. Further, this paradigm resulted in a breakdown of the normal sharp segregation of somatosensory areas of the hand leading to locally shifted receptive field topography with many digit fields overlapping. The authors concluded that cortical plasticity and learning-based dedifferentiation of sensory feedback information from the hand could contribute to the genesis of occupationally derived repetitive strain injuries and produce focal dystonia.

With functional imaging it is possible to examine both the primary motor and sensory cortical representation in larger mammals and humans. Further, plastic changes induced by normal learning (12,13,27) can be examined using PET or fMRI. Studies in patients recovering from acute cerebral injury (i.e., subcortical cerebral infarction) can also be examined for reorganizational changes that coincide with reacquisition of function in the face of injury (37).

Thus, functional imaging can be used to test the hypothesis put forth by Byl and colleagues (3) in human subjects with specific types of focal or generalized dystonia. Namely, comparison of representative primary somatosensory areas in patients with the syndrome can be compared objectively and quantitatively with normal subjects during the performance of fine motor control movements or other motor tasks. Such studies should lead to an objective measure by which the evaluation of this hypothesis can be tested and either validated or refuted.

CONCLUSION

Functional imaging is a rapidly developing set of methodologies of proven value in investigating normal brain function, organization, and task-related activity as well as pathologic states that can alter these variables. When used with the appropriate behavioral paradigms and analysis methods, such techniques can be extremely valuable in investigating the underlying pathophysiology of movement disorders, in general, and dystonic syndromes, in particular. The use of a wake-sleep paradigm may be particularly instructive in identifying the underlying neuronal networks that subserve these pathologic states. Further, such methods can be employed to validate or refute hypotheses put forth about the cause of acquired dystonic syndromes including the concept that learning-induced dedifferentiation of somatosensory cortex may be a contributing factor.

ACKNOWLEDGMENTS

We would like to thank Simon Cherry, Ph.D., for his assistance with three-dimensional PET reconstructions; Daniel Truong, M.D., for his referral of patients and for his suggestions to treat one patient with tetrabenazine; N. Satymurthy, Ph.D., and Jorge Barrio, Ph.D., for preparation of FDG; S. C. Huang, D.Sc., for the use of his software to calculate absolute glucose metabolic rates; Deborah Dorsey, R.N., for patient management; and Ron Sumida and Larry Pang for technical assistance. Thanks are also extended to the Benign Essential Blepharospasm Research Foundation, The Ahmanson Foundation, the Brain Mapping Medical Research Organization, and the Pierson-Lovelace Foundation for their generous support of Brain Mapping activities at UCLA.

REFERENCES

1. Altrocchi PH, Forno LS. Spontaneous oral-facial dyskinesia: neuropathology of a case. *Neurology* 1983;33:802–805.
2. Andersson U, Eckernas S-A, Hartvig P, Ulin J, Langstrom B, Haggstrom JE. Striatal binding of ^{11}C-NMSP studied with positron emission tomography in patients with persistent tardive dyskinesia: no evidence for altered dopamine D2 receptor binding. *J Neural Transm* 1990;79:215–226.
3. Byl NN, Merzenich MM, Jenkins WM. A primate genesis model of focal dystonia and repetitive strain injury: I. Learning-induced dedifferentiation of the representation of the hand in the primary somatosensory cortex in adult monkeys. *Neurology* 1996;47:508–520.
4. Ceballos-Baumann AO, Passingham RE, Marsden CD, Brooks DJ. Motor reorganization in acquired hemidystonia. *Ann Neurol* 1995;37:746–757.

5. Ceballos-Baumann AO, Passingham RE, Warner T, Playford ED, Marsden CD, Brooks DJ. Overactive prefrontal and underactive motor cortical areas in idiopathic dystonia. *Ann Neurol* 1995;37:364–372.

6. Chase TN, Tamminga CA, Burrows H. Positron emission tomographic studies of regional cerebral glucose metabolism in idiopathic dystonia. *Adv Neurol* 1988; 50:237–241.

7. Cherry SR, Dahlbom M, Hoffman EJ. 3D PET using a conventional multislice tomograph without septa. *J Comput Assist Tomogr* 1991;15:655–668.

8. Cherry SR, Woods RP, Hoffman EJ, Mazziotta JC. Improved detection of focal cerebral blood flow changes using three-dimensional positron emission tomography. *J Cereb Blood Flow Metab* 1993;13:630–638.

9. Eidelberg D, Moeller JR, Ishikawa T, et al. The metabolic topography of idiopathic torsion dystonia. *Brain* 1995;118:1473–1484.

10. Fox PT, Mintun MA, Raichle ME, Herscovitch P. A noninvasive approach to quantitative functional brain mapping with $H_2^{15}O$ and positron emission tomography. *J Cereb Blood Flow Metab* 1984;4:329–333.

11. Gilman S, Junck L, Young AB, et al. Cerebral metabolic activity in idiopathic dystonia studied with positron emission tomography. *Adv Neurol* 1988;50:231–236.

12. Grafton ST, Mazziotta JC, Presty S, Friston KJ, Frackowiak RSJ, Phelps ME. Functional anatomy of human procedural learning determined with regional cerebral blood flow and PET. *J Neurosci* 1992;12: 2542–2548.

13. Grafton ST, Mazziotta JC, Woods R, Phelps ME. Human functional anatomy of visually guided finger movements. *Brain* 1992;115:565–587.

14. Heiss WD, Pawlik G, Herholz K, Wagner R, Weinhard K. Regional cerebral glucose metabolism in man during wakefulness, sleep and dreaming. *Brain Res* 1985; 327:362–366.

15. Holmes CJ, Hoge R, Collins L, Evans A. Enhancement of T_1 MR images using registration for signal averaging. *NeuroImage* 1996;3:S28.

16. Holmes CJ, MacDonald D, Sled JG, Toga AW, Evans AC. Cortical peeling: CSF/gray/white matter boundaries visualized by nesting isosurfaces. In: Heinz K, Kikinis R, eds. *Visualization in Biomedical Computing*. New York: Springer, 1996:99–104.

17. Huang SC, Phelps ME, Hoffman EJ, et al. Noninvasive determination of local cerebral metabolic rate of glucose in man. *Am J Physiol* 1980;238: E69–E82.

18. Hutchinson M, Fife T, Woods R, Mazziotta JC. Glucose metabolism in craniocervical dystonia (Meige Syndrome). *Mov Disord (submitted)*.

19. Jankovic J, Ford J. Blepharospasm and orofacial-cervical dystonia: clinical and pharmacological findings in 100 patients. *Ann Neurol* 1983;13:402–411.

20. Jankovic J, Patel SC. Blepharospasm associated with brainstem lesions. *Neurology* 1983;33:1237–1240.

21. Karbe H, Holthoff VA, Rudolf J, Herholz K, Heiss WD. Positron emission tomography demonstrates frontal cortex and basal ganglia hypometabolism in dystonia. *Neurology* 1992;42:1540–1544.

22. Kullisevsky J, Marti MJ, Ferrer I, Tolosa E. Meige syndrome: neuropathology of a case. *Mov Disord* 1988;3:170–175.

23. Mazziotta JC, Huang SC, Phelps ME, Carson RE, MacDonald NS, Mahoney K. A noninvasive positron CT technique using oxygen-15 labeled water for the evaluation of neurobehavioral task batteries. *J Cereb Blood Flow Metab* 1985;5:70–78.

24. Meige H. Les convulsions de la face: une forme clinique de confulsion faciale, bilaterale et mediane. *Rev Neurol* 1910;10:437–443.

25. Playford ED, Fletcher NA, Sawle GV, Marsden CD, Brooks DJ. Striatal (^{18}F) dopa uptake in familial idiopathic dystonia. *Brain* 1993;116:1191–1199.

26. Perlmutter JS, Raichle ME. Pure hemidystonia with basal ganglion abnormalities on positron emission tomography. *Ann Neurol* 1984;15:228–233.

27. Raichle ME, Feiz JA, Videen TO. Practice-related changes in human brain functional anatomy during nonmotor learning. *Cereb Cortex* 1994;4:8–26.

28. Sawle GV, Leenders KL, Brooks DJ, et al. Dopa-responsive dystonia: (^{18}F)Dopa positron emission tomography. *Ann Neurol* 1991;30:24–30.

29. Schneider S, Feifel E, Ott D, Schumacher M, Lucking CH, Deuschl G. Prolonged MRI T_2 times of the lentiform nucleus in idiopathic spasmodic torticollis. *Neurology* 1994;44:846–850.

30. Snow B, Nygaard TG, Takahashi H, Calne DB. Positron emission tomographic studies of dopa-responsive dystonia and early-onset idiopathic parkinsonism. *Ann Neurol* 1993;34:734–738.

31. Stoessl AJ, Martin WR, Clark C, et al. PET studies of cerebral glucose metabolism in idiopathic torticollis. *Neurology* 1986;36:653–657.

32. Takahashi H, Levine RA, Galloway MP, Snow BJ, Calne DB, Nygaard TG. Biochemical and fluorodopa positron emission tomographic findings in an asymptomatic carrier of the gene for dopa-responsive dystonia. *Ann Neurol* 1994;35:354–356.

33. Toga AT, Mazziotta JC. *Brain mapping: the methods.* San Diego: Academic Press, 1996.

34. Tolosa E, Kulisevsky J, Fahn S. Meige syndrome: primary and secondary forms. *Adv Neurol* 1988;50: 509–515.

35. Tolosa E, Marti MJ. Blepharospasm-oromandibular dystonia syndrome (Meige's syndrome): clinical aspects. *Adv Neurol* 1988;49:73–84.

36. Weeks RA, Piccini P, Harding AE, Brooks DJ. Striatal D1 and D2 dopamine receptor loss in asymptomatic mutation carriers of Huntington's disease. *Ann Neurol* 1996;40:49–54.

37. Weiller C, Ramsay SC, Wise RJ, Friston KJ, Frackowiak RS. Individual patterns of functional reorganization in the human cerebral cortex after capsular infarction. *Ann Neurol* 1993;33:181–189.

38. Woods RP, Mazziotta JC, Cherry SR. MRI-PET registration with automated algorithm. *J Comput Assist Tomogr* 1993;17:536–546.

Dystonia 3: Advances in Neurology, Vol. 78,
edited by S. Fahn, C. D. Marsden, and M. DeLong
Lippincott–Raven Publishers, Philadelphia © 1998

17

Decreased [18F]Spiperone Binding in Putamen in Dystonia

*†Joel S. Perlmutter, *Mikula K. Stambuk, ‖Joanne Markham, *†‡Kevin J. Black, *Lori McGee-Minnich, ¶Joseph Jankovic, and †§Stephen M. Moerlein

Department of Neurology and Neurological Surgery, †Mallinckrodt Institute of Radiology, ‡Department of Psychiatry, §Department of Medicinal Chemistry, and ‖Institute for Biomedical Computing, Washington University School of Medicine, St. Louis, Missouri 63110; and ¶Department of Neurology, Parkinson's Disease Center and Movement Disorders Clinic, Baylor College of Medicine, Houston, Texas 77030.

Dystonia is a syndrome of repetitive or sustained involuntary muscle contractions that frequently produce twisting, repetitive movements and abnormal postures (7). Generalized idiopathic dystonia often begins in childhood, whereas focal dystonias more frequently start in adult life (7,14,28). There are several types of idiopathic focal dystonia including cranial dystonia and hand cramp. Cranial dystonia refers to involuntary spasms of facial muscles frequently affecting the eyelids and lower facial muscles. Dystonic hand cramp is produced by excessive co-contractions of agonist and antagonist muscles during specific tasks such as writing or typing (5,52). The idiopathic focal dystonias may share a common pathophysiology because there may be overlap of symptoms in some patients (19), but the precise etiologic relationship among the idiopathic focal dystonias remains unknown (32).

Multiple studies suggest that the putamen is a likely site of pathophysiology in dystonia. Several investigators described structural abnormalities in basal ganglia (6,15,29,44) mostly affecting the putamen in patients with secondary dystonias (4,10,25,26,35,49). We found abnormal hemodynamics in the putamen contralateral to the affected side of the body in a patient with posttraumatic paroxysmal hemidystonia despite completely normal brain magnetic resonance imaging (MRI), computed tomography (CT), and angiogram (40). More recently, MRI demonstrated abnormalities in the lentiform nucleus in idiopathic torticollis (50).

Abnormalities of dopaminergic pathways may play an important role in the pathophysiology of dystonia (3,11,24,34,43,45,46,48). The purpose of this study is to investigate whether there is an abnormality of D_2-like dopaminergic binding in putamen in patients with idiopathic focal dystonia. We limited the study to include only those with hand cramp and facial dystonia because these patients can lie in the positron emission tomography (PET) scanner without substantial movement or discomfort.

METHODS

Subjects

We studied 14 patients with cranial dystonia and seven with dystonic hand cramp (16 women, mean age, 59 ± 14 years, range 25 to 79) as well as 12 normals (six women, mean age, 53 ± 19 years, range 21 to 76). The patients did not have dystonia in other parts of the body. No subject had other neurologic or psychiatric disease; each had a Mini Mental State Examination score greater than 26 (8) and a

TABLE 1. *Subject characteristics*

Patient	Type of dystonia	Age (yr)	Gender	Duration (yr)	Medications	Time of last oral medicine (h)
1	Cranial	48	M	6	Trihexyphenidyl	6
2	Cranial	54	F	4.5	Hydralazine, clonazepam, levothyroxine btx/2 mo ago	6
3	Cranial	54	F	1.5	Estrogen, progesterone, diclofenac, indepamide, verapamil btx/2 wk ago	12 12
4	Cranial	46	F	4	None btx/5 mo ago	
5	Cranial	47	M	3	Aspirin btx/2 yr ago	24
6	Cranial	48	F	3	Clonazepam, orphenadrine btx/5 wk ago	24
7	Cranial	74	F	29	Cimetidine	24
8	Cranial	79	F	16	Hydrochlorothiazide btx/4 mo	24
9	Cranial	66	F	6	Salicylate btx/5 yr ago	24
10	Cranial	54	F	6	None btx/6 mo ago	
11	Cranial	54	F	1	Estrogen btx/5 wk ago	24
12	Cranial	73	M	1	Trihexyphenidyl	24
13	Cranial	77	F	12	None btx/4 wk ago	
14	Cranial	55	F	2.5	Estrogen, levothyroxine btx/4 mo ago	24
15	Hand	38	F	10	None	
16	Hand	50	M	3	None btx/3 mo ago	
17	Hand	59	F	15	Propoxyphene, atenolol	24
18	Hand	67	F	9	Quinapril btx/1 mo ago	24
19	Hand	68	M	26	None btx/3 yr ago	
20	Hand	25	F	4	None	
21	Hand	45	F	15	Levothyroxine, estrogen, progesterone	24
Mean		56	5M, 16F	8.5		
SD		14		7.9		
Range		25–79		1–29		
Normals						
22		21	M		None	
23		53	F		Nicotine patch	24
24		76	M		Hydrochlorothiazide, lovastatin, aspirin	24
25		24	F		None	
26		40	M		None	
27		24	F		Estrogen, progesterone	24
28		67	F		Gemfibrozil	24
29		60	F		None	
30		64	M		None	
31		72	M		None	
32		65	M		None	
33		63	F		Aspirin	24
Normals, mean		52	6F, 6M			
SD		20				
Range		21–76				

There was no statistically significant difference between the ages of the dystonics and normals ($p > 0.5$, two-tailed t test).

From ref. 42, with permission.

Hamilton Rating Scale for Depression score less than 6 (16). None were taking drugs known to affect dopamine receptors. Some patients had been treated with botulinum toxin A (btx) (Table 1). Each subject also had an MRI of the brain using the Siemens Vision 1.5 T Magnetom scanner. These studies were approved by the Human Studies Committee of Washington University and by the Radioactive Drug Research Committee (United States Food & Drug Administration). Each subject provided written informed consent.

Positron Emission Tomography

PET studies were done with the Siemens 953b in the two-dimensional mode with 31 simultaneous slices with 3.38-mm center-to-center slice separation (31,53). Attenuation factors were measured using rotating rod sources of [^{68}Ge]/[^{68}Ga]. Reconstructed transaxial resolution of the emission images was about 12 mm and axial resolution about 4.2 mm.

Protocol

Subjects had a 20-gauge catheter inserted into an arm vein for injection of radiopharmaceuticals and another one into a radial artery for sampling arterial blood. We placed radioopaque markers in the ears and then stabilized the head with a polyform mask molded to the subject's head. A lateral skull radiograph taken with a reference PET slice marked by a radioopaque wire provided a permanent record of the patient's position (9). The eyes were closed and the ears not further occluded. We measured regional cerebral blood volume (rCBV) with ^{15}O-labeled carbon monoxide and regional cerebral blood flow (rCBF) with ^{15}O-labeled water (17,30,47,58). Radioligand binding was measured with [^{18}F]spiperone ([^{18}F]SP). The free fraction (f_1; dimensionless) of [^{18}F]SP in arterial blood was measured for each subject using a centrifree technique (38). Three to 5 mCi of no-carrier-added [^{18}F]SP containing less than 1 μg of spiperone (specific activity greater than 2,000 Ci/mmole) was injected IV and PET started immediately. Scan lengths be-

gan at 60 seconds and increased to 10 minutes for a total of 3 hours (36). Frequent arterial blood samples were collected to measure total radioactivity and radiolabeled metabolites of [^{18}F]SP (38). Some of the patients had minimal blepharospasm during the scanning but no other movements were seen.

Data Analysis

An observer blinded to subject diagnosis identified all volumes of interest (VOIs). The coordinates of the center of putamen identified in a stereotactic brain atlas (55) were transferred to the appropriate single PET slice with a stereotactic technique (9). The VOI then was expanded to include activity on the slices immediately above and below. The regional values were averaged across the three slices and for the right and left putamen to reduce statistical noise. A single hemispheric cerebellar value was averaged from left- and right-sided regions identified on three PET slices. Regional values were sampled for all of the PET scans collected after injection of [^{18}F]SP and for the CBV and CBF images. We calculated radioligand binding using a tracer kinetic model previously described and validated (36–39). Briefly, we estimate the free fraction of radioligand in the cerebellum (f_2; dimensionless) as a measure of the nonspecific binding and assume that this value is the same in the putamen. Then we estimate the local permeability surface-area product (PS) for [^{18}F]SP at the blood-brain barrier, the combined forward-rate constant (CFRC) of [^{18}F]SP (this equals the apparent maximum number of specific binding sites times the association rate constant of [^{18}F]SP for the specific sites), as well as the dissociation rate constant of [^{18}F]SP- receptor complex.

RESULTS

No subject had a gross abnormality on MRI scan of the brain. Cerebellar CBV and CBF, putaminal CBV and CBF, and the measured free fraction of [^{18}F]SP in blood are listed in Table 2. There were no statistical differences between patients and normals. Estimated vari-

TABLE 2. *Measured variables used in tracer kinetic modeling*

	Cerebellar CBF (ml/[100 g·min])	Cerebellar CBV (ml/100 g)	Putaminal CBF (ml/[100 g·min])	Putaminal CBV (ml/100 g)	Free fraction in blood (f_1)
Dystonics					
Mean	71	2.8	80	4.6	0.051
SD	15	1.0	15	1.5	0.0175
(*n* = 21)					
Normals					
Mean	69	2.3	82	4.7	0.045
SD	10	0.7	14	1.2	0.0070
(*n* = 12)					

There were no statistically significant differences between dystonics and normals in any of these variables. f_1 is a dimensionless ratio. CBF and CBV were measured with PET and [^{15}O]-labeled water and carbon monoxide, respectively. The free fraction of [^{18}F]spiperone in arterial blood was measured using a microcentrifree technique as described in Methods.
From ref. 42, with permission.

ables including the free fraction of [^{18}F]SP in brain tissue, the cerebellar PS for [^{18}F]SP, PS for [^{18}F]SP in striatum, and the dissociation rate constant of [^{18}F]SP are given in Table 3. Only the CFRCs were significantly different between patients and controls, with dystonics about 29% lower than normals (p <0.05). There was no significant difference between the CFRC for dystonic hand cramp and cranial dystonia (p >0.2). It is important to note that a change in the CFRC is consistent with a change of the association-rate constant, the

TABLE 3. *PET measurements of [^{18}F]spiperone binding in putamen: variables determined with parameter estimation and the tracer kinetic model*

	Free fraction in tissue (f_2)	Cerebellar PS (sec^{-1})	Putaminal PS (sec^{-1})	Putaminal dissociation rate constant (sec^{-1})	Putaminal combined forward rate constant (sec^{-1})[a]
Dystonics					
Mean	0.0053	0.038	0.051	0.00013	0.20
SD	0.0017	0.0139	0.016	0.00007	0.07
Mean COV	3.3%	4.4%	3.4%	68%	29%
SD COV	0.9%	1.0%	0.9%	29%	11%
(*n* = 21)					
Normals					
Mean	0.0060	0.036	0.049	0.00017	0.28
SD	0.0034	0.0093	0.012	0.00011	0.14
Mean COV	3.4%	4.5%	4.3%	80%	43%
SD COV	1.1%	0.9%	1.2%	21%	24%
(*n* = 12)					

[a]p < 0.05 comparing dystonics to normals with two-tailed *t* test. There were no other significant differences between dystonics and normals.
Mean COV, the mean of the standard deviation of the variable estimate for each subject divided by the value of the estimated variable (this reflects the confidence of each individual value); SD (COV), the standard deviation of all of the subjects' COVs; PS, permeability surface-area product for [^{18}F]spiperone at the blood-brain barrier. f_2 is a dimensionless ratio. These variables were calculated using sequential PET measurements of regional radioactivity, PET measurements of regional CBF and CBV, blood measurements of the free fraction of [^{18}F]spiperone in blood, sequential measurements of total radioactivity, and radiolabeled metabolites of [^{18}F]spiperone in arterial blood with a three-compartment model that represents the *in vivo* behavior of [^{18}F]spiperone after intravenous injection. These variables were calculated for 1-cc tissue volume.
From ref. 42, with permission.

maximum number of specific binding sites (B_{max}), or both. The greater variance of the estimates for the dissociation rate constant limits the detection of statistical differences between groups.

DISCUSSION

We found decreased [¹⁸F]SP binding in putamen in patients with idiopathic dystonia affecting either the face or hand. This is the first demonstration of a receptor abnormality in idiopathic dystonia.

We must interpret our findings cautiously because [¹⁸F]SP specifically binds to D_2-like (about 74%) and to serotonergic S_2 sites [about 26% (39)]. It is also important to note that [¹⁸F]SP binding to D_2-like receptors could reflect binding to D_2 or D_3 specific sites, but less likely to D_4 binding sites because they are much less numerous in primate putamen (51).

Others have found reduced dopaminergic activity in dystonia consistent with the interpretation that reduced [¹⁸F]SP binding reflects a change in D_2-like binding. For example, there is a 15% mean reduction of [¹⁸F]dopa uptake in putamen in familial idiopathic dystonia (45). One patient with cranial dystonia had decreased cerebrospinal fluid homovanillic acid suggestive of decreased dopamine turnover (3); another patient with cranial dystonia had reduced dopamine in GPe (20); and there was reduced striatal dopamine in one patient with generalized dystonia (18). Patients with dopa-responsive dystonia (DRD) have a remarkable symptomatic response to levodopa. The more common autosomal-dominant DRD is associated with a deficiency of an enzyme required for biosynthesis of a cofactor for tyrosine hydroxylase (34), whereas the less common autosomal-recessive form is caused by a defect in tyrosine hydroxylase (23). Additionally, acute administration of neuroleptics that block D_2-like receptors may produce acute dystonic reactions (11,24,48). Dystonia may be an early symptom in some parkinsonian patients, suggesting that striatal dopamine deficiency may produce either dystonia or parkinsonism.

How do our findings fit with current models of basal ganglia function? One model describes multiple cortico-striato-pallido-thalamic-cortical loops with the cortical-striate input neurons of the motor loop predominantly projecting to putamen (1,2,12,13). Two major pathways project to the internal segment of the pallidum (GPi): (a) the direct pathway via inhibitory fibers connecting striatum and GPi, and (b) the indirect pathway including inhibitory neurons from striatum to the external segment of pallidum (GPe), inhibitory neurons projecting from GPe to subthalamic nucleus (STN), and excitatory neurons projecting from STN to GPi. The direct and indirect pathways converge on GPi, which then sends inhibitory neurons to ventral anterior thalamus that projects via excitatory neurons to cortical areas including premotor and motor regions. D_2-like receptors predominantly colocalize with and inhibit the striatopallidal neurons of the indirect pathway, whereas D_1 receptors colocalize with and facilitate the neurons of the direct pathway that project from striatum to GPi (12,13,22). We suggest that preferential decrease in D_2-mediated inhibition of the indirect pathway may produce dystonia. This is consistent with decreased [¹⁸F]SP binding in putamen as well as with our previous findings of a reduction in the vibration-induced blood flow responses in primary sensorimotor area (PSA) and supplementary motor area (56,57). The decreased blood flow response could reflect a local cortical change or an alteration in the cortico-striato-pallido-thalamic-cortical circuit. Decreased D_2-like inhibitory function in putamen could increase activity of the inhibitory putamen to GPe neurons, thereby decreasing activity of the inhibitory neurons projecting from GPe to STN. This could lead to increased activity of the excitatory neurons projecting from STN to GPi, increased activity of inhibitory neurons projecting from GPi to thalamus, and decreased activity of excitatory neurons projecting from thalamus to cortex. This might decrease reactivity in cortical areas when engaged by the motor loop through the basal ganglia. In support of this notion, we have reported that one patient with DRD had a reduced vibration-induced blood flow response in PSA that normalized after levodopa (41). It is possible that levodopa modified the PSA response by acting in the putamen, but other sites of action cannot be excluded.

Others have found functional changes in basal ganglia in either animal models or patients with dystonia but have not found selective changes in the indirect pathway or in D_2 receptors (21,27,33,54).

Our findings do not explain all types of dystonia. Patients with PD may develop at least three different patterns associated with dopa replacement therapy. Dystonia may occur when plasma dopa levels are low, so-called off-period dystonia, but also may occur when plasma levels peak. Finally, dystonia may occur as the effect of an individual dose begins or as it diminishes (46). Proposing pathophysiologic mechanisms for these three patterns of dystonia is difficult given the uncertainty of the relative influence of the different dopamine receptor subtypes on subsequent activities of the direct and indirect pathways.

In summary, we have found a decrease in [¹⁸F]SP binding in the putamen of patients with idiopathic adult-onset focal dystonias affecting the face or hand. There was no significant difference between patients with hand and facial dystonia, suggesting that there may be a common mechanism producing both conditions, consistent with the clinical impression that they share a similar pathophysiology (19). However, because we calculated [¹⁸F]SP binding for the entire putamen, our data do not exclude the possibility that different parts of putamen may have different degrees of decreased binding in the two types of dystonia. We propose that decreased function of D_2-like receptors in the indirect pathway may be the pathophysiologic correlate for at least some forms of idiopathic dystonia. Additional studies with more specific radioligands, including those for D_1 receptors, should help to clarify further the nature of this abnormality. It also would be interesting to determine the relative activity of the putaminal neurons projecting directly to GPi versus those projecting to GPe in animal models of dystonia.

ACKNOWLEDGMENTS

We appreciate useful discussions with Dr. Jonathan Mink and the expert technical assistance of the members of the Division of Radiological Sciences. We also thank Dr. William Hart for referral of some patients that participated in this study. This work has been supported by NIH grants NS31001, NS32318, and AA-07466 as well as by the Benign Essential Blepharospasm Foundation, the Greater St. Louis Chapter of the American Parkinson's Disease Association, the Clinical Hypotheses Research Section of the Charles A. Dana Foundation, the McDonnell Center for the Study of Higher Brain Function, the generous support of Mr. and Mrs. Jefferson Miller, and the Sam & Barbara Murphy Fund. A detailed report of these findings has just been reported in the *Journal of Neuroscience* (42).

REFERENCES

1. Alexander G, Crutcher M. Functional architecture of basal ganglia circuits: neural substrates of parallel processing. *Trends Neurosci* 1990;13:266–271.
2. Alexander G, DeLong MR, Strick P. Parallel organization of functionally segregated circuits linking basal ganglia and cortex. *Ann Rev Neurosci* 1986;9:357–381.
3. Ashizawa T, Patten B, Jankovic J. Meige's syndrome. *South Med J* 1980;73:863–866.
4. Bhatia K, Marsden CD. The behavioural and motor consequences of focal lesions of the basal ganglia in man. *Brain* 1994;117:859–876.
5. Cohen L, Hallett M. Hand cramps: clinical features and electromyographic patterns in a focal dystonia. *Neurology* 1988;38:1005–1012.
6. Demierre B, Rondot P. Dystonia caused by putamino-capsulo-caudate vascular lesions. *J Neurol Neurosurg Psychiatry* 1983;46:404–409.
7. Fahn S. Concept and classification of dystonia. *Adv Neurol* 1988;50:1–8.
8. Folstein M, Folstein S, McHugh P. "Mini-mental state": a practical method for grading the cognitive state of patients for the clinician. *J Psychiatr Res* 1975;12:189–198.
9. Fox P, Perlmutter J, Raichle M. A stereotactic method of anatomical localization for positron emission tomography. *J Comput Assist Tomogr* 1985;9:141–153.
10. Fross R, Martin W, Li D, et al. Lesions of the putamen: their relevance to dystonia. *Neurology* 1987;37:1125–1129.
11. Garver DL, Davis J, Dekirmenjian H, et al. Dystonic reactions following neuroleptics: time course and proposed mechanisms. *Psychopharmacologia* 1976;47:199–201.

12. Gerfen CR. The neostriatal mosaic: multiple levels of compartmental organization. *Trends Neurosci* 1992; 15:133–139.

13. Gerfen CR, Engber TM, Mahan LC, et al. D1 and D2 dopamine receptor-regulated gene expression of striatonigral and striatopallidal neurons. *Science* 1990;250: 1429–1432.

14. Greene P, Kang U, Fahn S. Spread of symptoms in idiopathic torsion dystonia. *Mov Disord* 1995;10:143–152.

15. Grimes J, Hassan M, Quarrington A, D'Alton J. Delayed-onset post-hemiplegic dystonia: CT demonstration of basal ganglia pathology. *Neurology* 1982;32: 1033–1035.

16. Hamilton M. A rating scale for depression. *J Neurol Neurosurg Psychiatry* 1960;23:56–62.

17. Herscovitch P, Markham J, Raichle M. Brain blood flow measured with intravenous $H_2^{15}O$: theory and error analysis. *J Nucl Med* 1983;24:782–789.

18. Hornykiewicz O, Kish SJ, Becker LE, Farley I, Shannak K. Brain neurotransmitters in dystonia musculorum deformans. *N Engl J Med* 1986;315:347–353.

19. Jankovic J, Leder S, Warner D, Schwartz K. Cervical dystonia: clinical findings and associated movement disorders. *Neurology* 1991;41:1088–1091.

20. Jankovic J, Svendeen CN, Bird ED. Brain Neurotransmitters in dystonia. *N Engl J Med* 1987;316:278–279.

21. Karbe H, Holthoff V, Rudolf J, Herholz K, Heiss W. Positron emission tomography demonstrates frontal cortex and basal ganglia hypometabolism in dystonia. *Neurology* 1992;42:1540–1544.

22. Keefe KA, Gerfen CR. D1-D2 dopamine receptor synergy in striatum: effects of intrastriatal infusions of dopamine agonists and antagonists on immediate early gene expression. *Neuroscience* 1995;66:903–913.

23. Knappskog PM, Flatmark T, Mallet J, Ludecke B, Bartholome K. Recessively inherited L-DOPA-responsive dystonia caused by a point mutation (Q381K) in the tyrosine hydroxylase gene. *Hum Mol Genet* 1995;4:1209–1212.

24. Kolbe H, Clow A, Jenner P, Marsden CD. Neuroleptic-induced acute dystonic reactions may be due to enhanced dopamine release on to supersensitive postsynaptic receptors. *Neurology* 1981;31:434–439.

25. Krauss J, Mohadjer M, Braus D, Wakhloo A, Nobbe F, Mundinger F. Dystonia following head trauma: a report of nine patients and review of the literature. *Mov Disord* 1992;7:263–272.

26. Lee M, Rinne J. Dystonia after head trauma. *Neurology* 1994;44:1374–1378.

27. Leenders K, Hartvig P, Forsgren L, et al. Striatal [11C]-N-methyl-spiperone binding in patients with focal dystonia (torticollis) using positron emission tomography. *J Neurol Transm* 1993;5:79–87.

28. Marsden C, Harrison M. Idiopathic torsion dystonia (dystonia musculorum deformans). *Brain* 1974;97: 793–810.

29. Marsden C, Obeso J, Zarranz J, Lang AE. The anatomical basis of symptomatic hemidystonia. *Brain* 1985; 108:463–483.

30. Martin W, Powers W, Raichle M. Cerebral blood volume measured with inhaled $C^{15}O$ and positron emission tomography. *J Cereb Blood Flow Metab* 1987; 7:421–426.

31. Mazoyer B, Trebossen R, Deutch R, Casey M, Blohm K. Physical characteristics of the ECAT 953B/31: a new high resolution brain positron tomograph. *IEEE Trans Med Imaging* 1991;10:499–504.

32. Micheli S, Fernandez-Pardal M, Quesada P, Brannan T, Obeso J. Variable onset of adult inherited focal dystonia: a problem for genetic studies. *Mov Disord* 1994; 9:64–68.

33. Mitchell I, Luguin R, Boyce S, et al. Neural mechanisms of dystonia: evidence from a 2-deoxyglucose uptake study in a primate model of dopamine agonist-induced dystonia. *Mov Disord* 1990;5:49–54.

34. Nygaard T. Dopa-responsive dystonia. *Curr Opin Neurol* 1995;8:310–313.

35. Obeso J, Gimenez-Roldan S. Clinicopathological correlation in symptomatic dystonia. *Adv Neurol* 1988; 50:113–122.

36. Perlmutter J, Kilbourn M, Raichle M, Welch M. MPTP-induced up-regulation of in vivo dopaminergic radioligand-receptor binding in humans. *Neurology* 1987;37:1575–1579.

37. Perlmutter J, Kilbourn M, Welch M, Raichle M. Nonsteady-state measurement of in vivo receptor binding with positron emission tomography: "dose-response" analysis. *J Neurosci* 1989;9:2344–2352.

38. Perlmutter J, Larson K, Raichle M, et al. Strategies for the in vivo measurement of receptor binding using positron emission tomography. *J Cereb Blood Flow Metab* 1986;6:154–169.

39. Perlmutter J, Moerlein S, Huang D-R, Todd R. Nonsteady-state measurement of in vivo radioligand binding with positron emission tomography: specificity analysis and comparison with in vitro binding. *J Neurosci* 1991;11:1381–1389.

40. Perlmutter JS, Raichle ME. Pure hemidystonia with basal ganglion abnormalities on positron emission tomography. *Ann Neurol* 1984;15:228–233.

41. Perlmutter JS, Raichle ME. Regional blood flow in dystonia: an exploratory study. In: Fahn S, Marsden CD, Calne DB, eds. Dystonia 2: *Advances in neurology*. Vol. 50. New York: Raven Press, 1988:255–264.

42. Perlmutter JS, Stambuk MK, Markham J, et al. Decreased [18F]spiperone binding in putamen in idiopathic focal dystonia. *J Neurosci* 1997 17:834–842.

43. Perlmutter JS, Tempel LW, Lich L. A new animal model of dystonia. *Soc Neurosci Abstr* 1993;19:1052.

44. Pettigrew L, Jankovic J. Hemidystonia: a report of 22 patients and a review of the literature. *J Neurol Neurosurg Psychiatry* 1985;48:650–657.

45. Playford E, Fletcher N, Sawle G, Marsden CD, Brooks D. Striatal [18F]dopa uptake in familial idiopathic dystonia. *Brain* 1993;116:1191–1199.

46. Poewe WH, Lees AJ, Stern GM. Dystonia in Parkinson disease: clinical and pharmacological features. *Ann Neurol* 1988;23:73–78.

47. Raichle M, Martin W, Herscovitch P, Mintun M, Markham J. Brain blood flow measured with intravenous $H_2^{15}O$. II. Implementation and validation. *J Nucl Med* 1983;24:790–798.

48. Rupniak N, Jenner P, Marsden CD. Acute dystonia induced by neuroleptic drugs. *Psychopharmacol* 1986; 88:403–419.

49. Rutledge J, Hilal S, Silver A, Defendini R, Fahn S. Magnetic resonance imaging of dystonic states. *Adv Neurol* 1988;50:265–275.

50. Schneider S, Feifel E, Ott D, Schumacher M, Lucking C, Deuschl G. Prolonged MRI T_2 times of the

lentiform nucleus in idiopathic spasmodic torticollis. *Neurology* 1994;44:846–850.

51. Seeman P, Guan HC, Van Tol H, Niznik H. Low density of dopamine D4 receptors in Parkinson's, schizophrenia and control brain striata. *Synapse* 1993;14:247–253.

52. Sheehy M, Marsden C. Writer's cramp—a focal dystonia. *Brain* 1982;105:461–480.

53. Spinks TJ, Jones T, Gilardi MC, Heather JD. Physical performance of the latest generation of commercial positron scanner. *IEEE Trans Nucl Sci* 1988;35:721–725.

54. Stoessl A, Martin W, Clark C, et al. PET studies of cerebral glucose metabolism in idiopathic torticollis. *Neurology* 1986;36:653–657.

55. Talairach J, Tournoux P. *Co-planar stereotaxic atlas of the human brain. New York: Theime Verlag, 1988.*

56. Tempel L, Perlmutter J. Abnormal vibration-induced cerebral blood flow responses in dystonia. *Brain* 1990;113:691–707.

57. Tempel LW, Perlmutter JS. Abnormal cortical responses to vibration in patients with writer's cramp. *Neurology* 1993;43:2252–2257.

58. Videen TO, Perlmutter JS, Herscovitch P, Raichle ME. Brain blood volume, flow and oxygen utilization measured with O-15 radiotracers and positron emission tomography: revised metabolic computations. *J Cereb Blood Flow Metab* 1987;7:513–516.

Dystonia 3: Advances in Neurology, Vol. 78,
edited by S. Fahn, C. D. Marsden, and M. DeLong.
Lippincott–Raven Publishers, Philadelphia © 1998.

18

Medical Therapy and Botulinum Toxin in Dystonia

Joseph Jankovic

Department of Neurology, Parkinson's Disease Center and Movement Disorders Clinic, Baylor College of Medicine, Houston, Texas 77030.

Symptomatic treatment of dystonia has markedly improved during the last decade, largely as a result of wider availability of and improved skills in the administration of botulinum toxin (BTX) and as a result of reemergence of neurosurgery as a therapeutic modality in patients with medically intractable dystonia. Refinements in stereotactic surgery, particularly thalamotomy, pallidotomy, and deep brain stimulation, as well as intrathecal infusion of baclofen have contributed to the growing role of surgery in the treatment of movement disorders, including dystonia. Because these approaches are reviewed elsewhere in the volume, this chapter focuses only on pharmacologic therapy.

One of the chief principles in the treatment of dystonia is the search for a secondary cause of dystonia in order to institute therapy specifically designed to treat or cure the underlying cause. In most cases of dystonia, however, no specific cause can be identified and the treatment is merely symptomatic, designed to improve patient's posture and function and to relieve associated pain. Frequently a troublesome symptom, dystonia can in rare instances be so severe that it may compromise respiration and the muscular spasms can cause muscle breakdown and a life-threatening hyperthermia and myoglobinuria. Proper and timely therapeutic intervention in such cases of "dystonic storms" can be lifesaving (67,88,117).

Although many therapeutic modalities have been reported to be effective in the treatment of dystonia, quantitative assessment may be difficult for the following reasons: (a) dystonia and its effects on function are difficult to quantitate and, therefore, most trials utilize crude clinical rating scales many of which have not been properly evaluated or validated, (b) dystonia is a syndrome with different etiologies, anatomic distributions, and heterogeneous clinical manifestations producing variable disability, (c) some patients, perhaps up to 15%, may have spontaneous, albeit transient, remissions, (d) the vast majority of therapeutic trials in dystonia are not double-blind, placebo-controlled, and (e) most studies, even those that have been otherwise well designed and controlled, have used small sample sizes, which makes the results difficult to interpret, particularly in view of a large placebo effect demonstrated in dystonia (81).

For these and other reasons, the selection of a particular choice of therapy is largely guided by personal clinical experience and by empirical trials (Table 1) (42,61). The age of the patient, the anatomic distribution of dystonia, and the potential risk of adverse effects are also important determinants of choice of therapy. The identification of a specific cause of dystonia, such as drug-induced dystonias or Wilson's disease, may lead to a treatment that is targeted

---

TABLE 1. *Therapy of dystonia*

Principles

Identify a specifically treatable cause—e.g., Wilson's disease, drugs, structural

Educate patient and family—genetic counseling

Therapy for idiopathic dystonia is symptomatic, not protective

Select pharmacologic therapy according to severity, age, type, and distribution

Surgical therapy should be reserved for disabling dystonia resistant to medications and/or BTX injections

Guide to therapeutic options

Carbidopa/levodopa 25/100 1/2 tab b.i.d. (rarely more than 3 tabs/day), particularly in childhood-onset dystonia; effective in DRD, biopterin deficiency, and dystonia-parkinsonism disorders

Anticholinergics—e.g., trihexyphenidyl: 2 mg b.i.d. and may increase up to 80 to 140 mg/d

Baclofen: 5 mg b.i.d. and may increase up to 60 to 160 mg/d; consider intrathecal infusion

Other: carbamazepine, benzodiazepines, tetrabenazine (with/without lithium and/or DRBD)

Botulinum toxin—for focal and segmental dystonia

Surgery: peripheral denervation, thalamotomy, pallidotomy deep brain stimulation

---

to the particular etiology. It is therefore prudent to search for identifiable causes of dystonia, particularly when some atypical features are present. It is beyond the scope of this chapter to discuss the diagnostic approaches to patients with dystonia; this topic is covered elsewhere in this volume and in other reviews (57,61).

PHYSICAL AND SUPPORTIVE THERAPY

Before reviewing pharmacologic and surgical therapy of dystonia, it is important to emphasize the role of patient education and supportive care as these are integral components of a comprehensive approach to patients with dystonia. Physical therapy and well-fitted braces are designed primarily to improve posture and to prevent contractures. Although braces are often poorly tolerated, particularly by children, in some cases they may be used as a substitute for a "sensory trick." For example, in some of our patients with cervical dystonia we were able to construct neck-head braces that seem to provide sensory input by touching certain portions of the neck or head in a fashion

similar to the patient's own sensory trick, thus enabling the patient to maintain a desirable head position. Various hand devices have been developed in an attempt to help patients with writer's cramp to use their hands more effectively and comfortably (100). Some patients find various muscle relaxation techniques and sensory feedback therapy useful adjuncts to medical or surgical treatments.

DOPAMINERGIC THERAPY

Pharmacologic treatment of dystonia is largely based on empirical, rather than scientific, rationale. Unlike Parkinson's disease, in which therapy with levodopa replacement is based on the finding of depletion of dopamine in the brains of parkinsonian animals and humans, our knowledge of biochemical alterations in idiopathic dystonia is very limited. One exception is the dopa-responsive dystonia (DRD) in which the biochemical and genetic mechanisms have been elucidated by studies of postmortem brains and by molecular DNA and biomechanical studies. Decreased neuromelanin in the substantia nigra with otherwise normal nigral cell count and morphology and normal tyrosine hydroxylase immunoreactivity were found in one brain of a patient with classic DRD (99). There was a marked reduction in dopamine in the substantia nigra and in striatum. These findings suggested that in DRD the primary abnormality was a defect in dopamine synthesis. This proposal is supported by the finding of a mutation in the GTP cyclohydrolase I gene on chromosome 14q, which indirectly regulates the production of tetrahydrobiopterin, a cofactor for tyrosine hydroxylase, the rate-limiting enzyme in the synthesis of dopamine (51,108).

DRD usually presents in childhood with dystonia, mild parkinsonian features, and pseudopyramidal signs (hypertonicity and hyperreflexia) predominantly involving the legs. A family history of dystonia or Parkinson's disease is common. At least one-half of the patients have diurnal fluctuations with marked progression of their symptoms toward the end of the day and relief after sleep. Many patients with this form of dystonia are initially misdiagnosed as having cerebral palsy. Some patients with DRD are not diagnosed until adulthood and family members of patients with typical DRD may present with adult-onset levodopa-responsive parkinsonism (48). The combination of levodopa-responsive dystonia and parkinsonism, inherited in an autosomal-dominant pattern, was also reported in a family characterized by rapidly evolving dystonia (over a period of days to weeks) starting between ages 14 and 45 (15,29). The take-home message from these reports is that a therapeutic trial of levodopa should be considered in all patients with childhood-onset dystonia, whether they have classic features of DRD or not.

Most patients with DRD improve dramatically even with small doses of levodopa (100 mg of levodopa with 25 mg of decarboxylase inhibitor), but some may require doses of levodopa as high as 1,000 mg/day. In contrast to patients with juvenile Parkinson's disease (52), DRD patients usually do not develop levodopa-induced fluctuations or dyskinesias. If no clinically evident improvement is noted after 3 months of therapy, the diagnosis of DRD is unlikely and levodopa can be discontinued. In addition to levodopa, patients with DRD also improve with dopamine agonists, with anticholinergic drugs, and with carbamazepine (89). In contrast to patients with DRD, patients with idiopathic or other types of dystonia rarely improve with dopaminergic therapy (79). Although dopaminergic therapy is remarkably effective in DRD, this strategy is not useful in the treatment of idiopathic dystonia. Apomorphine, however, perhaps by decreasing dopamine as well as serotonin turnover and release, may ameliorate dystonia (123).

ANTIDOPAMINERGIC THERAPY

Although used extensively in the past, most clinical trials have produced mixed results with dopamine receptor blocking drugs (DRBDs). Because of the poor response and the possibility of undesirable side effects, particularly sedation, parkinsonism, and tardive dyskinesia, the use of DRBDs in the treatment of dystonia

should be discouraged (56). Although antidopaminergic drugs have been reported to be beneficial in the treatment of dystonia, the potential clinical benefit is usually limited by the development of side effects. Dopamine-depleting drugs, however, such as tetrabenazine, have been found useful in some patients with dystonia, particularly in those with tardive dystonia (58,66). Tetrabenazine has the advantage over other antidopaminergic drugs in that it does not cause tardive dyskinesia, although it may cause transient acute dystonic reaction (74). The drug is not readily available in the United States, but it is dispensed by prescription under the trade name "Nitoman" in other countries, including the United Kingdom. It is possible that some of the new atypical neuroleptic drugs will be useful not only as antipsychotics, but also in the treatment of hyperkinetic movement disorders. Risperidone, a D_2 dopamine receptor blocking drug with a high affinity for $5HT_2$ receptors, has been reported to be useful in a 4-week trial of five patients with various forms of dystonia (123). Unfortunately, this drug may cause not only dose-related parkinsonism, but also persistent tardive syndrome. Clozapine, a D_4 dopamine receptor blocker with relatively low affinity for the D_2 receptors and high affinity for the $5-HT_{2A}$ receptors, has been reported to ameliorate the symptoms of tardive dystonia (112). The treatment of tardive dystonia and other tardive syndromes is discussed elsewhere in this volume and in other reviews (56), and will not be reviewed here.

ANTICHOLINERGIC THERAPY

Anticholinergic medications such as trihexyphenidyl have been found to be most useful in the treatment of generalized and segmental dystonia (46,53). In the experience of Greene et al. (46), patients with blepharospasm, generalized dystonia, tonic (in contrast to clonic) dystonia, and with onset of dystonia at age younger than 19 years seemed to respond better to anticholinergic drugs than other subgroups, but this difference did not reach statistical significance. Except for short duration of symptoms before onset of therapy, there was no other variable, such as gender or severity, that reliably predicted a favorable response. This therapy is generally well tolerated when the dose is increased slowly. We recommend starting with a 2-mg preparation, 1/2 tablet at bedtime and slowly advancing the dose up to 60 to 100 mg/day over the next 6 months as needed. Some patients experience dose-related drowsiness, confusion, memory difficulty, and hallucinations. In one study of 20 cognitively intact patients with dystonia, only 12 of whom could tolerate 15 to 74 of daily trihexyphenidyl, drug-induced impairments of recall and slowing of mentation was noted particularly in the older patients (109). Diphenhydramine, an anticholinergic with histamine H_1 antagonist properties, has been reported to have an antidystonic effect in three of five patients (113). The drug, however, was not effective in ten other patients with cervical dystonia and it was associated with sedation and other anticholinergic side effects in most patients. Further studies are needed to determine whether the antihistamine drugs are better than the conventional anticholinergics in the treatment of dystonia. Pyridostigmine and possibly cisapride, peripherally acting anticholinesterase agents, and eye drops of pilocarpine (a muscarinic agonist) often ameliorate at least some of the peripheral side effects such as dry mouth, urinary retention, and blurred vision.

OTHER PHARMACOLOGIC THERAPIES

Many patients with dystonia require a combination of several medications and treatments. Benzodiazepines (e.g., clonazepam, lorazepam) may provide additional benefit for patients whose response to anticholinergic drugs is unsatisfactory. Clonazepam may be useful in patients with blepharospasm and with myoclonic dystonia. Baclofen may be helpful for oromandibular dystonia, but it is only minimally effective for generalized dystonia. This $GABA_b$ autoreceptor agonist has been found in one retrospective study to produce substantial and sustained improvement in 29% of children at a

mean dose of 92 mg/day (range, 40 to 180) (41). Although initially effective in 28 of 60 (47%) adults with cranial dystonia, only 18% continued baclofen at a mean dose of 105 mg/day after a mean of 30.6 months (34). Narayan et al. (88) first suggested that intrathecal baclofen may be effective in the treatment of dystonia in 1981 in a report of an 18-year-old man with severe cervical and truncal dystonic spasms who was refractory to all forms of oral therapy and to large doses of paraspinal BTX injections. Muscle paralyzing agents were necessary to relieve these spasms, which compromised his respiration. Within a few hours after the institution of intrathecal baclofen infusion the patient's dystonia markedly improved and he was able to be discharged from the intensive care unit within 1 to 2 days. The subsequent experience with intrathecal infusions has been quite encouraging and studies are currently in progress to evaluate further this form of therapy in patients with dystonia and other motor disorders (93). In some patients treated with intrathecal baclofen for spasticity, the benefits persisted even after the infusion was stopped (30). Ford et al. (37) reviewed the experience with intrathecal baclofen in 25 patients and concluded that this form of therapy may be "more effective when dystonia is associated with spasticity or pain." It is not yet clear whether intrathecal baclofen can induce lasting remissions in patients with dystonia. This approach will be reviewed in more detail elsewhere in this volume.

Peripheral deafferentation with anesthetic was previously reported to improve tremor (95), but this approach may be also useful in the treatment of focal dystonia (76). An injection of 5 to 10 ml of 0.5% lidocaine into the target muscle improved focal dystonia for up to 24 hours. This short effect can be extended for up to several weeks if ethanol is simultaneously injected. The observation that blocking muscle spindle afferents reduces dystonia suggests that somatosensory input is important in the pathogenesis of dystonia (47,77). Local electromyography (EMG)-guided injections of phenol is currently investigated as a potential treatment of cervical dystonia (Massey, personal communication). Chemomyectomy with muscle-necrotizing drugs, such as doxorubicin, has been tried in some patients with blepharospasm and hemifacial spasm (120) but, because of severe local irritation, it is doubtful that this approach will be adopted into clinical practice.

Attacks of kinesigenic paroxysmal dystonia may be controlled with anticonvulsants (e.g., carbamazapine, phenytoin) (27). The nonkinesigenic forms of paroxysmal dystonia are less responsive to pharmacologic therapy, although clonazepam and acetazolamide may be beneficial.

BOTULINUM TOXIN

The introduction of BTX into clinical practice in the 1980s revolutionized the treatment of dystonia. The most potent biologic toxin, BTX has become a powerful therapeutic tool in the treatment of a variety of neurologic, ophthalmic, and other disorders manifested by abnormal, excessive, or inappropriate muscle contractions (20,59,62). In December 1989, after extensive laboratory and clinical testing, the Food and Drug Administration (FDA) approved this biologic as a therapeutic agent in patients with strabismus, blepharospasm, and other facial nerve disorders, including hemifacial spasm.

The therapeutic value of BTX is due to its ability to cause chemodenervation and to produce local paralysis when injected into a muscle. Of the seven immunologically distinct toxins, type A has been studied most intensely and has been used most widely, but the clinical applications of other types of toxins, including B, C, and F, are also being explored (43,84,87, 106).

BTX-A, currently used most for therapeutic purposes, is harvested from a culture medium after fermentation of a high toxin producing strain of *Clostridium botulinum,* which lyses and liberates the toxin into the culture (103). The toxin is then extracted, precipitated, purified, and finally crystallized with ammonium sulfate. The crystalline toxin is diluted from milligram to nanogram concentrations, freeze-dried, and dispensed as a white powder in small vials containing 100 mouse units (U) of the toxin. When isolated from bacterial cultures, BTX is noncovalently associated with nontoxic macromolecules, such as hemagglutinin. These nontoxic proteins enhance toxicity by protecting the neurotoxin from proteolytic enzymes in the gut, but they apparently have no effect on the potency of the toxin if injected parenterally.

The therapeutic effects of BTX are thought to be primarily due to its action at the neuromuscular junction, although its effects on the peripheral cholinergic autonomic nervous system are also being explored for therapeutic purposes. The mechanisms of action of the different types of BTX are becoming elucidated. The seven antigenically distinct toxins share structurally homologous subunits. Synthesized as single chain polypeptides (molecular weight of 150 kD), these toxin molecules have relatively little potency until they are cleaved by trypsin or bacterial enzymes into a heavy chain (100 K) and light chain (50 K). When linked by a disulfide bond, these dichains exert their paralytic action by preventing the release of acetylcholine (ACh). BTX, therefore, does not affect the synthesis or storage of ACh, but it does interfere with the release from the presynaptic terminal. While the heavy chain of the toxin binds to the presynaptic cholinergic terminal, the light chain acts as a zinc-dependent protease that selectively cleaves proteins that are critical for fusion of the presynaptic vesicle with the presynaptic membrane (104). Thus, the light chains of BTX-A and E cleave SNAP-25 (synaptosome associated protein), a protein needed for synaptic vesicle targeting and fusion with the presynaptic membrane (107). The light chains of BTX-B, D, and F prevent the quantal release of ACh by proteolytically cleaving synaptobrevin-2, also known as VAMP (vesicle associated membrane protein), an integral protein of the synaptic vesicle membrane (104). Type C cleaves syntaxin, a plasma membrane associated protein (50) (Table 2).

The primary effect of BTX is to induce paralysis of injected skeletal muscles, especially the most actively contracting muscles.

TABLE 2. *Botulinum neurotoxins*

Neurotoxin	Substrate	Localization
BTX—A, E	SNAP-25	Presynaptic plasma membrane
BTX— B, D, F	VAMP/ synaptobrevin	Synaptic vesicle membrane
BTX—C	Syntaxin	Presynaptic plasma membrane

BTX paralyzes not only the extrafusal fibers, but also the intrafusal fibers, thus decreasing the activity of Ib muscle afferents (35). This may explain the effect of BTX on reciprocal inhibition. In untreated patients with dystonia the second phase of reciprocal inhibition is usually decreased. BTX "corrects" the abnormal reciprocal inhibition by increasing the second phase, possibly through its effect on the muscle afferents (96). Although the effect on intrafusal fibers may contribute in part to the beneficial action of BTX in patients with dystonia, this does not seem to be its main action because BTX is effective in facial dystonia even though the facial muscles apparently do not have spindles.

Measuring variations in fiber diameter and using acetylcholine-esterase staining as indexes of denervation, Borodic et al. (12) showed that BTX diffuses up to 4.5 cm from the site of a single injection (10 U injected in the rabbit longissimus dorsi). Because the size of the denervation field is largely determined by the dose (and volume), multiple point injections along the affected muscle rather than a single point injection should, therefore, contain the biologic effects of the toxin in the targeted muscle (13). Blackie and Lees (9) also showed that frequency of dysphagia could be reduced by 50% when multiple rather than single injections are used.

It is important to note that the biologic activity of BOTOX, distributed by Allergan Pharmaceuticals (originally named Oculinum), is different from the toxin produced in the United Kingdom or in Japan. The standard unit for measuring potency of BOTOX® is derived from a mouse assay: 1 U of BTX is the amount of toxin found to kill 50% (LD50) of a group of mice. When administered intravenously or intramuscularly to monkeys, the LD50 for the U.S. toxin was estimated to be 40 U/kg, about 3,000 U when extracted to a 75-kg man (105). The dosages used in human therapeutic applications are markedly lower, representing 1% to 10% of this lethal dose. The toxin produced by using anion-exchange chromatography and RNase treatment and supplied by the Vaccine and Research Laboratory, Porton Down, Salisbury (Dysport) in the United Kingdom has different potency than BOTOX®. One ng of the U.K. toxin contains approximately 40 mouse U, whereas 1 ng of the U.S. toxin contains approximately 4 mouse U. Using quantitative analysis of regional paralysis produced by local injections into the gastrocnemius muscles of mice, Pearce et al. (92) estimated the potency ratio between Dysport and BOTOX® to be 4.2 to 1. Subsequent studies suggest that the true dose ratio of Dysport to BOTOX® is 2.5 to 1.

A small percentage of patients receiving repeated injections develop antibodies against BTX, causing them to be completely resistant to the effects of subsequent BTX injections (44,72). In one study, 24 of 559 (4.3%) patients treated for CD developed BTX antibodies (44). The authors suggested that the true prevalence of antibodies may be more than 7%. In addition to patients with BTX antibodies, they studied eight patients from a cohort of 76 (10.5%) who stopped responding to BTX treatments. These BTX-resistant patients had a shorter interval between injections, more "boosters," and a higher dose at the "nonbooster" injection as compared with nonresistant patients treated during the same period. As a result of this experience clinicians are warned against using booster injections and are encouraged to extend the interval between treatment as long as possible, certainly at least 1 month, and to use the smallest possible doses. In addition to high dosages, we also found that young age is a potential risk factor for the development of immunoresistance to BTX-A (72). Some of the patients who developed BTX-A antibodies have benefited from injections by immunologically distinct preparations, such as BTX-F and BTX-B (43,84,86). After 1 to 3 years some patients become antibody negative and when reinjected with the same type of toxin they may again experience transient benefit (102). The preliminary data suggest that BTX-B provides clinical effects similar to BTX-A, but the benefits of BTX-F seem to last only 1 month. It is likely that future research will result in the development of new and more effective neuromuscular blocking agents that provide therapeutic chemodenervation with long-term benefits and at lower cost.

Despite its proven therapeutic value, there are still many unresolved issues and concerns about BTX. These include lack of standardization of biologic activity of the different preparations of BTX, poor understanding of toxin antigenicity, variations in the methods of injection, and inadequate assays for BTX antibodies. Training guidelines for the use of botulinum toxin have been established (3). Clinicians interested in using BTX chemodenervation in their practice must have a knowledge of the disorders they treat, the involved anatomy, and be skilled in the technique of administration of BTX so that they can exercise proper precautions to minimize the potential risks associated with BTX. Possible contraindications to the use of BTX include the presence of myasthenia gravis (33), Eaton-Lambert syndrome, motor neuron disease, aminoglycoside antibiotics, and pregnancy. Besides occasional complications, usually related to local weakness, a major limitation of BTX therapy is its high cost. Several studies analyzing the cost effectiveness of BTX treatment, however, have demonstrated that the loss of productivity as a result of untreated dystonia and the cost of medications or surgery more than justify the financial expense of BTX treatments.

This review focuses on the use of BTX in the treatment of dystonia. The therapeutic impact of BTX, however, extends to many other disorders including strabismus, spasticity, tremors, tics, achalasia, spastic bladder, peripheral autonomic disorders, and even some cosmetic conditions (Table 3) (62). It is likely that the applications of BTX therapy will continue to expand in the future.

TABLE 3. *Clinical applications of botulinum toxin*

Focal dystonia
  Blepharospasm
  Lid "apraxia"
  Oromandibular-facial-lingual dystonia
  Cervical dystonia (torticollis)
  Laryngeal dystonia (spasmodic dysphonia)
  Task-specific dystonia (occupational cramps)
  Other focal dystonias (idiopathic, secondary)
Other involuntary movements
  Voice, head, and limb tremor
  Palatal myoclonus
  Hemifacial spasm
  Tics
Inappropriate contractions
  Strabismus
  Nystagmus
  Myokymia
  Bruxism (TMJ)
  Stuttering
  Painful rigidity
  Muscle contraction headaches
  Lumbosacral strain and back spasms
  Radiculopathy with secondary muscle spasm
  Spasticity
  Spastic bladder
  Achalasia (esophageal, pelvirectal)
  Other spasmic disorders
Other potential applications
  Protective ptosis
  Cosmetic (wrinkles, facial asymmetry)
  Debarking dogs
  Disorders of cholinergic autonomic nervous system
    (e.g., hyperhydrosis, sialorrhea, pain)
  Other

BLEPHAROSPASM

The effectiveness of BTX in blepharospasm was first demonstrated in a double-blind, placebo-controlled trial in 1987 (65). In a subsequent report of our experience with BTX in 477 patients with various dystonias and hemifacial spasm, Jankovic et al. (75) reviewed the results in 90 patients injected with BTX for blepharospasm. Moderate or marked improvement was noted in 94% of the blepharospasm patients. The average latency from the time of the injection to the onset of improvement was 4.2 days, the average duration of maximum benefit was 12.4 weeks, but the total benefit lasted considerably longer, average 15.7 weeks. Although 41% of all treatment sessions were followed by some side effects (ptosis, blurring of vision or diplopia, tearing, and local hematoma), only 2% affected patients' functioning. Complications usually improved spontaneously in less than 2 weeks. These results are consistent with those of other studies (32). There is no apparent decline in benefit and the frequency of complications actually decreases after repeat BTX treatments (70). Reasons for the gradual enhancement in efficacy and reduction in the frequency of complications with repeat treatments include greater experience and improvements in the injection technique. For example, one controlled study showed that an injection into the pretarsal rather than preseptal portion of the orbicularis oculi is associated with significantly lower frequency of ptosis (55). Ptosis can be prevented also by injecting initially only the lateral and medial portion of the upper lid, thus avoiding the midline levator muscle. We usually initially inject 5 U in each site in the upper lid and 5 U in the lower lid laterally only.

The functional improvement, experienced by the vast majority of patients after BTX injection, is difficult to express numerically. Many could not work, drive, watch TV, or read prior to the injections. As a result of reduced eyelid and eyebrow spasms, most can now function normally. In addition to the observed functional improvement, there is usually a meaningful amelioration of discomfort and, because of less embarrassment, the patients' self-esteem also frequently improves. BTX injections are now considered by many as the treatment of choice for blepharospasm (2,4). In addition to idiopathic blepharospasm, BTX injections have been used effectively in the treatment of blepharospasm induced by drugs (e.g., levodopa in parkinsonian patients or neuroleptics in patients with tardive dystonia), dystonic eyelid and facial tics in patients with Tourette's syndrome, and in patients in whom blepharospasm was associated with "apraxia of eyelid opening" (6,54,55,80).

OROMANDIBULAR DYSTONIA

Oromandibular dystonia is among the most challenging forms of focal dystonia to treat with BTX; it rarely improves with medica-

tions, there are no surgical treatments, and BTX therapy can be complicated by swallowing problems. The masseter (and possibly temporalis) muscles are usually injected in patients with jaw-closure dystonia. In patients with jaw-opening dystonia either the submental muscle complex or the lateral pterygoid muscles are injected. A meaningful reduction in the oromandibular-lingual spasms and an improvement in chewing and speech was achieved in more than 70% of all patients. Patients with dystonic jaw closure respond better than those with jaw-opening dystonia. Temporary swallowing problem, noted in less than 20% of all treatment sessions, was the most frequent complication. BTX injections provide the most effective relief of oromandibular dystonia and early treatment with BTX may prevent dental and other complications, including the TMJ syndrome and other oral and dental problems (11). Oromandibular involuntary movements caused by hemimasticatory spasms and other disorders such as Satoyoshi's syndrome have also been successfully treated with BTX (85).

LARYNGEAL DYSTONIA (SPASMODIC DYSPHONIA)

Until the introduction of BTX, the therapy of spasmodic dysphonia has been disappointing. The anticholinergic and benzodiazepine drugs only rarely provide meaningful improvement in voice quality. Unilateral transection of the recurrent laryngeal nerve, although effective in most patients, frequently causes unacceptable complications and the voice symptoms often recur (26). Several studies have established the efficacy and safety of BTX in the treatment of laryngeal dystonia and this approach is considered by most to be the treatment of choice for spasmodic dysphonia (16,75,84). Before a patient can be considered a potential candidate for BTX injections, however, the diagnosis of spasmodic dysphonia must be confirmed by detailed neurologic, otolaryngologic, and voice assessment and documented by video and voice recordings. There are three approaches currently used in the BTX treatment of spasmodic dysphonia: (a) unilateral EMG-guided injection of 5 to 30 U (75), (b) bilateral approach, injecting with EMG guidance 1.25 U to 4 U in each vocal fold (16), and (c) an injection via indirect laryngoscopy without EMG (36). Irrespective of the technique, most investigators report about 75% to 95% improvement in voice symptoms. One controlled study, however, concluded that unilateral injections "may provide both superior and longer lasting benefits" than bilateral injections (1). The dosage can be adjusted depending on the severity of glottal spasms and the response to previous injections. Adverse experiences include transient breathy hypophonia, hoarseness, and rare dysphagia with aspiration. Although more complicated and less effective, BTX injections into the posterior cricoarytenoid muscle with the EMG needle placed posterior to the thyroid lamina may be used in the treatment of the abductor form of spasmodic dysphonia (16). Using a multidisciplinary team approach, consisting of an otolaryngologist experienced in laryngeal injections and a neurologist knowledgeable about motor disorders of speech and voice, BTX injections can provide effective relief for most patients with spasmodic dysphonia (2,5). BTX may be useful in the treatment of voice tremor and stuttering (17,83).

CERVICAL DYSTONIA

The goal of therapy of cervical dystonia is not only to improve abnormal posture of the head and associated neck pain, but also to prevent the development of secondary complications such as contractures, cervical radiculopathy, and cervical myelopathy (110,119). The efficacy and safety of BTX in the treatment of cervical dystonia has been demonstrated in several controlled and open trials (9,45,60,68, 94). In one double-blind, placebo-controlled study of 55 patients with cervical dystonia, 61% improved after BTX injection (45). BTX has been found to be superior not only to placebo, but also to trihexyphenidyl (14). Open-label studies generally report a more dramatic improvement, partly because of a "placebo effect" and, more important, because of greater flexibility in selecting the proper dosage and site of injection. Most trials report that about 90% of patients experience improvement in function and control of head-neck and in pain. The average latency between injection and the onset of improvement (and muscle atrophy) is 1 week and the average duration of maximum improvement is 3 to 4 months. On the average, the injections are repeated every 4 to 6 months. Patients with long-duration dystonia have been found to respond less well than those treated relatively early, possibly because prolonged dystonia produced contractures (73). In one study, 28% of patients experienced some complication such as swallowing difficulties, neck weakness, and nausea sometime during the course of their treatment (some patients had up to 12 visits in 5 years). Dysphagia, the most common complication, was encountered in 14% of all 659 visits, but in only five instances was this problem severe enough to require changing to a soft or liquid diet. Complications are usually related to focal weakness, although distant and systemic subclinical and clinical effects, such as generalized weakness and malaise, rarely occur possibly as a result of blood distribution or retrograde axonal transport to the spinal motor neurons (38). Most complications resolve spontaneously, usually within 2 weeks. An injection into one or both sternocleidomastoid muscles was most frequently associated with dysphagia (13,23,60, 73). One study showed that dosages as small as 20 units administered as a single injection into the sternocleidomastoid muscle completely eliminated muscle activity and could produce neck weakness and dysphagia (19). In an analysis of patients who received five or more injections we found that the beneficial response was maintained and the frequency of complications with repeat injections actually declined (70). Results similar to those obtained with BTX type A have been obtained in patients treated for cervical dystonia with BTX type B (115). A standardized rating scale, the Toronto Western Spasmodic Torticollis Rating Scale (TWSTRS), is used in most clinical trials of cervical dystonia (24).

The most important determinants of a favorable response to BTX treatments are a proper selection of the involved muscles and an appropriate dosage. EMG may be helpful in some patients with obese necks or in whom the involved muscles are difficult to identify by palpation (31,39). One study attempted to determine the usefulness of EMG-assisted BTX injections and found that the percentage of patients showing any improvement after BTX was similar whether the injections were assisted by EMG or not (22). They also noted that "a significantly greater magnitude of improvement" was present in patients treated with the EMG-assisted method and that there was "a significantly greater number of patients with marked benefit" in the group randomly assigned to the EMG-assisted method of treatment. Because the majority (70% to 79%) of patients were previously treated with BTX, some may have been experiencing residual effects from previous injections, making the interpretation of the results difficult. Furthermore, the patients who were treated without EMG assistance received a higher dose, indicating more severe dystonia, thus possibly explaining lesser degree of observed improvement. The general consensus among most BTX users is that EMG is not needed in the vast majority of patients, except in rare instances when the muscles cannot be adequately palpated or the patient does not obtain adequate relief of symptoms with the conventional approach.

WRITER'S CRAMPS AND OTHER LIMB DYSTONIAS

Treatments of writer's cramps with muscle relaxation techniques, physical and occupational therapy, and medical and surgical therapies have been disappointing. Several open (6,71,78,97,98,101,121) and double-blind controlled (21,114,122) trials have concluded that BTX injections into selected hand and forearm muscles probably provide the most effective relief in patients with these task-specific occupational dystonias. In some studies fine wire electrodes were used to localize bursts of muscle activation during the task and the toxin was injected through a hollow EMG needle into the belly of the most active muscle (21). Similar beneficial results, however, were obtained in other studies without complex EMG studies (101). Several lines of evidence support the notion that an intramuscular injection of BTX into the forearm muscles corrects the abnormal reciprocal inhibition (96).

We studied the effects of BTX in 46 patients with hand dystonia who were injected into forearm muscles in 130 treatment sessions (71). The average age was 49.4 years and the dystonic symptoms were present for an average of 8.6 years. After careful examination and palpation of the forearm muscles during writing, the toxin was injected into either the wrist flexors (116 injections) or the wrist extensors (52 injections). The average baseline severity of dystonia was 3.5 on a 0 to 4 (4 = maximum) rating scale. The average peak effect response for all treatment sessions was 2.3 (0 = no response to 4 = maximum benefit). The latency from injection to onset of effect averaged 5.6 days and the benefit lasted an average of 9.2 weeks. Temporary hand weakness, the chief complication of this treatment, occurred in 54% of patients and in 34% of all treatment sessions. However, nearly all patients preferred the temporary weakness, which was usually mild, to the disabling writer's cramps. In addition to improving writer's cramps, BTX may provide relief in other task-specific disorders affecting typists, draftsmen, musicians, sportsmen, and other people who depend on skilled movements of their hands.

Other focal distal dystonias, besides those involving the hands, may be amenable to treatment with BTX. Patients with foot dystonia as a manifestation of idiopathic torsion dystonia and patients with parkinsonism who may experience foot dystonia as an early symptom of their disease, or more commonly, as a complication of levodopa therapy, may benefit from local BTX injections (90). BTX injections into the foot-toe flexors or extensors may not only alleviate the disability, pain, and discomfort often associated with such dystonia, but may also improve gait. Whether BTX injections will play an important role in the treatment of recurrent painful physiologic foot and calf cramps is yet to be determined.

OTHER INDICATIONS FOR BOTULINUM TOXIN

Hemifacial spasm is not considered a form of dystonia, even though it can cause blepharospasm and facial spasms. The chief difference between facial dystonia and hemifacial spasm is that the latter is consistently unilateral. Hemifacial spasm is defined as a neurologic disorder manifested by involuntary, recurrent twitches of the eyelids, perinasal, perioral, zygomaticus, platysma, and other muscles of only one side of the face (28). It is an example of a peripherally induced movement disorder and may be classified as segmental myoclonus in which the muscular contractions result from an irritative lesion of the ipsilateral facial nerve. The condition is not only annoying, but also socially embarrassing, and in some patients it causes unilateral blepharospasm that can interfere with vision. Hemifacial spasm is usually due to a compression or irritation of the facial nerve by an aberrant artery or abnormal vasculature around the brainstem. Although microvascular decompression of the facial nerve has a high success rate, this surgical treatment is associated with certain risks, such as permanent facial paralysis, deafness, stroke, and death. Therefore, local injections of BTX into involved facial muscles offers a useful alternative to surgical therapy. Nearly all patients improve, the complications are minimal and transient, and the approach can be individualized by injecting only those muscles whose contractions are most disturbing to the patient (75). In our experience, the average duration of improvement of hemifacial spasm was 5 months, longer than in any of the dystonic disorders. Except for transient facial weakness and ptosis there are usually no other complications. Along with blepharospasm, the FDA has approved BTX injections also for hemifacial spasm.

Tremor, an oscillatory movement produced by alternating or synchronous contractions of antagonistic muscles, is the most common movement disorder (82). Although propranolol, primidone, and other antitremor medications are usually satisfactory, when high-amplitude essential tremor significantly impairs activities of daily living, pharmacotherapy alone is not sufficient. In severe cases, neurosurgical treatment (thalamotomy, pallidotomy, or thalamic stimulation) may provide satisfactory relief.

Some form of tremor is present in about one-half of all dystonic patients (64). The observation that some patients treated for focal dystonia with BTX noted improvement in their tremor led to trials of BTX specifically for tremor (69). In a pilot study of 51 patients with disabling tremors of head-neck (42 patients) and hand (ten patients), we noted moderate to marked functional improvement and a reduction in the amplitude of the tremor in 67% of patients. The average duration of improvement was 10.5 weeks. Local weakness, lasting up to 3 weeks, occurred after the injection in 60% of patients with hand tremor and in 10% of those with head-neck tremor. Nearly all patients, however, preferred having mild weakness over disabling tremor. Other open and controlled studies subsequently reported benefit from BTX in patients with hand and head tremor (74,91,111).

Motor and phonic tics are usually manifestations of Tourette's syndrome, a familial neurobehavioral disorder. Tics are rarely disabling and they usually improve with antidopaminergic drugs. Some patients, however, have troublesome tics that may cause functional blindness or local discomfort. We have treated ten patients, five with disabling blinking and blepharospasm and five with painful dystonic tics involving the neck muscles, with BTX injections (54). All patients noted moderate to marked improvement in the intensity of tics and lessening of the premonitory "tension" that preceded the tics. The improvement lasted 2 to 20 weeks and, except for transient ptosis in two patients, there were no other complications.

Spasticity, rigidity, and *stiff-person syndrome* are examples of hypertonic disorders effectively treated with local injections of BTX (11,25,40,49).

SUMMARY

Patients with segmental or generalized dystonia beginning in childhood or adolescence should be initially tried on levodopa/carbidopa up to 1,000 mg of levodopa per day. If this therapy is successful, it should be maintained at a lowest possible dose. If ineffective after 3 months, than a high-dose anticholinergic (e.g., trihexyphenidyl, diphenhydramine) therapy should be instituted and the dosage increased to the highest tolerated level. If the results are poor, than baclofen, benzodiazepines, carbamazepine, and tetrabenazine should be tried. Some patients may require "triple therapy" consisting of an anticholinergic agent (e.g., trihexyphenidyl), monoamine depleting drug (e.g., tetrabenazine), and a dopamine receptor blocking drug (e.g., fluphenazine, pimozide, risperidol, or clozapine). Tetrabenazine alone or with anticholinergic drugs is particularly useful in the treatment of tardive dystonia. In some patients BTX injections may be helpful to control the most disabling symptom of the segmental or generalized dystonia. In most patients with adult-onset dystonia the distribution is usually focal and, therefore, BTX injections are usually considered the treatment of choice. In some patients this treatment may need to be supplemented by other drugs noted above or by surgical peripheral denervation. Thalamotomy should be reserved only for patients whose symptoms continue to be disabling despite optimal medical therapy or pallidotomy (89A). Any form of therapy should, of course, be preceded by a thorough evaluation designed to rule out secondary causes of dystonia. Finally, it is important to emphasize that patient education and counseling are essential components of a comprehensive therapeutic approach to all patients with dystonia.

ACKNOWLEDGMENTS

Parts of this manuscript have been included in: Jankovic J. Treatment of dystonia. In: Watts RL, Koller WC eds. Movement disorders: Neurologic principles and practice. New York: McGraw Hill, 1997 443–454.

REFERENCES

1. Adams SG, Hunt EJ, Charles DA, Lang AE. Unilateral versus bilateral botulinum toxin injections in spasmodic dysphonia: acoustic and perceptual results. *J Otolaryngol* 1993;22:171–175.
2. American Academy of Neurology. Assessment: the clinical usefulness of botulinum toxin-A in treating neurologic disorders. Report of the Therapeutics and Technology Assessment Subcommittee of the American Academy of Neurology. *Neurology* 1990;40: 1332–1336.
3. American Academy of Neurology. Training guidelines for the use of botulinum toxin for the treatment of neurologic disorders. Report of the Therapeutics and Technology Assessment Subcommittee of the American Academy of Neurology. *Neurology* 1994; 2401–2403.
4. American Academy of Ophthalmology. Botulinum toxin therapy of eye muscle disorders. Safety and effectiveness. *Ophthalmology* 1989;96(Part 2):37–41.
5. American Academy of Otolaryngology. Position statement on the clinical usefulness of botulinum toxin in the treatment of spasmodic dysphonia. *Arch Otolaryngol Head Neck Surg Bull* 1990;9:8.
6. Aramideh M, Ongerboer de Visser BW, Koelman JHTM, Speelman JD. Motor persistence of orbicularis oculi muscle in eyelid-opening disorders. *Neurology* 1995;45:897–902.
7. Bates AK, Halliday BL, Bailey CS, et al. Surgical treatment of essential blepharospasm. *Br J Ophthalmol* 1991;75:487–491.
8. Black JD, Dolly JO. Selective location of acceptors for botulinum neurotoxin A in the central and peripheral nervous systems. *Neuroscience* 1987;23:767–779.
9. Blackie JD, Lees AJ. Botulinum toxin treatment in spasmodic torticollis. *J Neurol Neurosurg Psychiatry* 1990;53:640–643.
10. Blasi J, Chapman ER, Link E, et al. Botulinum neurotoxin A selectively cleaves the synaptic protein SNAP-25. *Nature* 1993;365:160–163.
11. Blitzer A, Brin MF. Laryngeal dystonia: A series with botulinum toxin therapy. *Ann Otol Rhinol Laryngol* 1991;100:85–90.
12. Borodic GE, Ferrante R, Pearce LB, Smith K. Histologic assessment of dose-related diffusion and muscle fiber response after therapeutic botulinum A toxin injections. *Mov Disord* 1994;9:31–39.
13. Borodic GE, Pearce LB, Smith K, Joseph M. Botulinum A toxin for spasmodic torticollis: multiple vs single injection points per muscle. *Head Neck* 1992;14:33–37.
14. Brans JWM, Lindeboom R, Snoek JW, et al. Botulinum toxin versus trihexyphenidyl in cervical dystonia: a prospective, randomized, double-blind controlled trial. *Neurology* 1996;46:1066–1072.
15. Brashear A, Farlow MR, Butler IJ, et al. Variable phenotype of rapid-onset dystonia-parkinsonism. *Mov Disord* 1996;11:151–156.

16. Brin MF, Blitzer A, Stewart C, Fahn S. Treatment of spasmodic dysphonia (laryngeal dystonia) with local injections of botulinum toxin: review and technical aspects. In: Blitzer A, Brin MF, Sasaki CT, Fahn S, Harris KS (eds). *Neurologic disorders of the larynx.* New York: Thieme Medical Publishers, 1992:214–228.

17. Brin MF, Stewart C, Blitzer A, et al. Laryngeal botulinum toxin injections for disabling stuttering in adults. *Neurology* 1994;44:2262–2266.

18. Bucher SF, Seelos KC, Dodel RC, et al. Pallidal lesions. Structural and functional magnetic resonance imaging. *Arch Neurol* 1996;53:682–686.

19. Buchman AS, Comella CL, Stebbins GT, et al. Determining a dose-effect curve for botulinum toxin in the sternocleidomastoid muscle in cervical dystonia. *Clin Neuropharmacol* 1994;17:188–193.

20. Clarke CE. Therapeutic potential of botulinum toxin in neurologic disorders. *Q J Med* 1992;82:197–205.

21. Cole R, Hallett M, Cohen LG. Double-blind trial of botulinum toxin for treatment of focal hand dystonia. *Mov Disord* 1995;10:466–471.

22. Comella CL, Buchman AS, Tanner CM, et al. Botulinum toxin injection for spasmodic torticollis: increased magnitude of benefit with electromyographic assistance. *Neurology* 1992;42:878–882.

23. Comella CL, Tanner CM, DeFoor-Hill L, Smith C. Dysphagia after botulinum toxin injections for spasmodic torticollis. Clinical and radiologic findings. *Neurology* 1992;42:1307–1310.

24. Consky ES, Lang AE. Clinical assessments of patients with cervical dystonia. In: Jankovic J, Hallett M, eds. *Therapy with botulinum toxin.* New York: Marcel Dekker, 1994:211–237.

25. Davis D, Jabbari B. Significant improvement of stiff-person syndrome after paraspinal injection of botulinum toxin A. *Mov Disord* 1993;8:371–373.

26. Dedo HH, Izdebski K. Intermediate results of 306 recurrent laryngeal nerve sections for spastic dysphonia. *Laryngoscope* 1983;93:9–15.

27. Demirkiran M, Jankovic J. Paroxysmal dyskinesias: clinical features and classification. *Ann Neurol* 1995;38:571–579.

28. Digre K, Corbett JJ. Hemifacial spasm: differential diagnosis, mechanism, and treatment. In: Jankovic J, Tolosa E, eds. *Facial dyskinesias. Advances of neurology.* Vol. 49. New York: Raven Press, 1988:151–176.

29. Dobyns WB, Ozelius LJ, Kramer PL, et al. Rapid-onset dystonia-parkinsonism. *Neurology* 1993;43:2596–2602.

30. Dressnandt J, Conrad B. Lasting reduction of severe spasticity after ending chronic treatment with intrathecal baclofen. *J Neurol Neurosurg Psychiatry* 1996;60:168–173.

31. Dubinsky RM, Gray CS, Vetere-Overfield B, Koller WC. Electromyographic guidance of botulinum toxin treatment in cervical dystonia. *Clin Neuropharmacol* 1991;14:262–267.

32. Elston JS. Botulinum toxin for blepharospasm. In: Jankovic J, Hallett M, eds. Therapy with botulinum toxin. New York: Marcel Dekker, 1993 191–198.

33. Emerson J. Botulinum toxin for spasmodic torticollis in a patient with myasthenia gravis. *Mov Disord* 1994;9:367.

34. Fahn S, Henning WA, Bressman S, et al. Long-term usefulness of baclofen in the treatment of essential blepharospasm. *Adv Ophthalmol Plast Reconstr Surg* 1985;4:219–226.

35. Filippi GM, Errico P, Samtarelli R, et al. Botulinum A toxin effects on rat jaw muscle spindles. *Acta Otolaryngol (Stockh)* 1993;113:400–404.

36. Ford CN, Bless DM, Lowery JD. Indirect laryngoscopic approach for injection of botulinum toxin in spasmodic dysphonia. *Otolaryngol Head Neck Surg* 1990;103:752–758.

37. Ford B, Greene P, Louis ED, et al. Use of intrathecal baclofen in the treatment of patients with dystonia. *Arch Neurol* 1965;53:1241–1246.

38. Garner CG, Straube A, Witt TN, et al. Time course effects of local injections of botulinum toxin. *Mov Disord* 1993;8:33–37.

39. Gelb DJ, Yoshimura DM, Olney RK, et al. Change in pattern of muscle activity following botulinum toxin injections for torticollis. *Ann Neurol* 1991;29:370–376.

40. Grazko M, Polo KB, Jabbari B. Botulinum toxin A for spasticity, muscle spasms, and rigidity. *Neurology* 1995;45:712–717.

41. Greene P. Baclofen in the treatment of dystonia. *Clin Neuropharmacol* 1992;15:276–288.

42. Greene P. Medical and surgical therapy of idiopathic torsion dystonia. In: Kurlan R, ed. *Treatment of movement disorders.* Philadelphia, PA: JB Lippincott Co, 1995:153–181.

43. Greene P, Fahn S. Treatment of torticollis with injections of botulinum toxin type F in patients with antibodies to botulinum toxin type A. *Mov Disord* 1992;7[Suppl 1]:134.

44. Greene P, Fahn S, Diamond B. Development of resistance to botulinum toxin type A in patients with torticollis. *Mov Disord* 1994;9:213–217.

45. Greene P, Kang U, Fahn S, Brin MF, Moskowitz C, Flaster E. Double-blind, placebo controlled trial of botulinum toxin injection for the treatment of spasmodic torticollis. *Neurology* 1990;40:1213–1218.

46. Greene P, Shale H, Fahn S. Analysis of open-label trials in torsion dystonia using high dosage of anticholinergics and other drugs. *Mov Disord* 1988;3:46–60.

47. Hallett M. Is dystonia a sensory disorder? *Ann Neurol* 1995;38:139–140.

48. Harwood G, Hierons R, Fletcher NA, Marsden CD. Lessons from a remarkable family with dopa-responsive dystonia. *J Neurol Neurosurg Psychiatry* 1994;57:460–463.

49. Hesse S, Lücke D, Malezic M, et al. Botulinum toxin treatment for lower limb extensor spasticity in chronic hemiparetic patients. *J Neurol Neurosurg Psychiatry* 1994;57:1321–1324.

50. Huttner W. Snappy exocytoxins. *Nature* 1993;365:104–105.

51. Ichinose H, Ohye T, Takahi E, et al. Hereditary progressive dystonia with marked diurnal fluctuation caused by mutations in the GTP cyclohydrolase I gene. *Nat Genet* 1994;8:236–242.

52. Ishikawa A, Miyatake T. A family with hereditary juvenile dystonia-parkinsonism. *Mov Disord* 1995;10:482–488.

53. Jabbari B, Scherokman B, Gunderson CH, et al. Treatment of movement disorders with trihexyphenidyl. *Mov Disord* 1989;4:202–212.

54. Jankovic J. Botulinum toxin in the treatment of dystonic tics. *Mov Disord* 1994;9:347–349a.

55. Jankovic J. Apraxia of eyelid opening (Letter to the editor). *Mov Disord* 1995 10:686–687.

56. Jankovic J. Tardive syndromes and other drug-induced movement disorders. *Clin Neuropharmacol* 1995;18:197–214.

57. Jankovic J. Treatment of dystonia. In: Watts RL, Koller WC. *Movement disorders: neurologic principles and practice.* New York: McGraw Hill, 1997 443–454.

58. Jankovic J, Beach J. Long-term effects of tetrabenazine in hyperkinetic movement disorders. *Neurology* 1997 48:358–362.

59. Jankovic J, Brin MF. Therapeutic uses of botulinum toxin. *N Engl J Med* 1991;324:1186–1194.

60. Jankovic J, Brin MF, Comella C. *Handbook of botulinum toxin treatment for cervical dystonia.* New York: Churchill Livingstone, 1994.

61. Jankovic J, Fahn S. Dystonic disorders. In: Jankovic J, Tolosa E, eds. *Parkinson's disease and movement disorders.* 2nd ed. Baltimore: Williams & Wilkins, 1993:337–374.

62. Jankovic J, Hallett M, eds. Therapy with botulinum toxin. New York: Marcel Dekker, 1994:1–608.

63. Jankovic J, Hamilton W, Grossman RG. Thalamic surgery for movement disorders. In: Obeso JA, DeLong M, Ohye C, Marsden CD. *Advances in understanding the basal ganglia and new surgical approaches for Parkinson's disease. Advances in Neurology.* New York: Raven Press, 1997; 74:221–233.

64. Jankovic J, Leder S, Warner D, Schwartz K. Cervical dystonia: clinical findings and associated movement disorders. *Neurology* 1991;41:1088–1091.

65. Jankovic J, Orman J. Botulinum A toxin for cranial-cervical dystonia: a double-blind, placebo-controlled study. *Neurology* 1987;37:616–623.

66. Jankovic J, Orman J. Tetrabenazine treatment in dystonia, chorea, tics and other dyskinesias. *Neurology* 1988;38:391–394.

67. Jankovic J, Penn A. Severe dystonia and myoglobinuria. *Neurology* 1982;32:1195–1197.

68. Jankovic J, Schwartz K. Botulinum toxin injections for cervical dystonia. *Neurology* 1990;41:277–280.

69. Jankovic J, Schwartz K. Botulinum toxin treatment of tremors. *Neurology* 1991;41:1185–1188c.

70. Jankovic J, Schwartz K. Longitudinal follow-up of botulinum toxin injections for treatment of blepharospasm and cervical dystonia. *Neurology* 1993; 43:834–836.

71. Jankovic J, Schwartz K. The use of botulinum toxin in the treatment of hand dystonias. *J Hand Surg* 1993;18A:883–887.

72. Jankovic J, Schwartz K. Response and immunoresistance to botulinum toxin injections. *Neurology* 1995; 45:1743–1746.

73. Jankovic J, Schwartz KS. Clinical correlates of response to botulinum toxin injections. *Arch Neurol* 1991;48:1253–1256a.

74. Jankovic J, Schwartz K, Clemence W, Aswad A, Mordaunt J. A randomized, double-blind, placebo-controlled study to evaluate botulinum toxin type A in essential hand tremor. *Mov Disord* 1996;11:250–256.

75. Jankovic J, Schwartz K, Donovan DT. Botulinum toxin treatment of cranial-cervical dystonia, spasmodic dysphonia, other focal dystonias and hemifacial spasm. *J Neurol Neurosurg Psychiatry* 1990;53: 633–639.

76. Kaji R, Kohara N, Katayama M, et al. Muscle afferent block by intramuscular injection of lidocaine for the treatment of writer's cramp. *Muscle Nerve* 1995;18:234–235.

77. Kaji R, Rothwell JC, Katayama M, et al. Tonic vibration reflex and muscle afferent block in writer's cramp. *Ann Neurol* 1995;38:155–162.

78. Karp BI, Cole RA, Cohen LG, et al. Long-term botulinum toxin treatment of focal hand dystonia. *Neurology* 1994;44:70–76.

79. Lang AE. Dopamine agonists and antagonists in the treatment of idiopathic dystonia. In: Fahn S, Marsden CD, Calne DB, eds. *Dystonia: advances in neurology.* Vol. 50. New York: Raven Press, 1988:561–570.

80. Lepore V, Defazio G, Acquistapance D, et al. Botulinum A toxin for the so-called apraxia of lid opening. *Mov Disord* 1995;10:525–526.

81. Lindeboom R, de Haan RJ, Brans JWM, Speelman JD. Treatment outcomes in cervical dystonia: a clinimetric study. *Mov Disord* 1996;11:371–376.

82. Lou JS, Jankovic J. Essential tremor: clinical correlates in 350 patients. *Neurology* 1991;41:234–238.

83. Ludlow CL. Treatment of speech and voice disorders with botulinum toxin. *JAMA* 1990;264:2671–2675.

84. Ludlow CL, Hallett M, Rhew K, et al. Therapeutic use of type F botulinum toxin. *N Engl J Med* 1992; 326:349–350.

85. Merello M, Garcia H, Nogues M, Leiguarda R. Masticatory muscle spasm in non-Japanese patient with Satoyoshi syndrome successfully treated with botulinum toxin. *Mov Disord* 1994;9:104–105.

86. Mezaki T, Kaji R, Hamano T, Nagamine T, et al. Optimisation of botulinum treatment for cervical and axial dystonias: experience with Japanese type A toxin. *J Neurol Neurosurg Psychiatry* 1994;57:1535–1537.

87. Mezaki T, Kaji R, Kohara N, et al. Comparison of therapeutic efficacies of type A and F botulinum toxins for blepharospasm: a double-blind, controlled study. *Neurology* 1995;45:506–508.

88. Narayan RK, Loubser PG, Jankovic J, et al. Intrathecal baclofen for intractable axial dystonia. *Neurology* 1991;41:1141–1142.

89. Nygaard TG, Marsden CD, Fahn S. Dopa-responsive dystonia: Long-term treatment response and prognosis. *Neurology* 1991;41:174–181.

89A. Ondo WG, Desaloms M, Jankovic J, Grossman R, Surgical pallidotomy for the treatment of generalized dystonia. *Mov Disord* 1998 *(in press).*

90. Pacchetti C, Albani G, Martignoni E, et al. "Off" painful dystonia in Parkinson's disease treated with botulinum toxin. *Mov Disord* 1995;10:333–336.

91. Pahwa R, Busenbark K, Swanson-Hyland EF, et al. Botulinum toxin treatment of essential head tremor. *Neurology* 1995;45:822–824.

92. Pearce LB, Borodic GE, First E, MacCallum R. Measurement of botulinum activity: evaluation of the lethality assay. *Toxicol Appl Pharmacol* 1994;128: 69–77.

93. Penn RD, Gianino JM, York MM. Intrathecal baclofen for motor disorders. *Mov Disord* 1995;10: 675–677.

94. Poewe W, Schlosky L, Kleedorfer B, et al. Treatment of spasmodic torticollis with local injections of botulinum toxin. *J Neurol* 1992;239:21–25.

95. Pozos RS, Iaizo PA. Effects of topical anesthesia on essential tremor. *Electromyogr Clin Neurophysiol* 1992;32:369–372.

96. Priori A, Berardelli A, Mercuri B, Mafredi M. Physiological effects produced by botulinum toxin treatment of upper limb dystonia. Changes in reciprocal inhibition between forearm muscles. *Brain* 1995;118: 801–807.

97. Pullman SL, Greene P, Fahns S, Pederson SF. Approach to the treatment of limb disorders with botulinum toxin. *Arch Neurol* 1996;53:617–624.

98. Quirk JA, Sheean GL, Marsden CD, Lees AJ. Treatment of nonoccupational limb and trunk dystonia with botulinum toxin. *Mov Disord* 1996;11:377–383.

99. Rajput AH, Gibb WRG, Zhong XH, et al. DOPA-responsive dystonia—pathological and biochemical observations in a case. *Ann Neurol* 1994;35:396–402.

100. Ranawaya R, Lang A. Usefulness of a writing device in writer's cramp. *Neurology* 1991;41:1136–1138.

101. Rivest J, Lees AJ, Marsden CD. Writer's cramp: treatment with botulinum toxin injections. *Mov Disord* 1990;6:55–59.

102. Sankhla C, Jankovic J, Duane D. Variability of immunologic and clinical response in dystonic patients immunoresistant to botulinum toxin injections. *Mov Disord* 1997 13:150–154.

103. Schantz EJ, Johnson EA. Properties and use of botulinum toxin and other microbial neurotoxins in medicine. *Microbiol Rev* 1992;56:80–99.

104. Schiavo G, Rossetto O, Catsicas S, et al. Identification of the nerve terminal targets of botulinum neurotoxin serotypes A, D, and E. *J Biol Chem* 1993;265: 23794–23797.

105. Scott AB, Suzuki D. Systemic toxicity of botulinum toxin by intramuscular injection in the monkey. *Mov Disord* 1988;3:333–335.

106. Sheean GL, Lees AJ. Botulinum toxin F in the treatment of torticollis clinically resistant to botulinum toxin A. *J Neurol Neurosurg Psychiatry* 1995;59:601–607.

107. Sölner T, Whiteheart SW, Brunner M, et al. SNAP receptors implicated in vesicle targeting and fusion. *Nature* 1993;362:318–324.

108. Nygaard TG, Wooten GF, Dopa-responsive dystonia. Some pieces of the puzzle are still missing. *Neurology* 1998; 50:853–855.

109. Taylor AE, Lang AE, Saint-Cyr JA, et al. Cognitive processes in idiopathic dystonia treated with high-dose anticholinergic therapy: implications for treatment strategies. *Clin Neuropharmacol* 1991;14:62–77.

110. Treves T, Korczyn AD. Progressive dystonia and paraparesis in cerebral palsy. *Eur Neurol* 1986;25: 148–153.

111. Trosch RM, Pullman SL. Botulinum toxin A injections for the treatment of hand tremors. *Mov Disord* 1994;9:601–609.

112. Trugman JM, Leadbetter R, Zalis M, et al. Treatment of severe axial tardive dystonia with clozapine: case report and hypothesis. *Mov Disord* 1994;9:441–446.

113. Truong DD, Sandromi P, van der Noort S, Matsumoto RR. Diphenhydramine is effective in the treatment of idiopathic dystonia. *Arch Neurol* 1995; 52:405–407.

114. Tsui JKC, Bhatt M, Calne S, Calne DB. Botulinum toxin in treatment of writer's cramp: a double-blind study. *Neurology* 1993;43:183–185.

115. Tsui JKC, Hayward M, Mak EKM, Schulzer M. Botulinum toxin type B in the treatment of cervical dystonia: a pilot study. *Neurology* 1995;45:2109–2110.

116. Tsui JKC, O'Brien C. Clinical trials for spasticity. In: Jankovic J, Hallet M, eds. *Therapy with botulinum toxin.* New York: Marcel Dekker, 1994:523–534.

117. Vaamonde J, Narbona J, Weiser R, et al. Dystonic storms: a practical management problem. *Clin Neuropharmacol* 1994;17:344–347.

118. Valls-Sole J, Tolosa ES, Marti MJ, Allam N. Treatment with botulinum toxin injections does not change brainstem interneuronal excitability in patients with cervical dystonia. *Clin Neuropharmacol* 1994;17:229–235.

119. Waterston JA, Swash M, Watkins ES. Idiopathic dystonia and cervical spondylotic myelopathy. *J Neurol Neurosurg Psychiatry* 1989;52:1424–1426.

120. Wirtschafeter JD. Clinical doxorubicin chemomyectomy. An experimental treatment for benign essential blepharospasm and hemifacial spasm. *Ophthalmology* 1991;98:357–366.

121. Wissel J, Kabus C, Wenzel R. Botulinum toxin in writer's cramp: objective response evaluation in 31 patients. *J Neurol Neurosurg Psychiatry* 1996;61: 172–175.

122. Yoshimura DM, Aminoff MJ, Olney RK. Botulinum toxin therapy for limb dystonias. *Neurology* 1992;42: 627–630.

123. Zudas A, Cianchetti C. Efficacy of risperidone in idiopathic segmental dystonia. *Lancet* 1996;347:127–128.

Dystonia 3: Advances in Neurology, Vol. 78,
edited by S. Fahn, C. D. Marsden, and M. DeLong.
Lippincott–Raven Publishers, Philadelphia © 1998.

19

Surgical Treatment of Dystonia

Anthony E. Lang

Department of Neurology, The Toronto Hospital-University of Toronto, Toronto, Ontario,
M5T 2S8 Canada.

Surgery for dystonia has a long and complex history. Numerous surgical interventions have been attempted, in large part because of the significant disability caused by dystonia and its general resistance to a wide variety of medical therapies. These probably began with attempts to disable the abnormally contracting muscle when Minnius, in 1641, sectioned the sternocleidomastoid muscle in spasmodic torticollis (52). This century saw the application of a variety of central procedures culminating in the use of stereotactic lesions of various sites in the basal ganglia and thalamus. The purpose of this review is to summarize the current state of surgical procedures for various forms of dystonia. My emphasis will be to review developments that have occurred in the past 10 years, since the last International Congress on Dystonia. Where appropriate I will compare and contrast recent reports with some of the larger series appearing before that time.

"PERIPHERAL" SURGICAL PROCEDURES FOR DYSTONIA

Blepharospasm

Before botulinum toxin therapy revolutionized the management of this disabling form of focal dystonia, a number of surgical therapies had been attempted, often without much sustained benefit. Peripheral facial neurectomy was the most common of these, utilizing various techniques including alcohol injections, surgical sectioning, selective peripheral nerve avulsion, and percutaneous nerve thermolysis. These techniques resulted in a high recurrence rate and a wide variety of complications including paralytic ectropion, lagophthalmos, epiphora, exaggeration of upper lid dermatochalasis, lip paresis, dropping of the mouth, and loss of facial expression (4,27,45). A very high proportion of these patients also required secondary surgical procedures either because of inadequate effect or to correct one or more of the complications of the original procedure. In response to these unsatisfactory results, Gillum and Anderson (30) introduced a myectomy or extirpation procedure that entailed removing the upper orbicularis oculi, procerus and corrugator muscles, as well as the facial nerves in the postorbital facia combined with a browplasty with resectioning of the lower portion of the frontalis muscle and reinforcement of the levator aponeurosis. If necessary a lower myectomy resecting the tarsal, septal, and orbital portions of the orbicularis oculi in combination with a tarsal tuck procedure is performed as a secondary approach in patients obtaining incomplete benefit from the upper myectomy. The need for this second procedure has varied from 22% to 35% (28,40,45). Side effects of the myectomy include numbness of the forehead, chronic lymphedema of the periorbital region, and, less often, exposure keratitis, ptosis, or lid retraction and ectropion and lower lid retraction with the lower myectomy. In their review Patel and Anderson (48) report "improved visual disability in approximately 90% of cases of blepharospasm" with more than 400 myectomies over a 12-year period. When compared with facial nerve avulsion, myectomy has resulted in superior benefit, better patient acceptance, and a much lower need for secondary surgical procedures [required 4.5 times more frequently following facial nerve avulsion in a study by McCord et al. (45)].

Manual Dystonia

Recently, Charness et al. (16) have reported a 40% incidence of compressive ulnar neuropathy detected electrophysiologically in musicians with task-specific dystonia with 77% of patients who had flexion dystonia of the fourth and fifth digits demonstrating these abnormalities. This report suggests the possibility of a pronounced improvement of symptoms in response to ulnar nerve decompression when conservative management fails. This interesting observation clearly requires further evaluation and confirmation.

Cervical Dystonia

There have probably been a wider variety of surgical techniques attempted for cervical dystonia than in any other form of dystonia. Most of these have involved some form of "peripheral" intervention. Table 1 lists the various operations on the peripheral nervous system that have been applied to cervical dystonia.

Sectioning of the overactive muscle, most notably the sternocleidomastoid, represented

TABLE 1. *Peripheral surgeries for cervical dystonia*

Myotomies
Section of spinal accessory nerve (SAN)
Bilateral anterior cervical rhizotomies plus selective
  SAN section
Rhizotomies/SAN section plus
  thalamotomy/pallidotomy
Selective peripheral denervation (ramisectomy plus
  SAN section)
Epidural cervical cord stimulation[a]
Microvascular decompression of SAN roots

[a]This technique, discussed at the last International Congress on Dystonia, has been abandoned due to lack of efficacy.

the earliest attempt to surgically correct cervical dystonia. This approach has generally been abandoned due to lack of efficacy. However, Chen et al. (17) have recently reported excellent results in 13 of 15 patients with retrocollis using a posterior cervical myotomy procedure partially resecting the upper part of the trapezius, parts of the splenius and semispinalis capitis and semispinalis cervicis muscles bilaterally.

The most widely applied surgical technique for cervical dystonia has been bilateral anterior cervical rhizotomies usually combined with selective section of the spinal accessory nerve. This technique was reviewed by Gauthier et al. (29) at the last International Congress. Table 2 reviews the results of a number of the larger or more important series since Dandy introduced one form of the technique. As can be seen, most authors claim satisfactory response in over 60% of patients. However, long-term follow-up performed by Meares (47) in the late 1960s indicated that patients treated surgically fared considerably worse than those not operated on. More recently Hernesniemi and Keränen (35) found that none of their 12 patients obtained a good response. Five experienced fair benefit and the remainder were described

TABLE 2. *Ventral rhizotomies for cervical dystonia*

Authors and year	No.	% "Improved"
Dandy, 1930 (21)	8	87
Patterson and Little, 1943 (49)	16	56
Putnam et al., 1949 (52)	18	89
Poppen and Martinez-Niochet, 1951 (51)	36	61
McKenzie, 1955 (46)	12	83
Hamby, 1969 (32)	50	87
Wycis and Gildenberg, 1969 (62)	26	84
Meares, 1971 (47)	8	13
Stejskal, 1975 (58)	15	13
Tasker, 1976 (59)	47	55
Walsh, 1976 (61)	33	79
Fabinyi and Dutton, 1980 (23)	20	90
Gauthier et al., 1988 (29)	24	75
Hernesniemi and Keränen, 1990 (35)	12	0
Friedman et al., 1993 (26)	58	85

as having a poor or very poor outcome. Complications of anterior rhizotomies can be quite significant and disabling, including neck and shoulder weakness, neck instability (occasionally requiring a fusion procedure), limitation of voluntary neck movements, pain in the neck and shoulders, and dysphagia in more than 30% of patients. Recently Horner et al. (36) evaluated special swallowing studies performed before and after rhizotomy. Following surgery 95.1% showed radiologic swallowing abnormalities that were rated as moderate to severe in one-third of the patients. By subjective report one-half of these patients had a gradual improvement over 4 to 24 weeks after surgery. In general, the swallowing disturbances represented an aggravation of preexisting pharyngeal dysfunction secondary to the C1-3 rhizotomies and sectioning of the spinal accessory nerve.

Because of the overall disappointing results, and particularly the high complication rate of anterior rhizotomies in cervical dystonia, Bertrand et al. (7,8) introduced a selective peripheral denervation procedure (ramisectomy). This entails the variable sectioning of the posterior rami from C1-6 (on one or both sides depending on the clinical features) combined with sectioning of the spinal accessory nerve. Table 3 summarizes results from a number of recent reports using this technique. In general, the procedure is well tolerated. Complications include almost universal sensory loss over the distribution of the greater occipital nerve as well as less frequent trapezius paresis, dysphagia, occipital neuralgia, and hyperesthesia in the territory of the greater auricular nerve. Less

complex forms of dystonic head posturing respond better. For example, the excellent or very good responses obtained in 87% of Bouvier's cases were all in patients with rotational deviation (10). Laterocollis and retrocollis cases are reported to be less responsive. Braun and colleagues (12,13) have also found that secondary nonresponders to botulinum toxin (probably those who have developed antibodies to the toxin) are predictably much more favorably affected by the peripheral denervation procedure than are those with primary nonresponse. This latter group is probably composed of a mixture of patients with greater degrees of musculoskeletal contributions (e.g., contractures, ankylosis), deeper muscle involvement, and central neck postural disturbances that might be expected to be equally resistant to chemical and surgical denervation.

In 1986 Freckmann et al. (25) reported follow-up results of 33 patients who underwent bilateral lysis of spinal accessory nerve roots with sections of anastomoses between these and the dorsal roots of C1 and C2, division of the dorsal root of C1 and sometimes C2, combined with attempts to free the roots from adhesions and vascular contacts. All patients were said to have "proof of neurogenic lesions within the accessory nerve" on electromyography (EMG). At least 20 of these 33 patients were felt to be improved with excellent or good results obtained in 12. Benefit was often delayed up to 6 to 9 months after the procedure. Comparing the findings at operation to 100 postmortem evaluations the authors claimed a much higher occurrence of anastomoses between the spinal accessory nerve and the dorsal

TABLE 3. *Peripheral denervation for cervical dystonia*

	Bouvier, 1989 (10)	Arce and Russo, 1992 (3)	Bertrand and Lenz, 1992 (9)	Braun et al., 1976	Davis et al., 1991 (22)
No. of cases	108[a]	55	260	69	9
Excellent	32 (30%)	39 (71%)	106 (40%)	11 (16%)	?
Very good/good	62 (57%)	10 (18%)	124 (48%)	22 (32%)	?
Combined	94 (87%)	49 (89%)	230 (88%)	33 (48%)	5 (56%)
Fair	?	—	27 (10%)	19 (28%)	?
Poor	?	6 (11%)	3 (1%)	17 (24%)	?

[a]All rotational (60% of total of 180 patients); laterocollis and retrocollis less responsive.

root of C1 (87 versus 46%) (24). They hypothesized that the cervical dystonia resulted from a disordered proprioceptive input caused by mechanical irritation of the anastomoses between the spinal accessory nerve roots and the dorsal roots of C1/2. Benefit was obtained in patients with "purely horizontal torticollis" and not in those with combined forms, which they felt more likely represented "dystonia of central origin."

Although Freckmann et al. denied the validity of the notion that neurovascular contacts of the spinal accessory nerve root might cause cervical dystonia as in hemifacial spasm or trigeminal neuralgia, a number of subsequent authors have reported beneficial results from various microvascular decompression procedures. These have sometimes been combined with nerve section procedures. For example, Shima et al. (55) decompressed the 11th nerve by transposing the compressing artery [typically the vertebral or the posterior inferior cerebellar artery (PICA)] and sectioned the first and/or second cervical branches of the 11th nerve. These authors claimed that it is possible to distinguish clinically between dystonic torticollis and "spasmodic torticollis of 11th nerve origin" suggesting that the former is accentuated on standing and usually relieved in the supine position whereas the latter is reduced on standing and exaggerated on lying down (confirmed on simultaneous EMG assessment). Aksik (1) performed decompression of the accessory nerve with no root transection. In contrast to the findings of others performing similar procedures (25,39,53) this author was unable to find electrophysiologic evidence of compression of the accessory nerve. Remarkably, all 22 patients in the study were said to have evidence of abnormalities at operation including 19 (86%) with "chronic productive arachnoiditis," 13 of whom had compression of the accessory nerve by adhesions. The remainder had vascular or dentate ligament compression or accessory nerve neurinomas. Equally remarkably, 36% of patients were said to be cured and another 41% had significant improvement. Benefit usually occurred gradually over many months following surgery. Finally, Jho and Jannetta (39) recently reported their results of microvascular decompression in 20 patients with spasmodic torticollis. These authors found that the most common compressing blood vessels were the vertebral artery and/or the PICA. No nerve section was performed. Sixty-five percent of their patients were said to be "cured" (although it is admitted that most still had "some subtle tendency to move their necks to the prior abnormal position when they relaxed their head in the neutral position"), 20% were improved with minimal spasms, 5% had persistent moderate spasms, and only 10% were considered minimally improved or unchanged. Table 4 summarizes the results of microvascular decompression/lysis procedures. Proponents of

TABLE 4. *Microvascular decompression/lysis for cervical dystonia*

	Freckmann et al., 1986 (25)	Shima et al., 1988 (55)	Aksik, 1993 (1)	Jho and Jannetta, 1995 (39)
No.	33	7	22	20 (follow-up 17)
Excellent includes "cured"	5 (15%)	3 (43%)	17 (77%)	13 (65%)
Good	10 (30%)	2 (29%)	—	4 (20%)
Improved	12 (36%)	—	—	1 (5%)
Unchanged	3 (9%)	2 (29%)	5 (23%)	2 (10%)
Worse	2 (6%)	—		
Comments	1 surgical death Horizontal best 21/22 Combined forms poor: 5/9	Gradual improvement over 5 months 1 partial recurrence—adhesions	Neurinomas: 1 recurrence, 2 no improvement. Previous stereotactic surgery/retrocollis—poor response	Improvement gradual over 6 mo—2 yr

the microvascular decompression procedure emphasize the low complication rate (occasional persistent cerebrospinal fluid leak and rare stroke). They argue that, given the low complication rate, this procedure should be the first surgical approach for cervical dystonia (in properly selected cases) and that failures could go on to the selective peripheral denervation procedure of Bertrand. However, Bertrand himself has stated that previous failed microvascular decompression procedures have resulted in sufficient scarring from the laminectomy to interfere with successful outcome from peripheral denervation (9).

Comment

There are numerous problems with the reports of peripheral surgery for cervical dystonia, making it difficult to interpret and particularly accept the sometimes striking beneficial results reported. The variability and inconsistency of both electrophysiologic "evidence" of compressive neuropathy (e.g., spinal accessory nerve) and the reported intraoperative findings (e.g., anastamoses, arachnoiditis, vascular compression) is particularly concerning. Formal prospective blinded evaluations of patients undergoing these procedures compared to nonsurgical controls are sorely needed. In many cases, patients have not received a trial of botulinum toxin therapy before going on to surgery. Many of the reports in the literature have simply accepted patient statements of response rather than formally evaluating them. When clinical evaluations have been used, validated rating scales have not been applied and formal definitions of the responses reported are often lacking. As indicated, the evaluations have never been "blinded." Follow-up has often been brief or quite variable. Several studies have claimed that the best candidates for surgery are those with a short duration of symptoms. This "predictive factor" combined with short follow-up fails to take into account the potential for spontaneous remissions to account for a certain proportion of patients who have apparently responded well. Finally, there is a lack of long-term follow-up with respect to potential

musculoskeletal complications of earlier neck surgery (e.g., cervical spondylosis). With more patients developing secondary response failure from botulinum toxin type A due to antibody formation and the much shorter duration of effect of alternative serotypes (e.g., botulinum toxin types B and F), there is an increasing need for properly designed objective evaluations of these surgical techniques by neurologists experienced in the care and management of patients with cervical dystonia.

STEREOTACTIC SURGERY FOR DYSTONIA

Over the past 50 years, functional neurosurgeons have attempted to treat dystonia by placing lesions in a number of sites including the internal capsule, dentate nucleus, cerebral peduncle, putamen, subthalamus (including the zona incerta), globus pallidus, and thalamus. Synthesis and interpretation of this literature is exceedingly difficult. The patients treated are not uniform with respect to etiology, distribution, or subtype of movements. Differing surgical methodologies are often used, even when dealing with a single location of lesions (e.g., thalamus) and procedures often vary from patient to patient. For example, the number of lesions placed, the use of repeat procedures, the expansion of the lesions to involve two or more contiguous regions, and the combination of lesions in various sites [e.g., ventrolateral (VL) thalamus plus globus pallidus interna (GPi) or centrum medianum (CM)]. As with peripheral surgeries for cervical dystonia, the nature of postoperative evaluations has varied tremendously. With rare exception (see, e.g., References 2 and 60), reports have failed to define the methods of evaluation and have not used a validated rating scale. The timing of assessment with respect to surgery has varied tremendously. Finally, there has been little or no attempt to evaluate size and location of the lesions postoperatively with imaging and correlate these features with the clinical outcome [this is primarily because most reports predate the availability of modern imaging techniques such as magnetic resonance imaging (MRI)].

Current stereotactic surgical techniques for dystonia include electrocoagulation, gamma knife radiosurgery, and high-frequency deep brain stimulation. The majority of reports available in the literature have utilized cryosurgery, particularly thalamotomy. In 1985, Laitinen (42) surveyed a number of neurosurgeons asking them to indicate the location of thalamic lesions they used in the treatment of Parkinson's disease. There was considerable variability in target location from surgeon to surgeon, suggesting to Laitinen that a successful operation only required interruption of the pallido-thalamo-cortical pathway anywhere along its course; however, it is important to point out that the ventralis intermedius (Vim) nucleus of the thalamus does not receive pallidal output. The location of thalamic lesions used in the treatment of dystonia has also varied considerably. Cooper (18) usually combined lesions in the posterior half of the ventral lateral tier with another lesion in CM and sometimes one in the pulvinar. Tasker et al. (60) placed their lesions in (Vim) ±ventralis oralis posterior (Vop). Yamashiro and Tasker (63) found that patients obtaining the best responses had larger lesions with expansion rostrally and dorsally from the Vim. Andrew et al. (2) also lesioned the Vim as well as the more posterior ventralis caudalis externus (Vce) and ventralis caudalis internus (Vci) and CM. Grossman and colleagues (15) tended to make a more anterior VL lesion that involved Vop with extension, as necessary, rostrally into ventralis oralis anterior (Voa). Jeanmonod et al. (38) emphasized the role of the medial thalamic nuclei in the development of low-threshold calcium spikes, which they claimed result in the development of a variety of positive neurologic symptoms, including dystonia. These authors have espoused lesioning medial thalamic nuclei rather than the more "specific" thalamic nuclei targeted by other surgeons. Finally, some surgeons prefer to lesion the zona incerta near Voa/Vop rather than lesioning the thalamic nuclei themselves (e.g., A. Struppler, personal communication).

Cooper (18) championed the application of thalamic lesioning for dystonia. He claimed an overall moderate to marked improvement in 69.7% of 208 patients with idiopathic dystonia followed for a mean of 7.9 years. A further 18.3% were unchanged; however, on the basis of the natural history of the illness Cooper predicted that 84% of patients would have been expected to worsen without surgical intervention. Unfortunately, these striking results have not been duplicated by subsequent investigators. Even at the time of Cooper's report, skepticism of these striking results was evident (see the question posed by Dr. Hurtig, Reference 18, p. 449) and review of photographs of at least one of Cooper's patients suggests the possible inclusion of some cases with psychogenic dystonia (19). Tasker provided a detailed account of his own experience with thalamotomy at the last International Dystonia Symposium comparing his results with previous reports. Table 5 summarizes the reported series of thalamotomy for primary dystonia since Cooper's 1976 paper. Table 6 summarizes the results of three series that separated results of cases with secondary dystonia from those with primary dystonia. Review of the reports listed in Tables 5 and 6 allows a few generalizations. Most authors have found that phasic movements respond as well as tonic posturing and Andrew et al. (2) commented that "rapid distal movements" responded quite favorably. Limb dystonia has responded much more favorably than axial involvement. For example, Tasker et al. (60) obtained more than 50% improvement in 34% of involved limbs versus 13% for trunk and neck dystonia. In general, hemidystonia has responded well (2). Although the recent report of Cardoso et al. (15) described a better response in patients with generalized dystonia than in those with hemidystonia, this may have been a factor of the weighting of their scale for degree of disability and the shorter follow-up in the generalized dystonia group. Generally patients with progressive disease have obtained a poorer long-term response. For example, in 13 of 20 idiopathic torsion dystonia patients operated on by Tasker whom he felt had progressive disease at the time of surgery, only four had greater than 50% improvement on long-term follow up (60). Cardoso et al. (15)

TABLE 5. *Summary of thalamotomy for primary dystonia since Cooper's 1976 report*

	Cooper, 1976 (18)	Gros et al., 1976 (31)	Andrew et al., 1983 (2)		Burzaco, 1985 (14)	Tasker et al., 1988 (60)	Cardoso et al., 1995 (15)		Markova et al., 1996 (44)
Distribution	Gen = 208	n = 25	Gen = 10	Other = 10	Gen = 13	Gen = 20	Gen = 5	Seg = 2	n = 86 total (Gen + CD) Gen n = ?
Bilateral procedures	B~½	B = 7				B = 10	B = 1		
Worse/same	30.3%	~30%		50%		21%	20%	100%	31%
Slight improvement	45.2%	10%				26%			13.5%
Moderate improvement		~30%		~50%	69%	14%	60%		
Marked improvement	24.5%	33%				32%	20%	Combined 42.9%	55.5%
Significant complications	? 2% mortality, 18% speech in B	16%	3 deaths in 1st year (1 surgical)			25%; 10% (2) speech (both B)	35% immediate; persistent 6%		For entire group (i.e., Gen + CD) 12 transient hemiparesis, "supranuclear syndrome," 2 deaths

B, bilateral; Gen, generalized; Seg, segmental; CD, cervical dystonia. Data provided is often incomplete or responses are difficult to categorize. Percentages not aligned with one response category are combined figures for the category above and below (e.g. Cooper: 45.2% of patients had slight or moderate improvement).

TABLE 6. *Thalamotomy for secondary dystonia*

	Andrew et al., 1983 (2)		Tasker, 1988 (60)		Cardoso et al., 1995 (15)
Distribution and number	Hemi = 12	Other = 7 (6B)	Hemi = 13	Other^a = 21 (6B)	Hemi = 9 Other = 1
Worse/same		~70%	8%	19%	30%
Slight improvement			8%	24%	10%
Moderate improvement			38%	24%	50%
	100%	~30%			
Marked improvement			46%	33%	10%
Significant complications	8%	1 death	21%		Transient 35%

^{a}Includes "dystonia musculorum deformans" in retarded children (n = 5).
Hemi, hemidystonia; B, bilateral surgery.

found that the initial benefit obtained in patients with primary dystonia diminished by 43% at 32.9 months of follow-up compared to 30% in the secondary dystonia group at 41 months. This difference was probably due to the more progressive nature of the primary dystonia group; secondary dystonia patients were more stable, nine out of ten having hemidystonia due to a static lesion. Cooper (18) had originally found that Ashkenazi Jewish patients with positive family history obtained a much better response than non-Jewish patients with a positive family history of dystonia (he felt that this was predominantly related to a greater degree of limb involvement in the former and more trunk involvement in the latter). Subsequent studies have failed to demonstrate any different response in familial versus nonfamilial idiopathic dystonia. Finally, manual dexterity may improve twice as often in primary dystonia than secondary dystonia probably due to the coexistence of other motor dysfunction in the latter (e.g., pyramidal and cerebellar abnormalities) (60).

One of the major limiting factors to the use of thalamotomy in generalized dystonia or spasmodic torticollis has been the high proportion of patients developing disabling speech dysfunction following bilateral procedures. Cooper (18) reported a 20% incidence of these problems. Andrew et al. (2) found that 56% of their patients with bilateral thalamotomy developed dysarthria/dysphonia compared with 11% after unilateral surgery. Bertrand (6) reported a 10% incidence. Four of ten of the idiopathic torsion patients of Tasker et al. undergoing bilateral procedures developed speech difficulties; in two of these they felt that this may have been due to progressive dystonia rather than the surgery. Four of five of their secondary dystonia patients developed speech dysfunction, which was significant in two (60). Various predictive factors have been emphasized by these authors. In the report of Andrew et al., nine of ten patients with preoperative dystonic dysarthria/dysphonia experienced worsening of speech dysfunction (eight of these had undergone bilateral procedures). Further emphasizing the role of bilateral procedures, these authors found that 20 of 45 patients without preexisting speech abnormalities experienced new speech dysfunction with 19 of these 20 having undergone bilateral operations. Speelman and van Manen (57) found that unilateral thalamotomy was often sufficient to cause significant worsening of speech abnormalities in patients with cerebral palsy. The specific location of the lesion in the thalamus may also play a role in causing speech difficulties. Hassler and Hess in 1954 (34) emphasized the need to lesion Voi, especially in cases of torticollis because of its head and face representation, and later Hassler and Dieckmann (33) added a lesion in the H1 bundle of Forel because of its influence on turning of the head in animal experiments. However, Tasker et al. (60) and Bertrand (6) believed that this resulted in a greater degree of speech abnormality (due to the proximity of the corticobulbar fibers in the internal capsule) and this partially accounts for the localization of their lesions more posteriorly in Vim.

Recently Petzinger et al. (50) have attempted to define predictive factors for persistent speech abnormalities following thalamotomy by evaluating 31 patients who had undergone bilateral procedures (mostly by Cooper) compared to 15 unoperated idiopathic torsion dystonia patients selected for the presence of speech involvement. The severity and quality of speech disturbances found in the two groups were quite similar. More severe speech deficits in the surgical group were seen in patients with a greater number of left-sided lesions and who were younger at the time of surgery. In a smaller group who underwent MRI scanning, the presence of speech abnormalities did not correlate with the extent of brain injury found on imaging.

Table 7 summarizes the results of thalamotomy for cervical dystonia obtained from a small number of series since Cooper's report of 160 cases in 1977 (20). Sufficient data are lacking in most of these reports [with the exception of that by Andrew et al. (2)] and so the numbers can serve only as a very rough guide to the overall response rate. In general, the variable efficacy combined with a high incidence of speech complications has encouraged most surgeons to abandon stereotactic procedures for isolated cervical dystonia.

The ameliorative effects of posteroventral medial pallidotomy on dystonia in Parkinson's disease (all types: off-period, diphasic, and peak-dose dystonia, as well as dystonia unrelated to levodopa) almost certainly will encourage a renewal of interest in lesioning this site for other forms of dystonia. There is very little in the literature on the response of dystonia to pallidotomy. Cooper and others had found that the addition of pallidal lesions did not provide further benefit in patients undergoing thalamotomy. As pointed out by Laitinen et al. (43), lesions performed in the GPi at that time were located more anterior, medial, and dorsal to the site that Leksell had defined was much more effective in relieving the features of Parkin-

son's disease. We now know that this posterior, ventral, and lateral location is the site of the sensorimotor GPi. In 1985, Burzaco (14) reported results of pallidotomy (lesioning a region close but not identical to the "modern" pallidotomy site) versus thalamotomy. In general, the response rate was equivalent; however, he found that recovery of speech disturbances (seen in 14% of pallidotomies versus 17% of thalamotomy cases) was much more complete in the pallidotomy group. He also felt that the pallidotomy patients obtained better long-term results; however, the data supporting this statement were not provided. Iacono et al. (37) have recently reported a striking response to simultaneous bilateral lesions of the ansa lenticularis in a patient with primary generalized dystonia. Vitek et al. (Chapter 21 of this volume) have obtained marked improvement in three patients following unilateral posterior ventral medial pallidotomy although follow-up has been quite short. (See Addendum).

In preparation for the current symposium, with the assistance of Dr. Andres Lozano and Dr. Ron Tasker, a number of neurosurgeons were polled requesting information on each of the patients with dystonia that they had operated on over the past 10 years. This included age, sex, duration of dystonia, distribution of dystonia, etiology, other clinical information, whether electrocoagulation or deep brain stimulation was used, the location of the surgical procedure (a 15.0-mm parasagittal map of the thalamus and another 20.0-mm parasagittal map of the GPi were provided), whether unilateral or bilateral procedures were used, and the initial and final outcomes obtained applying a standardized rating scale from -1 to 4. Unfortunately, the response rate was rather low (30%). Five surgeons responded that they had not operated on dystonic patients over the past 10 years. The results of Iacono et al. and Vitek et al. reported at the International Symposium were combined with those of five other surgeons (N. Barbaro, D.A. Bosch, J. Henderson, D. Kondziolka, and A. Struppler). Tables 8 and 9 summarize the results of these small numbers of patients providing the site of the lesions in

TABLE 7. *Thalamotomy for cervical dystonia*

	Cooper, 1977 (20)	Bertrand et al., 1978 (8)	Andrew et al., 1983 (2)	Burzaco, 1985 (14)	Markova et al., 1996[b] (44)
	$N = 160$ B = all	$N = 13$ B = 3; + GP = 6; + P = 6 2 (1 B + GP, 1B)	$N = 20$ B = 15 33%B		$N = ?$ (total = 86)
Worse/same			100% U[a]	$N = 7$	
Slight improvement		1 (U)			10.8%
Moderate improvement		8 (1 U, 2 U + P, 1 U + GP, 2 U + GP + P, 1 B + GP, 1 B + GP + P)	67%B	57%	
Marked improvement	60%	2 (1 U, 1 U + GP)	0 U		60.2%
Significant complications	20% speech	1 poor result due to pseudobulbar complications	56% speech		

[a]Two patients obtained significant relief from limb tremor.
B, bilateral; U, unilateral; GP, unilateral pallidotomy; P, peripheral surgery.
[b]See Table 5 for additional details.

TABLE 8. *Recent results of functional surgery in primary dystonia*

Response (0–4)	Gen	Segm	CD	Other
4	GPi 3			
3	zi 2, GPi 1	GPi 3, VL 1		VL1 (hand)
2				
1				
0			zi 1	GPi + VL1 (hemi), GPi 1 (sp. dysph.)

Results of stereotactic surgery in 14 cases of primary dystonia from six surgeons (N. Barbaro, R. Bakay, D. Bosch, R. Iacono, D. Kondziolka, A. Struppler). Responses scores (-1 to 4) are as follows: -1 = Dystonia worse (none rated as worsened by surgery); 0 = no effect; 1 = mild improvement in movement disorder but no improvement in function; 2 = moderate in improvement in movement disorder but minimal or no improvement in function; 3 = moderate improvement in movement disorder and function; 4 = marked improvement in movement disorder and function.

Gen, generalized; Segm, segmental; CD, cervical dystonia; GPi, globus pallidus interna; VL, ventrolateral thalamus; zi, zona incerta. Numbers following the site of the lesion indicate number of patients in each response category who received that particular lesion. Hemi, hemidystonia (said to be idiopathic); sp. dysph., spasmodic dysphonia.

each case. As one can see, the results remain quite variable and it is difficult to deduce any definite conclusions from this experience.

Deep Brain Stimulation

In general, the current techniques of high-frequency deep brain stimulation used in Parkinson's disease have not been studied in dystonia. Variable results have been reported in the older literature that were modest at best. Patient populations have been quite mixed. Patients with cerebral palsy with severe spasticity and patients with thalamic pain combined with abnormal movements predominated (with deep brain stimulation used primarily for the spasticity and pain components, respectively). The site of stimulation has varied widely including the dentate nucleus, posterior thalamus, VL thalamus, pulvinar, internal capsule, and zona

incerta (56). It has generally been stated that choreoathetosis often improved in patients treated for deafferentation pain. "Torsion dystonia" was found to obtain less benefit and indeed VL surgery was known to even induce dystonia or athetosis. There are only two reports of the application of modern high-frequency Vim stimulation in dystonia. In 1993, Sellal et al. (54) reported striking benefit in a single patient with hemidystonia due to a thalamic lesion. Interestingly, prior to surgery this patient experienced a pronounced reduction in dystonic postures in response to sensory stimulation of the affected limb. In 1996, Benabid et al. (5) reported only mild benefit in two cases of familial idiopathic dystonia. Clearly further study of this technique is required. One of the major advantages would be a significant reduction in the occurrence of persistent speech dysfunction in patients undergoing bilateral proce-

TABLE 9. *Recent results of functional surgery in secondary dystonia*

Response (0–4)	Generalized	Segmental	Hemi
4			zi 1
3	VL 1		VL2, GPi 1
2	zi 1, VL 1, GPi 1	GPi 1	VL 1
1	GPi 1	zi 1	VL 1
0	zi 1 (initial response = 3), GPi 1		

Results of stereotactic surgery in 15 cases of secondary dystonia (variable etiologies) from six surgeons (N. Barbaro, D. Bosch, J. Henderson, R. Iacono, D. Kondziolka, A. Struppler). See footnote for Table 8 for details.

dures. The preferable sites for stimulation and the number of electrodes required will need careful evaluation. Theoretically, the method of implanting the four channel electrodes might differ from that used for tremor, for example attempting to span Vim and Vop in hopes of providing a larger field of stimulation. This might better replicate the larger lesions extending more rostrally and dorsally that Yamashiro and Tasker (63) found most effective.

CONCLUSIONS

There are a number of lessons to be learned in evaluating the earlier literature on dystonia surgery that need to be considered in planning for the future. Initial reports of striking benefits often have not been replicated in subsequent studies. Short-term follow-up is of limited value because early benefits, which are sometimes profound, are often lost. The absence of controlled clinical trials is of major concern, especially in light of Stejskal's 1975 report (58) in which five patients with cervical dystonia who underwent ventriculography only (without a further stereotactic procedure) obtained as good a response as the 51 others who had peripheral or stereotactic operations. Sometimes perplexing responses to surgery are seen. For example, Bertrand had one patient who obtained striking benefit from a unilateral thalamotomy. However, when a contralateral thalamotomy and pallidotomy was performed 1 year later for persistent symptoms on the other side, not only was this procedure ineffective but all original benefit was lost and the abnormal movements reappeared on the originally operated side (C. Bertrand, personal communication).

Much of the older literature is limited by inaccuracy of the sites of the lesions as well as the large size of the lesions performed. There is probably sufficient data to support the use of thalamotomy in carefully selected cases; however, there is still some controversy as to the best site of the lesion within the thalamus. Most reports describing the effects of pallidotomy were prior to the use of microrecording and modern imaging. The lesions were typically anterior, medial, and dorsal to the sensorimotor GPi. Very preliminary data suggest that posteroventral medial pallidotomy may play a role in the management of dystonia. However, evaluation of this technique should be carried out only in centers combining considerable experience in the evaluation and management of dystonia with expertise in the functional neurosurgery of movement disorders. The role of deep brain stimulation also needs to be explored further. There should be strong consideration given to a formal multiinstitutional program designed to answer critical outstanding questions such as the roles of medial pallidotomy and deep brain stimulation in the management of dystonia.

Finally, it is clear that modern functional surgery for movement disorders requires extensive imaging and physiologic testing both to optimally localize the intended lesion(s) and to reduce the potential complications such as hemianopia, hemiplegia, and hemisensory abnormalities. There have been a small number of recent reports describing the use of gamma knife thalamotomy or pallidotomy for movement disorders. For example, Kwon and Whang (41) reported a patient with hemidystonia due to tuberculous meningitis treated with gamma knife radiosurgery directed at the posteroventral globus pallidus. Although dystonia improved slowly over the next 16 months, the patient also developed a homonymous hemianopia. The availability of the technique cannot justify its utilization if better results with fewer complications are obtainable with other approaches (as is clearly the case here using current stereotactic techniques). It is my opinion that the use of gamma knife radiosurgery is not a reasonable alternative in the management of dystonia aside from exceptional circumstances when other alternatives are unavailable.

ADDENDUM

Since this chapter was completed further experience with posteroventral medial pallidotomy has been reported. Our group described striking improvement in a young Jewish boy with severe gereralized idiopathic dystonia treated with bilateral pallidotomy (Lozano et al, 1997). Subsequently, Ondo and colleagues (1998) reported marked improvements in 6 of

8 patients treated with pallidotomy with the other 2 benefitting but to a lesser extent.

ACKNOWLEDGMENT

Thanks to Dr. A. Lozano for his helpful comments.

REFERENCES

1. Aksik I. Microneural decompression operations in the treatment of some forms of cranial rhizopathy. *Acta Neurochir (Wien)* 1993;125:64–74.
2. Andrew J, Fowler CL, Harrison MJG. Stereotaxic thalamotomy in 55 cases of dystonia. *Brain* 1983;106: 981–1000.
3. Arce C, Russo L. Selective peripheral denervation: a surgical alternative in the treatment for spasmodic torticollis. Review of fifty-five patients. *Mov Disord* 1992;7:128.
4. Bates AK, Halliday BL, Bailey CS, Collin JRO, Bird AC. Surgical management of essential blepharospasm. *Br J Ophthalmol* 1991;75:487–490.
5. Benabid AL, Pollak P, Gao DM, et al. Chronic electrical stimulation of the ventralis intermedius nucleus of the thalamus as a treatment of movement disorders. *J Neurosurg* 1996;84:203–214.
6. Bertrand C. The treatment of spasmodic torticollis with particular reference to thalamotomy. In: Morley TP, ed. *Current controversies in neurosurgery.* Philadelphia: WB Saunders, 1976:455–459.
7. Bertrand C, Molina-Negro P, Bouvier G, Gorczyca W. Observations and analysis of results in 131 cases of spasmodic torticollis after selective denervation. *Appl Neurophysiol* 1987;50:319–323.
8. Bertrand C, Molina-Negro P, Martinez SN. Combined stereotactic and peripheral surgical approach for spasmodic torticollis. *Appl Neurophysiol* 1978;41:122–133.
9. Bertrand CM, Lenz FA. Surgical treatment of dystonias. In: Tsui J, Calne DB, eds. *Handbook of dystonia.* New York: Marcel Dekker, 1995:329–345.
10. Bouvier G. The use of selective denervation for spasmodic torticollis in cervical dystonias. *Can J Neurol Sci* 1989;16:242.
11. Braun V, Neff U, Richter HP. Selective peripheral denervation for the treatment of spasmodic torticollis. *Mov Disord* 1996;11:208.
12. Braun V, Richter H, Schroder JM. Selective peripheral denervation for spasmodic torticollis: is the outcome predictable? *J Neurol* 1995;242:504–507.
13. Braun V, Richter H-P. Selective peripheral denervation for the treatment of spasmodic torticollis. *Neurosurgery* 1994;35:58–62.
14. Burzaco J. Stereotactic pallidotomy in extrapyramidal disorders: Session VI: Motor disorders. Proc. 9th Meeting World Soc. Stereotactic and Functional Neurosurgery, Toronto, 1985. *Appl Neurophysiol* 1985;48: 283–287.
15. Cardoso F, Jankovic J, Grossman RG, Hamilton WJ. Outcome after stereotactic thalamotomy for dystonia and hemiballismus. *Neurosurgery* 1995;36:501–508.
16. Charness ME, Ross MH, Shefner JM. Ulnar neuropathy and dystonic flexion of the fourth and fifth digits: clinical correlation in musicians. *Muscle Nerve* 1996; 19:431–437.
17. Chen XK, Ji SX, Zhu H, Ma AB. Operative treatment of bilateral retrocollis. *Acta Neurochir (Wein)* 1991; 113:180–183.
18. Cooper IS. 20-Year follow-up study of the neurosurgical treatment of dystonia musculorum deformans. *Adv Neurol* 1976;14:423–452.
19. Cooper IS. Dystonia: surgical approaches to treatment and physiological implications. In: Yahr MD, ed. *The basal ganglia: research publications: Association for Research in Nervous and Mental Disease.* New York: Raven Press, 1976;369–384.
20. Cooper IS. Neurosurgical treatment of the dyskinesias. *Clin Neurosurg* 1977;24:367–390.
21. Dandy W. An operation for the treatment of spasmodic torticollis. *Arch Surg* 1930;20:1021–1032.
22. Davis DH, Ahlskog JE, Litchy WJ. Selective peripheral denervation for torticollis: preliminary results. *Mayo Clin Proc* 1991;66:365–371.
23. Fabinyi G, Dutton J. The surgical treatment of spasmodic torticollis. *Aust NZ J Surg* 1980;50:155–157.
24. Freckmann N, Hagenah R. Relationship between the spinal accessory nerve root and the posterior root of the first cervical nerve in spasmodic-torticollis and common autopsy cases. *Zentralbl Neurochir* 1986;47: 134–138.
25. Freckmann N, Hagenah R, Herrmann H-D, Muller D. Bilateral microsurgical lysis of the spinal accessory nerve roots for treatment of spasmodic torticollis. *Acta Neurochir (Wien)* 1986;83:47–53.
26. Friedman AH, Nashold BS, Jr, Sharp R, Caputi F, Arruda J. Treatment of spasmodic torticollis with intradural selective rhizotomies. *J Neurosurg* 1993;78:46–53.
27. Frueh BR, Callahan A, Dortzbach RK, et al. The effects of differential section of the VII nerve on patients with intractable blepharospasm. *Trans Am Acad Ophthalmol* 1976;81:595–602.
28. Frueh BR, Musch DC, Bersani TA. Effects of eyelid protractor excision for the treatment of benign essential blepharospasm. *Am J Ophthalmol* 1992;113:681–686.
29. Gauthier S, Perot P, Bertrand G. Role of surgical anterior rhizotomies in the management of spasmodic torticollis. In: Fahn S, Marden CD, Calne DB, eds. *Dystonia 2. Advances in neurology,* New York: Raven Press, 1988:633–636.
30. Gillum WN, Anderson RL. Blepharospasm surgery. An anatomical approach. *Arch Ophthalmol* 1981;99: 1056–1062.
31. Gros C, Frerebeau PH, Perez-Domingues E, Bazin M, Privat JM. Long term results of stereotaxic surgery for infantile dystonia and dyskinesia. *Neurochirurgia* 1976;19:171–178.
32. Hamby W. Spasmodic torticollis. Results after cervical rhizotomy in 50 cases. *J Neurosurg* 1969;31: 323–326.
33. Hassler R, Dieckmann G. Stereotactic treatment of different kinds of spasmodic torticollis. *Confin Neurol* 1970;32:135–143.
34. Hassler R, Hess WR. Experimentell und anatomische befunde uber die Drehbewegungen und ihre nervosen Apparate. *Arch Psychiatr Nervenkr* 1954;192:488–526.

35. Hernesniemi J, Keränen T. Long-term outcome after surgery for spasmodic torticollis. *Acta Neurochir (Wein)* 1990;103:128–130.

36. Horner J, Riski JE, Ovelmen-Levitt J, Nashold BS, Jr. Swallowing in torticollis before and after rhizotomy. *Dysphagia* 1992;7:117–125.

37. Iacono RP, Kuniyoshi SM, Lonser RR, Maeda G, Inae AM, Ashwal S. Simultaneous bilateral pallidoansotomy for idiopathic dystonia musculorum deformans. *Pediatr Neurol* 1996;14:145–148.

38. Jeanmonod D, Magnin M, Morel A. Low-threshold calcium spike bursts in the human thalamus. Common physiopathology for sensory, motor and limbic positive symptoms. *Brain* 1996;119:363–375.

39. Jho HD, Jannetta PJ. Microvascular decompression for spasmodic torticollis. *Acta Neurochir (Wien)* 1995; 134:21–26.

40. Jones TW, Waller RR, Samples JR. Myectomy for essential blepharospasm. *Mayo Clin Proc* 1985;60:663–666.

41. Kwon Y, Whang CJ. Stereotactic gamma knife radiosurgery for the treatment of dystonia. *Stereotact Funct Neurosurg* 1995;64:222–227.

42. Laitinen LV. Brain targets in surgery for Parkinson's disease. *J Neurosurg* 1985;62:349–351.

43. Laitinen LV, Bergenheim AT, Hariz MI. Leksell's posteroventral pallidotomy in the treatment of Parkinson's disease. *J Neurosurg* 1992;76:53–61.

43A. Lozano AM, Kumar R, Gross RE et al. Globus palidus internus pallidotomy for generalized dystonia *Mov Disord* 1997; 12:865–870.

44. Markova ED, Sungurov EB, Peresedov VV, Ivanova-Smolenskaya IA. Medical and neurosurgical treatment of torsion dystonia. *Mov Disord* 1996;11:228.

45. McCord CD, Coles WH, Shore JW, Spector R, Putnam J. Treatment of essential blepharospasm. I. Comparison of facial nerve avulsion and eyebrow-eyelid muscle stripping procedure. *Arch Ophthalmol* 1984;102: 266–268.

46. McKenzie KG. The surgical treatment of spasmodic torticollis. *Clin Neurosurg* 1955;2:37–43.

47. Meares R. Natural history of spasmodic torticollis and effect of surgery. *Lancet* 1971;2:149–151.

47A. Ondo WO, Desalomas M, Jankovic J, Grossman RG. Pallidotomy for generalized dystonia. *Mov Disord* 1998; 13: *(in press)*.

48. Patel BCK, Anderson RL. Diagnosis and management of essential blepharospasm. *Ophthalmic Pract* 1993; 11:293–302.

49. Patterson RM, Little SC. Spasmodic torticollis. *J Nerv Ment Dis* 1943;98:559–571.

50. Petzinger GM, Stewart C, Khandji AG, et al: Thalamotomies and speech impairment in idiopathic torsion dystonia (ITD). *Mov Disord* 1996;11:229.

51. Poppen JL, Martinez-Niochet A. Spasmodic torticollis. *Surg Clin N Am* 1951;31:883–890.

52. Putnam TJ, Herz E, Glaser GH. Spasmodic torticollis. *Arch Neurol Psychiatry* 1949;61:240–247.

53. Saito S, Moller AR, Jannetta PJ, Jho HD. Abnormal response from the sternocleidomastoid muscle in patients with spasmodic torticollis: observations during microvascular decompression operations. *Acta Neurochir (Wien)* 1993;124:92–98.

54. Sellal F, Hirsch E, Barth P, Blond S, Marescaux C. A case of symptomatic hemidystonia improved by ventroposterolateral thalamic electrostimulation. *Mov Disord* 1993;8:515–518.

55. Shima F, Fukui M, Kitamura K, Kuromatsu C, Okamura T. Diagnosis and surgical treatment of spasmodic torticollis of 11th nerve origin. *Neurosurgery* 1988;22:358–363.

56. Siegfried J, Rea GL. Deep brain stimulation for the treatment of motor disorders. In: Dade Lunsford L, ed. *Modern stereotactic neurosurgery.* Boston: Martinus Nijhoff, 1988:409–412.

57. Speelman JD, van Manen J. Cerebral palsy and stereotactic neurosurgery: long term results. *J Neurol Neurosurg Psychiatry* 1989;52:23–30.

58. Stejskal L. Therapeutic results in axial hyperkinesias including torticollis. The effect of the plane of deviation. *J Neurol Sci* 1975;25:481–490.

59. Tasker RR. The treatment of spasmodic torticollis by peripheral denervation: The McKenzie operation. In: Morley TP, ed. *Current controversies in neurosurgery.* Philadelphia: W.B. Saunders, 1976:448–454.

60. Tasker RR, Doorly T, Yamashiro K. Thalamotomy in generalized dystonia. In: Fahn S, ed. *Dystonia 2. Advances in neurology.* New York: Raven Press, 1988: 615–631.

61. Walsh LS. Spasmodic torticollis. *Inst Neurol Madras Proc* 1976;6:36–41.

62. Wycis HT, Gildenberg PL. *Long range evaluation of the surgical treatment of spasmodic torticollis.* Amsterdam: Excerpta Medica, 1969:193–197.

63. Yamashiro K, Tasker RR. Stereotactic thalamotomy for dystonic patients. *Sterotact Funct Neurosurg* 1993; 60:81–8

Dystonia 3: Advances in Neurology, Vol. 78,
edited by S. Fahn, C. D. Marsden, and M. DeLong.
Lippincott–Raven Publishers, Philadelphia © 1998.

20

Intrathecal Baclofen in the Treatment of Dystonia

*Blair Ford, *Paul E. Greene, *‡Elan D. Louis, *Susan B. Bressman,
†Robert R. Goodman, §Mitchell F. Brin, *Saud Sadiq, and *Stanley Fahn

*Departments of *Neurology and †Neurosurgery, Neurological Institute, College of Physicians and
Surgeons, Columbia University, New York, New York 10032; ‡Gertrude H. Sergievsky Center,
Columbia University, New York, New York 10032; and the §Department of Neurology, Mount
Sinai Medical Center, New York, New York 10029.*

MECHANISM OF ACTION

Intrathecal baclofen (ITB) is a highly effective and reliable treatment for severe spasticity of spinal origin. There has been recent interest in applying this technique to other disorders of increased muscular tone, including dystonia. Baclofen (beta-4-chlorophenyl-gamma-aminobutyric acid) is a synthetic analog of gamma-amino butyric acid, or GABA, the ubiquitous inhibitory neurotransmitter in the mammalian central nervous system (CNS). Acting on presynaptic $GABA_B$ receptors by reducing calcium influx and increasing potassium conductance, baclofen inhibits the release of several neurotransmitters, including the excitatory amino acids glutamate and aspartate (36). $GABA_B$ receptors are distributed throughout the CNS. In the spinal cord, $GABA_B$ receptors are concentrated heavily in superficial layers of the dorsal horn, lamina I, II, III, and IV (47). In the brain, the highest concentrations of GABA are in the substantia nigra and putamen (18). Physiologically, baclofen reduces the excitability of spinal cord neurons and interneurons, and has many additional effects in the brain that are potentially relevant to its use in disorders of increased muscular tone (21).

PHARMACOKINETICS

In clinical practice, oral baclofen has long been regarded as a drug of choice for spasticity of spinal origin (13,56). Baclofen has also been considered to be one of the most effective agents for treating dystonia (17). However, treatment with oral baclofen is often limited due to adverse effects, such as nausea and sedation. Baclofen does not easily cross the blood-brain barrier, and high systemic doses are required to achieve an effective CNS concentration for disorders of increased muscular tone (26). Moreover, baclofen is uniformly distributed between the spinal cord and supraspinal centers when administered orally.

With the development of intrathecal catheter delivery systems, it was found that microgram quantities of baclofen, injected directly into the lumbar subarachnoid space, could produce important reductions in spasticity without causing the sedation that may occur using oral baclofen. The onset of action is generally 30 to 60 minutes after an intrathecal bolus dose (48). The peak effect occurs about 4 hours after the bolus injection, with a gradual tapering 6 to 8 hours after the bolus, although individual variation occurs (37,48). When injected into the lumbar cistern, baclofen diffuses rostrally with cerebrospinal fluid (CSF) flow, but a concentration gradient is established, giving a lumbar cistern to cisterna magna ratio of approximately 4:1 (28). This preferential accumulation of baclofen in the region of the lower spinal cord underlies its potent effect on spasticity, with relative freedom of adverse CNS effects, such as drowsiness. On pharmacokinetic grounds, therefore, ITB has the ideal profile for a treatment of spasticity of spinal origin.

ITB has been used in the treatment of spasticity of spinal origin for more than 10 years. It has passed the test of rigorously designed clinical trials (45), and its beneficial effect is well-documented in more than 1,000 patients worldwide (1,4,11,13,30–32,40,42,45). For individuals with spasticity of spinal origin, standard bolus test injections of ITB reliably identify patients who will receive long-term benefit from a continuous ITB infusion, delivered by implantable pump (7,30,40). Indications for pump implantation exist as well as dosing guidelines for continuous ITB infusion (42,54).

TECHNICAL ISSUES

The technical instructions for ITB test dosing are described in the literature (42,45), the clinical reference guide (54), as well as the package insert (Lioresal Intrathecal, Medtronic Inc., Minneapolis, MN). The drug is diluted to obtain an initial single bolus dose of 50 μg. Under sterile conditions, using topical anesthesia, the drug is injected into the lumbar cistern over a period of not less than 1 minute. If multiple, escalating intrathecal test doses are contemplated on successive days, the drug may be delivered into the subarachnoid space through a temporary spinal catheter. During the test dosing period, concomitant oral medications for dystonia should not be changed. Following a test dose injection, the patient should be observed for clinical changes and adverse effects over the ensuing 4 to 8 hours.

In patients with spasticity of spinal origin, clear reductions in motor tone can be produced by the standard ITB test doses at 50, 75, or 100

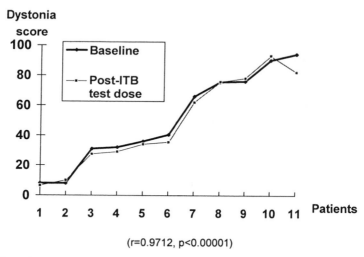

(r=0.9712, p<0.00001)

FIG. 1 Dystonia rating scale (20) scores before and after ITB test doses in patients who underwent implantation of pump. Baseline and post-ITB dystonia rating scale scores (9) of videotaped examinations represent the mean of two blinded observers. Rating scales scores were similar between investigators ($r = 0.9712$, $p < 0.00001$). A decrease in score after ITB test dosing represents an improvement, and an increase in score denotes a worsening. The patients are arranged in order of increasing severity of dystonia at the baseline (pretest dose) session. In patient 4 with generalized dystonia, due to incomplete videotaping, only cranial dystonia and speech were rated out of a possible maximum score of 24; for all other individuals, the dystonia rating scale maximum score was 120.

μg. In selected cases, ITB bolus doses exceeding 100 μg can be safely given in patients with severe, refractory spasticity, if warranted (6,41). The decision to implant a pump has been facilitated by the use of rating scales for spasticity. A decline in the Ashworth scale (see Table 1) of one or two points indicates that the patient will benefit from long-term administration of ITB (11,42).

EXPANDING THE INDICATIONS FOR INTRATHECAL BACLOFEN

The success of ITB in the treatment of spasticity of spinal origin led to treatment attempts using this technique in spasticity of cerebral origin (3,4,12), central pain (23), and miscellaneous motor disorders, including stiff person syndrome (14,44,52), tetanus (8), and others (43). Because oral baclofen can be an effective agent for dystonia (21), the use of ITB in dystonia is a logical application of this technique. In contrast to its use in spasticity, there remains limited clinical experience with ITB in dystonia patients. Many important questions need to be answered regarding the treatment of dystonia with ITB, pertaining both to the testing procedure and to chronic treatment using continuous baclofen infusion. As in spasticity, the implantation of a pump into an individual is a step not easily reversed. Ideally, the testing procedure should be able to detect those patients most likely to have a good long-term outcome from ITB continuous infusion.

INTRATHECAL BACLOFEN IN DYSTONIA

The important clinical issues regarding ITB for patients with dystonia are:

1. Who should be considered for ITB test dose trials?
2. What is the efficacy of ITB in dystonia?
3. How to predict the long-term clinical response to ITB before pump implantation?
4. Safety issues and complication rates.

The first case report of ITB treatment for dystonia was published in 1991 (39), describing treatment in an 18-year-old man with severe, predominantly axial dystonia due to birth injury. A report published the same year documented reduced muscle spasms and hypertonia in a patient with Hallervorden-Spatz disease (Reference 15, case 3). In a case of postencephalitic dystonia (53), a single test dose of 50 μg ITB appeared to reduce spasticity but increase dystonic movements. A larger series of patients with various motor disturbances included several individuals with dystonia, including posttraumatic hemidystonia, focal foot dystonia, cerebral palsy with athetosis, Wilson's disease, stiff person syndrome, anoxic encephalopathy, and painful legs/moving toes syndrome (43). The authors noted that spasticity tended to reduce in these patients, even when the effect of ITB on dystonia was not marked. Another report described improvement in a patient with severe tardive axial dystonia, followed for 6 months after ITB therapy (16).

Collectively, these reports established the feasibility of using ITB in dystonia, but none provided a systematic evaluation of the actual efficacy of treatment, adverse effects, or long-term consequences. The only published series of ITB treatment for dystonia is an open-label retrospective analysis of the experience at the Center for Dystonia, Columbia-Presbyterian Medical Center (20). Twenty-five patients with dystonia underwent open-label test doses of ITB, of whom 13 individuals were implanted with a pump for continuous infusion. Baseline and post-ITB test dose videotapes of ten of these individuals were evaluated by blinded observers, many months after pump implantation. Although mean rating scale scores improved in six of these ten individuals, there was no statistically significant change in scores for the group as a whole ($p < 0.097$) (Fig. 1). Five patients had parkinsonism and dystonia, and in none was improvement in parkinsonism or postural stability observed following a test dose of ITB.

The lack of significant change in the dystonia rating scale scores suggests that ITB produces little visible change in dystonia that can be detected by a blinded observer. In this context, it can be difficult to separate a placebo response from a medication effect. In addition, serial evaluations may be confounded by daily fluctuations in the dystonia that are unrelated to medication effect. In one report of ITB for spasticity, the placebo effect of ITB test doses accounted for an improvement of about 15% (24). In patients with spasticity, it is possible to distinguish a placebo effect from a medication response because the clinical effect, easily quantified using standard rating scales, is more consistent and exceeds in magnitude that which can be considered due to placebo. If placebo test doses are contemplated for dystonia, we recommend that the first dose be the placebo, against which all subsequent responses can be measured. In the Columbia study (20), two of seven placebo injections produced a clinically apparent benefit.

DIFFERENTIAL EFFECT OF BACLOFEN ON SPASTICITY AND DYSTONIA

Investigators have observed a disparity between the effect of ITB on spasticity and dystonia when the two conditions occur together. In a report of 37 patients with cerebral palsy (4), ranging in age from 5 to 27 years, seven patients had "considerable athetosis" in addition to spasticity. The mean daily dose of continuous ITB for the group as a whole did not exceed 325 μg. The authors documented a significant, sustained reduction in spasticity, quantified using the Ashworth scale (Table 1), but noted no improvement in athetosis. A similar observation was made in a series of patients with motor disorders treated with ITB (43).

Is the reverse situation true? When dystonia dominates the clinical picture, does the presence of spasticity predict a good response to ITB? Patients in the Columbia study (20) had idiopathic dystonia ($n = 13$), dystonia secondary to a diffuse encephalopathy ($n = 7$), and dystonia associated with parkinsonism ($n = 5$); five individuals had undergone previous thalamotomy for dystonia. In addition to dystonia, 18 of the 26 (69%) patients had superimposed painful spasms and signs of spasticity, defined

TABLE 1. *Ashworth rating scale for spasticity*

1	No increase in tone
2	Slight increase in tone, giving a "catch" when affected part is moved in flexion or extension
3	More marked increase in tone, but affected part easily flexed
4	Considerable increase in tone; passive movement difficult
5	Affected part rigid in flexion or extension

(See ref. 45.)

as the presence of velocity-dependent increases in tonic stretch reflexes ("clasp-knife hypertonia"), exaggerated stretch reflexes, and extensor plantar responses. Based on treating neurologists' examinations at the time of the first ITB test dose, 17 of 25 (68%) patients had spasticity or painful spasms, in addition to dystonia. In 12 of these 17 patients (67%), ITB bolus gave clinical benefit; 11 underwent pump implantation. By contrast, only three of eight (37.5%) patients without spasticity improved after a test injection of ITB. This outcome difference between patients with and without spasticity was not statistically significant ($p = 0.13$, Fisher's exact test), perhaps due to insufficient numbers. The odds ratio for the association between spasticity and benefit from a test dose was 3.57 but the confidence intervals were wide (95% CI = 0.67 to 19.05).

In large series of patients with spasticity, the response rate to ITB is high, even when symptoms are refractory to high doses of oral baclofen (1,7), approaching 100%. In one double-blind, placebo-controlled study of 140 patients with spinal spasticity, all individuals responded to a mean bolus ITB dose of 42.8 μg (38). By contrast, the response rate to ITB test doses is lower in dystonia than in spasticity. In the Columbia series (20), only 13 of the 25 patients (52%) with severe dystonia were judged to have sufficient benefit to justify pump implantation. In addition, a higher dose of ITB is often needed to produce a clinical response in dystonia. In the Columbia study (20), 25 patients underwent a total of 65 test doses of ITB, ranging from 25 to 250 μg, with a mean dose of 116 μg. The manufacturer's suggested upper limit of 100 μg for treatment of spasticity was exceeded in 26 test doses administered to 14 dystonia patients. In three of these patients, a favorable response to a dose exceeding 100 μg was the determining factor in the decision to implant a pump.

TEST DOSE—ADVERSE EFFECTS

The test dose procedure is generally very safe, but may produce a number of mild, reversible adverse effects. In the Columbia series (20), 18 of 65 ITB test doses were complicated by minor symptoms that included drowsiness, leg numbness, weakness, headache, or light-headedness. Serious complications may occur when using test doses exceeding the recommended upper limits, and may be especially likely in patients of small body size. After receiving a dose of 125 μg, one adult male patient weighing 90 pounds experienced respiratory depression, requiring oxygen by mask and observation in the intensive care unit. He had developed mild drowsiness following an injection of 75 μg ITB and diazepam 20 mg i.v. given 1 day earlier. Another individual devel-

oped respiratory depression after receiving a dose of 200 μg; a bolus injection of 150 μg 1 day earlier had given some benefit with no side effects. The overall complication rate was 20.5% for test bolus doses below or equal to 100 μg, and 46% for doses exceeding 100 μg, a significant difference (*p* <0.03, odds ratio = 3.19, 95% CI = 1.10 to 9.32) (Fig. 2). If high doses of ITB appear warranted, we now recommend dose increments of no more than 25% of the previous ITB bolus, unless the testing is conducted in an intensive care setting. The test dosing should be administered through a spinal catheter that remains in place so that CSF removal can be performed for excessive drowsiness. Intravenous access should be maintained so that physostigmine may be given if needed.

LONG-TERM EFFECTS OF CONTINUOUS INTRATHECAL BACLOFEN

In spasticity of spinal origin, continuous treatment with ITB provides long-term reduction in motor tone and relief of muscles spasm (1,41,42,45). In one series, 64 patients implanted with pumps had spasticity rating scale scores that remained constant over a mean follow-up interval of 30 months (42). A similar result was obtained in a different series of 75 patients followed for 19 months (11). The authors in both reports stated that most patients elected to continue ITB treatment once it was started, but no analysis of long-term functional outcome was provided. A sustained functional improvement in a variety of daily living tasks and ability to transfer was described in another report of 18 patients with spinal spasticity (6). Spasticity is not the only determinant of disability in affected individuals, however. Persisting deficits in weakness and coordination may continue to reduce a patient's functional capacity even when the spasticity is greatly reduced by ITB, but this aspect of ITB treatment outcome has not been emphasized (5).

In patients with cerebral palsy, the spasticity rating scale scores predictably improve using chronic ITB (4). The effect of ITB on functional capacity depends on the severity and distribu-

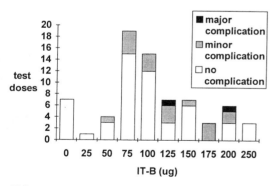

FIG. 2. Graph of adverse effects resulting from test bolus injections of ITB in patients with dystonia (20). Minor complications included mild drowsiness, lightheadedness, nausea, and other reversible symptoms. Major complications included respiratory depression and coma, requiring monitoring or ventilatory support in the intensive care unit. All complications were reversible. The incidence of complications for ITB doses exceeding 100 μg was statistically significant (*p* <.03), as compared to doses equal or below 100 μg.

TABLE 2. *Follow-up data on patients with dystonia receiving ITB by implantable pump[a]*

Patient	Dystonia etiology and distribution	Follow-up duration (mos.)	Baseline dystonia rating scale score[b]	Global dystonia score		Disability score	
				Before pump	After pump[d]	Before pump	After pump[d]
1	Idiopathic, childhood-onset, generalized	27	75.5	3	3	3	3
2	Secondary dystonia, diagnosis uncertain, childhood-onset generalized	32	66	3	3	3	3
3	Idiopathic, childhood onset, generalized	16	8	1	0	1	0
4	Idiopathic, childhood onset, generalized, s/p R thalamotomy	24	14.5[c]	3	3	1	1
5	Idiopathic, childhood onset, bilateral leg involvement	20	8	1	1	1	0
6	Idiopathic, adult-onset, generalized, s/p R thalamotomy	19	31	2	2	1	1
7	Idiopathic, childhood onset, generalized s/p, bilateral thalamotomy	30	76	3	3	3	3
8	Postanoxic/drug over-dose, generalized	18	40.5	2	2	3	2
9	Postencephalitic, generalized, s/p R thalamotomy	25	36	2	2	2	2
10	Childhood CP/delayed onset dystonia, generalized	26	16[e]	2	2	1	1
11	Idiopathic, adult-onset, segmental craniofacial	18	51[f]	2	2	1	1

[a]Table includes only those patients followed for more than 6 months after pump implantation. Of the three implanted individuals not included here, one developed a skin erosion requiring pump removal at 2 months, and his pump was not reimplanted. The other two patients had pumps implanted too recently for adequate follow-up data.

[b]The dystonia rating scale score has a maximum possible score of 120 (ref. 40).

[c]This baseline dystonia scale score includes only cranial structures and speech due to incomplete videotaping, and the maximum possible score is 24.

Oral medications after ITB pump implanted	Patient's response to question, "Do you think the ITB is providing a sustained benefit?"	Peak dose ITB (μg/d)	Long-term outcome and complications
Unchanged	No	1,200	Outcome: loss of efficacy, switched to intrathecal morphine, subsequently underwent thalamotomy Complications: none
Unchanged	No	1,350	Outcome: loss of efficacy, switched to intrathecal morphine Complications: overdose due to 800 μg flush, respiratory arrest requiring intubation
Reduced	Yes	880	Outcome: continuing good effect Complications: spinal headache requiring blood patch
Unchanged	No	900	Outcome: no clear effect Complications: respiratory depression requiring monitoring in NICU
Reduced	Yes	1,840	Outcome: continuing good effect but some loss of efficacy requiring escalation of ITB dose Complications: CSF leak along catheter requiring blood patch
Off oral meds, receiving botulinum toxin A	Yes	1,500	Outcome: continuing relief from severe spasms Complications: overdose at 1,500 μg/d, admitted to hospital; withdrawal spasms due to pump delivery rate inconsistency; catheter tip-induced spinal myoclonus, resolved with retraction of catheter
Unchanged	Yes	807	Outcome: continuing modest benefit Complications: none
Unchanged	Yes	500	Outcome: continuing benefit, but declining efficacy Complications: overdose with respiratory arrest after catheter tip replaced due to fibrosis
Off meds	No	900	Outcome: loss of benefit Complications: none
Reduced	Yes	480	Outcome: continuing good effect Complications: none
Unchanged, receiving botulinum toxin A	No	400	Outcome: lack of sustained benefit Complications: overdose with generalized hypotonia requiring emergency evaluation and stopping ITB infusion for 24 hours; lack of sustained benefit

[d]Global dystonia scores and disability scores after pump implantation were obtained at the most recent follow-up contact.
[e]Only available baseline videotape was 3 years before ITB testing and pump implantation
[f]Only available baseline videotape was 2 years before ITB testing and pump implantation

tion of the motor deficit as well as baseline function (4). In the largest reported series, a group of 37 patients with cerebral palsy was divided into a functional group ($n = 25$), all capable of self-care, and a dependent group ($n = 12$), requiring assistance for daily activities. Patients in the functional group showed improvements in spasticity, as expected, in addition to fine hand coordination and functional capacity. In the group of more disabled patients, spasticity also improved, but with no benefit in manual activity or functional capacity; in neither group was the ability to transfer improved.

LONG-TERM EFFECTS IN DYSTONIA

Little is known regarding the long-term effect of ITB on dystonia. In the Columbia study (20), 13 patients with dystonia underwent pump implantation, and 11 were followed for more than 6 months. The results are listed in Table 2. The interval between pump implantation and the most recent contact ranged between 18 and 32 months, with a mean of 21 months. Each patient or caregiver was asked whether they considered the ITB to be having a continuing beneficial effect. In six patients there was sustained benefit, but in five others the ITB had lost its effectiveness. Two individuals experienced a complete loss of ITB efficacy, and were switched to intrathecal morphine; one of these subsequently underwent a thalamotomy for intractable dystonia.

The long-term effect of ITB on functional capacity was measured using simple global ratings for dystonia and disability (Table 3). Functional capacity improved in only two of 11 cases (19%), even though important aspects of the condition, such as pain or spasms, were helped. Overall, the two individuals with the best outcomes (patients 3 and 5) had the mildest dystonia in the group. Due to limitations of sample size, no statistical correlation between dystonia severity and long-term benefit could be made. Improvements in speech have been noted in patients with cerebral palsy treated with ITB (3), and this was observed during the initial treatment of patient 11 (20),

TABLE 3. *Rating scales pertaining to functional outcomes in patients treated with chronic ITB infusion*

Global Dystonia Score
  0—No dystonia present
  1—Mild dystonia with little impairment
  2—Moderate dystonia with obvious or pronounced movements or spasms
  3—Severe dystonia preventing ambulation or the performance of daily living activities
Disability Score
  0—Not disabled, leading a normal life
  1—Mild disability but continuing full-time household duties or work outside the home
  2—Moderate disability with impairment in daily living activities, but still independent
  3—Severe disability, with loss of independence for daily living activities

who had segmental craniofacial and laryngeal dystonia.

An important outcome variable in dystonia patients treated using ITB is the need for concomitant oral medication or botulinum toxin injections. ITB treatment may enable an individual experiencing a chronic adverse medication effect to reduce or eliminate the offending agent. Five of 11 (45%) implanted patients in the Columbia series were able to reduce or stop their previous oral medications, whereas the other six (54%) continued at the original doses.

THE PROBLEM OF TOLERANCE

Tolerance to the beneficial effect of ITB frequently complicates long-term administration in patients with spasticity (1,2,6,7,9,12,35,41,42,45), perhaps due to a downregulation of spinal $GABA_B$ receptors (29). Increasing the infusion rate is often effective in regaining clinical benefit, but this increases the incidence of complications, such as baclofen overdose. Many centers use drug holidays and intermittent intrathecal morphine (1) or fentanyl administration (10) to desensitize patients to the ITB. Declining efficacy of ITB treatment has been observed in long-term treatment for spasticity, necessitating increases in dosing over time. In spasticity, it is rare for the medication to become completely ineffective, however, and that occurrence suggests a device malfunction (50).

In the Columbia patients with dystonia, tolerance appeared to develop in every patient, including those who derived sustained benefit from ITB. The mean peak dose of ITB in patients followed for more than 3 months was 948.7 μg/day; the highest dose to date is 2,015 μg/day. In patients with dystonia, several factors may contribute to the need for escalating dosing, including the development of pharmacologic tolerance, the result of tapering of oral medications, possible disease progression (22), and the continuing desire by both patient and physician to optimize treatment. As we and others have observed, however, increasing the infusion rate unfortunately decreases the margin for safety should a complication occur. We have not employed drug holidays from ITB for suspected tolerance, but in two patients, baclofen was replaced by intrathecal morphine, providing a benefit at least as marked as ITB.

COMPLICATIONS OF CHRONIC INTRATHECAL BACLOFEN THERAPY

Complications are an inevitable consequence of chronic ITB infusion by implantable pump. Even at specialized centers with broad clinical experience using intrathecal drug delivery systems, the incidence of severe, life-threatening complications is well-documented (49,55). Complications may result from ITB overdosage (6,15) or abrupt underdosage (35, 51) of any cause. Pump malfunction, programming error, infection, and catheter problems have all been reported. In one study, 40% of 102 patients experienced catheter-associated complications at an increasing rate over 80 months (46). Complications requiring pump removal occurred in nine of 21 (43%) patients (41) in one series. In another report, 26 of 46 (56%) patients required operations to correct complications or pump failure (55). Procedures and algorithms to evaluate suspected pump malfunction are described in the clinical reference manual (54) as well as in several published reports (6,15,35,49,50,51,55).

In the Columbia experience (20), complications of chronic ITB treatment included the development of CSF leaks and spinal headaches, requiring blood patches, in two patients. To date, five of the 13 (38%) implanted patients have experienced severe complications, all requiring hospitalization: baclofen overdose with respiratory depression ($n = 4$), fibrosis of catheter tip requiring replacement ($n = 1$), catheter-induced spinal myoclonus and skin erosion requiring pump removal ($n = 1$), and acute baclofen withdrawal ($n = 1$). All complications reversed promptly once identified and treated; the patient with acute baclofen withdrawal responded to a bolus of ITB, and did not require dantrolene (25). Adverse events are particularly likely at higher daily doses of ITB, when the margin for error is smaller, and a sudden reduction in infusion is more likely to precipitate baclofen withdrawal, a potentially fatal condition (27,33,34,55). This underscores the recommendation that ITB programs be conducted only at centers with adequate clinical experience and resources, including intensive care unit, radiologic and neurosurgical support, as well as outpatient monitoring capacity.

CONCLUSION

Intrathecal baclofen is an effective therapy in patients with severe spasticity of spinal origin. To date, its role as a possible treatment for dystonia has been reported in approximately 50 patients with dystonia, including an open-label series that retrospectively analyzed the effect of ITB on dystonia using rating scales and measures of functional outcome (20). The main observation is that ITB is not as effective in patients with dystonia as compared to those with spasticity. In patients with severe generalized dystonia, the response rate to test doses of ITB is low, even with doses exceeding the manufacturer's recommended upper limit. The patients in the Columbia dystonia series who remained satisfied with the long-term effects of ITB described benefit in terms of reduced painful spasms, ease of transfers, and other issues pertaining to quality of life. These improvements, not obtainable by oral medication, were important to the patients and their caretakers but did not fundamentally reduce the overall level of dependence.

In complex dystonia patients who have additional features of pain, spasms, and spasticity, it is possible that ITB has varying effects on the different clinical elements. Because ITB reduces spasticity and can decrease spasm-related pain, we believe that dystonia patients with these features may represent a group that is more likely to benefit from the technique. Reported improvement in patients with spasticity and dystonia due to head injury or cerebral palsy supports this supposition (3). This remains an important issue for ongoing study. ITB may be helpful in treating dystonic storm, a life-threatening condition of fulminant dystonia (14). Additional guidelines for ITB testing and patient selection are listed in Table 4.

In evaluating a potential new treatment for dystonia, open-label testing can provide valuable information regarding patient selection procedures, treatment efficacy, safety, and guidelines. In future prospective evaluations of ITB in dystonia, additional scales that quantify factors such as pain, spasticity, and painful dystonic spasms are recommended. A critical task is to refine selection criteria for ITB treatment by identifying individuals with dystonia who respond to test doses. Dystonia in adults tends to be poorly responsive to treatments of all types (21). To date, most reported dystonia patients treated using ITB have been severely afflicted, a population that is the most challenging to help. It is possible that patients with milder degrees of dystonia might have a superior response to ITB, as did patients 3 and 5 in the Columbia series (20). This has not been systematically evaluated because the implantation of a pump, with its risks of complications, is more difficult to justify in these individuals.

The two central issues regarding ITB remain unresolved: (a) Can effective long-term treatment with continuous ITB be safely carried out in dystonia?, and (b) Can the testing procedure

TABLE 4. *Suggested guidelines for use of ITB in patients with dystonia, based on the experience at the Center for Dystonia, Columbia-Presbyterian Medical Center*

Candidates for ITB test dosing
  Dystonia associated with spasticity
  Dystonia with superimposed painful dystonic spasms
  Severe, continuous dystonic movements ("dystonic storm")
  ? Mild dystonia
Procedures for ITB test dose trials
  1. Test doses should be administered in hospital setting on consecutive days.
  2. Make a careful baseline examination.
  3. Quantify the clinical response to each test dose using dystonia rating scale, Ashworth and spasm scales, pain scales, and measures of activity of daily living capacity.
  4. Increase the ITB test doses on consecutive days using increments of no higher than 25%.
  5. If ITB test doses greatly exceeding 100 μg, or if risk of oversedation and respiratory depression seems present, consider performing the test dosing in an intensive care setting.
  6. During test dose trials, consider giving rechallenge ITB doses to assess reproducibility of effect and to confirm a positive response.
  7. Consider using a placebo injection, after obtaining informed consent. The effect of a placebo injection may be most clear when it is administered as the first of the series of injections.
Management of suspected drug tolerance during chronic ITB infusion
  1. Ascertain that pump is functioning correctly by checking reservoir and programming features.
  2. Evaluate possible catheter malfunction with X-rays and dye studies.
  3. If tolerance to drug effect appears most likely, increasing the infusion rate may alleviate the problem for a period of time.
  4. Consider addition or increase in oral medications, including baclofen, benzodiazepines, anticholinergics, and dantrolene.
  5. Add ITB morphine to infusion, or replace ITB with intrathecal morphine.
  6. Gradually decrease and discontinue ITB, substituting with oral medications, to provide a drug holiday for several weeks, before gradually reintroducing the treatment at a lower infusion rate.

identify patients who will experience a sustained benefit from continuous ITB? The role of ITB in dystonia may ultimately be determined through a comparison of ITB and the best available alternatives, including oral medication and surgery, taking into account relevant additional clinical features such as spasticity and pain.

ACKNOWLEDGMENT

This work was supported by the dystonia Medical Research Foundation. It was presented at the Third International Dystonia Meeting, October 1996, Miami, Florida.

REFERENCES

1. Abel NA, Smith RA. Intrathecal baclofen for treatment of intractable spinal spasticity. *Arch Phys Med Rehabil* 1994;75:54–58.
2. Akman MN, Loubser PG, Donovan WH, O'Neill RN, Rossi CD. Intrathecal baclofen: does tolerance occur? *Paraplegia* 1993;31:516–520.
3. Albright AE. Baclofen in the treatment of cerebral palsy. *J Child Neurol* 1996;11:77–83.
4. Albright AL, Barron WB, Fasick MP, Polinko P, Janosky J. Continuous intrathecal baclofen for spasticity of cerebral origin. *JAMA* 1993;270:2475–2477.
5. Armstrong RW. Intrathecal baclofen and spasticity: what do we know and what do we need to know? *Dev Med Child Neurol* 1992;34:739–745.
6. Azouvi P, Mane M, Thiebaut J-B, Denys P, Remy-Neris O, Bussel B. Intrathecal baclofen administration for control of severe spinal spasticity: functional improvement and long-term follow-up. *Arch Phys Med Rehabil* 1996;77:35–39.
7. Becker WJ, Harris CJ, Long ML, Ablett DP, Klein GM, DeForge DA. Long-term intrathecal baclofen therapy in patients with intractable spasticity. *Can J Neurol Sci* 1995;22:208–217.
8. Brock H, Moosbauer W, Gabriel C, Necek S. Treatment of severe tetanus by continuous intrathecal infusion of baclofen [Letter]. *J Neurol Neurosurg Psychiatr* 1995;59:193–194.
9. Burke RE, Fahn S, Marsden CD, Bressman SB, Moskowitz C, Friedman J. Validity and reliability of a rating scale for the primary torsion dystonias. *Neurology* 1985;35:73–77.
10. Chabal C, Jacobson L, Terman G. Intrathecal fentanyl alleviates spasticity in the presence of tolerance to intrathecal baclofen. *Anesthesiology* 1992;76:312–314.
11. Coffey RJ, Cahill D, Steers W, et al. Intrathecal baclofen for intractable spasticity of spinal origin: results of a long-term multicenter study. *J Neurosurg* 1993;78:226–232.
12. Concalves J, Garcia-March G, Sanchez-Ledesma MJ, Onzain I, Broseta J. Management of intractable spasticity of supraspinal origin by chronic cervical intrathecal infusion of baclofen. *Stereotact Funct Neurosurg* 1994;62:108–112.
13. Davidoff RA. Antispasticity drugs: mechanism of action. *Ann Neurol* 1985;17:107–116.
14. Dalvi A, Fahn S, Ford B. Intrathecal baclofen in the treatment of dystonic storm. *Mov Disord* 1998 *(in press)*.
15. Delhaas EM, Brouwers JRB. Intrathecal baclofen overdose: report of seven events and review of the literature. *Int J Clin Pharmacol Ther Toxicol* 1991;29:274–280.
16. Dressler D, Oeljeschlager R-O, Ruther E. Severe tardive dystonia: treatment with continuous intrathecal baclofen administration. *Mov Disord* 1997;12:585–587.
17. Fahn S. Systemic therapy of dystonia. *Can J Neurol Sci* 1987;14:528–532.
18. Fahn S, Cote LJ. Regional distribution of GABA in the brain of the Rhesus monkey. *J Neurochem* 1968;15:209.
19. Ford B, Fahn S. Intrathecal baclofen [Letter]. *Neurology* 1994;44:1367–1368.
20. Ford B, Greene P, Louis ED, et al. Treatment of dystonia using intrathecal baclofen. *Arch Neurol* 1996;1241–1246.
21. Greene P. Baclofen in the treatment of dystonia. *Clin Neuropharmacol* 1992;15:276–288.
22. Greene P, Kang UJ, Fahn S. Spread of symptoms in idiopathic torsion dystonia. *Mov Disord* 1995;10:143–152.
23. Herman RM, D'Luzansky SC, Ippolito R. Intrathecal baclofen suppresses central pain in patients with spinal lesions. *Clin J Pain* 1992;8:338–345.
24. Hugenholtz H, Nelson RF, Dehoux E, Bickerton R. Intrathecal baclofen for intractable spinal spasticity—a double-blind cross-over comparison with placebo in 6 patients. *Can J Neurol Sci* 1992;19:188–195.
25. Khorasani A, Peruzzi WT. Dantrolene treatment for abrupt intrathecal baclofen withdrawal. *Anest Analg* 1995;80:1054–1070.
26. Knutsson E, Lindblom U, Beissinger RL, Martenson A. Plasma and cerebrospinal fluid levels of baclofen at optimal therpeutic responses in spastic paresis. *J Neurol Sci* 1974;23:473–484.
27. Kofler M, Arturo LA. Prolonged seizure activity after baclofen withdrawal. *Neurology* 1992;42:697–698.
28. Kroin JS, Ali A, York M, Penn RD. The distribution of medication along the spinal canal after chronic intrathecal administration. *Neurosurgery* 1993;33:226–230.
29. Kroin JS, Penn RD. Intrathecal baclofen down-regulates $GABA_B$ receptors in the rat substantia gelatinosa. *J Neurosurg* 1993;79:544–549.
30. Lazorthes Y, Sallerin-Caute B, Verdie J, Bastide R, Carillo J. Chronic intrathecal baclofen administration for control of severe spasticity. *J Neurosurg* 1990;72:393–402.
31. Lewis KS, Mueller WM. Intrathecal baclofen for severe spasticity secondary to spinal cord injury. *Ann Pharmacol* 1993;27:767–773.
32. Loubster PG, Narayan RK, Sandin KJ, et al. Continuous infusion of intrathecal baclofen: long-term effects on spasticity in spinal cord injury. *Paraplegia* 1991;29:48–64.
33. Mandac BR, Hurvitz EA, Nelson VS. Hyperthermia associated with baclofen withdrawal and increased spasticity. *Arch Phys Med Rehabil* 1993;74:96–97.

34. Meinck HM, Tronnier V, Rieke K, Wirtz CR, Flugel D, Schwab S. Intrathecal baclofen treatment for stiff-man syndrome: pump failure may be fatal. *Neurology* 1994;44:2209–2210.

35. Meythaler JM, Steers WD, Tuel SM, Cross LL, Haworth CS. Continuous intrathecal baclofen in spinal cord spasticity. *Am J Phys Med Rehabil* 1992;71:321–327.

36. Misgeld U, Bijak M, Jarolimek W. A physiological role for GABA$_B$ receptors and the effects of baclofen in the mammalian central nervous system. *Prog Neurobiol* 1995;46:423–462.

37. Muller H, Zierski J, Dralle D, Kraub D, Mart-Schler E. Pharmacokinetics of intrathecal baclofen. In: Muller H, Zierski J, Penn R, eds. *Local spinal therapy of spasticity.* Berlin: Springer, 1988:155–214.

38. Nance P, Schryvers O, Schmidt B, Dubo H, Loveridge B, Fewer D. Intrathecal baclofen therapy for adults with spinal spasticity: therapeutic efficacy and effect on hospital admissions. *Can J Neurol Sci* 1995;22:22–29.

39. Narayan RK, Loubster PG, Jankovic J, Donovan WH, Bontke CF. Intrathecal baclofen for intractable axial dystonia. *Neurology* 1991;41:1141–1142.

40. Ochs GA. Intrathecal baclofen. *Baillieres Clin Neurol* 1993;2:73–86.

41. Patterson V, Watt M, Byrnes D, Crowe D, Lee A. Management of severe spasticity with intrathecal baclofen delivered by a manually operated pump. *J Neurol Neurosurg Psychiatr* 1994;57:582–558.

42. Penn RD. Intrathecal baclofen for spasticity of spinal origin: seven years of experience. *J Neurosurg* 1992;77:236–240.

43. Penn RD, Gianino JM, York MM. Intrathecal baclofen for motor disorders. *Mov Disord* 1995;10:675–677.

44. Penn RD, Mangieri EA. Stiff-man syndrome treated with intrathecal baclofen. *Neurology* 1993;43:2412.

45. Penn RD, Savoy S, Corcos D, et al. Intrathecal baclofen for severe spinal spasticity: a double blind crossover study. *N Engl J Med* 1989;320:1517–1521.

46. Penn RD, York MM, Paice JA. Catheter systems for intrathecal drug delivery. *J Neurosurg* 1995;83:215–217.

47. Price GW, Wilkin GP, Turnbull MJ, Bowery NG. Are baclofen-sensitive GABAB receptors present on primary afferent terminals of the spinal cord? *Nature* 1984;307:71–74.

48. Sallerin-Caute B, Lazorthes Y, Monserrat B, Cros J, Bastide R. CSF baclofen levels after intrathecal administration in severe spasticity. *Eur J Clin Pharmacol* 1991;40:363–365.

49. Saltuari L, Kronenberg M, Marosi MJ, et al. Indication, efficiency and complications of intrathecal pump supported baclofen treatment in spinal spasticity. *Acta Neurol* 1992;14:187–194.

50. Schurch B. Errors and limitations of the multimodality checking method of defective spinal intrathecal pump systems. *Paraplegia* 1993;31:611–615.

51. Seigfried RN, Jacobson L, Chabal C. Development of an acute withdrawal syndrome following the cessation on intrathecal baclofen in a patient with spasticity. *Anesthesiology* 1992;5:1048–1050.

52. Silbert PL, Matsumoto JY, McManis PG, Stolp-Smith KA, Elliott BA, McEvoy KM. Intrathecal baclofen therapy in stiff-man syndrome: a double blind, placebo-controlled trial. *Neurology* 1995;45:1893–1897.

53. Silbert PL, Stewart-Wynne EG. Increased dystonia after intrathecal baclofen [Letter]. *Neurology* 1992;42:1639–1640.

54. SynchroMed Infusion System. *Clinical reference guide.* Minneapolis, MN: Medtronic, Inc., 1993.

55. Teddy P, Jamous A, Gardner B, Wang D, Silver J. Complications of intrathecal baclofen delivery. *Br J Neurosurg* 1992;6:115–118.

56. Young RR, Delwaide PJ. Spasticity. *N Engl J Med* 1981;304:28–33 (Part I); *N Engl J Med* 1981;304:96–99 (Part II).

Dystonia 3: Advances in Neurology, Vol. 78,
edited by S. Fahn, C. D. Marsden, and M. DeLong.
Lippincott–Raven Publishers, Philadelphia © 1998.

21

GPi Pallidotomy for Dystonia: Clinical Outcome and Neuronal Activity

*Jerrold L. Vitek, *J. Zhang, *M. Evatt, *Klaus Mewes, *Mahlon R. DeLong,
†Takao Hashimoto, *S. Triche, and ‡R. A. E. Bakay

*Department of Neurology, Emory University School of Medicine, Atlanta, Georgia 30322;
†Department of Medicine (Neurology), Shinshu University School of Medicine, 3-1-1 Asahi,
Matsumoto 390-8621, Japan; and ‡Emory University School of Medicine, Department of
Neurosurgery, The Emory Clinic, Atlanta, Georgia 30322.

Dystonia is a movement disorder characterized by sustained or intermittent muscle activity leading to altered voluntary movement and abnormal postures. Dystonia is both a symptom and a disease. Primary dystonia is generally considered a hereditary disorder presenting in both generalized and focal forms. The observation that dystonia may occur as a presenting symptom of Parkinson's disease (PD) has led to speculation that dystonia may be similar pathophysiologically to PD. Dystonia, however, also appears in Parkinson's patients as a complication of treatment with L-dopa, suggesting that at least some forms of dystonia could pathophysiologically resemble a hyperkinetic disorder. Hypokinetic disorders appear to result from increased mean discharge rates of neurons in the internal segment of the globus pallidus (GPi), whereas hyperkinetic disorders are associated with decreased mean discharge rates in GPi (10,15,16,30). Although 2-deoxyglucose (2-DG) studies in N-methyl-4-phenyl-1,2,3,6,-tetra hydropyridine (MPTP) primates with levodopa-induced dystonia and positron emission tomography (PET) studies in humans with dystonia suggest a lowered rate of neuronal discharge in GPi (20), at present, there is no evidence at the neuronal level to support or refute either concept.

Medical therapy has been variably effective in alleviating dystonia (13). Although some patients may benefit significantly from high-dose anticholinergics or from various combinations of anticholinergics, dopamine-depleting drugs, or dopamine blockers, most patients either do not benefit substantially or are unable to tolerate the drugs in high enough doses because of developing debilitating side effects. Although a variety of surgical approaches have been tried for various types of dystonia, the results have been quite variable (1,6,25). Due to the inconsistent benefit of these procedures they are rarely used in the treatment of dystonia.

Pallidotomy has been used for a number of movement disorders including dystonia (5, 7,8,14,19,21). As with dystonia, pallidotomy for PD had been associated with significant variability in outcome, precluding its use as a consistently reliable alternative for patients refractory to medical therapy (5,14). Recently, however, because of a better understanding of the rationale for surgery, improved techniques, and more consistently good outcomes, there has been a resurgence in enthusiasm for pallidotomy in the treatment of PD (2,11,18,27). Our own experience with pallidotomy for PD has indicated that it provides substantial benefit to the vast majority of patients with advanced idiopathic PD, but that these benefits are critically dependent on lesion location (27,29). We have also observed almost complete amelioration of dystonic symptoms in PD patients with prominent drug-induced or "off" dystonia who have undergone pallidotomy. Based on this experience and previous reports of symptomatic benefit to dystonic patients following pallidal lesions (5,6,14) we performed pallidotomy in three patients with primary dystonia. We report here the clinical outcomes and the characteristics of neuronal activity recorded from the pallidum during the course of microelectrode mapping prior to pallidotomy.

PATIENT SELECTION/CLINICAL PROTOCOL

Three patients with disabling, medically intractable primary generalized dystonia were evaluated at selected intervals pre- and postoperatively using the Burke-Fahn-Marsden Dystonia Rating Scales Movement (FMDRS-M) and Disability (FMDRS-D). In addition the activity patterns of select muscle groups were studied with surface electromyography (EMG)

during rest or the execution of simple movements at each clinic evaluation. High-resolution magnetic resonance images were used to reconstruct the lesions and confirm their location within the posterior (sensorimotor) portion of the pallidum.

RESULTS OF CLINICAL AND QUANTITATIVE ASSESSMENTS

Clinical Outcome

Dystonic symptoms were alleviated intraoperatively immediately after lesioning. Postoperative clinical evaluations using the BFMDRS-M and BFMDRS-D revealed significant improvement. Postoperative evaluations for these three patients were carried out at 1 week, and at 1 and 2 months, respectively. Comparison of postsurgical assessments with preoperative baseline scores reveals marked improvement in the BFMDRS-M and BFMDRS-D in all three patients as shown in Figs. 1 and 2, respectively. Preoperative BFMDRS-M and BFMDRS-D scores were determined for each patient twice before surgery and averaged 34,

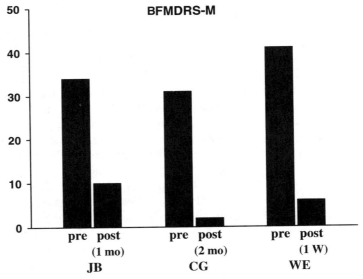

FIG. 1. Fahn-Marsden Dystonia Rating Scale for Movement (FMDRS-M) for three patients pre- and postpallidotomy.

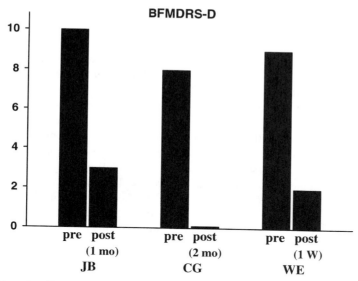

FIG. 2. Fahn-Marsden Dystonia Rating Scale for Disability (FMDRS-D) for three patients pre- and postpallidotomy.

31, and 41, and 10, 8, and 8.5, respectively. Postoperatively the BFMDRS-M and BFMDRS-D were reduced to 10, 5, and 6, and 3, 0, and 2, respectively. Overall the postoperative FMDRS-M and BFMDRS-D mean scores in these patients improved 80% and 72%, respectively. Coincident with the dramatic reduction in movement and disability scores, each patient reported marked improvement in motor function associated with significant subjective improvement in all activities of daily living. The most severely affected patient with axial dystonia was able to achieve relief from his dystonia preoperatively only by lying on his right side. He is now able to sit, stand, and walk with minimal torsional movement, predominantly involving the neck, which was mostly due to the activity of muscles on the side ipsilateral to his pallidotomy. Following pallidotomy he has been able to sit in a chair, go shopping, and perform fine motor tasks previously impossible for him.

Objective Testing of Electromyographic Activity

Preoperatively, all three patients underwent systematic assessment of spontaneous muscle activity under different postures and during simple movements. All three patients demonstrated intermittent posturing of the limbs at rest or with arms held outstretched. This was associated with intermittent and often times sustained EMG activity in agonist and antagonist muscle groups. During simple movements requiring reciprocal activation and inactivation of agonist-antagonist muscle groups, we routinely observed excessive and altered temporal patterning of muscle activity. There was routinely an "overflow" of activation into normally quiescent muscle groups. Following pallidotomy, in accordance with the clinical benefit we observed a marked reduction of EMG activity in the affected body regions present during rest preoperatively and a more "normal" pattern of activation during movement with decreased coactivation of agonist-antagonist muscle groups.

ELECTROPHYSIOLOGIC MAPPING/LESIONING TECHNIQUE

The technique of single cell recording, mapping, and lesioning is the same as that for pallidotomy for PD (28). This technique offers a reliable method for accurately identifying and defining the sensorimotor territory of GPi prior to lesioning. Different patterns of neural activity within the striatum, external and internal segments of the globus pallidus, GPe and GPi, are identified together with nearby critical structures (i.e., optic tract and internal capsule), and are used to generate a physiologic map of the region. During the mapping procedures in these patients we collected neuronal activity in GPe and GPi. These data were analyzed "off" line to determine mean firing rates and assess patterns of neural activity and receptive field properties.

Neuronal Activity

A total of 68 cells were collected from the pallidum in the course of performing microelectrode-guided pallidotomy in three patients with idiopathic generalized dystonia. Forty cells from GPe and 28 from GPi were studied. Mean discharge rates in GPe were 38 ± 24 Hz whereas those in GPi were 48 ± 18 Hz. Although there are no data from normal humans for comparison, the rates in GPe and GPi were reduced compared to that found in patients with PD but slightly faster than that found in a patient with hemiballismus. Figure 3 demonstrates the mean discharge rates in GPe and GPi for patients with dystonia compared to those with PD and hemiballismus.

Patterns of neuronal activity in GPe and GPi were also significantly different from those reported in normal animals. Unlike the tonic activity reported in normal primates, neuronal activity in GPi displayed irregular grouped discharges. This pattern was observed in the majority of cells in GPe and GPi and was similar to that observed in patients with PD and hemiballismus (see Fig. 4). In each case there are irregularly grouped discharges superimposed on varying tonic rates of activity. In patients with hemiballismus and dystonia the pattern of neuronal activity in GPi was similar to that within GPe with periods of activity interspersed with pauses and a tendency for irregularly grouped discharges.

Receptive fields in the dystonic patients were significantly widened compared to that

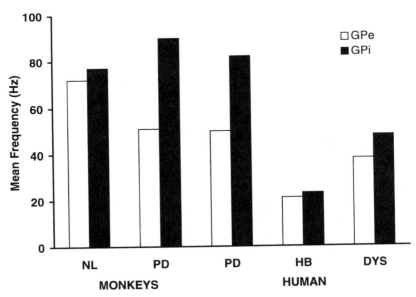

FIG. 3.   Mean discharge frequencies for neurons in GPe and GPi in normal (NL) and Parkinsonian monkeys (PD), and humans with Parkinson's disease (PD), hemiballismus (HB), and dystonia (DYS).

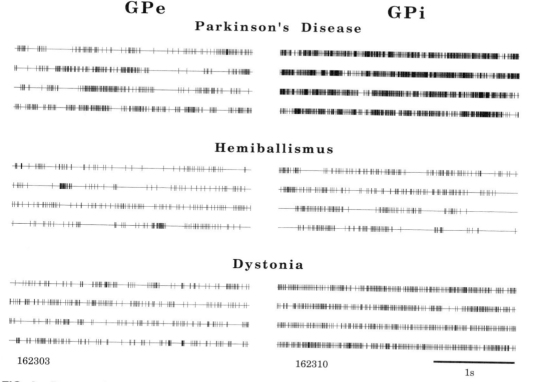

FIG. 4. Rasters of spontaneous neuronal activity for neurons in GPe and GPi from patients with Parkinson's disease, hemiballismus, and dystonia.

reported in intact animals. Of 65 neurons examined for their receptive field properties, 28 (43%) responded to passive manipulation or active movement of the limbs, face, or trunk. Of these, 19 (29%) responded to movement of multiple joints in one or more limbs, 13 (20%) to manipulation of more than one limb, and 7 (11%) to manipulation of the ipsilateral as well as the contralateral limb.

MODEL FOR DYSTONIA

The finding of lowered mean discharge rates in GPe and GPi together with increased phasic responses to peripheral manipulations strongly suggests overactivity in *both* the direct and indirect pathways, as shown in Fig. 5. Increased striatal inhibitory input to GPe and GPi would account for the lowering of mean discharge rates in these nuclei. Studies in MPTP-treated primates with levodopa-induced dystonia and PET studies in patients with dystonia have shown increased levels of metabolism in GP, consistent with increased input over the direct pathway (12,20). The increased phasic responses to peripheral manipulation could be accounted for by excessive input over the subthalamopallidal (excitatory) portion of the indirect pathway. Evidence that the subthalamic nucleus is the major source of peripheral input to GPi has been obtained in studies examining somatosensory responsiveness in GPi before and after STN lesions (15,16). In addition to the decrease in mean discharge frequency in GPi in patients with dystonia, there is also an alteration in the *pattern* of neuronal activity in GPi with a change from continuous firing to irregularly grouped discharges. Conceivably in-

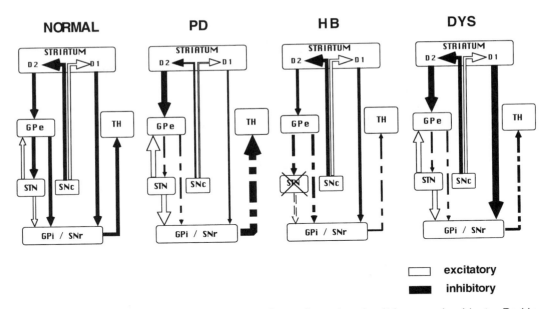

FIG. 5. Schematic representation of the basal ganglia motor circuit in normal subjects, Parkinson's disease (PD), hemiballismus (HB), and dystonia (DYS). Inhibitory connections are represented by filled arrows and excitatory projections by open arrows. The relative amount (rate) of neuronal activity is represented by the thickness of the arrows. The interrupted lines represent altered patterns of neuronal activity. GPe, globus pallidus pars externa; GPi, globus pallidus pars interna; STN, subthalamic nucleus; SNc, substantia nigra pars compacts; SNr, substantia nigra pars reticulata; TH, thalamus. D1 and D2 represent dopamine receptor subtypes.

creased synchronization of discharge between GPi neurons may be an important feature of dystonia as well, accounting for the loss of reciprocal inhibition and the overflow phenomenon. Thus, we propose that dystonia results from a combination of decreased discharge rates, altered patterns, and responses of neurons in GPi to phasic inputs and possibly excessive synchronization of neuronal activity within basal ganglia, brainstem, thalamic, and cortical circuits. The etiology of such neural activity may be varied, but its removal or inactivation would likely lead to a "normalization" of activity in these circuits coincident with alleviation of dystonic symptoms.

RELEVANCE TO CURRENT MODELS OF HYPO- AND HYPERKINETIC MOVEMENT DISORDERS

Based on the simplistic model of hypo- and hyperkinetic movement disorders one would predict that lesions in the sensorimotor pallidum that disrupt the pallidothalamic "motor" circuit would alleviate parkinsonian signs, yet one would also predict that such lesions would lead to disinhibition of the motor thalamus, and result in dyskinesias. Similarly, the model also predicts that a lesion in the thalamus should worsen parkinsonian motor signs, because the etiology of altered movement in PD is proposed to occur as a result of excessive inhibition of the motor thalamus. Lesions within the motor thalamus, however, do not exacerbate or induce parkinsonian motor signs, as predicted by the model, but instead are reported to improve or abolish parkinsonian tremor and rigidity, suggesting that a decrease in activity of thalamic neurons cannot, by itself, account for the development of parkinsonian motor signs.

Alternatively, these motor signs may occur, in part, due to an *altered* pattern of neuronal activity. This altered pattern of thalamocortical activity may, in turn, disrupt the *normal opera-*

tion of cortico-cortical circuits involved in motor control (23,24). Our observations of increased bursting and rhythmic oscillatory patterns of activity within the thalamus in parkinsonian monkeys, the clear improvement in most parkinsonian motor signs following thalamotomy, together with the altered patterns and responses of pallidal neurons to phasic inputs in patients with idiopathic dystonia and PD lend direct support to this hypothesis (28, 31). The fact that patients with dystonia or dyskinesia, in which mean discharge rates are reduced in GPi, improve following both pallidotomy and thalamotomy strongly suggests that altered neuronal activity contributes significantly to and may be the underlying basis for the development of the altered movement associated with these movement disorders. This altered neuronal activity may result in changes in spatial-temporal patterning of cortical output, essentially introducing noise into cortical signals leading to a lower signal-to-noise ratio and an increase in the likelihood of errors in transmission of information through the neural circuitry.

Such errors could have a varied phenotypic expression dependent on the particular combination and degree of changes in mean discharge rate, the particular alteration in pattern and phasic responses of neuronal activity, the degree of synchronization of neurons, and which cortical-subcortical systems are most affected. It is not difficult to relate such changes in cortical output to the development of overflow or action dystonia. Other forms of dystonia (i.e., that occurring during rest) could develop as a result of a progressive increase in the amount and degree of synchrony of spontaneous neuronal activity in the pallidum, leading to a progressively lower threshold for activation of brainstem and/or cortical regions associated with movement, eventually precipitating muscle activity at rest. Thus, the beneficial effect of pallidotomy or thalamotomy for dystonia may lie in its effectively interrupting the flow of altered neuronal activity and leading to a "normalization" of cortical and subcortical activity and improvement in cortical signal processing.

RELEVANCE TO THE TREATMENT OF DYSTONIA

From a therapeutic standpoint, the amelioration of dystonia by GPi lesions is extremely important, because other surgical treatments for dystonia (i.e., cervical rhizotomy and thalamotomy) have been associated with considerable variability in outcome with complication rates varying from 16% to 50%. Rhizotomy is not an option for patients with limb or trunk dystonia, and is variably effective for patients with torticollis (17). Thalamotomy has been reported effective in alleviating both primary and secondary dystonia; however, the benefits vary from none to marked with approximately one-third showing marked benefit, one-third mild to moderate, and one-third with no or little benefit (25). This variable outcome likely stems from lack of a common target with most targeting various combinations of Vim, Vop, and Voa, CM or pulvinar (1,6,32). The complication rate associated with thalamotomy may partially stem from the problems associated with target localization and the functional heterogeneity of this structure with adjacent thalamic nuclei subserving functions involving language, memory, attention, and sensation. Given the complicated onion-skin somatotopy of the motor thalamus a large lesion is generally required to involve the necessary portions of the motor thalamus. These types of lesions are more likely to be associated with a greater risk for a complication occurring secondary to encroachment on adjacent thalamic subnuclei or corticospinal tract. Pallidotomy offers a considerable advantage over thalamotomy. The pallidal target (i.e., sensorimotor portion of GPi) is clearly defined and relatively free of complications often associated with thalamotomy such as language disorders, gait ataxia, and sensory loss. In addition, lesions within the GPi, which is upstream from the thalamus, could also remove altered neuronal input to brainstem regions, that is, pedunculopontine nucleus (PPN) and the midbrain extrapyramidal area (MEA), which may also be involved in mediating the disordered movement associated with dystonia. Thus, the fact that the sensorimotor portion of GPi is a well-defined target with a potentially greater, more widespread effect on dystonic symptoms, makes it a more attractive target to lesion for patients with dystonia. Thus, improved understanding of the pathophysiologic basis underlying the development of dystonia provides a foundation for the development of new treatment strategies employing either current ablative methods or through the development of new innovative techniques such as deep brain stimulation.

DEEP BRAIN STIMULATION AS AN ALTERNATIVE APPROACH TO THE TREATMENT OF DYSTONIA

Patients with generalized dystonia at increased risk of complications associated with bilateral pallidotomy may benefit by deep brain stimulation (DBS) on the unoperated side. The effects of DBS are reversible and provide a method in which patients who require bilateral procedures to gain optimum functional benefit may safely do so without the accentuated risk of complications currently associated with bilateral ablative procedures. Chronic DBS has been used predominantly for the treatment of parkinsonian, essential, and cerebellar outflow tremors (3,26). To date there is only one report of DBS for the treatment of dystonia (22). DBS, however, allows greater flexibility by allowing a variety of pulse widths, stimulation frequencies, current intensities, and lead combinations (using a multipolar lead), which can be used to optimize the beneficial effect. Similarly, if untoward side effects occur, stimulation parameters can be adjusted to minimize them. Although the physiologic basis underlying the beneficial effect of DBS is unclear, one potential mechanism is by inhibiting or "jamming" rhythmic neuronal activity. This could occur by desynchronizing (4), or blocking transmission of neuronal activity (9). Alternatively, if stimulation can be used to activate projection neurons, stimulation within the GPe could potentially be a more effective site for DBS in both dystonia and PD. Normalization of activity within GPe would theoretically have far greater effects on amelioration of

dystonia and parkinsonian motor signs because it can potentially affect all the major output areas, including the subthalamic nucleus (STN), substantia nigra pars reticulata (SNr), as well as GPi, as compared to only a few as with ablation or stimulation of STN or GPi.

OVERVIEW

In summary, our preliminary data have demonstrated the beneficial effect of inactivation of the sensorimotor portion of GPi in patients with dystonia. Pallidotomy results in marked improvement in motor functioning and dystonic symptoms with a significant reduction in disability. This benefit is even more striking when one considers the generally poor response of the vast majority of these patients to medical therapy. Furthermore, the neural data gathered during the course of these procedures provides new insight into the pathophysiology of dystonia. The process whereby a lesion can restore functioning and reverse symptoms such as dystonia is not intuitively obvious. In the case of PD and now dystonia, however, it is becoming increasingly clear that the signs and symptoms of these disorders result from both altered patterns and rates of neural activity. It is that alteration of the pallidofugal pathway that results in a disruption and inhibition of structures innervated by this system (i.e., thalamocortical and midbrain tegmental targets). These systems, it appears, are unable to function normally when subjected to the abnormal and altered inhibitory input from the pallidum. Removal of this input appears to restore the functional integrity of the thalamic and midbrain regions. Thus, as in PD, the rationale for ablation of the sensorimotor portion of GPi in dystonia is to remove abnormal activity that causes other portions of the central nervous system to malfunction. Removal of this altered activity has been demonstrated to lead to improvement in movement. Thus, while the movements may differ significantly between hypokinetic and hyperkinetic disorders, the response to lesioning is the same (i.e., cessation of the abnormal movement). Hence, the role of ablative surgery (e.g., pallidotomy), can be viewed as a process whereby an unregulated, disruptive circuit is removed, thus allowing the remaining structures and circuits to function more normally.

REFERENCES

1. Andrew J, Fowler CJ, Harrison MJG. Stereotaxic thalamotomy in 55 cases of dystonia. *Brain* 1983;106: 981–1000.
2. Baron MS, Vitek JL, Bakay RAE, et al. Treatment of advanced Parkinson's disease with microelectrode-guided pallidotomy: 1 year pilot-study results. (Pallidotomy for advanced PD). *Ann Neurol* 1996 *(submitted).*
3. Benabid AL, Pollak P, Seigneuret E, Hoffman D, Gay E, Perret J. Chronic VIM thalamic stimulation in Parkinson's disease, essential tremor and extra-pyramidal dyskinesias. *Acta Neurochir* 1993;58:39–44.
4. Blond S, Caparros-Lefebvre D, Parker F, et al. Control of tremor and involuntary movement disorders by chronic stereotactic stimulation of the ventral intermediate thalamic nucleus. *J Neurosurg* 1991;77:62–68.
5. Burzaco J. Stereotactic pallidotomy in extrapyramidal disorders. *Appl Neurophysiol* 1985;48:283–287.
6. Cooper IS. 20-year followup study of the neurosurgical treatment of dystonia musculorum deformans. *Adv Neurol* 1976;14:423–452.
7. Cooper IS, Bravo G. Chemopallidectomy and chemothalamectomy. *J Neurosurg* 1958;3:244–250.
8. Cooper IS, Poloukhine N. The globus pallidus as a surgical target. *J Am Geriatr Soc* 1956;4:1182–1207.
9. Deiber M, Pollak P, Passingham R, et al. Thalamic stimulation and suppression of parkinsonian tremor. Evidence of a cerebellar deactivation using positron emission tomography. *Brain* 1993;116:267–279.
10. DeLong MR. Primate models of movement disorders of basal ganglia origin. *Trends Neurosci* 1990;13:281–285.
11. Dogali M, Fazzine E, Kolodny E, et al. Stereotactic ventral pallidotomy for Parkinson's disease. *Neurology* 1995;45:753–761.
12. Eidelberg D. Metabolic brain networks in idiopathic torsion dystonia. Abstract presented at the Third International Dystonia Symposium, 1996.
13. Fahn S. Drug treatment of hyperkinetic movement disorders. *Semin Neurol* 1987;7:192–208.
14. Gross C, Frerebeau PH, Perez-Dominguez E, Bazin M, Privat JM. Long term results of stereotaxic surgery for infantile dystonia and dyskinesia. *Neurochirurgia* 1976;19:171–178.
15. Hamada I, DeLong MR. Excitotoxic acid lesions of the primate subthalamic nucleus result in transient dyskinesias of the contralateral limbs. *J Neurophysiol* 1992;68:1850–1858.
16. Hamada I, DeLong MR. Excitotoxic acid lesions of the primate subthalamic nucleus result in reduced pallidal neuronal activity during active holding. *J Neurophysiol* 1992;68:1859–1866.
17. Hamby WB, Schiffer S. Spasmodic torticollis; results after cervical rhizotomy in 80 cases. *Clin Neurosurg* 1970;17:28–37.
18. Lozano AM, Lang AE, Galvez-Jimenez N, et al. Effect of GPi pallidotomy on motor function in Parkinson's disease. *Lancet* 1995;346:1383–1387.
19. Meyers R. Surgical interruption of the pallidofugal fibres: its effect on the syndrome paralysis agitans and technical considerations in its application. *NY State J Med* 1942;42:317–325.
20. Mitchell IJ, Boyce S, Sambrook MA, Crossman AR. A 2-deoxyglucose study of the effects of dopamine agonists on the parkinsonian primate brain. *Brain* 1992; 115:809–824.
21. Narabayashi H, Okuma T. Procaine oil blocking of the globus pallidus for the treatment of rigidity and tremor of parkinsonism. *Psychiat Neurol Jpn* 1954;56:471–495.
22. Sellal F, Hirsch E, Barth P, Blond S, Marescaux C. A case of symptomatic hemidystonia improved by ventrosposterolateral thalamic electrostimulation. *Mov Disord* 1993;4:515–518.
23. Steriade M. Basic mechanisms of sleep generation. *Neurology* 1992;42[Suppl 6]:9–18.
24. Steriade M, McCarley RW. *Brainstem control of wakefulness and sleep.* New York: Plenum Press, 1990.
25. Tasker RR, Doorly T, Yamashiro K. Thalamotomy in generalized dystonia. *Adv Neurol* 1988;50:615–631.
26. Vitek JL, Ashe J, DeLong MR, Alexander GE. Physiologic properties and somatotopic organization of the primate motor thalamus. *J Neurophysiol* 1994;71: 1498–1513.
27. Vitek JL, Bakay RAE, DeLong MR. GPi pallidotomy for medically intractable Parkinson's disease. *Adv Neurol (in press)* (Abstr).
28. Vitek JL, Bakay RAE, Hashimoto T, et al. Microelectrode-guided pallidotomy: technical approach and application for treatment of medically intractable Parkinson's Disease. *J Neurosurg* 1996.
29. Vitek JL, Hashimoto T, Baron MS, et al. Lesion location related to outcome in microelectrode-guided pallidotomy. *Ann Neurol* 1994;36:279 (Abstr).
30. Vitek JL, Kaneoke Y, Hashimoto T, Bakay RAE, DeLong MR. Neuronal activity in the pallidum of a patient with hemiballismus. *Am Neurol Assoc* 1995 (Abstr).
31. Vitek JL, Zhang J, DeLong MR, Mewes K, Bakay RAE. Neuronal activity in the pallidum in patients with medically intractable dystonia. Abstract presented at the Third International Dystonia Symposium, 1996.
32. Yamashiro K, Tasker RR. Stereotactic thalamotomy for dystonic patients. *Stereotact Funct Neurosurg* 1993; 60:81–85.

Dystonia 3: Advances in Neurology, Vol. 78,
edited by S. Fahn, C. D. Marsden, and M. DeLong.
Lippincott–Raven Publishers, Philadelphia © 1998.

22

Experience with Stereotactics for Dystonia: Case Examples

*†Robert P. Iacono, †Sandra M. Kuniyoshi, and †Tony Schoonenberg

Neuroscience and †Movement Disorders Center, Loma Linda University Medical Center, Loma Linda, California 92354.

Stereotactic surgical interventions in dystonia have in the past been applied to a variable population of patients with widely differing diagnoses and disease expression. These operations have included targeting various nuclei of the thalamus including Voa, Vop, Vim, centromedian (CM), the subthalamic areas H_1, H_2, and zona incerta, the internal nucleus of the pallidum, and the dentate nuclei of the cerebellum (2,4,5,10,15). The choice of targets for dystonia, as for stereotactics in general, has been empiric, broadly based on past evidence of the efficacy of these targets for movement disorders in general, with no described discrimination of different targets for different presentations or diagnosis (4,17). Historically, however, it appears that the results of these operations are exquisitely sensitive to target and technique, as evidenced by their having fallen out of clinical use, following reports of unsatisfactory results of some operations, compounded by the inability of surgeons to easily reproduce another surgeon's successful rendition of the operation (5,16,19).

In addition to the diversity of surgical targets and techniques available, the spectrum of dystonia varies widely, and has been broadly divided into generalized young-onset dystonia in which axial and hyperkinetic symptoms predominate and focal adult-onset dystonia, which are generally appendicular, focal, cranial, and typically involve the distal aspect on one or two limbs (2,9,20,23). By comparison, we have di-

vided Parkinson's disease (PD) symptoms into predominantly axial akinetic postural instability versus hyperkinetic appendicular tremor and dyskinesia dominant expressions (14). Our conceptualization of motor control referable to dominance of movement disorder expression involves the differential influence of the basal ganglionic thalamocorticospinal system and the basal ganglionic to brainstem spinal system (11). The former is implicated in movement disorders of discretely innervated structures such as the face, larynx, and fingers and the latter, of axial, proximal musculature. Involved in this schema is the additional supposition that direct pallidal efferents to brainstem areas, such as the pedunculopontine nucleus (PPN), influence reticulospinal pathways (6,21). This is of primary importance in axial/akinetic symptoms in PD and truncal/proximal musculature abnormalities, including the lower extremities, in generalized dystonia. This is evidenced by the susceptibility of appendicular and hyperkinetic symptoms such as tremor and chorea to thalamotomy (i.e., modulation of the basal ganglionic thalamocortical system) whereas predominantly axial symptoms affecting postural stability and gait are uniquely improved by posteroventral pallidotomy. However, pallidotomy has less influence on tremor and distal extremity dexterity (e.g., rapid repetitive movements of individual digits) than thalamotomy (14).

The failure of thalamotomy to consistently alleviate the symptoms of primary generalized dystonia as reported by Yamashiro and Tasker in 25 patients in 1993, and others stands in contrast to our pallidotomy dystonic case reported here (4,12,20,24). Although Cooper and others report numerous good results for dystonia with both pallidotomy and thalamotomy, the actual targets obtained and a correlation with results is less clear-cut as these operations were accomplished before magnetic resonance imaging (MRI) or computed tomography (CT) were available to evaluate pre- and postoperative targets (5,10, 16). Of the few patients treated for writer's

cramp with stereotactics, thalamotomy has been shown to be particularly successful, suggesting the significant influence of the thalamus in putatively cortically mediated dystonias (22). The few additional cases reported here serve to stress the limited utility, and to broaden the knowledge base of stereotactics for dystonia.

METHODS

Our technique, as published elsewhere, involves MRI/ventriculographic calculation of

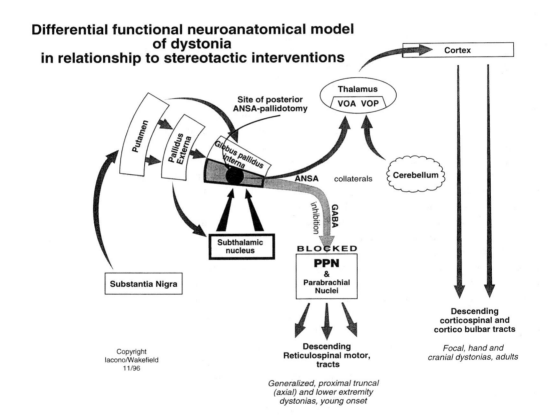

Differential functional neuroanatomical model of dystonia in relationship to stereotactic interventions

Copyright
Iacono/Wakefield
11/96

FIG. 1. Differential functional neuroanatomic model of dystonia in relationship to stereotactic intervention. Basal ganglionic output via the internal pallidum's ansa lenticularis' pallidal-tegmental bundle projects extrapyramidal influences directly to brainstem motor centers such as the pedunculopontine nucleus (PPN) (8,14). The PPN, in turn, is related to the reticularis gigantocellularis, ventralis, and magnocellular tegmental field, which control axial and proximal appendicular musculature via medioventral descending reticulospinal tracts (8,21). Unlike thalamotomy, which interrupts the pallidal/cerebellar/thalamic cortical output, pallidotomy may also influence control of otherwise inaccessible axial muscles involved in generalized dystonia.

anatomic target with stimulation-derived confirmation of anatomic target for both thalamotomy and pallidotomy (14). The PV pallidotomy target includes that subjacent portion of the ansa lenticularis and the posteroventral part of the somatomotor internal pallidum limited to locations below the intercommissural plane. A 1.8 ×2 mm lesion electrode is employed with 60° to 80° C lesions of 3 to 6 mm in diameter over a 5-mm trajectory 20° off sagittal 50° to 55° above the baseline ending 18 to 20 mm lateral, 15 to 16 mm anterior of the posterior commissure, and 1 mm below the floor of the third ventricle, in the ansa lenticularis. This position is verified by impedance and macroelectrode stimulation parameters that have been calibrated against microelectrode verification and postmortem specimens; combining these parameters with the intraoperative ventriculographic verifications makes this method extremely reliable and reproducible.

SIX CASE REPORTS

Meige's Syndrome

A 59-year-old woman presented with a 20-year history of blepharospasm, oral-facial dyskinesia, spasmodic dysphonia, anterocollis, and torticollis, all refractory to medication (18). The patient also demonstrated periods of hyperventilation, clenching of teeth, contraction of the platysma associated with spasms of torticollis, and choking. She had no prior exposure to neuroleptics and family history was negative for any neurologic disease. All symptoms were sustained throughout the day and exacerbated by emotional factors. Sequential botulinum toxin injections were initially helpful for blepharospasm, but soon failed. She underwent orbicularis myotomies with improvements. She underwent bilateral ansa-pallidotomy and afterward showed increasing improvement over 2 weeks. Stable improvement at 1 year included a 70% reduction in neck dystonia and oral-facial dyskinesia. The spasmodic dysphonia was not significantly improved.

Idiopathic Torsion Dystonia

A 17-year-old Russian male presented with end-stage idiopathic torsion dystonia (ITD) after a 10-year progressive history. He was cachexic with continuous generalized choreic and dystonic movements involving trunk and extremities. This case has been previously individually reported in detail (12). Radio frequency 80°C lesions were created bilaterally, confined to the most ventral posterior pallidum and ansa lenticularis. All hyperkinesias and dystonia resolved. The patient showed marked flaccidity for 1 week. The patient became fully functional, capable of self-care, and ambulatory after 2 months. At 2-year follow-up, there was no evidence of dystonia, and the patient demonstrated normal muscle control in all extremities. All medications were able to be discontinued, and the patient resumed a normal life with no evidence of any recurrence of symptoms.

Spasmodic Dysphonia with Left Lower Extremity Dystonia

A 48-year-old man with a 15-year history of spasmodic dysphonia and left lower extremity dystonia was diagnosed initially as atypical parkinsonism and experienced partial improvement of bradykinesia, left lower extremity dystonia, but not dysphonia to levodopa therapy. Unilateral pallidotomy was performed with improvement of the leg symptoms but no change in either speech or the spasmodic dysphonia (1).

Writer's Cramp

A 71-year-old Jewish man presented with a 30-year history of task-specific induced high-amplitude intention tremor of the right hand and arm associated with mild ipsilateral torticollis. He was unable to use the right hand for most fine movements, and unable to accomplish any legible writing. Because of the predominant appendicular nature of the dystonia/tremor, it was decided to perform thalamotomy, involving a trajectory to incorporate the ventroposterior Vim nucleus through the

Vop nucleus ending in the Voa nucleus. The 1.8 × 2.0 mm electrode was employed to create lesions of 60° to 70° C for 60 seconds, the probe withdrawn in sequence a total of 6 mm. At the completion of the operation all intention tremor was eliminated and hand dexterity and writing was reported to be normal. Torticollis was improved but remained symptomatic, with follow-up of 6 months.

Torticollis

A 47-year-old woman with an 18-year history of torticollis had failed medical and botulinum toxin therapy. She underwent contralateral posteroventral pallidotomy showing gradual improvement of 70% over 4 weeks. Improvement was stable at 6 and 12 months.

Cerebral Palsy with Dystonia

A 24-year-old Chinese male presented with cerebral palsy with dystonic components and bilateral choreic movements involving the neck and legs as well as significant and otherwise typical spasticity (3). A right posteroventral pallidotomy was performed with reported improvement in activities of daily living. Followed at 3 and 6 months this improvement was not found to be clinically significant.

There were no complications, either surgical or neurologic, following any of these procedures.

DISCUSSION

Stereotactic procedures such as thalamotomy and pallidotomy have a history of being applied to the spectrum of dystonia with widely varying results. Much of the clinical acumen required for successful application of stereotactics, as the successes themselves, has been forgotten. Cooper reported 226 cases of ITD having undergone 122 bilateral or 104 unilateral procedures, both pallidotomy and various thalamic targets (5). Average follow-up of 8 years revealed good results in 69%, 12% worse, and 2% mortality. Stereotactics for spasmodic torticollis have been reported by

many authors, including Hassler et al. (92 cases) and Kandel (162 cases) (10,16). Targets have included the VL or Voa nuclei of the thalamus, with success in these series of up to 67%. Numerous reports from that era also documented efforts to treat cerebral palsy with various stereotactic procedures, however, with much less success (3,7,10). At least one case of writer's cramp treated by VL destruction with success has been reported. Shima (Communication at 6th Annual Seminar of Kyushu-Yamaguchi Functional Neurosurgery, July 1996; Fumio Shima, Department of Clinical Neurophysiology, Kyushu University, Fukuoka, Japan) has recently performed 66 cases of stereotactic operations for dystonia including 46 Voa thalamotomies and 20 PVPs. Patients had ITD ($n = 40$), Meige's syndrome ($n = 15$), and writer's cramp ($n = 8$). Some of the operations were bilateral, including Voa/Vop thalamotomy. Analysis of these cases revealed a therapeutic advantage of pallidotomy for childhood-onset generalized dystonia and of thalamotomy for adult-onset focal dystonia. Our reported small series is also suggestive of this trend, with the additional evidence of the failure of pallidal and thalamic lesions in improving dysphonia and cerebral palsy-related dystonia (one case each).

The mechanism of ansa pallidotomy that we have proposed emphasizes the unique influence of the posteroventral pallidum via the ansa lenticularis in the pallido-tegmental bundle on axial and postural symptoms. Anatomic studies show involvement of brainstem, especially pedunculopontine influences on reticulospinal axial motor control as we have proposed (6,14,21). The nucleus reticularis gigantocellularis responds specifically to PPN inputs and modulates proximal axial musculature and the spinal locomotor apparatus (8). The concept that pallidotomy may therefore directly influence the putative brainstem-spinal abnormalities that occur in generalized dystonia in particular, distinguishes this procedure from thalamotomy with limited influence in these problems (2). Thus, the applicability of thalamotomy for adult, focal, facial, and distal appendicular dystonias and pallidotomy for juvenile, axial, proximal, and generalized dystonia based on this model is proposed, (see Fig. 1). Due to this conceptualization, the PVP operation is targeted to the posteroventral-most internal pallidum and subjacent ansa lenticularis contiguous with the superior optic-tract border. This ansa pallidotomy has as its goal interrupting pallidal brainstem efferents based on the above premise. In PD, axial, akinetic, and postural problems are similarly addressed (14).

Another advantage of pallidotomy, and specifically ansa pallidotomy confined to the posteroventral-most pallidum, is the ability to operate bilaterally without risk of speech, cognitive, or pseudobulbar-like symptoms associated with bilateral thalamotomy (5,7,10). This is likely due to the discrete nature of these ventral pallidal and ansa lesions, which spare the more anterodorsal aspects of the sensorimotor pallidum, which putatively projects heavily to thalamic nuclei, including VL and CM (6,21). Bilateral operations have historically been required in ITD and other generalized dystonias (5,10,13).

Following the operation for ITD and writer's cramp, all medications were discontinued. These patients experienced excellent results despite the long-standing, severe, and progressive nature of their problem, demonstrating the reversibility and potentially nonstructural nature of these illnesses. As per our experience with tremor and dystonia of Parkinson's disease and reports from the classic period of stereotactics, it is likely that many of these benefits will be permanent (5,16).

CONCLUSIONS

Stereotactic techniques are therapeutically valuable when applied to both focal and generalized dystonia. Pallidotomy is especially applicable to generalized dystonia such as ITD due to its putative influences on brainstem axial muscular control and the ability to safely perform this operation bilaterally. Classic thalamotomy of Vim/Vop and Voa targets cannot ordinarily be performed bilaterally, but remains useful for focal adult-onset dystonia that

manifests unilateral distal appendicular symptoms. The stereotactic interventions are exquisitely sensitive to target and technique. The wide spectrum of dystonia diagnoses and expression suggests the need for a case-by-case, surgeon-by-surgeon scrutiny of the indications and results of stereotactics for dystonia. Clear discrimination of the optimal target for the varying expressions of dystonia may reveal the predominant pathways involved in the mechanistic reversal of dystonia symptoms and provide insight into the pathophysiologic mechanisms of these movement disorders.

REFERENCES

1. Aminoff M, Dedo H, Izdebski K. Clinical aspects of spasmodic dysphonia. *J Neurol Neurosurg Psychiatr* 1978;41:361–365.
2. Andrew J. Stereotaxic thalamotomy in 55 cases of dystonia. *Brain* 1983;106:981–1000.
3. Broggi GLA, Bono R, Giorgi C, Nardocci N, Franzini A. Long term results of stereotactic thalamotomy for cerebral palsy. *Neurosurgery* 1983;12:195–202.
4. Cardoso F, Jancovic J, Grossman G, Hamilton W. Outcome after stereotactic thalamotomy for dystonia and hemiballismus. *Neurosurgery* 1995;36:501–507.
5. Cooper I. 20-year follow up study of the neurosurgical treatment of dystonia musculorum deformans. *Adv Neurol* 1976;14:170–177.
6. Crossman A, Jackson A. Nucleus tegmenta pedunculopontinus: efferent connections with special reference to the basal ganglia, studied in the rat by anterograde and retrograde transport of horseradish peroxidase. *Neuroscience* 1983;10:725–765.
7. Frank F, Fabrizi A, Frank-Ricci R, Gaist G. Stereotaxis and abnormal movements. *Acta Neurochir* 1987; 39:66–69.
8. Garcia-Rill E. The basal ganglia and the locomotor regions. *Brain Res Rev* 1986;11:47–63.
9. Greene P, Kang U, Fahn S. Spread of symptoms in idiopathic torsion dystonia. *Mov Disord* 1995;10:143–152.
10. Hassler R, Riechert T, Mundinger F. Physiological observations in stereotaxic operations in extrapyramidal motor disturbances. *Brain* 1960;83:337–351.
11. Iacono R, Lonser R, Morenski J. Stereotactic surgery for Parkinson's disease. *Mov Disord* 1994;9:470–473.
12. Iacono RP, Kuniyoshi S, Lonser RR, Maeda G, Inae AM, Ashwal S. Simultaneous bilateral pallidoansotomy for idiopathic dystonia musculorum deformans. *Pediatr Neurol* 1996;14:145–148.
13. Iacono RP, Lonser RR, Yamada S. Contemporaneous bilateral postero-ventral pallidotomy for early onset "juvenile type" Parkinson's disease. *Acta Neurochir* 1994;131:247–252.
14. Iacono RP, Shima F, Lonser RR, Kuniyoshi S, Maeda G, Yamada S. Results, indications, and physiology of posteroventral pallidotomy for patients with Parkinson's disease. *Neurosurgery* 1995;36:1118–1127.

15. Kandel E. Dystonia musculorum deformans. In: Walker A, ed. *Functional and stereotactic neurosurgery.* New York: Plenum, 1981:241–266.

16. Kandel E. Spasmodic torticollis. In: Walker A, ed. *Functional and stereotactic neurosurgery,* New York: Plenum, 1981:267–288.

17. Lenz FA, Martin R, Kwan HC, Tasker RR, Dostrovsky JO. Thalamic single-unit activity occurring in patients with hemidystonia. *Stereotact Funct Neurosurg* 1990; 54–55:159–162.

18. Mark W, Sage J, Dickson D. Meige syndrome in the spectrum of Lewy Body disease. *Neurology* 1994;44: 1432–1436.

19. Marsden C. Blepharospasm, oromandibular dystonia syndrome (Brueghels Syndrome). 1976;39:1204.

20. Marsden C, Harrison M. Idiopathic torsion dystonia (dystonia musculorum deformans). A review of forty-two patients. *Brain* 1974;97:793–810.

21. Parent A, *Basal ganglia: pallidotegmental projections.* Carpenter's Human Neuroanatomy. 9th ed. Chap. 19. Baltimore: Williams & Wilkins, 1996:834–837 (see also fig. A&B, p.835).

22. Siegfried J, Crowell R, Perrett E. Cure of tremulous writer's cramp by stereotaxic thalamotomy. *J Neurosurg* 1969;30:182–185.

23. Tasker R, Doorly T, Yamashiro K. Thalamotomy in generalized dystonia. *Adv Neurol* 1988;50:615–631.

24. Yamashiro K, Tasker RR. Stereotactic thalamotomy for dystonic patients. *Stereotact Funct Neurosurg* 1993;60:81–85.

Dystonia 3: Advances in Neurology, Vol. 78,
edited by S. Fahn, C. D. Marsden, and M. DeLong.
Lippincott–Raven Publishers, Philadelphia © 1998.

23

Botulinum Toxin Type B: An Open-Label, Dose-Escalation, Safety and Preliminary Efficacy Study in Cervical Dystonia Patients

*Paul A. Cullis, †Christopher F. O'Brien, ‡Daniel D. Truong, §Martin Koller, ‖Timothy P. Villegas, and §J. D. Wallace

*Department of Neurology, Wayne State University School of Medicine, Detroit, Michigan 48093; †Colorado Neurological Institute, Englewood, Colorado 80110; ‡Parkinson's and Movement Disorders Program, Long Beach, California 90806; §Athena Neurosciences, Inc., South San Francisco, California 94080; and ‖Pharmaceutical Research Associates, Charlottesville, Virginia 22903.

Cervical dystonia (CD) is a focal dystonia characterized by involuntary, dystonic contractions of neck and/or shoulder muscles that result in turning or tilting movements of the head, with or without sustained abnormal head postures. There is often pain or discomfort and tremor of the head may be present. Oral medications do not usually provide sustained relief (2,3).

Chemodenervation with botulinum toxin type A has been shown to be an effective treatment for CD (6). *Clostridium botulinum* produces at least seven serologically distinct neurotoxins designated A through G (8). Types A, B, E, and F have been associated with human poisoning (5). Botulinum toxin produces its effect by preventing the release of acetylcholine (ACh) from presynaptic nerve terminals at the neuromuscular junction. The different serotypes affect different intracellular docking proteins involved in the release of ACh. Type A cleaves SNAP-25 and type B (Neurobloc™) cleaves synaptobrevin (VAMP) (4). A previous pilot study had shown that low doses of Neurobloc™ could be administered safely in patients with CD (7). The objectives of this open-label study were to evaluate the safety and tolerability of increasing doses of Neurobloc™ in

patients with CD; to determine the occurrence of dose-limiting side effects; to evaluate and provide preliminary evidence for efficacy and dose-response of Neurobloc™ in patients with CD; and to provide information on the immunogenicity of Neurobloc™.

METHODS

Subjects

This was a three-center, open-label, dose-escalation study. Twenty-eight patients with a clinical diagnosis of CD received injections of Neurobloc™ into two to four superficial neck and shoulder muscles. All of the patients were either naive or still responsive to botulinum toxin A treatment. Patients who did not obtain significant clinical benefit from initial low doses of Neurobloc™ were eligible for subsequent higher doses. Patients who experienced clinical benefit received subsequent injections only when their improvement from their baseline Toronto Western Spasmodic Torticollis Rating Scale (TWSTRS)-Severity Scale score fell below 10%. Intervals between injections were not fixed, but could occur as frequently as every 2 weeks, depending on the patient's change from baseline in the TWSTRS-Severity Scale score. Doses were to increase by a factor of 1.25 for successively enrolled patients and 1.5 for repeat doses in the same patient. After the initial eight patients, who could receive multiple doses, the subsequent 20 patients received single doses up to 12,000 Units (U). All 28 patients completed the study. Patients ranged in age from 32 to 74 years, with a mean age of 50.9 years. Nineteen patients (68%) were women and nine patients (32%) were men.

Assessments

Efficacy variables included TWSTRS scores (1), which consisted of Severity Scale, Disability Scale, Pain Scale and Total Scale scores, Analog Pain Assessments, and Patient and Investigator Global Assessments. The Patient Analog Pain Scale was measured by the patient making a mark along a 100-mm line labeled at its extremes as "No Pain" and "Worst Ever Pain." The Physician and Patient Global Assessment Scales (Visual Analog Scales) were completed by the patient and the investigator independently making a mark along a 100-mm line labeled at its extremes as "Not Improved" and "Much Improved." Safety variables included adverse events, clinical laboratory values, vital signs, and physical and neurologic examinations. Because this was an open-label, nonrandomized study, no inferential analyses were performed. Patients received between one and three doses of Neurobloc™, and each dosing session was considered to be a separate set of data. The 40 dosing sessions were categorized into one of four dose groups (100 to 899 U, 900 to 2,399 U, 2,400 to 5,999 U, and 6,000 to 12,000 U) in summary tables (Table 1). The primary measure of effectiveness was improvement from baseline to Week 4 in the TWSTRS-Severity Scale score by at least 25%. An enzyme-linked immunosorbent assay (ELISA) method was developed at Athena Neurosciences, Inc., South San Francisco, California, to assess any antibody production to Neurobloc™ during the course of the study.

TABLE 1. *Mean improvement baseline to Week 4 by TWSTRS scores by dose group*

| TWSTRS | Neurobloc™ dose group in units | | | |
	100–899	900–2,399	2,400–5,999	6,000–12,000
Severity	3.0	2.9	5.4	5.3
Disability	1.5	0.9	3.1	1.9
Pain	2.0	1.1	3.0	2.8
Total	6.5	4.9	11.5	10.0

Drug Supply and Injection Technique

Neurobloc™ was supplied by Athena Neurosciences, Inc., and stored in a refrigerator at 2° to 8°C. Neurobloc™ was injected into two to four involved muscles based on clinical assessment and head position under electromyographic (EMG) guidance. The total dose was divided among one to three injection sites in each of the two to four selected muscles. Injection volume was between 0.10 and 1.0 ml for each site. Injections were performed by a neurologist trained in the therapeutic use of botulinum toxin in patients with cervical dystonia (P.A.C., C.F.O., and D.D.T.).

RESULTS

Efficacy

Response to Treatment

Twenty-eight patients participated in the study from 28 to 177 days, with a mean time in the study of 71.9 days. Patients were treated with one to three doses of study medication, with eight patients (29%) receiving two or more doses. Patients who did not obtain significant clinical benefit (at least a 25% improvement in TWSTRS-Severity Scale) from the initial low doses were eligible for subsequent higher doses. Cumulative doses ranged from 1,430 to 12,000 U and individual doses ranged from 300 to 12,000 U of Neurobloc™. There were 40 total doses given to the 28 patients. Response to treatment, which was defined as a 25% improvement in TWSTRS-Severity Scale score, generally increased as dose increased. The percentage of patients who responded to treatment

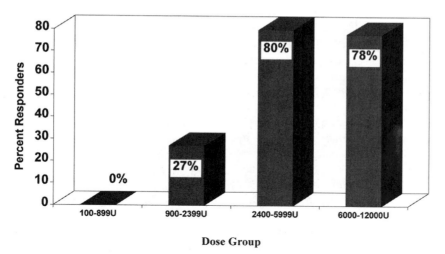

FIG. 1. Percent responders by dose group at Week 4.

was greater in the two higher dose groups than in the two lower dose groups (Fig. 1).

Improvement in TWSTRS Scores

Changes in the TWSTRS-Severity Scale score were greater and generally of longer duration for the higher doses of Neurobloc™ than for the lower doses. Table 1 shows the mean improvement in TWSTRS scores for each dose group. Improvement in TWSTRS scores occurred at all doses but was greatest at the higher doses. The mean percent improvement in the TWSTRS-Severity Scale scores from baseline to Week 4 was likewise greatest at the higher doses of Neurobloc™ (Fig. 2). The effectiveness of Neurobloc™ was supported by the TWSTRS-Disability Scale, -Pain Scale, and -Total Scale scores. Likewise, Patient and Investigator Global Assessment scores generally indicated greater effectiveness at higher doses.

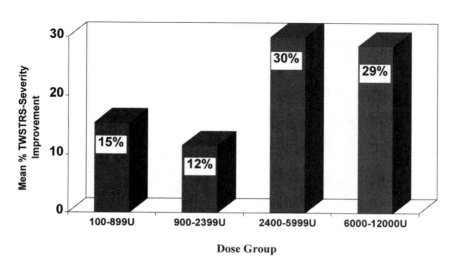

FIG. 2. Mean percent improvement in TWSTRS-severity scale scores at Week 4.

Safety

Neurobloc™ was safe and well tolerated. No patients experienced a serious adverse event or withdrew from the study because of an adverse event. Eleven patients (39%) experienced at least one adverse event that was considered by the investigator to be related to the study medication. Those adverse events experienced by more than one patient and considered related to treatment were neck pain (four patients; 14%), injection site pain (four patients; 14%), asthenia (two patients; 7%), and dysphagia (two patients; 7%). No dose-response relationship was apparent for adverse events in this study and no clinically significant abnormalities or trends in clinical laboratory evaluations were noted.

DISCUSSION

Neurobloc™ was safe and well tolerated at doses from 300 to 12,000 U. No dose-limiting side effects were identified. Adverse events that were considered related to treatment with Neurobloc™ were mild or moderate in intensity and generally resolved quickly. Adverse events did not appear to be related to dose. The effectiveness of Neurobloc™ was demonstrated by using the TWSTRS-Severity Scale score. Greater effectiveness occurred at higher doses of Neurobloc™ than at lower doses. No Neurobloc™ antibodies developed during the study. Although we did not formally study the duration of effect, it appeared similar, clinically, to that seen with commercially available preparations of botulinum toxin A. Our study clearly suggests that Neurobloc™ is safe and well tolerated and warrants double-blind, placebo-controlled trials to evaluate its potential efficacy in treating CD.

ACKNOWLEDGMENTS

We acknowledge the contributions of Pharmaceutical Research Associates, Inc., Charlottesville, Virginia, for their assistance with the management of this study and with the preparation of this paper. We also gratefully acknowledge the help of the following study coordinators: Jan Chrzan, Kerry Duncan, and Anna Graces.

This clinical research project was supported by grants from Athena Neurosciences, Inc., South San Francisco, California.

REFERENCES

1. Consky ES, Lang AE. Clinical assessment of patients with cervical dystonia. In: Jankovic J, Hallet M, eds. *Therapy with botulinum toxin.* New York: Marcel Dekker Inc, 1994:211–237.
2. Cullis PA. Spasmodic torticollis. In: Johnson RT, ed. *Current therapy in neurologic disease.* Vol. 2. Toronto: BC Decker, 1987:238–241.
3. Cullis PA, Walker P. The treatment of spasmodic torticollis. In: Quinn NP, Jenner PG, eds. *Disorders of movement.* London: Academic Press, 1989:295–301.
4. Jahn R, Niemann H. Molecular mechanisms of Clostridial neurotoxins. *Ann NY Acad Sci* 1994;733: 245–255.
5. Smith LDS. The occurrence of *Clostridium botulinum* and *Clostridium tetani* in the soil of the United States. *Health Lab Sci* 1978;15:74–80.
6. Tsui JKC, Eisen A, Calne D. Botulinum toxin in spasmodic torticollis. *Adv Neurol* 1988;50:593–597.
7. Tsui JKC, Haywood M, Mak EKM, Schulzer M. Botulinum toxin type B in the treatment of cervical dystonia: a pilot study. *Neurology* 1995;45:2109–2111.
8. Weber JT, Hatheway CL, St. Louis ME. Botulism. In: Hoeprich PD, Jordan MC, Ronald AR, eds. *Infectious diseases: a treatise of infectious processes.* 5th ed. Philadelphia: JB Lippincott, 1994;1185–1194

Dystonia 3: Advances in Neurology, Vol. 78,
edited by S. Fahn, C. D. Marsden, and M. DeLong.
Lippincott–Raven Publishers, Philadelphia © 1998.

24

Dose Standardization of Botulinum Toxin

*Peter Y. K. Van den Bergh and †Dominique F. Lison

*Service de Neurologie, Cliniques Universitaires St-Luc, Brussels, Belgium; and †Unité de
Toxicologie Industrielle et Médecine du Travail, Ecole de Santé Publique,
University of Louvain, Brussels, Belgium.*

Two preparations of botulinum toxin type A are commercially available, Dysport (Speywood Pharmaceuticals Ltd., Maidenhead, Berkshire SL64UH, UK) and Botox (Allergan, Inc., Irvine, CA, US). The biologic potency of the toxin preparations has traditionally been expressed in units, 1 unit (U) being defined as the median lethal intraperitoneal dose (LD_{50}) in mice (33). Interestingly, Dysport and Botox U are not equivalent. The difference in clinical potency becomes evident when comparing doses as used by various investigators to treat focal dystonia. It has been estimated empirically that 4 to 5 Dysport U are equivalent to 1 Botox U (9,27). Although one can question the appropriateness of the mouse lethality assay to determine the biologic potency of botulinum toxin for its use in a clinical setting, the assay is accepted as valid and useful (33). The unit disparity therefore appears paradoxical. It poses practical problems of dosage, especially in Europe, where Dysport and Botox are both available. Differences in mouse lethality assay methodology, as developed by Speywood Pharmaceuticals and Allergan may be responsible for this discrepancy. However, methodologic differences have been reported to lead to a Botox/Dysport potency ratio of approximately 2/1 (19,29), which is clearly smaller than the estimated clinical potency ratio of 4–5/1 (9,27). To try to understand the reason for this discordance, we compared the biologic potency of Botox and Dysport by using the mouse lethal-

ity assay and by determining the optimal doses to treat patients with focal movement disorders.

MATERIALS AND METHODS

Mouse Lethality Assays

Botox and Dysport were reconstituted in sterile, preservative-free, normal saline. Female, 25 g NMRI mice (Iffa Credo, Brussels, Belgium) were injected intraperitoneally with 200 µl of freshly prepared 0.25 to 8 U dilutions of the toxins and observed for 4 days. The death rate was determined for each dose and LD_{50} estimates were calculated by probit analysis (17). Dysport and Botox were tested in four and three independent experiments, respectively.

Patients

The optimal dose of Botox was determined in patients with hemifacial spasm ($n = 10$) and cervical dystonia ($n = 10$), who had been successfully treated with Dysport for 2 to 7 years. All patients were stable responders to Dysport with respect to improvement rate, dosage, and relapse intervals. Based on the proposed 1/4–5 dose equivalence for Botox/Dysport, the starting dose of Botox was set at one-fourth of the Dysport dose, which had been used to treat these patients. Optimal dosage was reached in two to three injection sessions within 1 month.

Treatment and assessment procedures were as described previously (37).

Statistical Analysis

To determine whether differences between results were significant, the data were subjected to the Student's unpaired *t* test.

RESULTS

Mouse Lethality Assays

LD_{50} values (mean $\pm$SD) of 2.57 $\pm$0.91 U and 0.90 $\pm$0.19 U were obtained for Dysport and Botox, respectively. The biologic potency of Botox appeared to be 2.86 times greater than that of Dysport ($p = 0.0068$).

Patients

To obtain improvement rates (mean $\pm$ SD) of 73.7 $\pm$ 21.3% with Dysport and 71.5 $\pm$ 18.5% with Botox ($p = 0.8$) for hemifacial spasm, a dose (mean $\pm$ SD) of 43.8 $\pm$ 12.7 U of Dysport and 18.8 $\pm$ 6.7 U of Botox was needed (p <0.001; potency ratio of 2.33). The duration of benefit was 3.95 $\pm$ 2.0 months with Dysport and 3.44 $\pm$ 2.14 months with Botox ($p > 0.5$). To obtain improvement rates (mean $\pm$ SD) of 72.8 $\pm$ 17.9% with Dysport and 65.7 $\pm$ 18.9% with Botox ($p = 0.4$) for cervical dystonia, a dose (mean $\pm$ SD) of 362.6 $\pm$ 130.2 U of Dysport and 145.5 $\pm$ 48.5 U of Botox was needed (p <0.001; potency ratio of 2.49). The duration of the benefit was 2.9 $\pm$ 0.7 months with Dysport and 2.6 $\pm$ 1.0 months with Botox ($p > 0.5$). None of the patients developed dysphagia after treatment with either Dysport or Botox.

DISCUSSION AND CONCLUSION

The unit disparity between the two commercially available botulinum toxin type A preparations, Dysport and Botox, is a matter of concern, because of the resulting confusion with regard to dose equivalence in patient treatment. Our mouse lethality assay results indicate that the biologic potency of Botox exceeds that of

Dysport by a factor of 2 to 3, which is in agreement with results from other investigators (19,29). Hambleton and Pickett (19) have suggested that the Botox mouse lethality assay method underestimates true toxin potency, because, unlike the Dysport method, it does not include gelatin buffer as a protein stabilizer. Other factors may play a role, however, because Pearce et al. (29), comparing toxin potencies by using the Botox mouse lethality assay with the inclusion of gelatin buffer, still found an approximately twofold difference between Dysport and Botox units. Although the reason for this difference remains unresolved, it seems clearly related to differences in mouse lethality assay methodology.

When comparing doses of Dysport and Botox, as used in various studies on the treatment of focal movement disorders, the clinical potency of Botox seems to exceed that of Dysport not by a factor of 2 to 3, which would be explained by the different mouse lethality assay methods, but by a factor of 4 to 5 (9,27). We have proposed two main reasons that might possibly explain this discordance (37). First, the chemical properties and biologic activities of the two toxin preparations are different. It is possible, therefore, that the motor endplate binding and tissue diffusion properties are dissimilar. Secondly, Dysport is typically diluted at 200 U/ml, Botox at 25 to 100 U/ml. This concentration factor may account for differences in diffusion and paralysis, hence clinical outcome. However, our present results, showing a 2–3/1 potency ratio for Botox/Dysport not only in the mouse lethality assay, but also in the clinical setting of patient treatment, disagree with the clinical potency ratio of 4–5/1, estimated by others (9,27).

We propose that this estimated clinical potency of 4–5/1 is related to a tendency to use higher than necessary Dysport doses. Comparison of treatment results of different investigators, although difficult and potentially misleading, because of differences in assessment procedures and injection techniques, are supportive of this proposal. To treat blepharospasm (Fig. 1), published mean Botox doses vary between 25 and 100 U, the dose range be-

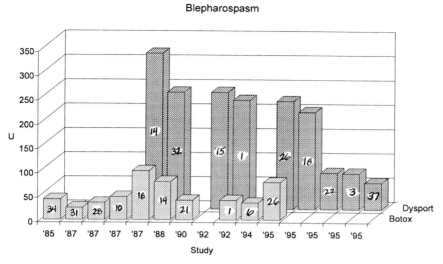

FIG. 1. Mean doses of Botox and Dysport in the treatment of blepharospasm. Numbers within columns refer to reference numbers.

ing similar in early and recent studies. In contrast, mean doses of Dysport have decreased from 200 to 320 U in earlier studies to 55 to 75 U in more recent studies. Because most investigators have used a mean Botox dose of 25 to 40 U, a Dysport/Botox dose equivalence of 2–3/1

appears to be a reasonable estimate. To treat cervical dystonia (Fig. 2), published mean Botox doses vary between 83 and 370 U, lower and higher doses being used both in early and recent studies. In contrast again, mean doses of Dysport have steadily decreased over time

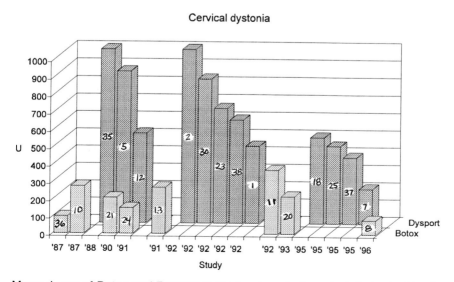

FIG. 2. Mean doses of Botox and Dysport in the treatment of cervical dystonia. Numbers within columns refer to reference numbers.

TABLE 1. *Incidence of botulinum toxin type A-related dysphagia in cervical dystonia*

Year	Ref.	Botox dose (U)[a]	Dysphagia (%)		Ref.	Dysport dose (U)[a]	Dysphagia (%)	
			Patients	Visits			Patients	Visits
1987	36	100	2	2				
1987	10	276	0	0				
1988					35	1,000	90	90
1990	21	209	23	13	5	875	52	28
1991	24	150	0	0	12	520	25	—
1991	13	269	24	11				
1992	11	370	31	31	2	1,000	74	44
1992					30	832	57	22
1992					38	600	—	32
1992					1	448	18	18
1995					37	385	7	2
1995					7	204	25	9
1996	8	83	2	2				
1996	*b	145	0	0	*b	362	0	0

[a]Mean doses.
[b]Present study.

from 1,000 U to as low as 204 U. Another indicator of dose appropriateness is the frequency of occurrence of botulinum toxin-related dysphagia in cervical dystonia, which is clearly dose-dependent (Table 1). With mean Botox doses of 83 to 150 U, dysphagia has been reported to occur in 0 to 2% of treatment sessions. With mean Dysport doses of 204 to 385 U, dysphagia complicated 0 to 9% of treatment sessions. These comparative data on cervical dystonia treatment are also suggestive of a Dysport/Botox dose equivalence of 2–3/1.

We conclude that the discrepancy between clinical dose equivalence and mouse lethality assay results may be more apparent than real and that the difference in potency between Botox and Dysport may be due only to different Allergan and Speywood Pharmaceuticals mouse lethality assay methods.

REFERENCES

1. Albanese A, Colosimo C, Caretta D, Dickmann A, Bentivoglio AR, Tonali P. Botulinum toxin as a treatment for blepharospasm, spasmodic torticollis and hemifacial spasm. *Eur Neurol* 1992;32:112–117.
2. Anderson TJ, Rivest J, Stell R, et al. Botulinum toxin treatment of spasmodic torticollis. *J R Soc Med* 1992;85:524–529.
3. Aramideh M, Ongerboer de Visser BW, Brans JWM, Koelman JHTM, Speelman JD. Pretarsal application of botulinum toxin for treatment of blepharospasm. *J Neurol Neurosurg Psychiatry* 1995;59:309–311.
4. Biglan AW, May M, Bowers RA. Management of facial spasm with *Clostridium botulinum* toxin, type A (Oculinum). *Arch Otolaryngol Head Neck Surg* 1988;114:1407–1412.
5. Blackie JD, Lees AJ. Botulinum toxin treatment in spasmodic torticollis. *J Neurol Neurosurg Psychiatry* 1990;53:640–643.
6. Borodic GE. Hemifacial spasm: evaluation and management, with emphasis on botulinum toxin therapy. In: Jankovic J, Hallett M, eds. *Therapy with botulinum toxin.* New York: Marcel Dekker, 1994:331–351.
7. Brans JWM, de Boer IP, Aramideh M, Ongerboer de Visser BW, Speelman JD. Botulinum toxin in cervical dystonia: low dosage with electromyographic guidance. *J Neurol* 1995;242:529–534.
8. Brans JWM, Lindeboom R, Aramideh M, Speelman JD. *Mov Disord* 1996;11[Suppl 1]:224.
9. Brin MF, Blitzer A. Botulinum toxin: dangerous terminology errors. *J R Soc Med* 1993;86:493–494.
10. Brin MF, Fahn S, Moskowitz C, et al. Localized injections of botulinum toxin for the treatment of focal dystonia and hemifacial spasm. *Mov Disord* 1987;2:237–254.
11. Comella CL, Buchman AS, Tanner CM, Brown-Toms MC, Goetz CG. Botulinum toxin injection for spasmodic torticollis: increased benefit with electromyographic assistance. *Neurology* 1992;42:878–882.
12. D'Costa, Abbott RJ. Low dose botulinum toxin in spasmodic torticollis. *J R Soc Med* 1991;84:650–651.
13. Dubinsky RM, Gray CS, Vetere-Overfield B, Koller WC. Electromyographic guidance of botulinum toxin treatment in cervical dystonia. *Clin Neuropharmacol* 1991;12:262–267.
14. Elston JS. Long-term results of treatment of idiopathic blepharospasm with botulinum toxin injections. *Br J Opthalmol* 1987;71:664–668.
15. Elston JS. Management of blepharospasm and hemifacial spasm. *J Neurol* 1992;239:5–8.

16. Engstrom PF, Arnoult JB, Mazow ML, et al. Effectiveness of botulinum toxin therapy for essential blepharospasm. *Opthalmology* 1987;94:971–975.

17. Finney DJ. *Probit analysis*. 3rd ed. Cambridge: Cambridge University Press, 1971.

18. Guevara CO, Sindern E, Malin JP. Experience with botulinum toxin therapy after 3 years. *Mov Disord* 1995;10:372.

19. Hambleton P, Pickett AM. Potency equivalence of botulinum toxin preparations. *J R Soc Med* 1994;87:719.

20. Jankovic J, Schwartz K. Longitudinal experience with botulinum toxin injections for treatment of blepharospasm and cervical dystonia. *Neurology* 1993; 43:834–836.

21. Jankovic J, Schwartz K, Donovan DT. Botulinum toxin treatment of cranial-cervical dystonia, spasmodic dysphonia, other focal dystonias and hemifacial spasm. *J Neurol Neurosurg Psychiatry* 1990;53:633–639.

22. Kloss TM. Two year follow up in 65 patients with dystonia and hemifacial spasm treated with botulinum toxin. *Mov Disord* 1995;10:383.

23. Lees AJ, Turjanski N, Rivest J, Whurr R, Lorch M, Brookes G. Treatment of cervical dystonia, hand spasms, and laryngeal dystonia with botulinum toxin. *J Neurol* 1992;239:1–4.

24. Lorentz IT, Subramaniam SS, Yiannikas C. Treatment of idiopathic spasmodic torticollis with botulinum toxin A: a double-blind study on twenty-three patients. *Mov Disord* 1991;6:145–150.

25. Maciejek C, Niezgodzinska-Maciejek A. The clinical usefulness of Dysport in patients with spasmodic torticollis and writer's cramp. *Mov Disord* 1995;10:373.

26. Marion MH, Sheehy M, Sangla S, Soulayrol S. Dose standardisation of botulinum toxin. *J R Soc Med* 1995;59:102–103.

27. Marsden CD. Author's reply. *J R Soc Med* 1993;86:494.

28. Mauriello JA, Coniaris H, Haupt EJ. Use of botulinum toxin in the treatment of one hundred patients with facial dyskinesias. *Ophthalmology* 1987;94: 976–979.

29. Pearce LB, Borodic GE, First ER, McCallum RD. Measurement of botulinum toxin activity: evaluation of the lethality assay. *Toxicol Appl Pharmacol* 1994; 128:69–77.

30. Poewe W, Schelosky L, Kleedorfer B, Heinen F, Wagner M, Deuschl G. Treatment of spasmodic torticollis with local injections of botulinum toxin. *J Neurol* 1992;239:21–25.

31. Ruusuvaara P, Setälä K. Long-term treatment of involuntary facial spasms using botulinum toxin. *Acta Ophthalmologica* 1990;68:331–338.

32. Saraux H. Traitement des blépharospasmes et des hémispasmes faciaux par injection de toxine botulique. *J Fr Ophthalmol* 1988;11:237–240.

33. Schantz EJ, Kautter DA. Standardized assay for *Clostridium botulinum* toxins. *J Assoc Off Anal Chem* 1978;61:96–99.

34. Scott AB, Kennedy RA, Stubbs HA: Botulinum A toxin injection as a treatment for blepharospasm. *Arch Ophthalmol* 1985;103:347–350.

35. Stell R, Thompson PD, Marsden CD. Botulinum toxin in spasmodic torticollis. *J Neurol Neurosurg Psychiatry* 1988;51:920–923.

36. Tsui JK, Fross RD, Calne S, Calne DB. Local treatment of spasmodic torticollis with botulinum toxin. *Can J Neurol Sci* 1987;14:533–535.

37. Van den Bergh P, Francart J, Mourin S, Kollmann P, Laterre EC. Five-year experience in the treatment of focal movement disorders with low-dose Dysport™ botulinum toxin. *Muscle Nerve* 1995;18:720–729.

38. Wissel J, Poewe W. Dystonia—a clinical, neuropathological and therapeutic review. *J Neural Transm Suppl* 1992;38:91–104.

Dystonia 3: Advances in Neurology, Vol. 78,
edited by S. Fahn, C. D. Marsden, and M. DeLong.
Lippincott–Raven Publishers, Philadelphia © 1998.

25

Laryngeal Dystonia (Spasmodic Dysphonia): Observations of 901 Patients and Treatment with Botulinum Toxin

*Mitchell F. Brin, †Andrew Blitzer, and *‡Celia Stewart

Department of Neurology, Mount Sinai Medical Center, New York, New York 10029; †Head and Neck Surgical Associates, The Roosevelt Hospital, New York, New York 10016; and ‡Department of Speech-Language Pathology and Audiology, New York University, New York, New York 10003.

Idiopathic spasmodic dysphonia (SD) and laryngeal dystonia are clinical terms used to describe an action-induced laryngeal movement disorder (29). In 1871, Traube (79) coined the term "spastic dysphonia" when describing a patient with nervous hoarseness. The affliction has been described as though the patient were "trying to talk wilst being choked," (36) or "stuttering with the vocal cords" (8). Although Aronson (3,4) documented that Minnesota Multiphasic Personality Inventory (MMPI) and psychiatric interviews did not discriminate between patients with SD and those in the normal population, many patients are still referred to psychiatrists for treatment because the correct diagnosis is not made when the patient initially presents for treatment.

Several lines of evidence have supported the notion that SD is a form of dystonia. Fraenkel (42,43) and Gowers (48) compared the involuntary movements in SD to those of other dystonias. However, in the earlier works, a psychogenic etiology was proposed (19). Nevertheless, SD had been compared to other focal dystonias such as occupational writer's cramp (42,43) and oromandibular dystonia (46). Jacome and Yanez (51) associated SD with Meige disease, or segmental-cranial dystonia; other authors subsequently have concurred (12,47,

67). In 1982, Marsden and Sheehy (67) stated that "all evidence points to the conclusion that blepharospasm and oromandibular dystonia seen in Meige disease is another manifestation of adult-onset torsion dystonia, [and] since dysphonia may occur in the same syndrome, it is quite likely that dysphonia itself may be the sole manifestation of dystonia." We also noted that many of the phenomenologic, clinical, and laboratory features of patients with focal "spastic dysphonia" were similar to the dysphonia found in many patients with focal, segmental, and more generalized disease (12). Both the clinical examination and electromyographic (EMG) (18) characteristics led us to the conclusion that most cases of dysphonia clinically diagnosed as "spastic dysphonia" are focal forms of cranial dystonia. Because of these observations, we have recommended the terminology "spasmodic dysphonia" or "laryngeal dystonia" rather than "spastic dysphonia," particularly in view of the absence of classic spastic signs in those affected with the disorder.

Long-term treatment of SD was unrewarding until we initiated the program of local injections of botulinum toxin type A (BTX-A, BTX). As a result of our BTX treatment program, heretofore unrecognized and undiagnosed patients came for treatment. We now review some of the clinical and treatment findings in our population of patients with laryngeal dystonia.

METHODS

Patient Sample

Patients are ascertained by referral to one of the authors. Patients with dystonia, including those with laryngeal dystonia, come to our centers primarily to obtain treatment or participate in research studies. Patients who were ascertained specifically for genetic research are not reported, unless they underwent a patient-care evaluation and/or treatment. For this analysis, we have included only patients that have been evaluated and treated by the authors.

Diagnostic Evaluations

Detailed neurologic evaluations are performed on all patients with suspected dystonia. This includes a comprehensive neurologic examination, including examining the patient performing postures and tasks that may bring out the signs of dystonia (38). In order to confirm the diagnosis of the laryngeal movement disorder, patients also undergo a detailed otolaryngologic and speech-language assessment. Videotapes (38) and voice recordings are performed before treatment; fiberoptic laryngoscopy is performed to evaluate for any anatomic abnormalities and to confirm abnormal vocal cord motion with talking and other gestures. Phonatory characteristics are documented using the Unified Spasmodic Dysphonia Rating Scale (78).

Although computed tomography (CT) and magnetic resonance imaging (MRI) examinations had been requested for many patients in the past, subsequent to 1990, most patients did not undergo neuroimaging unless the physical or diagnostic examination suggested a symptomatic etiology, or there were extenuating circumstances. For most cases, routine screening blood studies including chemistries, blood count, ceruloplasmin, antinuclear antibodies,

thyroid function, and erythrocyte sedimentation rate were performed.

Patients with a diagnosis of dystonia are classified according to primary and secondary diagnosis. The primary diagnosis represents the most likely etiologic diagnosis, after a consensus discussion among the examiners. For a patient to have primary dystonia, there should not be any evidence by history, examination, or laboratory studies of any secondary cause for the dystonic symptoms, with the exception of precipitation by trauma (52). Therefore, there must be a normal perinatal and early developmental history, no prior history of neurologic illness, or exposure to drugs known to cause acquired dystonia (e.g., phenothiazines). There must also be normal intellectual, pyramidal, cerebellar and sensory examinations, and diagnostic studies (34,66). Patients who have abnormalities noted above are classified as having symptomatic or secondary dystonia.

Within the category of primary dystonia includes that group of patients with known genetic etiologies, whereby the fundamental clinical features are dystonia. This includes patients with disease linked to chromosomes 8, 9, and X.

The secondary diagnosis represents the next most likely diagnosis, if an alternate diagnosis is entertained. In the case of dystonia whereby symptoms are deemed to be triggered by a physical trauma (including a throat infection), a flag is set in the database.

Two distinct types of SD have been proposed (3): *adductor:* due to irregular hyperadduction of the vocal folds; and *abductor:* due to intermittent abduction of the vocal folds. Some patients appear to have a combination of the two. Patients with *add*uctor SD exhibit a choked, strained-strangled voice quality with abrupt initiation and termination of voicing resulting in short breaks in phonation. Patients with *abd*uctor SD exhibit a breathy, effortful voice quality with abrupt termination of voicing resulting in aphonic whispered segments of speech. The assignment of "adductor" versus "abductor" is based on the phonatory examination and direct visualization of the vocal folds during speech and phonatory tasks.

Database Storage and Statistical Management

Research clinical and treatment information is stored in a FoxPro relational database management system on a Novell network. Patient demographic information is entered into the Master module; visit clinical information is entered as a single record. Recurring records are added to the BTX therapeutic module for each treatment and follow-up visit. This module captures muscles injected, dose, dilution, adverse effects of therapy, duration of benefit, and a global rating of the pre- and postinjection functional status (24). Although the authors are currently at separate institutions in New York, we continue to store treatment information on a centralized server. Patient data were imported into SPSS Version 7 for the current analysis and graphic development.

Botulinum Toxin Treatment Strategies

Adductor Spasmodic Dysphonia

At the time of the first injections in 1984, no one had ever injected the vocalis muscle complex with BTX (11,13,31,33). We had already investigated patients with percutaneous EMG of the vocalis muscles (18), and this technique was applied to the vocalis muscles. We established the method of laryngeal injections utilizing a monopolar Teflon-coated EMG needle with an exposed tip (Fig. 1). The needle is placed into the thyroarytenoid (TA) vocalis complex by impaling the muscle through the cricothyroid membrane, using a previously described technique (18) (Fig. 2). The muscle is identified by the interference pattern on the EMG; phonation augments the response. Once the muscle is identified, the syringe barrel is withdrawn slightly to ensure that the needle tip is not within a vessel, and then the toxin is gently injected.

The patient is asked to try not to cough or swallow when the needle is in the airway or the TA muscle. An unusual patient has an uncontrollable cough and gag reflex. In this situation, 0.3 ml of 1% xylocaine without epinephrine is injected into the airway through the cricothy-

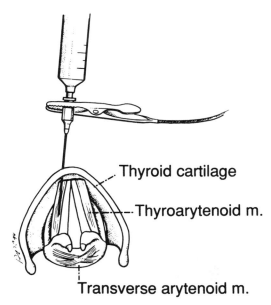

FIG. 1. The Teflon-coated EMG needle is placed through the cricothyroid membrane into the thyroartenoid muscle. BTX is injected through the needle into the target muscle.

roid membrane, and the patient is instructed to cough the solution to aerosolize it to coat the laryngeal musculature. This technique, however, may interfere slightly with the EMG interference pattern. In many cases, local anesthetic is not required after the first or second injection procedure.

In addition to generally accepted precautions (1), it is not recommended that patients be injected into the vocal cords just prior to surgery requiring (or at risk for) general anesthesia. The vocalis muscles are important in protecting the airway, and any weakness afforded by injection of BTX may leave the airway relatively vulnerable postoperatively.

Xylocaine injections into the recurrent laryngeal nerve are not performed before therapy with BTX; experience has demonstrated that failure to respond to xylocaine injections does not predict response to therapy with BTX.

Because of concern regarding potential complications, our first patient was injected as a hospital inpatient with intensive care monitoring; this proved unnecessary, and unless other-

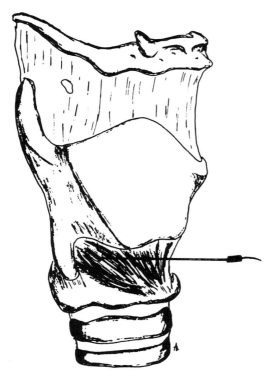

FIG. 2. Lateral view of an EMG needle placed through the cricothyroid membrane.

wise hospitalized, all patients are injected in the outpatient department. The calculation of the dose to be injected evolved as we gained experience with injecting this small muscle. Aiming to minimize the total dose of injected toxin, we initially embarked on a first-treatment program of injecting TA muscles with small doses of 3.75 U/0.1 ml; there was a substantial benefit (14). Side effects included breathy hypophonia and clinically insignificant aspiration. Both were transient, and most patients were free of side effects within the first 2 weeks. Nevertheless, we encountered some patients with prolonged severe breathy hypophonia lasting up to a few weeks. Therefore, we began to treat patients with lower doses of 1.0 to 1.25 units BTX/vocal cord (total dose 2.0 to 2.5 Units/session, Fig. 3) typically compromising duration of benefit. At these lower doses, we rarely have treatment failures.

Follow-up therapy is carefully individualized for each patient. Patients develop a "portfolio" as their response to therapy is carefully charted. If the first treatment was satisfactory, then the same dose is administered at follow-up. However, if there was excessive breathy hypophonia or aspiration, then the dose is reduced. Doses as low as 0.10 U/0.1 ml have

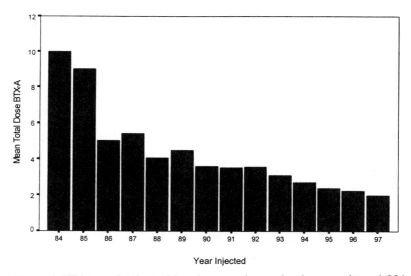

FIG. 3. Total dose of BTX type A injected into laryngeal muscles by year ($N = 4,621$ treatment sessions).

been injected into each TA muscle. In some cases, lower doses are associated with fewer adverse effects, but also an unacceptable shortened duration of benefit. Therefore, some patients are injected with low doses, but more frequently. In other cases, 1.25 to 2.5 U (in 0.1 ml) are administered into one TA, and on follow-up, the opposite TA is injected. This approach is successful in select patients, because on follow-up, they have residual weakness of the opposing TA complex. In all cases, the patient is counseled that different strategies may be required to identify the best individualized chronic treatment program.

Abductor Spasmodic Dysphonia

We have reported our technique in treating abductor SD with BTX (16,28). We were initially reluctant to initiate treating the posterior cricoarytenoid muscle (PCA) with BTX because of our concern that the airway may be compromised. Nevertheless, a severely disabled patient, experiencing employment difficulties, urged initiation of therapy. We initially attempted impaling the PCA per-orally; this was technically difficult and there was no benefit. Therefore, a percutaneous approach was adopted. Our initial two patients were treated in the hospital; all subsequent patients have been treated in the outpatient setting.

In most cases, we initiate therapy by weakening one PCA muscle with 3.75 U in 0.15 ml. In approximately 25% of patients, weakening or paralyzing just one PCA allowed for significant voice improvement. The other patients may have little or no benefit, despite production of an abductor paresis or paralysis with a unilaterally medialized vocal cord. These patients need additional toxin injections and treatment is performed no sooner than 2 weeks subsequent to the first injection. For those who still have abduction on the initial side, an additional 2.5 to 3.75 U is given to paralyze that PCA. If the PCA is already paralyzed, and the voice is not improved, conservative serial doses of 0.675 to 2.5 U in 0.1 ml are given into the contralateral PCA. No further injections are given if there has been stridor, or if the glottic

chink has been significantly narrowed. When both of the patient's PCA muscles have been treated and are weakened, and there is narrowing of the glottic chink and/or patients have significant tremor, 2.5 U of BTX in 0.1 ml are injected into the cricothyroid muscle.

RESULTS

Demographics

Between July 1983 and August 1996, 1,448 patients with dystonia were evaluated. Patient ascertainment is shown in Fig. 4. Demographic and select laboratory information on these patients is presented in Tables 1 and 2.

The interval between onset of symptoms of dystonia, as reported by the patient, and diagnosis by one of the authors declined for all cases of dystonia evaluated, including cases of laryngeal dystonia (Table 3, Fig. 5). These observations mirror increased awareness of dystonia, which was popularized, in part, by the presence of effective treatment with botulinum toxin.

The primary and secondary etiologies are outlined in Table 4.

We have identified eight patients with paradoxical motion of the vocal cords on inspiration resulting in a narrowed obstructed airway and stridor (25,30,49,58,64). These patients (six idiopathic; one tardive, one anoxic/toxic) had inappropriate adduction of the vocal cords

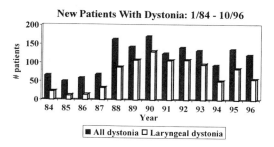

FIG. 4. Patient ascertainment. Note that new patient visits increased with more routine availability of BTX therapy in the mid-1980s.

TABLE 1. *Laryngeal dystonia*

	All dystonia		Laryngeal dystonia			
	Primary dystonia	Secondary dystonia	Primary dystonia	Secondary dystonia	Primary, laryngeal onset	Primary, laryngeal focal
	N = 1448		*N* = 901			
N	1,129	319	744	157	606	492
Age onset (±SD)	39.3 ± 17.0	37.0 ± 20.5	39.0 ± 16.2	40.1 ± 20.9	40.3 ± 15.0	40.6 ± 14.3
F	717 (63.5)	215 (67.4)	471 (63.3)	109 (69.4)	388 (64.0)	313 (63.3)
Jewish	360 (27.8)	74 (23.2)	152 (20.4)	33 (21.0)	116 (19.1)	86 (17.5)
+ Fam Hx (%)	174 (15.4)	24 (7.5)	90 (12.1)	14 (8.9)	64 (10.6)	48 (9.8)
Trauma (%)	156 (13.8)		119 (16.0)		95 (15.7)	82 (16.7)
Focal (%)	740 (65.5)	132 (41.4)	492 (66.1)	83 (52.9)	504 (83.2)	492 (100)
Seg Cran (%)	201 (17.8)	51 (16.0)	161 (21.6)	32 (20.4)	74 (12.2)	
All Seg (%)	107 (9.5)	60 (18.8)	51 (6.9)	17 (10.8)	21 (3.5)	
Gnlized (%)	81 (7.2)	76 (23.8)	40 (5.4)	25 (15.9)	7 (1.2)	
% Adductor			82.9	72.4	81.9	82.6

Non-Jew, non Jewish; + Fam Hx, positive family history of dystonia; Seg Cran, segmental cranial; All Seg, all segmentals and hemidystonia; Gnlized, generalized.

TABLE 2. *Laryngeal dystonia: antinuclear antibodies (N = 181)*

	Total	ANA negative	ANA = 1:40	ANA > 1:40
All patients	181	145	11	25
Female	123	96	8	19
Familial1	14	9	2	3

TABLE 3. *Interval between onset of symptoms and diagnosis by one of the authors, January 1983–October 1996[a]*

Dystonia	Number of cases	Year of diagnosis	Interval between symptom onset and diagnosis (yr ± SEM)
All cases of dystonia	9	1983	17.6 ± 7.0
	161	1989	11.0 ± 0.9
	63	1996	8.8 ± 1.5
	1321	1983–1996	9.9 ± 0.3
Dystonia with larynx involved	2	1983	30 ± 18.0
	118	1989	11.5 ± 1.1
	27	1996	8.1 ± 2.2
	835	1983–1996	10.2 ± 0.4
Dystonia with larynx onset	1[b]	1984	21
	102	1989	10.9 ± 1.2
	10	1996	7.4 ± 2.1
	673	1984–1996	9.4 ± 0.4

[a]We are reporting only those cases in whom an age at onset is known with clinical certainty.
[b]No cases of laryngeal-onset dystonia diagnosed in 1983; only one case diagnosed in 1984.

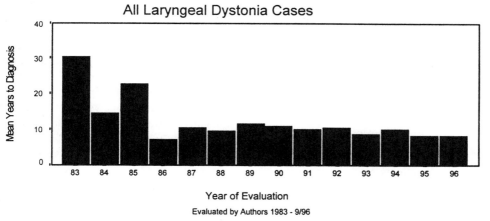

FIG. 5. The interval to diagnosis of dystonia declined during the mid-1980s. This decline corresponded with the increased awareness of the condition, associated with the availability of therapy.

during quiet respiration resulting in stridor. Symptoms frequently improved with speaking. The average age at onset of the idiopathic cases was 48.5 years (range 27 to 64); the tardive began at 61 years and the anoxic/toxic case began at 22 years. Three (one idiopathic, each of the secondary cases) had laryngeal onset of their dystonia; four had blepharospasm at onset; one began in the left arm.

Respiratory obstruction was mild to severe; gas exchange was impaired in one and one had required tracheostomy. Diaphragmatic syner-

gism was evaluated by video cinefluoroscopy and respiratory inductance plethysmography. Patients had a primary respiratory dysrhythmia with inappropriate, dysynergistic, fragmented, diaphragmatic contractions and inappropriate inspiratory (apneustic?) pauses. Spouses complained bitterly of disruption of sleep; sleep studies were abnormal, but respirations dramatically normalized with relief of obstruction in deep sleep stages. Patients complained of daytime excess fatigability interfering with normal work performance. Four were offered

TABLE 4. *Primary clinical etiology of dystonia*

| | All dystonia (%) | Laryngeal dystonia | | |
		All laryngeals (%)	Laryngeal onset (%)	Laryngeal focal (%)
N	1,398	872	694	566
Primary dystonia	1,078 (77.1)	709 (81.3)	584 (84.1)	480 (84.8)
Secondary factors				
Peripheral trauma	160	109	93	81
Essential tremor	214	124	94	66
Perinatal injury	15 (1.1)	6 (0.7)	0	0
Head injury	17 (1.2)	6 (0.7)	1 (0.1)	1 (0.2)
Encephalitis	3 (0.2)	1 (0.1)	0	0
Stroke	10 (0.7)	1 (0.1)	1 (0.1)	1 (0.2)
Tardive	48 (3.4)	24 (2.8)	12 (1.7)	7 (1.2)
Psychogenic	18 (1.3)	2 (0.2)	1 (0.1)	1 (0.2)
Brain tumor	1 (0.1)	0	0	0
Metabolic	2 (0.1)	1 (0.1)	0	0
Essential tremor	38 (2.7)	37 (4.2)	31	27 (4.8)
Symptomatic, other known diagnosis	52 (3.7)	35 (4.0)	31 (4.3)	29 (5.1)
Symptomatic, unknown diagnosis	116 (8.3)	50 (5.7)	24 (3.5)	19 (3.4)

vocalis muscle injections of BTX with an outstanding relief of laryngeal symptoms; however, the respiratory dysrhythmia continued.

Genetics

A family history of neurologic disease was explored in all patients with dystonia (Table 5). In some cases, the history was obvious, and in others, family studies and/or interviews by a genetic counselor elucidated the family history. One patient with abductor SD was the index case for one of our Amish/Mennonite families reported with disease associated with chromosome 8 (2). Familial cases are observed among Jewish and non-Jewish patients with disease associated with abnormalities on chromosome 9 (23,70), and African-Americans (personal observations).

TABLE 5. *Familial laryngeal dystonia (N = 90 patients)*

Onset	Age onset familial (*N*)	Age onset nonfamilial (*N*)
Larynx	36.4 ± 14 (64)	41.1 ± 15 (463)[a]
Other	21.1 ± 15 (26)	35.2 ± 20 (93)[a]
All cases	31.9 ± 16 (90)	40.0 ± 16 (556)[a]

[a]*p* < 0.05 compared to familials.

Often the family history is negative, only to be established by examinations of family members that may reveal family members with dystonia. For example, one young patient reported a negative family history. However, at the end of the consultation when her father was writing some notes, we identified his severe writer's cramp, which he had been taking for granted. The data we present likely represent a minimum estimate for familial disease in this population.

From a sample of 744 patients with primary dystonia and laryngeal involvement, 90 had a family history of dystonia (Table 5). Of these, 64 had onset in the larynx and 26 had onset in other body regions. The age at onset of those patients with laryngeal onset was later than those with onset in other body regions. In both groups, the age of onset of the genetic cases was statistically earlier than those without a family history.

Antinuclear Antibodies

There are sporadic reports of immunologic abnormalities in patients with cranial dystonia. We systematically performed antinuclear antibodies (ANA) evaluations on 181 consecutive

TABLE 6. *Botulinum toxin treatment*

Laryngeal spasms	N	Number of visits	Dose injected per session, Units ± SD (range)	Onset of effect, days ± SD	Peak effect, days ± SD	Duration benefit, wk ± SD	Initial PNF ± SD	Final PNF ± SD	Final–initial PNF ± SD
Adductor	639	4,621	3.096 ± 3.1 (0.005–30)	2.4 ± 4.3	9.0 ± 12.7	15.1 ± 12.3	52.4 ± 22.0	89.71 ± 13.0	37.33 ± 20.7[a]
Abductor	108	840	2.163 ± 1.07 (0.5–6.25)	4.1 ± 5.5	10.0 ± 12.5	10.5 ± 12.2	54.8 ± 21.9	66.7 ± 23.4	16.3 ± 11.7[a]

At the time of treatment, patients are instructed on completing the rating scales, and they are provided a worksheet to complete at home. They record the onset and duration of the toxin's effect. In addition, they track their "Percent of Normal Function" (PNF). This is a global visual scale where 100% is a normal voice, and 0% is an inability to phonate.

[a] $p < 0.05$.

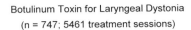

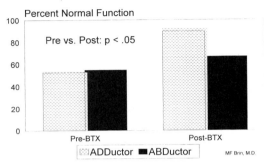

FIG. 6. BTX significantly improves function in patients with laryngeal dystonia. See text and Table 6 for details.

primary laryngeal patients, and report the data in Table 2. The significance of these findings is not known. Among the 181 patients with laryngeal dystonia, 25 (13.8%) had ANA elevations greater than 1:40. Among the 123 women with laryngeal dystonia, 19 (15.4%) had ANA elevations.

Therapy with Botulinum Toxin

The results of therapy with BTX are found in Table 6 and Figure 6. At the time of treatment, patients are instructed on completing the rating scales, and they are provided a worksheet to complete at home. They record the onset and duration of the toxin's effect. In addition, they track their "Percent of Normal Function" (PNF). This is a global visual analog scale where 100% is a normal voice, and 0% is an in-

ability to phonate. When they return for a follow-up evaluation, patients return the rating scale forms and also provide information on adverse events (Table 7).

DISCUSSION

This report represents the largest series of personally examined and treated patients with laryngeal dystonia. Our demographic data are likely skewed due to ascertainment biased by the availability of effective treatment with BTX. Subsequent to more routine availability of BTX in the mid-1980s, patient accrual increased (Fig. 4) and interval to diagnosis decreased (Fig. 5).

The most common etiology of laryngeal dystonia, in our series, was primary disease. It is remarkable that there were very few cases of psychogenic laryngeal dystonia, as compared to the larger group of patients with dystonia. It is possible that psychogenic laryngeal involvement is treated in the community by speech-language pathologists prior to referral to a tertiary care center. Alternatively, although we use accepted criteria for establishing a psychogenic etiology (40), we may be underdiagnosing patients with psychogenic etiologies. When evaluating patients with a suspected psychogenic etiology, we will often perform a videoscopic swallowing assessment whereby we utilize a thoreus filter to better define laryngeal movement. We have often observed unusual laryngeal or diaphragmatic movements (21) suggesting an organic cause.

Tardive dystonia is diagnosed when dystonic symptoms occur within 6 months of exposure

TABLE 7. *Common adverse events after treatment with botulinum toxin*

Laryngeal spasms	Patient symptom	Number of observations (% of all treatment sessions)	Average severity ± SD	Average duration (wk ± SD)	Median duration (wk)	Range of duration (wk)
Adductor	Breathiness	2,200 (47.6)	2.0 ± 0.8	3.2 ± 2.8	2.5	0.1–45
	Aspiration	274 (5.9)	1.6 ± 0.7	2.2 ± 2.1	2.0	0.1–13
	Dysphagia	688 (14.9)	1.5 ± 0.7	2.2 ± 2.1	2.0	0.1–21
Abductor	Stridor	58 (6.9)	1.6 ± 0.7	3.1 ± 2.9	2.0	0.1–12
	Dysphagia	94 (11.2)	1.48 ± 0.7	2.2 ± 2.7	1.3	0.1–16

to a neuroleptic (35,54). Although tardive dystonia is represented in our series, the percent of cases with laryngeal involvement is less than that seen in the larger series of dystonia. It is our impression that tardive laryngeal dystonia is generally underdiagnosed in the community population. A specific phenotype is seen in tardive patients with more generalized symptoms: striking axial involvement with arching, abduction of the arms, and posterior displacement of the shoulders with an abundance of midline cranial involvement. Often when consulting on a psychiatric ward, we will see additional patients with laryngeal disease. These patients, in general, are not referred for treatment, and therefore are not equivalently represented in our sample.

Dystonia may be precipitated by peripheral trauma (31,52,65). We accept a traumatic contribution if there is an anatomic relationship between the site of trauma and site of dystonia onset, the interval between the injury and onset or aggravation of dystonia is within 12 months, and typically if there is an interval of pain. Most often, the patient experiences pain at the site of the injury, and as that pain resolves, dystonic symptoms become increasingly apparent, as if the resolution of pain transitions into dystonic signs. Of the larger group of dystonia patients, 14.8% have peripheral trauma as an inciting cause; similar percentages are observed among the laryngeal group. The physical trauma is typically blunt trauma, and not surgical. In the larynx, the most common type of injury is a symptomatic viral sore throat, which must be differentiated from the hoarseness that is often experienced at the onset of SD. However, we have observed patients develop SD after intubation, and subsequent to direct physical trauma to the larynx or neck.

Patients often report the onset of SD after an emotionally traumatic or stressful event. Although stress may aggravate dystonic symptoms, there are no data available to support the notion that stress can trigger dystonia. The report of a prior stressful event may represent recall bias. Nevertheless, some case histories are striking. Stress may alter the immune system (20,39,50,77) and therefore potentially modify

a person's susceptibility to infection (56); a viral sore throat appears to be the most common peripheral injury precipitating laryngeal dystonia.

The establishment of a clinical diagnosis of adductor or abductor spasms may be useful for planning treatment; there is no evidence that the fundamental pathophysiology causing dystonic spasms is different between the two groups. Most patients have predominant adductor or abductor spasms. However, some patients are mixed, and many have a vocal tremor (27).

Because many patients with SD present with a tremulous voice, the differential diagnosis between spasmodic vocal breaks due to essential tremor and those due to a dystonic tremor can be difficult; this topic has been reviewed elsewhere (27). In general, dystonic tremors are irregular and have a directional preponderance; symptoms are increased when the patient postures the affected body part in a position opposed to the primary dystonic contractions. For instance, patients with torticollis often have a head tremor that can be damped by placing the head into the preferred posture. Many patients with SD have an irregular vocal tremor that can be recorded both acoustically, electromyographically (18), and with accelerometry.

Patients with dystonic larynges presenting with the phonatory characteristics of SD may have vocal tremor (30,71,73). Acoustic evaluation and tremor physiology evaluation may be useful in establishing the diagnosis. The clinical distinction between primary dystonia causing symptoms of tremor, and the disease entity of essential tremor, may be difficult in many cases, particularly when a patient presents with symptoms of essential tremor in other body parts (55,59). Discriminating between tremulousness due to essential tremor (ET) or dystonia is particularly difficult when studying voice because (a) the laryngeal muscles of phonation, as a whole, are never available for study at complete rest: one or more muscles is contracting at a given moment; and (b) dystonic laryngeal muscles cannot twist or turn: the glottic muscles can only adduct or abduct in some inappropriate fashion, which may include the speed and rhythmicity of tremor, or myoclonus.

Patients with vocal ET can have breaks and hesitations in their speech pattern, likely due to either hyperadduction or hyperabduction of the vocal folds during contextual speech and/or phonatory tasks. Additional contribution to the choppy speech pattern may come from lingual tremor whereby the tongue beats up against the posterior pharyngeal wall and interrupts air flow. These patients present with the phenomenology of spasmodic dysphonia. In the clinic, we have found that asking the patient to speak or perform tasks with a whisper is often useful because of less muscle activation, and a subtle tremor may become discernible.

One could argue that if tremor characteristic of ET were present in other body parts, then the laryngeal movement disorder should be essential tremor, and not SD due to dystonia. This is not always the case, as limb tremor that has the clinical characteristics of ET is not uncommonly identified in patients with dystonia (55,60). It is likely that some patients with isolated phonatory tremor with strain strangle speech are initially misdiagnosed and sometimes later correctly categorized (7). A greater understanding of the pathophysiology of tremor, coupled with genetic studies may be required to make the absolute distinction.

Many patients with laryngeal dystonia have a family history of dystonia. Our data demonstrate that 12.1% (90/744) of the primary patients with laryngeal involvement have a positive family history. Familial cases had an earlier age at onset than the nonfamilial cases. Laryngeal involvement has been described for each chromosomal loci mapped for dystonia, including chromosome 9 (22), 8 (2), and 18 (57). It is noteworthy that the second Amish family reported by Almasy came to our attention for treatment of laryngeal dystonia.

The significance of the ANA abnormalities in this population is unknown. Cervical dystonia has been associated with thyroid abnormalities, suggesting an autoimmune contribution. We did not systematically assess the frequency of thyroid abnormalities in our patient population.

Physical methods and speech therapy temporize symptoms in some patients, but significantly help few. By the time patients presented to our center, most had failed speech therapy. In our treatment program, systemic pharmacotherapy provided little symptomatic relief. Dedo (37) described dramatic relief of symptoms by sectioning the recurrent laryngeal nerve. The initial favorable reports were temporized by Aronson's review of 33 patients (5,6) treated with surgery. By 3 years, only 36% of patients had some persistent improvement and only 1 of 33 achieved a persistent normal voice. Adverse effects included breathiness, hoarseness, diplophonia, and falsetto. Of the 64% with failed voices at 3 years, 48% were worse than before surgery. Failures were more common among women (77%) than men (36%).

We established the treatment approach with local injections of BTX (11,32), which have emerged as the most effective therapy for most patients with SD. Patients with adductor symptoms report a normal or nearly normal voice during therapy; abductor patients experience benefit, but less robust.

The Baylor and NIH Centers have injected higher doses (15 to 30 U BTX) into one vocalis complex in order to effect a unilateral paralysis (63,68) or weakness in adductor SD. All centers agree that regardless of technique, there is a dramatic improvement in symptoms (9,26, 44,53,63) in nonsurgical patients with an 80% to 100% improvement in speech function during therapy. Adverse experiences in both groups include transient breathy hypophonia or hoarseness (up to 50% of patients)[1] and clinically insignificant aspiration of fluids (up to 25% of patients). Less common complications include hyperventilation in fewer than 2% of patients, and in fewer than 1% each: brief coughing slight blood-tinged sputum, a viral-feeling sore throat, pruritus without a rash, and diplophonia. In over 1,000 cases of SD treated in this country, there have been no reported

---

[1]In New York, "breathiness" is probably overrated as *any* evidence of a hypophonic voice. This may explain why we have reported a higher percentage of patients with breathiness than in other series. Breathy aphonia is rare.

cases of documented pneumonia, although bronchitis rarely occurs.

Ford et al. (41) reported an indirect laryngoscopic approach for injecting the toxin into the vocal fold. They report that the technique has the advantage of being "familiar to the otolaryngologist and requires no special EMG equipment or training." The onset of response to toxin appears delayed (mean 9.1 days), but the degree of benefit and duration of efficacy appears comparable to the EMG techniques described above. Garcia Ruiz et al. (45) reported greater efficacy using the transoral approach. It is our experience that with increased experience, EMG-guided injections have a high rate of success. It is noteworthy that when the patient is initially treated, the muscle appears to be electrically active at multiple sites throughout the course of the muscle. On follow-up, the electrical recruitment pattern, an index of muscle contraction, may be patchy. EMG guidance has the advantage of controlled administration of treatment into the more actively contracting regions of the muscle.

Regardless of technique, BTX injections have several advantages over surgical therapy in the management of intractable disease. The patient is awake and there is no risk of anesthesia. Graded degrees of weakening can be achieved by varying the dose injected. Most adverse effects are transient and are due to an extension of the pharmacology of the toxin. If the patient has a strong response to therapy and too much weakness occurs, strength gradually returns. We anticipate that increasing knowledge of the molecular pathophysiology of SD will permit the development of new treatment strategies.

Patients with adductor SD, who have already undergone recurrent laryngeal nerve section and have a midline vocal cord, have a marked improvement from BTX therapy, but the degree of benefit is somewhat less than in the nonsurgical patient (10,62). When performing the EMG, a moderate to marked interference pattern is present on the surgical side in many patients, and some patients respond to injection of the "paralyzed" midline cord. Our experience is that the voice quality is better when the mobile cord is injected compared to the midline cord. In an early series, when injecting the functional cord, there was a mean postinjection function of 81% as compared to 59% when injecting the paralyzed cord (10). Similar to the nonsurgical cases, treatment is individualized; an occasional patient requires bilateral injections.

Abductor SD can be successfully treated with BTX (Tables 6 and 7) (9,16,28). However, because of the limitations and concerns about developing stridor, we are very cautious about totally weakening the PCA muscle. Most patients experience progressive improvement over time as the vocal cords become "tuned up," coming closer to the midline with successive treatments. Stridor, when it occurs, is typically mild and may be minimized by avoiding strenuous exercise. Nevertheless, for most patients, treatment is beneficial and side effects are short-lived.

An occasional patient has been noted to be worse after treatment (16). In some patients with subtle dystonic tremor prior to therapy, weakening the PCA muscle permits the vocal cord to move at higher amplitude and aggravates the tremor. An underlying unvoiced tremor becomes apparent when there is increased phonation and improved adduction.

For most patients, treating the PCA muscle is adequate. However, other muscles and alternative injection approaches should be considered. Ludlow et al. (61) reported hyperactivity of the cricothyroid muscles in patients with abductor spastic dysphonia. Ten patients in their series were found to have EMG bursts of the cricothyroid during voice breaks on speaking. They therefore postulated that these patients would benefit from BTX injection of the cricothyroid. They then gave these patients bilateral cricothyroid injections of 5 to 10 U/ side. When assessed by spectrographic analysis of speech rate, percent periodicity, and length of voiceless consonants, all patients had improvement. This treatment was not helpful in patients with only activation abnormalities of the PCA muscle. On a case-by-case basis, we have found that injection of the cricothyroid or strap muscles may result in a smoother voice pattern, particularly when tremor is present.

Rontal et al. (72) advocated approaching the PCA by passing the EMG injection needle through the cricothyroid membrane and then through the thyroarytenoid joint. However, this approach has resulted in arthritic changes in that joint, and is not generally recommended. When the larynx is difficult to rotate, we have adopted a transcricoid approach, passing the needle through the airway and through the cricoid cartilage. This approach has been useful in young individuals with soft cartilage, but there is a risk of blocking the lumen of the EMG injection needle with a cartilaginous fragment.

In a series of prospectively studied abductor patients, we examined preinjection factors that may correlate with result, and devised a staging system for abductor SD patients (15). Stage I patients are those with focal symptoms; stage II patients have segmental cranial or axial; stage III patients have a tremor with dystonia; and stage IV patients have a tremor with segmental axial/cranial and/or respiratory dyssynchrony. Our experience is that patients with simply focal abductor SD respond better to BTX therapy than those with more widespread disease and/or vocal tremor.

We have also treated three patients who failed anterior commissure release procedures performed elsewhere. These patients had intense adductor spasms with a postoperative foreshortened appearance of the larynx. These patients were treated initially with 2.5 U (in 0.1 ml) into each vocal cord. All experienced benefit but probably because of the laxity of the vocal cord from the release, most experienced a narrowed pitch range. They also experienced an extended period of breathy hypophonia. Problems with restricted pitch range have persisted, but breathy hypophonia has responded to treatment individualization.

We recommend that all patients receiving BTX therapy continue in speech therapy in order to relearn how to most effectively utilize their vocal muscles and breathing strategies after BTX therapy. Murry and Woodson (69) demonstrated a prolonged duration of benefit when speech therapy was added to the BTX treatment program. After a patient has completed an initial course of therapy, we urge them to return to the speech-language pathologist at regular intervals (2 to 3 times/year) to refresh the therapeutic exercises and recommendations.

Recently, BTX has been used to treat laryngeal adduction associated with vocal tics (74,76), in addition relieving obstruction due to cricopharyngeal muscle spasm (17,75).

Patient acceptance of this form of therapy is high. Compared with alternative methods of therapy, treatment with BTX is preferred by most patients with SD, and is currently offered as primary therapy. For all forms of SD, injections into the vocalis muscle should be performed by a physician trained in the anatomy and physiology of the larynx. Because reflex laryngeal stridor occasionally occurs during laryngeal EMG, it is recommended that injections be administered in an environment equipped to treat laryngeal stridor (1).

ACKNOWLEDGEMENTS

This work was supported by the Dystonia Medical Research Foundation, PHS DC-01139, and the Bachmann-Strauss Foundation.

REFERENCES

1. AAN. Assessment: the clinical usefulness of botulinum toxin-A in treating neurologic disorders. Report of the Therapeutics and Technology Assessment Subcommittee of the American Academy of Neurology. *Neurology* 1990;40:1332–1336.
2. Almasy L, Bressman SB, Kramer PL, et al. Idiopathic torsion dystonia linked to chromosome 8 in two Mennonite families. *Ann Neurol* 1996(*in press*).
3. Aronson AE, Brown JR, Litin EM, Pearson JS. Spastic dysphonia. I. Voice, neurologic, and psychiatric aspects. *J Speech Hear Disord* 1968;33: 203–218.
4. Aronson AE, Brown JR, Litin EM, Pearson JS. Spastic dysphonia. II. Comparison with essential (voice) tremor and other neurologic and psychogenic dysphonias. *J Speech Hear Disord* 1968;33:219–231.
5. Aronson AE, DeSanto LW. Adductor spastic dysphonia: 1 1/2 years after recurrent laryngeal nerve resection. *Ann Otol Rhinol Laryngol* 1981;90:2–6.

6. Aronson AE, De SLW. Adductor spastic dysphonia: three years after recurrent laryngeal nerve resection. *Laryngoscope* 1983;93:1–8.

7. Aronson AE, Hartman DE. Adductor spastic dysphonia as a sign of essential (voice) tremor. *J Speech Hear Disord* 1981;46:52–58.

8. Bellussi G. Le disfonie impercinetiche. *Atti Labor Fonet Univ Padova* 1952;3:1.

9. Blitzer A, Brin M. Laryngeal dystonia: a series with botulinum toxin therapy. *Ann Otol Rhinol Laryngol* 1991;100:85–89.

10. Blitzer A, Brin MF, Fahn S. Botulinum toxin therapy for recurrent laryngeal nerve section failure for adductor laryngeal dystonia. A L A 1989(abst).

11. Blitzer A, Brin MF, Fahn S, Lange D, Lovelace RE. Botulinum toxin (BOTOX) for the treatment of "spastic dysphonia" as part of a trial of toxin injections for the treatment of other cranial dystonias [Letter]. *Laryngoscope* 1986;96:1300–1301.

12. Blitzer A, Brin MF, Fahn S, Lovelace RE. Clinical and laboratory characteristics of focal laryngeal dystonia: study of 110 cases. *Laryngoscope* 1988;98:636–640.

13. Blitzer A, Brin MF, Fahn S, Lovelace RE. Localized injections of botulinum toxin for the treatment of focal laryngeal dystonia (spastic dysphonia). *Laryngoscope* 1988;98:193–197.

14. Blitzer A, Brin MF, Greene PE, Fahn S. Botulinum toxin injection for the treatment of oromandibular dystonia. *Ann Otol Rhinol Laryngol* 1989;98:93–97.

15. Blitzer A, Brin MF, Stewart C, Aviv JE, Fahn S. Abductor laryngeal dystonia: a series treated with botulinum toxin. *Laryngoscope* 1992;102:163–167.

16. Blitzer A, Brin MF, Stewart C, Fahn S. Abductor laryngeal dystonia: a series treated with botulinum toxin. *Am Laryngol Rhinol Otolog Soc* (Triological Soc) 1991(abst).

17. Blitzer A, Komisar A, Baredes S, Brin MF, Stewart C. Voice failure after tracheoesophageal puncture: Management with botulinum toxin. *Otolaryngol Head Neck Surg* 1995;113:668–670.

18. Blitzer A, Lovelace RE, Brin MF, Fahn S, Fink ME. Electromyographic findings in focal laryngeal dystonia (spastic dysphonia). *Ann Otol Rhinol Laryngol* 1985;94:591–594.

19. Bloch P, Rio. Neuro-psychiatric aspects of spastic dysphonia. *Folia Phoniatr (Basel)* 1965;17:310–364.

20. Bonneau RH, Sheridan JF, Feng N, Glaser R. Stress-induced modulation of the primary cellular immune response to herpes simplex virus infection is mediated by both adrenal-dependent and independent mechanisms. *J Neuroimmunol* 1993;42:167–176.

21. Braun N, Abd A, Baer J, Blitzer A, Stewart C, Brin M. Dyspnea in dystonia. A functional evaluation. *Chest* 1995;107:1309–1316.

22. Bressman SB, de Leon D, Kramer PL, et al. Dystonia in Ashkenazi Jews: clinical characterization of a founder mutation. *Ann Neurol* 1994;36:771–777.

23. Bressman SB, de Leon D, Kramer PL, et al. Dystonia in Ashkenazi Jews: clinical characterization of a founder mutation [published erratum appears in *Ann Neurol* 1995 Jan;37(1):140]. *Ann Neurol* 1994;36:771–777.

24. Brin MF. Interventional neurology: treatment of neurological conditions with local injection of botulinum toxin. *Arch Neurobiol (Madr)* 1991;54:173–189.

25. Brin MF, Blitzer A, Braun N, Stewart C, Fahn S. Respiratory and obstructive laryngeal dystonia treatment with botulinum toxin (Botox). *Neurology* 1991;41 [Suppl 1]:291(abst).

26. Brin MF, Blitzer A, Fahn S, Gould W, Lovelace RE. Adductor laryngeal dystonia (spastic dysphonia): treatment with local injections of botulinum toxin (Botox). *Mov Disord* 1989;4:287–296.

27. Brin MF, Blitzer A, Stewart C. Vocal tremor. In: Findley LJ, Koller WC, eds. *Handbook of tremor disorders*. New York: Marcel Dekker, 1995:495–520.

28. Brin MF, Blitzer A, Stewart C, Fahn S. Botulinum toxin: now for abductor laryngeal dystonia. *Neurology* 1990;40[suppl 1]:381(abst).

29. Brin MF, Blitzer A, Stewart C, Fahn S. Treatment of spasmodic dysphonia (laryngeal dystonia) with local injections of botulinum toxin: review and technical aspects. In: Blitzer A, Brin MF, Sasaki CT, Fahn S, Harris KS, eds. *Neurological disorders of the larynx*. New York: Thieme, 1992:214–228.

30. Brin MF, Fahn S, Blitzer A, Ramig LO, Stewart C. Movement disorders of the larynx. In: Blitzer A, Brin MF, Sasaki CT, Fahn S, Harris KS, eds. *Neurological disorders of the larynx*. New York: Thieme, 1992: 248–278.

31. Brin MF, Fahn S, Bressman SB, Burke RE. Dystonia precipitated by peripheral trauma. *Neurology* 1986; 36[Suppl 1]:119.

32. Brin MF, Fahn S, Moskowitz CB, et al. Injections of botulinum toxin for the treatment of focal dystonia. *Neurology* 1986;36[Suppl 1]:120(abst).

33. Brin MF, Fahn S, Moskowitz C, et al. Localized injections of botulinum toxin for the treatment of focal dystonia and hemifacial spasm. *Mov Disord* 1987;2:237–254.

34. Burke RE, Brin MF, Fahn S, Bressman SB, Moskowitz C. Analysis of the clinical course of non-Jewish, autosomal dominant torsion dystonia. *Mov Disord* 1986; 1:163–178.

35. Burke RE, Fahn S, Jankovic J, et al. Tardive dystonia: late onset and persistent dystonia caused by antipsychotic drugs. *Neurology* 1982;32:1335–1346.

36. Critchley M. Spastic dysphonia ("inspiratory speech"). *Brain* 1939;62:96–103.

37. Dedo HH. Recurrent laryngeal nerve section for spastic dysphonia. *Ann Otol Rhinol Laryngol* 1976;85: 451–459.

38. de Leon D, Moskowitz CB, Stewart C. Proposed guidelines for videotaping individuals with movement disorders. *J Neurosci Nurs* 1991;23:191–193.

39. Dobbs CM, Vasquez M, Glaser R, Sheridan JF. Mechanisms of stress-induced modulation of viral pathogenesis and immunity. *J Neuroimmunol* 1993;48:151–160.

40. Fahn S, Williams DT. Psychogenic dystonia. *Adv Neurol* 1988;50:431–455.

41. Ford CN, Bless DM, Lowery JD. Indirect laryngoscopic approach for injection of botulinum toxin in spasmodic dysphonia. *Otolaryngol Head Neck Surg* 1990;103:752–758.

42. Fraenkel B. Ueber beschaeftigungsneurosen der stimme. Leipzig:G Thieme, 1887.

43. Fraenkel B. Ueber die beschaeftigungsschwaeche der stimme: mogiphonie. *Dtsch Med Wochenschr* 1887; 13:121–123.

44. Gacek RR. Botulinum toxin for relief of spasmodic dysphonia. *Arch Otolaryngol Head Neck Surg* 1987; 113:1240.

45. Garcia Ruiz PJ, Cenjor Espanol C, Sanchez Pernaute R, et al. Laryngeal dystonia. Comparison of transcutaneous and transoral injection of botulinum toxin. [Distonia laringea. Tratamiento con toxina botulinica mediante tecnica transcutanea y transoral. Estudio comparativo]. *Neurologia* 1996;11:216–219.

46. Gerhardt P. *Bewegunggsstoerungen der stimmbaender. Nothnagels spezielle pathologie und therapie.* Vol. 13, 1896.

47. Golper LAC, Nutt JG, Rau MT, Coleman RO. Focal cranial dystonia. *J Speech Hear Disord* 1983;48:128–134.

48. Gowers WR. *Manual of diseases of the nervous system.* 3rd ed. London:Churchill, 1899:200.

49. Grillone GA, Blitzer A, Brin MF, Annino DJ Jr., Saint-Hilaire MH. Treatment of adductor laryngeal breathing dystonia with botulinum toxin type A. *Laryngoscope* 1994;104:30–32.

50. Hermann G, Tovar CA, Beck FM, Allen C, Sheridan JF. Restraint stress differentially affects the pathogenesis of an experimental influenza viral infection in three inbred strains of mice. *J Neuroimmunol* 1993; 47:83–93.

51. Jacome DE, Yanez GF. Spastic dysphonia and Meigs disease [Letter]. *Neurology* 1980;30:349.

52. Jankovic J. Post-traumatic movement disorders: central and peripheral mechanisms. *Neurology* 1994;44: 2006–2014.

53. Jankovic J, Schwartz K, Donovan DT. Botulinum toxin treatment of cranial-cervical dystonia, spasmodic dysphonia, other focal dystonias and hemifacial spasm. *J Neurol Neurosurg Psychiatry* 1990;53:633–639.

54. Kang UJ, Burke RE, Fahn S. Natural history and treatment of tardive dystonia. *Mov Disord* 1986;1:193–208.

55. Lang A, Quinn N, Marsden CD, et al. Essential tremor [Letter; Comment]. *Neurology* 1992;42:1432–1434.

56. Lee DJ, Meehan RT, Robinson C, Mabry TR, Smith ML. Immune responsiveness and risk of illness in U.S. Air Force Academy cadets during basic cadet training. *Aviat Space Environ Med* 1992;63:517–523.

57. Leube B, Rudnicki D, Ratzlaff T, Kessler KR, Benecke R, Auburger G. Idiopathic torsion dystonia: assignment of a gene to chromosome 18p in a German family with adult onset, autosomal dominant inheritance and purely focal distribution. *Hum Mol Genet* 1996;5:1673–1677.

58. Lew MF, Shindo M, Moskowitz C, et al. Adductor laryngeal "breathing dystonia" in a case of X-linked dystonia-parkinson syndrome. *Mov Disord* 1992;7: 301(abst).

59. Lou JS, Jankovic J. Essential tremor: clinical correlates in 350 patients. *Neurology* 1991;41:234–238.

60. Lou JS, Jankovic J. Essential tremor: clinical correlates in 350 patients [see comments]. *Neurology* 1991; 41:234–238.

61. Ludlow CL, Hallett M, Sedory SE, Fujita M, Naunton RF. The pathophysiology of spasmodic dysphonia and its modification by botulinum toxin. In: Berardelli A, Benecke R, Manfredi M, Marsden CM, eds. *Motor disturbances II.* New York: Academic Press, 1990: 273–288.

62. Ludlow CL, Naunton RF, Fujita M, Sedory SE. Spasmodic dysphonia: botulinum toxin injection after recurrent nerve surgery. *Otolaryngol Head Neck Surg* 1990;102:122–131.

63. Ludlow CL, Naunton RF, Sedory SE, Schulz GM, Hallett M. Effects of botulinum toxin injections on speech in adductor spasmodic dysphonia. *Neurology* 1988;38:1220–1225.

64. Marion MH, Klar R, Cohen M. Stridor and focal laryngeal dystonia. *Lancet* 1992;1:457–458.

65. Marsden CD. Peripheral movement disorders. In: Marsden CD, Fahn S, eds. *Movement disorders 3.* Oxford: Butterworth-Heinemann, 1994:406–417.

66. Marsden CD, Harrison MJG. Idiopathic torsion dystonia (dystonia musculorum deformans). A review of forty-two patients. *Brain* 1974;97:793–810.

67. Marsden CD, Sheehy MP. Spastic dysphonia, Meige disease, and torsion dystonia [Letter]. *Neurology* 1982; 32:1202–1203.

68. Miller RH, Woodson GE, Jankovic J. Botulinum toxin injection of the vocal fold for spasmodic dysphonia. A preliminary report. *Arch Otolaryngol Head Neck Surg* 1987;113:603–605.

69. Murry T, Woodson GE. Combined-modality treatment of adductor spasmodic dysphonia with botulinum toxin and voice therapy. *J Voice* 1995;9:460–465.

70. Ozelius L, Kramer PL, Moskowitz CB, et al. Human gene for torsion dystonia located on chromosome 9q32-q34. *Neuron* 1989;2:1427–1434.

71. Pool KD, Freeman FJ, Finitzo T, et al. Heterogeneity in spasmodic dysphonia. Neurologic and voice findings. *Arch Neurol* 1991;48:305–309.

72. Rontal M, Rontal E, Rolnick M, Merson R, Silverman B, Truong DD. A method for the treatment of abductor spasmodic dysphonia with botulinum toxin injections: a preliminary report. *Laryngoscope* 1991;101:911–914.

73. Rosenfield DB, Donovan DT, Sulek M, Viswanath NS, Inbody GP, Nudelman HB. Neurologic aspects of spasmodic dysphonia [See comments]. *J Otolaryngol* 1990;19:231–236.

74. Salloway S, Stewart CF, Israeli L, et al. Botulinum toxin for refractory vocal tics. *Mov Disord* 1996;11: 746–748.

75. Schneider I, Pototschnig C, Thumfart WF, Eckel HE. Treatment of dysfunction of the cricopharyngeal muscle with botulinum A toxin—introduction of a new, noninvasive method. *Ann Otol Rhinol Laryngol* 1994; 103:31–35.

76. Scott BL, Jankovic J, Donovan DT. Botulinum toxin injection into vocal cord in the treatment of malignant coprolalia associated with Tourette's syndrome. *Mov Disord* 1996;11:431–433.

77. Sternberg EM. Hypoimmune fatigue syndromes: diseases of the stess response? [Editorial] [Corrected] [Published erratum appears in *J Rheumatol* 1993 May; 20(5):925] [Comment]. *J Rheumatol* 1993;20:418–421.

78. Stewart CF, Allen EL, Tureen P, Diamond BE, Blitzer A, Brin MF. Adductor spasmodic dysphonia: standard evaluation of symptoms and severity. *J Voice* 1997; 11:95–103.

79. Traube L. Gesammelte Beitrage zur Pathologie und Physiologie. 2nd ed. Berlin: Verlag von August Hirschwald, 1871:674.

Dystonia 3: Advances in Neurology, Vol. 78,
edited by S. Fahn, C. D. Marsden and M. DeLong.
Lippincott–Raven Publishers, Philadelphia © 1998.

26

Dystonias Responding to Levodopa and Failure in Biopterin Metabolism

*Yoshiko Nomura, *†Kimiaki Uetake, *Shoko Yukishita, *‡Hiroaki Hagiwara,
*‡Tatsuroh Tanaka, *Ritsuho Tanaka, *Kei Hachimori, *‡Nobuyoshi
Nishiyama, and *Masaya Segawa

*Segawa Neurological Clinic for Children, Tokyo 101 0062, Japan; †Department of Pediatrics,
Hokkaido University School of Medicine, Tokyo 101 0062, Japan; and ‡Faculty of Pharmaceutical
Sciences, Department of Chemical Pharmacology, University of Tokyo, Tokyo, 113 Japan.

Hereditary progressive dystonia with marked diurnal fluctuation (HPD) is known to be a dominantly inherited postural dystonia with female predominance (33,37,40), caused by the abnormality of the gene of GTP cyclohydrolase I (GCH-I) located at chromosome 14q22.1-q22.2 (14).

HPD is characterized by the marked diurnal fluctuation of symptoms in childhood, in which postural dystonia aggravates toward evening and ameliorates nearly completely in the morning after sleep, and all symptoms respond to levodopa completely without any side effects (33,40). These effects are sustained and are observed without any relation to the severity and longevity of the disease or ages of the patients (37,39).

Dopa-responsive dystonia (DRD) was first proposed as a term including all dystonias that responded to levodopa (25); however, DRD diagnosed by the revised criteria (2,26)—strictly defined DRD—which is used broadly in journals, is identical to HPD. In this report HPD/DRD is used to denote the strictly defined DRD in the literature.

GCH-I is the first step and rate-limiting enzyme to synthesize tetrahydrobiopterin (BH_4) and the decrease of GCH-I leads to decreased BH_4 and failure of tyrosine hydroxylase (TH)

synthesis and eventually induces a decrease of dopamine (DA). The decreased BH_4 is also seen in other enzyme abnormalities concerned with the biosynthetic pathways of BH_4 (Fig. 1).

Among these, abnormalities of 6-pyruvoyl-tetrahydropterin synthase (PTPS) and dihydropteridine reductase (DHPR) are known to present dystonia with diurnal fluctuation responding to levodopa.

We compared the clinical symptoms of these disorders and showed the specificity of HPD/DRD among them.

SUBJECTS

Ten personal cases with HPD from five families who were proved to have the abnormal GCH-I gene were compared with the cases of other enzyme abnormalities of pteridine metabolism; one male patient had DHPR deficiency, one male patient had the dihydrobiopterin synthesis (DHBS) defect, and one female patient had PTPS deficiency. The patient with DHPR deficiency has been followed by one of the authors (K.U.) and the other patients were reported by Tanaka et al. (44) and Hanihara et al. (10), respectively.

Patients with HPD were diagnosed by their clinical characteristics. DHPR deficiency was

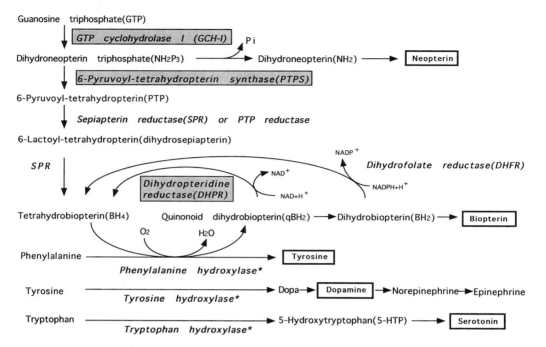

FIG. 1. Tetrahydrobiopterin (BH$_4$) biosynthetic pathway and aromatic amino acid hydroxylase system in biopterin deficient dystonia. Deficiencies of enzymes shadowed in the figure are discussed in the text.

diagnosed by enzymologic studies. The diagnosis of a DHBS defect was based on a high urinary concentration of neopterin and trace amounts of biopterin and normal DHPR activity, and the diagnosis of PTPS deficiency was based on a molecular genetic analysis.

RESULTS

Clinical Characteristics of Hereditary Progressive Dystonia with marked diurnal fluctuation (HPD) in Reference to Mutations of the GCH-I Gene

Gene analyses were performed in ten patients from five families and seven sporadic cases of HPD, all of whom have been followed at our clinic.

Among these the mutations of the gene were detected in five patients from three families and five sporadic cases including newly detected cases (13,14, Yukishita et al. to be published) (Table 1). In one sporadic patient, gene

analysis of her parents revealed the father having the same mutation as the proband (13). In others, including one family with four cases that has shown the linkage to chromosome 14q (3,43) and low GCH-I activities in the peripheral mononuclear blood cells in affected members (14), abnormalities have not been found in the coding region of the GCH-I gene.

The locations of the mutation show various areas involving exons 1, 2, 4, and 5 of the GCH-I gene, and there were five types of missense mutations, one nonsense mutation, and two frameshift mutations (Table 1). There was no correlation in the type and location of mutations among familial and clinically sporadic cases. However, given family members, either affected or asymptomatic carriers, showed identical mutation.

Clinical characteristics were evaluated to investigate whether there were differences among the patients whose mutation was identified in the coding regions (group A) and those whose

TABLE 1. *Mutation of GTP cyclohydrolase I in HPD*

Patient		Sex	Exon	Mutation		Age of onset (y, mo)	Plain levodopa vs. with inhibitor[d]
Family	Sa						
	Y Sa	F	1[a]	3 ins GG	Frameshift mutation	10	Plain levodopa
	H Sa	F				6	Plain levodopa
Family	K						
	M K	F	1[a]	Arg 88 Trp	Missense mutation	4, 11	With inhibitor
Family	Su						
	S Su	F	2[a]	Asp 134 Val	Missense mutation	8	Plain levodopa
	K Su	M				2, 7	(With inhibitor)
	A Su	F				1, 4	Plain levodopa
Patient							
	Y Y	F	1[b]	Leu 79 Pro	Missense mutation	3~4	With inhibitor
	R M	F	2[c]	Cys 141 Arg	Missense mutation	6	(With inhibitor)
	A I	F	4[b]	511 del 13bp	Frameshift mutation	7, 9	With inhibitor
	M S	F	4[c]	Gln 180 Stop	Nonsense mutation	8	Plain levodopa
	K N	M	5[a]	Gly 201 Glu	Missense mutation	8, 6	With inhibitor

[a]Data from Ref. 14.
[b]Data from Ref. 13.
[c]Yukishita et al. (to be published).
[d]Decarboxylase inhibitor, ( ): with inhibitor already prescribed by local physician.

genes have not been identified in the coding region (group B) and also among the loci of the mutation. Although each group consists of small numbers, the familial cases of group A showed the youngest age of onset, especially in the same generation of the proband. However, there seem to be no differences in the symptoms at onset between groups A and B. The degree of diurnal fluctuation of the symptoms did not differ significantly between groups A and B. However, all of them showed marked diurnal fluctuation in childhood which subsided with age, particularly in the third decade (23,37). The occurrence of postural tremor did not differ between the two groups, and in all patients who developed tremor it was after the second decade, and often after the fourth decade in both groups (37).

Regarding treatment, all patients were started with plain levodopa. However, some needed to change to levodopa with decarboxylase inhibitor, in an age-dependent manner in the early teens, because of a perceived decrease in the effectiveness of the plain levodopa (39). Cases in one family whose mutation is in exon 1, and

three sporadic cases whose mutation was in exon 1, 4, and 5 had to be changed from plain levodopa to that with decarboxylase inhibitor (Table 1). Among these patients one sporadic case had abnormality in exon 4 with a frameshift mutation and the rest were missense mutations. Those who had stable courses on plain levodopa included the family that had a missense mutation in exon 2 and frameshift in exon 1, and the sporadic case of nonsense mutation in exon 4. The family who is linked to chromosome 14q but with no mutation in the coding region revealed that three of four patients in this family needed to have the medication changed to levodopa with decarboxylase inhibitor.

GCH-I activity was evaluated in seven patients (six familial cases and one clinically sporadic case) and four of their parents (Table 2). The activity of GCH-I of peripheral mononuclear cells of HPD/DRD patients ranged from 2% to 20%, but those of the two nonmanifesting male carriers, both fathers of the patients, were 36% and 37% of normal controls (14).

There are no apparent differences in clinical features or mutation site according to the levels

TABLE 2. *GTP cyclohydrolase I (GCH-I) activity in HPD*

Name		Sex		GCH-1 activity[a] (pmol h^{-1} mg protein^{-1})	GCH-I mutation in coding region
Family Sa	Y Sa	F	Mother of proband, patient	0.9	Exon 1
	H Sa	F	Proband	3.6	Exon 1
Family K	M K	F	Proband	0.3	Exon 1
	Father	M	Nonmanifesting carrier	6.9	Exon 1
Family Su	A Su	F	Proband	1.5	Exon 2
	Father	M	Nonmanifesting carrier	6.7	Exon 2
	Mother	F	Healthy	22.7	—
Family T	T R	F	Proband	2.4	Not found, but linked to chromosome 14q
	K W	F	Cousin of proband, patient	1.9	Not found, but linked to chromosome 14q
	Father to KW	M	Healthy	16.2	—
Patient	K N	M	Sporadic case	2.4	Exon 5
Healthy controls					
Total	[N = 13]			18.8 ± 2.9 (9.0–46.1)	
Female	[N = 8]			15.3 ± 1.6	
Male	[N = 5]			24.3 ± 6.9	

_____ : HPD patient.
[a]Data from Ref. 14.
Activity: mean ± SEM; ( ): range of values.

of the activities of GCH-I in peripheral mono-nuclear blood cells. But one patient whose GCH-I activity was the lowest required lev-odopa with decarboxylase inhibitor from the beginning of the treatment at 5 years 9 months of age, after 2 months treatment with plain lev-odopa, and she experienced unstable respon-siveness to the medication at approximately 11 years of age, after menarche. The intelligence quotient of this patient was in the lower limits of the normal range, and the two aunts who also suffered from HPD showed insufficient re-sponse to plain levodopa.

A Case with Dihydropteridine Reductase (DHPR) Deficiency

The boy was a product of nonconsan-guineous marriage. There was no neurologic or metabolic disorders in the family. Prenatal, perinatal, and neonatal history was normal in-cluding a Guthrie screening test done on the fifth day after birth. Developmental milestones showed delay in motor function: sitting at 1 year and unassisted walking at 6 years of age. Past history did not show any specific diseases other than the present illness.

The present illness revealed that since the age of 2 months the boy developed opistho-tonic-like dystonic posture in action or while taking certain postures, which worsened to-ward the evening. Muscle tone at rest was hy-potonic at 3 years of age, an anticholinergic drug was administered but the symptoms wors-ened, and the treatment was changed to lev-odopa. The dystonia showed moderate im-provement but the effects were not stable. Mental retardation was also present. During the follow-up course, at around 14 years, he developed epilepsy. For mental retardation and epilepsy, levodopa showed no effects.

The blood amino acid analysis showed moder-ate elevation of the levels of phenylalanine. Plasma neopterin was normal and biopterin was abnormally high with a markedly decreased neopterin-biopterin ratio. Cerebrospinal fluid (CSF) neopterin was below normal and biopterin was within the normal range with a moderately decreased neopterin-biopterin ratio. Homovanil-

lic acid (HVA) and 5-hydroxyindole acetic acid (5-HIAA) levels in CSF were markedly de-creased.

DHPR activity of peripheral red blood cells (RBC), shown as a percentage of normal control, revealed 0% in the patient, 38% in the father, 43% in a younger sister, and 97% in an older brother. PTPS activity of RBC was normal.

The diagnosis of DHPR deficiency, with au-tosomal-recessive inheritance, was made.

A Case with Dihydrobiopterin Synthesis (DHBS) Defect

A man with a DHBS defect with mild clini-cal symptoms was reported by Tanaka et al. in 1987 (44). Family history revealed no consan-guinity or neurologic diseases. Prenatal and perinatal courses were uneventful. This patient showed psychomotor development to be de-layed from late infancy; he spoke at 1.5 years and walked at 2.5 years.

At around 10 years of age, difficulty in walking became apparent; he was unable to stand without support and speech was slurred. When he was seen at age 14 years, he showed mild mental retardation, dysarthria, limb hy-pertonicity, and hyperreflexia. Because of high serum phenylalanine and a positive urinary fer-ric chloride test his symptoms were thought to be consistent with phenylketonuria (PKU). On a low phenylalanine diet he did better until 20 years of age, when the dietary therapy was discontinued and symptoms showed gradual worsening. Around this time it was noticed that his symptoms improved after sleep. At 24 years of age, he had epileptic attacks, moderate men-tal retardation, forced laughing, dysphasia, and festinated and monotonous speech with de-layed initiation were noted. Limbs were ex-tremely stiff. Increased muscle tone, exagger-ated deep tendon reflex, and Babinski signs were noted bilaterally. He tended to lie in a posture with elbows flexed, and hips, knees, and ankles extended. Myoclonus was observed in the limbs. Initiation of motion was delayed and coordinated movement was not smooth. These motor symptoms including speech showed marked diurnal fluctuation; he was able to walk in the morning, but was unable even to sit at noon or in the evening.

Serum phenylalanine was abnormally high. Urinary 5-HIAA was abnormally low and HVA was also slightly low. HVA and 5-HIAA were markedly reduced in CSF, 5-HIAA more severely than HVA. Urinary neopterin was high and biopterin was low. DHPR activity in RBC was normal. Administration of BH_4 lowered serum phenylalanine and improved the motor symptoms. Levodopa further improved the motor symptoms.

The diagnosis of a DHBS defect was made based on laboratory findings with high neopterin and trace biopterin in urine, decreased HVA and 5-HIAA in CSF, and normal DHPR activity.

DHBS consists of three enzymes including PTPS, which, however, was not known when this case was reported. The biochemical data of the DHBS-deficient case presented here are compatible with PTPS deficiency. The identification of the enzyme deficiency and molecular genetic analysis are now under investigation.

A Case with 6-Pyruvoyl-Tetrahydropterin Synthase (PTPS) Deficiency

Recently, Hanihara et al. (10) presented a case with PTPS deficiency. This patient was a 44-year-old woman with generalized dystonia with marked diurnal fluctuation. Family history showed consanguinity in her parents and her sister is thought to have an identical disorder. The prenatal and perinatal history were normal. The history showed tonic-clonic seizure starting at 18 months of age and an abnormal crawling pattern using arms with legs fixed in an extended posture.

At 2 years, spasticity was observed in the lower extremities and the diagnosis of cerebral palsy was made. She began walking at age 4 years with unsteady scissors gait. Speech and intellect were normal. Diurnal fluctuation of motor ability was noted at 7 years of age; she was able to walk in the morning but not in the evening. She walked until the age of 27 years. At 30 years of age, when she presented for medical attention, she was noted to be mentally retarded. At age 41 years she was further evaluated, which revealed increased muscle tone and generalized dystonia of rigid neck, flexed elbows and wrists, and extended knees and ankles with pes equinovarus posture. Deep tendon reflexes were exaggerated but plantar responses were flexor. Blepharospasms, oromandibular dyskinesia, including bizarre tongue protrusion, were also observed. These were described by authors as Meige's syndrome plus double hemiplegic-like dystonia. Tremor was observed in the upper extremities. All of these symptoms showed diurnal fluctuation of amelioration in the morning after sleep and aggravation toward evening.

Serum phenylalanine level was mildly elevated and urinary neopterin was increased. HVA and 5-HIAA in CSF were within the normal range. The diagnosis of partial PTPS deficiency was made. Levodopa treatment showed dramatic improvement of dystonia, which has been continued. However, the effectiveness of levodopa was not complete as observed in HPD/DRD.

Molecular analyses showed a homozygous mutation in the PTPS gene. The clinical symptoms of this patient were mild and progression was very slow in spite of a homozygous mutation.

DISCUSSION

HPD was first described by Segawa et al. (40) in 1971 as inherited basal ganglia disease with marked diurnal fluctuation of symptoms and dramatic response to levodopa. Later, with the examination of a patient in her 50s, it was called "hereditary progressive dystonia with marked diurnal fluctuation," as a new dominantly inherited dystonia different from juvenile parkinsonism and Parkinson's disease (33).

Abnormality of pteridine metabolism in HPD was shown by the decrease of biopterin and neopterin levels in CSF, and a decrease of GCH-I was suspected as its etiology (5,6).

The genetic locus of HPD/DRD was first detected by Nygaard et al. (27), who mapped the locus for this disorder to the long arm of chromosome 14, a 22 cM region between D14S47

(14q11.2-q22) and D14S63 (14q11-q24.3) by linkage analysis, and Endo et al. (3) and Tanaka et al. (43) found the gene of HPD on the same locus as HPD/DRD. These findings further provoked the discovery of the mutation of the gene of GCH-I in HPD located in chromosome 14q22.1-q22.2 (14). Therefore, HPD is considered as dominantly inherited GCH-I deficiency.

On the other hand, GCH-I, PTPS, and DHPR deficiencies with recessive inheritance are known as variants of PKU. These variant PKUs, in contrast with classic PKU, which is recessive phenylalanine hydroxylase deficiency, reveals progressive neurologic symptoms despite dietary control of phenylalanine levels.

GCH-I, PTPS, and DHPR are involved with the biosynthesis and regeneration of BH_4. BH_4 is the natural cofactor of the aromatic acid oxidase (e.g., phenylalanine hydroxylase, tyrosine hydroxylase, and tryptophan hydroxylase), which converts phenylalanine to tyrosine, tyrosine to dopamine (DA), and tryptophan to serotonin (5HT), respectively (Fig. 1). BH_4 is also required as a cofactor of nitric oxide synthases. Thus a BH_4 defect results in deficiencies of both DA and 5HT accompanied by hyperphenylalaninemia.

Pathophysiology of Hereditary Progressive Dystonia with marked diurnal fluctuation (HPD): Dominant GCH-I Deficiency

The complete and sustained response to levodopa without any side effects suggested the pathophysiology of HPD as a functional disorder of the nigrostriatal (NS)-DA neuron without morphologic changes (37).

Clinical courses of HPD are characterized by onset in childhood and progression in the first two decades followed by a stationary stage after the fourth decade, which correlates well with the age-dependent variation of the TH activities in the terminal of NS-DA neurons (18,37). TH activities in the brain (18) as well as the secretion of DA at the terminal of the NS-DA system (28) are also known to show the circadian fluctuation: a decremental variation in the active period and an incremental one in the resting period. The pathophysiology of HPD was therefore suggested as a decrease of TH at the termi-

nal of the NS-DA neuron to the critical level of normal range but preserving the physiologic modulation (37). These were supported by polysomnographic analyses (35,38) and were confirmed by neuropathologic (29) and neurohistochemical studies (11,29) on an autopsied case of sporadic DRD that later was proven to have a mutation in the GCH-I gene (7). Further, normal (42) or subnormal (32) incorporation observed in ^{18}F-Dopa positron emission tomography (PET) studies suggests the lesion of HPD/DRD at the level of hydroxylation of tyrosine preserving its downstream normally in the dopamine metabolic pathway (42).

Similar age variation as TH is also observed in levels of urinary secretion of biopterin and neopterin (41), and neopterin, BH_4, dihydrobiopterin (BH_2), HVA, and 5-HIAA in CSF (12). Therefore, age variation and diurnal fluctuation observed in TH activity are considered to be modulated by GCH-I activity via BH_4 and consequently reflected in the level of DA and 5HT. It is also speculated that the relatively short half-life of BH_4 might explain the diurnal fluctuation of symptoms in HPD (14).

The affinity of BH_4 for TH is the lowest among hydroxylases which use BH_4 as cofactor (16,24). So with partial decrement of BH_4, DA synthesis is rather selectively involved in HPD.

Crossman and his colleagues examined MPTP monkeys in the state of peak dose dystonia and revealed no apparent involvement of the indirect striatal pathway and preservation of the ventral lateral (VL) nucleus of the thalamus and the pedunculopontine nucleus (PPN) without suppression (19,31). Furthermore the monkey could move with four limb locomotion (19). In reference to this experimental findings, we speculated that in HPD, the affected NS-DA neurons develop postural dystonia through the striatal direct pathway and its efferent, which does not inhibit PPN or VL nucleus of the thalamus.

Although it is not clarified in primate and human, a particular descending basal ganglia efferent to the reticulospinal tract via the mesopontine brainstem nucleus other than PPN is suggested for postural dystonia.

Histochemical studies on an autopsied case showed a decrease in DA content in the basal ganglia, similar to interregional distribution as Parkinson's disease (PD), but different from it in the subregional distribution with predominant decrement in the ventral portion (11,29).

In human striatum, particularly in the rostral caudate, the striosome/patches are more numerous in the medial/ventral portions of the nucleus, whereas in its dorsal/lateral portions the matrix compartment is more homogeneous (9). In reference to this compartmental substructure of the rostral caudate, the DA loss in the caudate head of idiopathic PD appears to be more pronounced in the matrix, and that of HPD/DRD in the striosome/patch compartment (11). Striosome/patch cells have D1 receptors, GABA, and substance P, and project to the medial globus pallidus as the direct pathway, whereas matrix cells have D2 receptors, GABA, and enkephalin and project to the lateral globus pallidus as the indirect pathway (8). During the developmental course of the striatum, the patch-striatonigral neurons mature earlier than the matrix-striatonigral neurons and project early to the substantia nigra (45).

The studies on MPTP monkeys revealed that there is no receptor supersensitivity in the state of peak dose dystonia (19). Polysomnographic studies on HPD also revealed no occurrence of receptor supersensitivities (36,38). These were confirmed by a C^{11} raclopride PET study that revealed no upward or downward regulation of the D2 receptor in HPD/DRD patients (17).

Therefore, in HPD, hypofunctioning terminals of NS-DA neurons involve mainly D1 receptors of the direct pathway, and the dysfunction of this system can develop the characteristic feature of dystonia in childhood as this pathway matures early in the developmental course.

Without morphologic abnormalities and normal preservation of aromatic amino acid decarboxylase, levodopa showed marked effect. Uninvolvement of the indirect pathways and normal preservation of the D2 receptors prevent the occurrence of levodopa-induced side effects and the development of action dystonia (34,35).

Uninvolvement of the PPN relates to the preservation of the locomotive activities in HPD until the advanced state (34,35).

Differences in functional maturation between direct and indirect pathways are observed in developmental age variations of voluntary saccadic eye movements. Both direct and indirect pathways have roles for generating voluntary saccades specific for each: the former for executing the saccades and the latter for peripheral suppression making the saccades more accurate (15). It is also shown that the former is involved mainly in the visually guided saccades and the latter in the memory-guided saccades (15).

The studies on developmental age variation of both types of voluntary saccade revealed marked age variation in memory saccades during the first one and half decades, in which the indirect pathways are in the state of suppression (Fukuda et al. to be published).

A ^{11}C raclopride PET study revealed an increase in the number of D2 receptors in the early 20s, which reduced to the "adult" level around the mid-20s (1).

These evidences from neurophysiology and neuroimaging imply that DA transmission in normal subjects is in the state of exaggeration at the D2 receptors in the first two decades. Therefore, in these years, particularly in the first one and half decades, the targets of the basal ganglia efferents, which are modulated by indirect pathways, are under insufficient suppression.

In the case of HPD, delay in the functional maturation of an indirect pathway and rather hyperactive D2 receptors that are present in childhood may minimize the manifestations of the direct pathway mediated symptoms of HPD in the early decades (Fig. 2). This may be another reason why the dystonia of HPD appears to progress in the first two decades without any apparent progressive decrement of the TH activity compared with normal levels.

The affinity of BH_4 for TH is the lowest among hydroxylases that use BH_4 as a cofactor (16,24). Therefore with partial decrement of BH_4, dopamine synthesis is rather selectively involved in HPD.

Pathophysiology of Recessive Failure of Pteridine Metabolism

Patients with abnormal pteridine metabolism discussed in this chapter have postural dystonia with diurnal fluctuation that responds to levodopa, but they show other features different

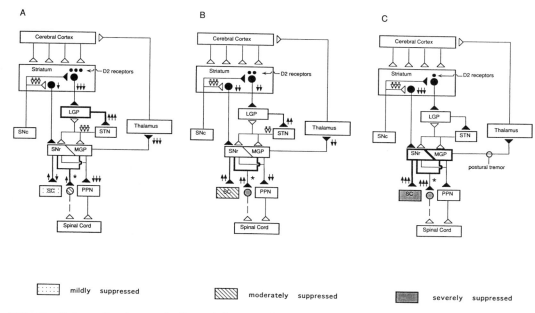

FIG. 2. Schematic demonstration of the possible pathophysiologies of HPD in the first three decades. As TH activities at the terminal is high in the 1st decade and decrease with age, the effects of its decrement in HPD is reduced in the early two decades. In the striatum, the numbers of DA-D_2 receptors are high, but decrease with age rapidly until the early 20s. As for the efferents of the basal ganglia, a particular descending pathway which does not inhibit PPN is suspected to be involved in the development of postural dystonia of HPD. This putative efferent projection is shown in the figure with the asterisk. A, B, C indicate 1st decade, middle of the 2nd decade, and early 3rd decade of HPD, respectively. Grades of the suppression of SC are indicated at the bottom of the figure. LGP, lateral globus pallidus; MGP, medial globus pallidus; STN, subthalamic nucleus; SNc, substantia nigra pars compacta; SNr, substantia nigra pars reticulata; SC, superior colliculus; PPN, pedunculopontine nuclei; black triangle or circle, inhibitory neuron; white triangle, excitatory terminal; black arrow, inhibitory process; white arrow; excitatory process.

than HPD, such as psychomotor retardation, seizure, myoclonus, hypotonia, spasticity, and abnormal locomotion, suggesting the involvement of neurons or neural systems other than the NS-DA neuron.

With homozygous mutant genes of PTPS or DHPR, marked decrease of the enzyme causes marked reduction of BH_4. Consequently, it provides a marked decrement of 5HT as well as DA.

5HT neurons modulate postural tone and locomotion by involving the midbrain centers for posture and locomotion (20) and also have important roles for the functional maturation of the cerebral cortex, early in the developmental course (4,21). Marked postural hypotonia and moderate mental deterioration observed in the patient with DHPR deficiency are considered to be related to hypofunction of 5HT neurons.

Abnormal interlimb coordination and mental deterioration in a male patient with the DHBS (PTPS) defect may also be caused by hypofunction of this neuron (Fig. 3). These are supported by the decrease of 5-HIAA in CSF observed in these cases. However, in the female patient with PTPS deficiency, there was no definite laboratory evidence suggesting hypofunctioning of the 5HT neuron. Homozygosity of mutant genes in this case might have some role for the involvement of 5HT neurons.

Characteristic Features of Dystonia Due to BH_4 Deficiency

Dystonia observed in disorders presented in this chapter is caused by abnormal BH_4 metabolism and all of them showed postural dystonia

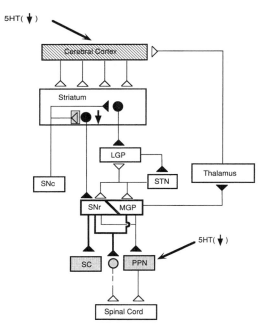

FIG. 3. Schematic demonstration of the possible pathophysiology of dystonia due to recessive DHPR and PTPS deficiencies. Both DA and 5HT are thought to be decreased in these disorders. Shadow indicates the suppressed nuclei or region. LGP, lateral globus pallidus; MGP, medial globus pallidus; STN, subthalamic nucleus; SNc, substantia nigra pars compacta; SNr, substantia nigra pars reticulata; SC, superior colliculus; PPN, pedunculopontine nuclei; black circle or triangle, inhibitory neuron; white triangle, excitatory terminal.

with diurnal fluctuation and responsiveness to levodopa; the same pathophysiology as HPD might be present although there are some similarities and dissimilarities among disorders (Table 3).

The onset of these disorders is mostly in childhood. HPD usually starts in early to mid-childhood with gait disturbance; those of recessive DHPR and PTPS deficiency start in late infancy to early toddler age. Reported patients with recessive GCH-I deficiencies developed marked exaggeration of muscle tone with severe opisthotonic posture and crossed lower extremities in infancy, in addition to hypotonia

of trunkal muscle, severe developmental retardation, and convulsions (22).

The dystonia in HPD is a postural dystonia involving mainly the extremities, lower more than upper, and with asymmetry. Although the one due to recessive DHPR deficiency is generalized dystonia with opisthotonus, the one due to recessive PTPS deficiency revealed to be also generalized dystonia with opisthotonus but this case showed blepharospasm and oromandibular dyskinesia. On the other hand, the dystonia observed in the case of DHBS (PTPS) deficiency seemed to have involved mainly the extremities.

These observations reveal that severe reduction of BH_4 due to recessively inherited disorders of pteridine metabolism causes dystonia more marked in severity and wider in its distribution. Marked reduction of BH_4 may also involve DA-D2 receptors and may reduce the effect of the developmental decrement of receptors. This consequently reduces the hypoactivity of the basal ganglia efferents modulated by indirect pathways and increases the effects of hypoactivity of the direct pathway related efferents, that is, exaggerated muscle tone or dystonia. The blepharospasm, orofacial dyskinesia, and plastic rigidity observed in recessive PTPS deficiency might suggest the decrease of DA activity involving D2 receptors and the indirect pathways. The late appearance of the symptoms may also be due to the developmental reduction of D2 receptors in adulthood. However, the opisthotonic posture observed in severely affected patients is not a feature observed in idiopathic PD, although it is observed in some patients with idiopathic dystonia that respond to stereotaxic operation with a different target from that for PD (Narabayashi H, to be published). Therefore, the involved neural pathways in the basal ganglia of these BH_4 deficiencies may differ from PD.

The diurnal fluctuation of symptoms are commonly present in all these dystonias with various degrees from moderate to marked. The onset of diurnal fluctuation of dystonia was in infancy in the patient with DHPR deficiency; in the patient with the DHBS (PTPS) defect the fluctuation was observed from 20 years of age;

TABLE 3. *Biopterin deficient dystonia and diurnal fluctuation of symptoms*

	Causative gene	Mode of inheritance	Age of onset	Dystonia	Symptoms other than dystonia	Diurnal fluctuation of symptoms	Onset of fluctuations
HPD (Segawa) Hanihara's case[a]	GCH-I PTPS	AD AR	Early childhood 18 mo	Postural dystonia of leg Generalized dystonia, orofacial dyskinesia	None Mental retardation Seizure	(++) (+)	Early childhood 7 yr
Tanaka's case[b]	DHBS (PTPS)		Infancy	Dystonia of limbs	Mental retardation Rigid spasticity Myoclonus	(+)	20 yr
KU's case (Uetake)	DHPR	AR	2 mo	Generalized dystonia	Psychomotor delay Seizure	(+)	2 mo

GCH-I, GTP cyclohydrolase I; PTPS, 6-pyruvoyl-tetrahydropterin synthase; DHPR, dihydropteridine reductase; DHBS, dihydrobiopterin synthesis; AD, autosomal dominant; AR, autosomal recessive.
[a]From Ref. 10, with permission.
[b]From Ref. 44, with permission.

and in another case of PTPS deficiency it was since age 7 years. However, the diurnal fluctuation was not described in cases with recessive GCH-I deficiency (22). These are in contrast to the typical diurnal fluctuation of HPD, which is marked in early childhood and becomes less obvious in the second decade.

As mentioned earlier, diurnal or circadian fluctuation is observed in the activity of TH in the whole brain (18) and dopamine secretion at the terminal of NS-DA neuron (28). The short half-life of BH_4 can cause decremental variation in the active period, manifesting as diurnal fluctuation in clinical symptoms (14). Therefore, diurnal fluctuation observed in these disorders with pteridine metabolism might be due to the fluctuation of BH_4 content and its effect on TH activity. That there is no apparent fluctuation in patients with recessive GCH-I deficiency (22) suggests the roles of GCH-I for the diurnal or circadian variation.

The late occurrence of diurnal fluctuation as observed in the patient with the DHBS (PTPS) defect might simply be related to the fact that the reduction of BH_4 was not so severe in this mild case and delayed the clinical manifestation of diurnal fluctuation to the early 20s when the physiologic decrement of BH_4 becomes greater. Normal preservation of GCH-I in these disorders might also involve this late occurrence of fluctuation.

Although the effectiveness of levodopa on dystonia was observed in all these cases, in cases with DHPR and PTPS deficiency it was not as marked as in HPD and did not last long, showing aggravation in the evening even with levodopa treatment. The levodopa effect on recessive GCH-I deficiency seems to be unappreciated. This may partly be due to the severity of BH_4 or DA depletion but may also relate to the mode of inheritance being recessive in contrast to HPD, which is dominant.

Female predominance observed in HPD is not observed in other disorders with pteridine metabolism, although the number of cases was limited. This sex preference might be due to a sex difference of the dopamine neuron, which is determined genetically (30).

Differences between Dominant and Recessive Inheritance

The differences in clinical features between HPD and DHPR or PTPS deficiencies might also be related to their mode of inheritance, whether it is dominant or recessive pteridine metabolism. Both recessive and dominant abnormalities are known only in the GCH-I gene and dominant cases of PTPS and DHPR deficiency have not been reported so far. In recessive disorders of enzymes for BH_4 synthesis, a marked decrease of BH_4 affects phenylalanine hydroxylase as well as TH, and consequently causes a decrement of 5HT in addition to DA. HPD, in contrast, is due to dominant inheritance involving the GCH-I gene and heterozygote of the GCH-I gene abnormality present as an HPD patient or a nonmanifesting carrier. This heterozygous abnormality causes partial decrement of GCH-I and may affect the DA synthesis rather selectively, because as discussed the affinity to BH_4 is lowest in tyrosine hydroxylase among hydroxylases that require BH_4 as a cofactor.

The levels of the GCH-I activities in HPD patients are below 20% of the normal range, while nonmanifesting male carriers showed 36% and 37% of normal controls (14). The heterozygotes of the patients with recessive GCH-I deficiency do not develop the symptoms of HPD, probably because the level of the GCH-I activity of the heterozygote is usually near 50%. It is important to consider the role of dominant negative theory in the case of HPD concerning the pathophysiology of these disorders of enzyme deficiencies (14). However it does not explain all cases.

It is uncommon, as pointed out by Tanaka (44), for a patient with DHBS deficiency to be diagnosed in adulthood with such mild symptoms. Similarly the PTPS deficient patient of Hanihara was diagnosed as partial PTPS deficiency and also showed relatively milder clinical features with HVA and 5-HIAA in CSF to be within the normal range. These cases suggest that a homozygous mutation of the PTPS gene (10) can be present as a partial deficiency of BH$_4$ activity and show a milder course, with dystonia characterized by diurnal fluctuation. However, the early occurrence of other neurologic symptoms in infancy and early childhood suggest that the homozygous occurrence of the affected gene may aggravate or accentuate the pathologic processes.

Furthermore, enzyme deficiency caused by recessive inheritance may cause a degenerative process, whereas that by dominant inheritance can remain stationary, manifesting as only a functional abnormality without a degenerative process. This may cause differences in clinical courses and responses to levodopa between HPD and other recessive disorders of pteridine metabolism.

REFERENCES

1. Antonini A, Leenders KL, Reist H, Thomann R, Beer H-F, Locher J. Effect of age on D$_2$ dopamine receptors in normal human brain measured by positron emission tomography and ^{11}C-raclopride. *Arch Neurol* 1993;50: 474–480.
2. Calne DB. Dopa-responsive dystonia. *Ann Neurol* 1994;35:381–382.
3. Endo K, Tanaka H, Saito M, et al. The gene for hereditary progressive dystonia with marked diurnal fluctuation (HPD) maps to chromosome 14q. In: Segawa M, Nomura Y, eds. *Age-related dopamine-dependent disorders, Monogr Neural Sci*, Vol. 14. Basel: Karger, 1995:120–125.
4. Fujimiya M, Kimura H, Maeda T. Postnatal development of serotonin nerve fibers in the somatosensory cortex of mice studied by immunohistochemistry. *J Comp Neurol* 1986;246:191–201.
5. Fujita S, Shintaku H. Etiology and pteridin metabolism abnormality of hereditary progressive dystonia with marked diurnal fluctuation (HPD: Segawa disease). *Med J Kushiro City Hosp* 1990;2:64–67.
6. Furukawa Y, Nishi K, Kondo T, Mizuno Y, Narabayashi H. CSF biopterin levels and clinical features of patients with juvenile parkinsonism. In: Narabayashi H, Nagatsu T, Yanagisawa N, et al., eds. *Advances in neurology*. Vol. 60, New York: Raven Press, 1993:562–567.
7. Furukawa Y, Shimadzu M, Rajput AH, et al. GTP-cyclohydrolase I gene mutations in hereditary progressive and dopa responsive dystonia. *Ann Neurol* 1996; 39:609–617.
8. Gibb WRG. Selective pathology, disease pathogenesis and function in the basal ganglia. In: Kimura J, Shibasaki H, eds. *Recent advances in clinical neurophysiology*. Amsterdam: Elsevier, 1996:1009–1015.
9. Graybiel AM, Ragsdale CW, Jr. Histochemically distinct compartments in the striatum of human, monkey and cat demonstrated by acetylthiocholinesterase staining. *Proc Natl Acad Sci* 1978;75:5723–5726.

10. Hanihara T, Inoue K, Kawanishi C, et al. 6-pyruvoyltetrahydropterin synthase deficiency presenting generalized dystonia with diurnal fluctuation of symptoms: a clinical and molecular study. *Mov Disord* 12:408–411,1997.
11. Hornykiewicz O. Striatal dopamine in dopa-responsive dystonia: comparison with idiopathic Parkinson's disease and other dopamine-dependent disorders. In: Segawa M, Nomura Y, eds. *Age-related dopamine-dependent disorders, Monogr Neural Sci.*, Vol. 14. Basel: Karger, 1995:101–108.
12. Hyland K, Surtees RAH, Heales SJR, Bowron A, Howells DW, Smith I. Cerebrospinal fluid concentrations of pterins and metabolites of serotonin and dopamine in a pediatric reference population. *Pediatr Res* 1993;34:10–14.
13. Ichinose H, Ohye T, Segawa M, et al. GTP cyclohydrolase I gene in hereditary progressive dystonia with marked diurnal fluctuation. *Neurosci Lett* 1995;196:5–8.
14. Ichinose H, Ohye T, Takahashi E, et al. Hereditary progressive dystonia with marked diurnal fluctuation caused by mutations in the GTP cyclohydrolase I gene. *Nat Genet* 1994;8:236–242.
15. Kato M, Hikosaka O. Function of the indirect pathway in the basal ganglion oculomotor system: visuo-oculomotor activities of external pallidum neurons. In: Segawa M, Nomura Y, eds. *Age-related dopamine-dependent disorders, Monogr Neural Sci.* Vol. 14. Basel: Karger, 1995:178–187.
16. Kato T, Yamaguchi T, Nagatsu T, et al. Effects of structures of tetrahydropterin cofactors on rat brain tryptophan hydroxylase. *Biochim Biophys Acta* 1980; 611:241–250.
17. Leenders KL, Antonini A, Meinck H-M, Weindl A. Striatal dopamine D2 receptors in dopa-responsive dystonia and Parkinson's disease. In: Segawa M, Nomura Y, eds. *Age-related dopamine-dependent disorders. Monogr Neural Sci.*, Vol. 14. Basel: Karger, 1995: 95–100.
18. McGeer EG, McGeer PL. Some characteristics of brain tyrosine hydroxylase. In: Mandel I, ed. *New concepts in neurotransmitter regulation*. New York, London: Plenum, 1973:53–68.
19. Mitchell IJ, Luquin R, Boyce S, et al. Neural mechanisms of dystonia: evidence from a 2-deoxyglucose uptake study in a primate model of dopamine agonist-induced dystonia. *Mov Disord* 1990;5:49–54.
20. Mori S, Matsuyama K, Kohyama J, Kobayashi Y, Takakuski K. Neuronal constituents of postural and locomotor control systems and their interactions in cats. *Brain Dev* 1992;14[Suppl]:S109–S120.
21. Morrison JH, Foote SL, Molliver ME, Bloom FE, Lidov HGW. Noradrenergic and serotonergic fibers innervate complementary layers in monkey primary visual cortex: an immunohistochemical study. *Proc Natl Acad Sci* 1982;79:2041–2405.
22. Neiderwieser A, Blau N, Wang M, Joller P, Atarés M, Cardesa-Garcia J. GTP cyclohydrolase I deficiency, a new enzyme defect causing hyperphenylalaninemia with neopterin, biopterin dopamine, and serotonin deficiencies and muscular hypotonia. *Eur J Pediatr* 1984; 141:208–214.
23. Nomura Y, Segawa M. Intrafamilial and interfamilial variations of symptoms of Japanese hereditary progressive dystonia with marked diurnal fluctuation. In:

Segawa M, ed. *Hereditary progressive dystonia with marked diurnal fluctuation*. Carnforth, UK: Parthenon, 1993:73–96.

24. Numata (Sudo) Y, Kato T, Nagatsu T, et al. Effects of stereochemical structures of tetrahydrobiopterin on tyrosine hydroxylase. *Biochim Biophys Acta* 1977;480: 104–112.

25. Nygaard TG, Marsden CD, Duvoisin RC. Dopa responsive dystonia. In: Fahn S, Marsden CD, Calne DB, eds. *Advances in neurology*, Vol. 50. New York: Raven Press, 1988:377–384.

26. Nygaard TG, Snow BJ, Fahn S, Calne DB. Dopa-responsive dystonia: clinical characteristics and definition. In: Segawa M, ed. *Hereditary progressive dystonia with marked diurnal fluctuation*. Carnforth, UK: Parthenon, 1993:21–35.

27. Nygaard TG, Wihelmsen KC, Risch NJ, et al. Linkage mapping of dopa-responsive dystonia (DRD) to chromosome 14q. *Nat Genet* 1993;5:386–391.

28. Phillips AG. Paper presented at the *Third International Basal Ganglia Society Meeting*, Gagliari, Italy, 1989.

29. Rajput AH, Gibb WRG, Zhong XH, et al. Dopa-responsive dystonia: pathological and biochemical observations in one case. *Ann Neurol* 1994;35:396–402.

30. Reisert I, Pilgrim C: Sexual differentiation of monoaminergic neuron genetic epigenetic. *Trends Neurosci* 1991;14:468–473.

31. Sambrook MA, Crossmann AR, Mitchell IJ. Experimental models of basal ganglia disease. In: Marsden CD, Fahn S, eds. *Movement disorders 3*. Oxford: Butterworth-Heinemann, 1994:28–45.

32. Sawle GV, Leenders KL, Brooks DJ, et al. Dopa-responsive dystonia: [F-18] Dopa positron emission tomography. *Ann Neurol* 1991;30:24–30.

33. Segawa M, Hosaka A, Miyagawa F, Nomura Y, Imai H. Hereditary progressive dystonia with marked diurnal fluctuation. In: Eldridge R, Fahn S, eds. *Advances in neurology*. Vol. 14. New York: Raven Press, 1976: 215–233.

34. Segawa M, Nomura Y. Hereditary progressive dystonia with marked diurnal fluctuation. In: Segawa M, ed. *Hereditary progressive dystonia with marked diurnal fluctuation*. Carnforth UK: Parthenon, 1993:3–19.

35. Segawa M, Nomura Y. Hereditary progressive dystonia with marked diurnal fluctuation and dopa-responsive dystonia: pathognomonic clinical features. In: Segawa M, Nomura Y, eds. *Age-related dopamine-dependent disorders, Monogr Neural Sci*. Vol. 14. Basel: Karger, 1995:10–24.

36. Segawa M, Nomura Y, Hikosaka O, et al. Roles of the basal ganglia and related structures in symptoms of dystonia. In: Carpenter MB, Jayaraman A, eds. *The basal ganglia II*. New York: Plenum, 1987:489–504.

37. Segawa M, Nomura Y, Kase M. Diurnally fluctuating hereditary progressive dystonia. In: Vinken PJ, Bruyn GW, Klawans HL, eds. *Handbook of clinical neurology, Vol. 5 (49):extrapyramidal disorders*. Amsterdam: Elsevier Biomedical, 1986:529–539.

38. Segawa M, Nomura Y, Tanaka S, et al. Hereditary progressive dystonia with marked diurnal fluctuation: consideration on its pathophysiology based on the characteristics of clinical and polysomnographical findings. In: Fahn S, Marsden CD, Calne DB, eds. *Advances in neurology*. Vol. 50. New York: Raven Press, 1988:367–376.

39. Segawa M, Nomura Y, Yamashita S, et al. Long term effects of L-Dopa on hereditary progressive dystonia with marked diurnal fluctuation. In: Berardelli A, Benecke R, Manfredi M, Marsden CD, eds. *Motor disturbance II*. London: Academic Press, 1990:305–318.

40. Segawa M, Ohmi K, Itoh S, Aoyama M, Hayakawa H. Childhood basal ganglia disease with remarkable response to L-Dopa, 'hereditary basal ganglia disease with marked diurnal fluctuation.' *Shinryo* (Tokyo) 1971; 24:667–672.

41. Shintaku H. Early diagnosis of 6-pyruvoyl-tetrahydropterin synthase deficiency. *Pteridines* 1994;5:18–27.

42. Snow BJ, Okada A, Martin WRW, Duvoisin RC, Calne DB. Positron-emission tomography scanning in dopa-responsive dystonia, parkinsonism-dystonia, and young-onset parkinsonism. In: Segawa M, ed. *Hereditary progressive dystonia with marked diurnal fluctuation*. Carnforth, UK: Parthenon, 1993:181–186.

43. Tanaka H, Endo K, Tsuji S, et al. The gene for hereditary progressive dystonia with marked diurnal fluctuation maps to chromosome 14q. *Ann Neurol* 1995;37: 405–408.

44. Tanaka K, Yoneda M, Nakajima T, Miyatake T, Owada M. Dihydrobiopterin synthesis defect: an adult with diurnal fluctuation of symptoms. *Neurology* 1987;37: 519–522.

45. van der Kooy D, Fishell G, Krushel LA. The development of striatal compartments: from proliferation to patches. In: Carpenter MB, Jayaraman A, eds. *The basal ganglia II*. New York: Plenum, 1987:81–9

Dystonia 3: Advances in Neurology, Vol. 78,
edited by S. Fahn, C. D. Marsden, and M. DeLong.
Lippincott–Raven Publishers, Philadelphia © 1998.

27

Molecular and Biochemical Aspects of Hereditary Progressive and Dopa-Responsive Dystonia

*Yoshiaki Furukawa, †Mitsunobu Shimadzu, ‡Oleh Hornykiewicz, and *Stephen J. Kish

Human Neurochemical Pathology Laboratory, Clarke Institute of Psychiatry, Toronto, Ontario M5T 1R8, Canada; †Department of Genetics, Mitsubishi Kagaku Bio-Clinical Laboratories, Inc., Itabashi-ku, Tokyo 174, Japan; and ‡Institute of Biochemical Pharmacology, University of Vienna, Vienna A-1090, Austria.

Dopa-responsive dystonia (DRD) is a disorder characterized by childhood-onset dystonia followed by parkinsonism, and a dramatic and sustained response to low doses of levodopa (L-dopa) (77). Segawa and coworkers (86) first suggested that this was a new disease entity and defined it as hereditary progressive dystonia (HPD) with marked diurnal fluctuation. HPD/DRD is inherited as an autosomal-dominant trait with sex-influenced low penetrance. Segawa and colleagues (87) hypothesized, from their clinical and polysomnographic studies, that the pathogenesis of HPD/DRD is a hypofunction of the nigrostriatal dopaminergic terminals, which is associated with reduction of tyrosine hydroxylase (TH) activity. There was, however, no evidence for a genetic linkage between HPD/DRD and the TH locus itself (17,95).

(6R)-L-Erythro-5,6,7,8-tetrahydrobiopterin (BH_4) is the natural cofactor for TH (9), tryptophan hydroxylase (58), and phenylalanine hydroxylase (44), and is synthesized as shown in Fig. 1. The former two enzymes catalyze the rate-limiting reactions in the synthesis of catecholamines (67) and serotonin (42,58), respectively. In the brain, BH_4 is highly localized in the striatum, especially in the nigrostriatal dopaminergic terminals (15,19,52,54,82). The intracellular content of BH_4 is usually near the Michaelis constant of TH, and thus BH_4 could limit TH activity in the nigrostriatal dopaminergic neurons (45,54,63). Therefore, this regulatory factor for TH was measured in cerebrospinal fluid (CSF) of HPD/DRD (16,18,25, 55,99) and an abnormality of GTP-cyclohydrolase I (GCH), which catalyzes the first step in the BH_4 biosynthetic pathway, was postulated (16,18,23,25).

This chapter summarizes recent advances in molecular and biochemical aspects in HPD/DRD with a special emphasis on our new data, namely, the status of BH_4 in the brain of genetically analyzed patients with HPD/DRD.

MOLECULAR ASPECTS

Linkage Analyses of HPD/DRD

After exclusion of the TH (17,95), DYT1 (51), or dopamine β-hydroxylase (84) gene as a causative gene for HPD/DRD, Nygaard et al. (78) mapped the HPD/DRD gene to chromosome 14q in three North American families of English or Welsh descent. Subsequently, this linkage was confirmed in at least one Japanese,

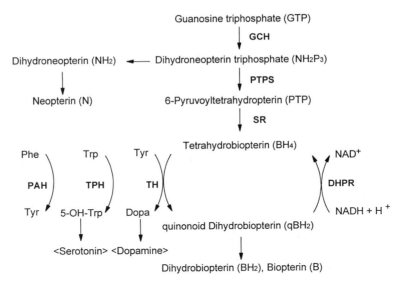

FIG. 1. Tetrahydrobiopterin (BH$_4$) biosynthetic pathway and BH$_4$-dependent hydroxylation of aromatic amino acids. Total biopterin (BP) includes BH$_4$, quinonoid dihydrobiopterin, dihydrobiopterin, and (oxidized) biopterin. Total neopterin (NP) consists of degradation products [dihydroneopterin and (oxidized) neopterin] of dihydroneopterin triphosphate. GCH, GTP-cyclohydrolase I; PTPS, 6-pyruvoyltetrahydropterin synthase; SR, sepiapterin reductase; DHPR, dihydropteridine reductase; TH, tyrosine hydroxylase; TPH, tryptophan hydroxylase; PAH, phenylalanine hydroxylase.

one German, one French-Canadian, and several English families (30,76,78,92). In contrast to early-onset dystonia in Ashkenazi Jews (10) and the X-linked form of dystonia-parkinsonism in Filipinos (28), HPD/DRD has a worldwide distribution and there is no evidence for an increased prevalence of this disease in any ethnic group. The prevalence of HPD/DRD in both Japan and England was estimated at 0.5 per million (78).

Mutations of the GCH Gene in HPD/DRD

Ichinose and colleagues (40) determined the chromosomal localization of GCH to 14q22.1-22.2 within the HPD/DRD locus, and discovered four independent mutations of the GCH gene in three familial and one sporadic Japanese HPD/DRD patients (Table 1). Subsequently, three different mutations of the GCH gene were found in Japanese patients (32,39). The human GCH gene is composed of six exons

spanning approximately 30 kilobases (38). We identified two novel nonsense mutations in exon 1 of the GCH gene and a new mutation at the 3'end of intron 1 in an autopsied case of English-Irish descent and two Japanese patients with HPD/DRD (27). This was the first report showing a mutation of the GCH gene in a non-Japanese HPD/DRD patient. The details of this clinically, pathologically, and biochemically examined case were reported by Rajput and co-workers (81). Our results suggested that the pathogenesis of HPD/DRD, among patients of different racial backgrounds, is an abnormality of GCH function due to mutations in the GCH gene. Bandmann et al. (4) and Jeon et al. (Chapter 31 of this volume) have also reported different mutations of this gene in British and Korean HPD/DRD patients, respectively. Recently, moreover, we have found a deletion [from nucleotide position 229 to 246, according to Togari et al. (94)] in exon 1 (Family 1) and a G-to-A transition at the splice acceptor site of intron 3

TABLE 1. *Mutations of the GTP-cyclohydrolase I gene in patients with hereditary progressive dystonia/dopa-responsive dystonia*

Study	Exon or Intron	Nucleotide change		Effect on coding sequence
Ichinose et al. (40)				
Family K	Exon 1	**C**GG	**T**GG	Missense mutation (Arg 88 Trp)
Family Su	Exon 2	G**A**C	G**T**C	Missense mutation (Asp 134 Val)
Family Sa	Exon 1	A^{1}TG GAG	A^{1}TG **GG** GAG	Frame shift change (G^3 ins GG)
Patient N	Exon 5	G**G**A	G**A**A	Missense mutation (Gly 201 Glu)
Hirano et al. (32)				
Patient	Intron 2	5'-**g**t	5'-**c**t	Defective splicing (Exon 2 skipping)
Ichinose et al. (39)				
Family I	Exon 4	A^{511}**TT GTA GAA ATC TAT** (13-bp del)		Frame shift change (T^{512} to A^{524} del)
Patient Y	Exon 1	C**T**G	C**C**G	Missense mutation (Leu 79 Pro)
Furukawa et al. (27)				
Patient 1	Exon 1	**G**AG	**T**AG	Nonsense mutation (Glu 65 Ter)
Patient 2	Intron 1	a**g**-3'	a**a**-3'	Defective splicing (Exon 2 skipping)
Patient 3	Exon 1	TC**A**	T**A**A	Nonsense mutation (Ser 114 Ter)
Bandmann et al. (4)				
Family Mo	Exon 1	C**G**G	C**C**G	Missense mutation (Arg 88 Pro)
Family Ro	Exon 3	C**A**T	C**C**T	Missense mutation (His 153 Pro)
Family Ha	Exon 6	C**G**A	**T**GA	Nonsense mutation (Arg 216 Ter)
Family Hu	Exon 6	A**A**A	A**G**A	Missense mutation (Lys 224 Arg)
Family Sm	Exon 6	T**T**C	T**C**C	Missense mutation (Phe 234 Ser)
Patient Be	Exon 5	**G**GG	**A**GG	Missense mutation (Gly 203 Arg)
Hirano et al. (31)				
Patient	Exon 2	CA**C**	CC**C**	Missense mutation (His 144 Pro)
Ueno et al. (96)				
Patient	Exon 1	A^{1}T**G**	A^{1}T**C**	Translation start point change (A^1 to A^{58} del)
Jeon et al. (Chapter 31, this volume)				
Family K	Exon 1	TCA	TG**A**	Nonsense mutation (Ser 114 Ter)
This study				
Family 1	Exon 1	T^{229}**CC ATC CTG AGC TCG CTG** (18-bp del)		In frame change (T^{229} to G^{246} del)
Family 2	Intron 3	a**g**-3'	a**a**-3'	Defective splicing

(Family 2) in the GCH gene among French-Canadian HPD/DRD families [Family 1 is followed by Dr. A. E. Lang (Toronto, Ontario) and Family 2 by Dr. A. Hunter (Ottawa, Ontario)]. Because the deletion in Family 1 was suspected from the direct sequencing (38,40), the polymerase chain reaction (PCR) products were subcloned into the pT7BlueT vector (Novagen) and then sequenced (27). Mutated sequences were confirmed on both identical and complementary strands.

As shown in Table 1, none of the mutations in the GCH gene in HPD/DRD reported to date (including this study) have been detected more than once, and all of the patients were heterozygous in terms of these mutations (4,27, 31,32,39,40,96, Chapter 31 of this volume). The mutations are distributed through all the exons. There are ten missense and four nonsense mutations, and one insertion as well as two deletions introducing frame shift or in frame change. A point mutation in the initiation codon, which changes the translation start point, has also been described. Furthermore, three significant point mutations in introns of the GCH gene have been found. We identified a G-to-A transition at the splice acceptor site of intron 1 and confirmed skipping of the entire exon 2 due to defective splicing [at nucleotide position 344-453 (94)] in the mature mRNA (27). This exon skipping shifts the translational reading frame and predicts a premature termination codon in exon 3. Interestingly, Hirano and associates (32) also reported the same skipping (whole exon 2) due to a G-to-C change at the splice donor site of intron 2. Both mutations abolish authentic AG and GT dinucleotides (i.e., the GT-AG rule (66), respectively). Bandmann et al. (4) discovered a G-to-C change located in the same codon as one of the mutations (Arg 88 Trp) reported by Ichinose et al. (40), but this change resulted in a different amino acid substitution (Arg 88 Pro). Recently, Jeon et al. (Chapter 31) have described a C-to-G change [at nucleotide position 341 (94)] causing a nonsense mutation (Ser 114 Ter). This is the same nucleotide position at which we found a C-to-A transversion resulting in the nonsense mutation with a different termination codon (27).

Recently, Nar and colleagues (69) reported the atomic structure of GCH from *Escherichia coli*. It was shown that GCH consists of ten identical subunits (homodecameric complex of 250 kD, a dimer of pentamers) and thus there are ten equivalent active sites (GTP binding pockets). They have suggested that His 112, His 113, and His 179 of *E. coli* GCH [corresponding to His 143, His 144, and His 210 of human GCH (62)], and the disulfide bridge between Cys 110 and Cys 181 (Cys 141 and Cys 212 of human GCH), mainly participate in catalysis at the active site. The structure-activity relationship of these amino acid residues lining the active site cavity was confirmed by measurements of the enzyme activity in the crude cell extracts of the recombinant mutant strains (70). However, none of the missense mutations in HPD/DRD, except for His 144 Pro (31), are localized in or around the active sites described above (see Table 1). Moreover, it has been shown that both Arg 88 Trp and Gly 201 Glu substitutions located outside of the GTP binding pockets can severely reduce the activity of human GCH (40). Therefore, further amino acids appear to be necessary for the complete enzyme activity, especially for human GCH.

We have also examined the GCH gene in the second autopsied case with HPD/DRD (followed by Dr. T. G. Nygaard), in which genomic DNA was extracted from brain tissue. The clinical details of this familial case, a 68-year-old Caucasian woman, are described elsewhere (75). In brief, she was the first born of identical twins. Although delivery was induced at 8 months due to maternal preeclampsia, she was normal until 12 years of age when she manifested inversion of the right foot. Her gait disturbance and equinovarus posturing gradually progressed, and postural dystonia of the left hand was also apparent after age 20. Diurnal fluctuation of the symptoms (aggravation of the symptoms toward evening and their alleviation in the morning after sleep) was observed. She was initially diagnosed as "hereditary dystonia-parkinsonism," and then successfully treated with low doses of L-dopa (100 mg/day with decarboxylase inhibitor) for more than a decade until her death due to breast cancer. Positron emission tomographic (PET) scanning using the tracer 6-fluorodopa (FD) demonstrated normal striatal FD uptake in this case (89). A preliminary neuropathologic investigation showed adequate numbers of preserved neurons with focal pigment loss and no evidence of Lewy body formation in the substantia nigra. In this HPD/DRD case, however, we could find no mutations in any of the exons and the splicing junctions of the GCH gene by DNA sequencing.

Ichinose and colleagues (39,40) studied sequencing of the GCH gene in a total of ten (eight probands and two sporadic cases) HPD/DRD families, clinically followed by Segawa and coworkers. In four probands (40%) out of these ten, they were unable to detect any mutations in the translated portion of the GCH gene. Bandmann et al. (4) have also reported that, in four familial and two sporadic cases (50%) from a total of 12 (nine familial and three sporadic cases) families, there were no mutations in the coding region of the GCH gene. Both studies included families, in whom linkage analyses showed cosegregation of the chromosome 14q region in affected members. In HPD/DRD families without mutations in the coding region, especially in the families with positive linkage to the HPD/DRD locus, it is possible to speculate that mutations are located outside the coding region but inside the 5′ regulatory, 3′ end, or intronic region of the GCH gene (38,73,94,101), or that this gene is deleted on one of the chromosomes. Another possibility is that mutations are localized in some regulatory gene(s) that has an influence on the GCH gene expression.

GCH mRNA Levels in HPD/DRD

Hirano and coworkers (32) first investigated quantitative reverse transcription PCR (RT-PCR) of non-phytohemagglutinin (PHA) stimulated lymphocytes mRNA from a 22-year-old male HPD/DRD patient and an asymptomatic carrier (his mother). Skipping of the entire exon 2 of the GCH gene due to a G-to-C change at the 5′ end of intron 2 was discovered in this family. Quantitative RT-PCR revealed that expression levels of normal GCH mRNA in terms of the ratio of wild-type GCH/β actin mRNA were low in the patient (0.62) and his asymptomatic mother (0.71) compared with controls (1.08 ±0.12; mean ±2 SD). Moreover, they indicated that the ratio of mutant/wild-type GCH mRNA in the patient (0.28) was higher than that in the asymptomatic carrier (0.083). Independently, our RT-PCR Southern blot analysis of PHA stimulated mononuclear blood cells, showed that the ratio of mutant/wild-type GCH mRNA (estimated by densitometer) was 0.17 in an HPD/DRD patient having the same exon 2 skipping (27). These results have suggested that the reason carriers do not manifest any symptoms (while they have one mutant allele) is partly explained by such a low level of the ratio of mutant/wild-type GCH mRNA compared with HPD/DRD patients. Recently, Hirano et al. (31) have examined another HPD/DRD family with His 144 Pro substitution of the GCH gene, and also found that the ratio of mutant/wild-type GCH mRNA in a female patient (0.97) was higher than that in an asymptomatic carrier (her father) (0.80). They attributed the disparity of degree of the differences between the ratios in the affected and asymptomatic persons in their two families to the mutation differences (i.e., the frame shift change as a result of the defective splicing and the missense mutation).

GCH Deficiency with Autosomal-Recessive Trait

At least 12 patients with GCH deficiency with autosomal-recessive (AR) trait have been listed in the international database of BH_4 deficiencies (6). These patients develop hyperphenylalaninemia and neurologic symptoms, including mental retardation, developmental delay, trunk hypotonia, limb hypertonia, tremors, and convulsions (6,7,13,38,71,72,85). Since identification of the GCH gene as a causative gene for HPD/DRD, there has been one report in which dystonic movement responding to L-dopa in AR GCH deficiency was described (7). Ichinose and associates (7,38) sequenced the GCH gene in two patients with AR GCH deficiency including the patient with dystonic movement and identified missense mutations on both alleles of each patient. These mutation sites were different from those discovered in HPD/DRD. One had a G-to-A transition causing an amino acid substitution of methionine at codon 211 with isoleucine (Met 211 Ile), and the other showed a G-to-A transition resulting in Arg 184 His. Introduction of these mutated enzymes into a prokaryotic expression system [the same system employed in the HPD/DRD study (40)] confirmed a complete loss of GCH activity, indicating that there was no qualitative difference between the mutations in AR GCH deficiency and those (Arg 88 Trp and Gly 201 Glu) in HPD/DRD (38,40). Interestingly, in contrast to most mutations in HPD/DRD, both mutations in AR GCH deficiency are located around amino acids relating to the GTP binding pockets [Arg 184 and Met 211 of human GCH correspond to Arg 153 and Tyr 180 of *E. coli* GCH, respectively (62)] proposed by Nar and coworkers (69,70).

Autosomal-Recessive Dystonias Responding to L-dopa

Lüdecke and colleagues (60) described a point mutation in exon 11 of the TH gene (C-to-A change resulting in Gln 381 Lys) in a Caucasian family with dystonia responding to L-dopa. In this family, two affected children were homozygous and the healthy parents as well as the normal sister were heterozygous for the mutation (AR inheritance). Subsequently, the same group (49) reported that the specific activity (being measured at tyrosine concentrations prevailing *in vivo*) of the mutated enzyme was approximately 15% of the wild-type form in the coupled *in vitro* transcription-translation assay system. Recently, Lüdecke et al. (61) have also identified a T-to-C transition in exon 5 (Leu 205 Pro) of the TH gene in a Greek girl (homozygote), who developed parkinsonism responding to L-dopa, ptosis, trunk hypotonia,

and myoclonic jerks, in her early infancy. Thus, there is a remarkable heterogeneity of clinical phenotypes in AR TH deficiency.

Marked diurnal fluctuation is one of the characteristics of HPD/DRD. However, at least three patients who showed dystonia responding to L-dopa with this phenomenon as a result of enzyme deficiency in the BH$_4$ synthesis, but not GCH deficiency, have been reported (16,29,93). An abnormal function of 6-pyruvoyltetrahydropterin synthase (PTPS), which catalyzes the second step in the BH$_4$ biosynthetic pathway (see Fig. 1), may be causative for these patients. Mutations of the PTPS gene have only been discovered to be recessive, and the gene structure consisting of six exons has been identified (2,29,43,48, 57,79). Recently, Hanihara et al. (29) have found an A-to-G transition in the PTPS gene introducing an amino acid substitution of isoleucine with valine at position 114 (Ile 114 Val) in one of the three dystonia patients mentioned above. The main clinical feature of this patient (a 44-year-old Japanese woman) was generalized dystonia with diurnal fluctuation, and other features, such as convulsions, mental retardation, and hyperphenylalaninemia, were mild despite no treatment until age 41. She showed dramatic and sustained response to L-dopa administration. In contrast, although Ashida et al. (2) reported the same point mutation (A-to-G change resulting in Ile 114 Val) in a Japanese boy, symptoms of this patient were relatively severe and there was no description of dystonia. Clinical manifestations of PTPS deficiency usually resemble those of AR GCH deficiency, and no correlation has yet been detected between mutations in this gene and various clinical phenotypes (1,2,29,43,48,57,79, 85). PTPS appears to have significant function in the BH$_4$ metabolism, especially in humans, and may be the rate-limiting enzyme in the BH$_4$ biosynthesis in the human, whereas in nonhuman mammals, GCH is considered to be the rate-limiting enzyme (7,38). There might be autosomal-dominant BH$_4$ deficient families, who develop dystonia responding to L-dopa but not hyperphenylalaninemia, due to mutations in the genes coding for BH$_4$ biosynthetic enzymes (especially, PTPS) other than GCH.

Other AR dystonias with diurnal fluctuation that respond to L-dopa (dihydropteridine reductase deficiency, etc.) appear in Chapter 26 of this volume.

BIOCHEMICAL ASPECTS

Blood Analyses

Because basal GCH activity in mononuclear blood cells is too low to be measured, Ichinose and colleagues (40) determined the enzyme activity after stimulation of the cells with PHA according to the method of Blau et al. (8). In six patients from four HPD/DRD families and one sporadic patient as well as two asymptomatic carriers, they measured the GCH activity. The HPD/DRD patients were found to have only 2% to 19% of mean control value, whereas the carriers showed 36% and 37%. Blau et al. (8) demonstrated that, in a family with AR GCH deficiency, no GCH activity in PHA stimulated mononuclear cells could be detected in a patient (homozygote), while the enzyme activities were reduced to 30% and 46% of controls in the asymptomatic father and mother (obligate heterozygotes), respectively. It was also confirmed that this patient had no GCH activity in the liver biopsy specimens (72).

Recently, Levine and coworkers (53) have established a new assay system of GCH activity by using lymphoblastoid cell lines. In affected members and asymptomatic carriers of a HPD/DRD family, the GCH activity in these cell lines was 20% to 50% of normal controls. Responses to different stimulations of the enzyme (i.e., PHA, interferon-γ plus lipopolysaccharide, etc.) in these cell lines detected from the family members and controls were variable (Chapter 29 of this volume).

Cerebrospinal Fluid Analyses

For the early and correct diagnosis of HPD/DRD, simultaneous measurement of CSF total biopterin (BP) and neopterin (NP) has been recommended (22,23,25,27). Total BP includes BH_4, quinonoid dihydrobiopterin, dihydrobiopterin and (oxidized) biopterin (see Fig. 1), and most of BP in the brain exists as BH_4 (19,54). Total NP consists of degradation products [dihydroneopterin and (oxidized) neopterin] of dihydroneopterin triphosphate, which is the first intermediate in the biosynthesis of BH_4 from GTP. More than 70% of NP in CSF exists as the dihydro form (34,35,97). Both BP and NP in CSF can be measured according to the method of Fukushima and Nixon (19), that is, iodine oxidation under acidic conditions and subsequent quantitation by reverse-phase high performance liquid chromatography with fluorescence detection.

It is known that BP is highly concentrated in the striatum (15,19,52,54,82), and that there is a positive correlation between levels of BP and TH activity in the caudate nucleus of controls and parkinsonian patients (68). A rostrocaudal gradient for BP value in CSF and a significant positive correlation between CSF BP and homovanillic acid levels have been demonstrated (21,24,59). It has been suggested, therefore, that BP in CSF is derived from the brain and that decreased CSF BP concentrations in patients with Parkinson's disease (PD) mainly reflect degeneration of the nigrostriatal dopaminergic neurons (21,24,25,59). Although increased CSF NP levels have received much attention as a sensitive biochemical marker for inflammation within the CNS (26,35), the functional significance of NP in the brain is still unknown. Sawada et al. (82) measured neopterin derivatives (including dihydroneopterin triphosphate after phosphatase treatment) in human brain, and found that neopterin derivatives were distributed differently from BP and not concentrated in monoaminergic neurons.

As shown in Table 2, there have been at least five reports in which both CSF BP and NP levels in each HPD/DRD patient were individually described, and all of the patients showed very low BP and NP concentrations (16,18,25,27,90). However, because CSF BP levels are also significantly reduced in patients with PD as well as early-onset parkinsonism, BP in CSF alone cannot be a biochemical marker for

TABLE 2. *CSF total biopterin (BP) and neopterin (NP) levels in patients with hereditary progressive dystonia/dopa-responsive dystonia*

Study	Sex	Age (yr) at onset	Age (yr) at CSF analysis	BP (pmol/ml)		NP (pmol/ml)	Normal values (pmol/ml)
Fink et al. (16)							
Case 1	F	<6	26	4.0		4.4	BP; 20.6 ± 1.4
Case 2	F	<5	31	4.2		4.8	NP; 22.6 ± 1.5
Case 3	M	1.5	8	2.2		3.3	(mean ± SD)
Case 4	M	1.5	5	3.2		2.4	
Fujita and Shintaku (18)							
Patient	F	5	19	3.6		3.4	BP; 10.0–26.0
							NP; 9.0–20.0
Furukawa et al. (25)							
Case 1	F	3	6	7.1		4.4	BP; 13.3 ± 0.5
Case 2	F	8	15	(9 A.M.)	5.9	4.3	NP; 25.9 ± 1.8
				(9 P.M.)	5.5	5.1	(mean ± SE)
Takahashi et al. (90)							
Case 3-1	F	3.5	12	3.3		3.3	BP; 20.6 ± 1.4
Case 3-2	M	<1.5	9	6.9		3.9	NP; 22.6 ± 1.5
Case 2-4 (carrier)	M	—	34	6.7		8.0	(mean ± SD)
Furukawa et al. (27)							
Patient 3	M	6	8	5.9		8.9	BP; 13.6 ± 0.6
							NP; 24.1 ± 1.6
							(mean ± SE)

HPD/DRD (21,22,24,25,56,59, 100). Fink and coworkers (16) first reported a decrease of CSF NP in HPD/DRD. Fujita and Shintaku (18) described an HPD/DRD patient who demonstrated decreased NP and BP concentrations in CSF, but not in serum or urine. Furukawa and colleagues (22) measured CSF NP levels in patients with essential tremor, PD, early-onset parkinsonism with dystonia, HPD/ DRD, and other types of dystonia (dopa-nonresponsive dystonia), and found a marked reduction of NP content in only the HPD/DRD patients. We have confirmed reduced CSF NP concentrations in genetically proven patients with HPD/DRD (27). It has been reported, moreover, that only AR GCH deficiency showed decreased CSF NP content among BH_4 deficiencies with AR trait (6,85), and that patients with AR GCH deficiency had no detectable GCH activity in liver biopsy specimens (7,72). Thus, CSF NP appears to reflect, at least in part, GCH activity in the brain, and the measurement of NP content in CSF may be useful for the diagnosis of HPD/DRD. However, because of the known influence of age (20,22,25, 27,36,55,56,88) and immune status (26,35,97, 98) on NP, it is necessary to have age-matched controls and exclude samples with infections, when a patient is diagnosed as HPD/DRD by using CSF NP data.

We compared mean CSF NP and BP concentrations in three HPD/DRD patients (6 to 15 years) with those in five normal age-matched controls (8 to 19 years) (25,27). At the time of CSF collection, none of the patients or the controls had inflammatory diseases, and all lumbar punctures were performed at 9 to 10 A.M. The 2nd to 4th ml of CSF was used for the analyses. The mean CSF NP level in the HPD/DRD patients (5.9 ±1.5 pmol/ml, mean ±SE; range, 4.3 to 8.9) was significantly lower than that in the age-matched controls (15.8 ±1.5; p <0.005 by Student's two-tailed t test; range, 13.0 to 21.1) (Fig. 2). The mean CSF BP level in the patients (6.3 ±0.4 pmol/ml; range, 5.9 to 7.1) was also significantly reduced compared with the controls (11.9 ±0.8; p <0.005; range, 9.9 to 14.4).

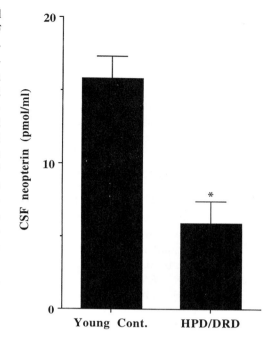

FIG. 2. The mean (±SE) total neopterin levels in CSF of three patients with hereditary progressive dystonia/dopa-responsive dystonia (HPD/DRD) and five age-matched young controls (Young Cont.) (25,27). *p <0.005, for the difference from the young controls (Student's two-tailed t test).

Brain Analyses

It is known that, in autopsied PD brains, loss of dopamine (DA) in the putamen is more severe than that in the caudate nucleus (5,46,47, 74), and that there exists a characteristic rostrocaudal pattern of DA loss in each striatal subdivision, that is, the rostral portion of the caudate is more severely affected than the caudal portion and the opposite rostrocaudal gradient is found in the putamen (46,47,74). In the first autopsied case with HPD/DRD (Case 1), Rajput and coworkers (81) showed the similar interregional caudate/putamen pattern and striatal subregional rostrocaudal patterns of DA loss, and also demonstrated decreased levels of TH protein as well as TH activity in the striatum. In contrast to PD, however, in the substantia nigra of HPD/DRD Case 1, TH protein content was well preserved and TH immunoreactivity was normal, despite the considerable reduction of DA content. The nigral cell populations appeared normal except for reduced melanin content.

We have measured BP and NP concentrations in the putamen of Case 1 and the second autopsied case (Case 2) with HPD/DRD. Because Case 1 was 19 years and Case 2 was 68 years, we also analyzed three young controls (mean age, 22.0 years) and three elderly controls (72.0 years) with no neurologic, psychiatric, or inflammatory disease. Both BP and NP levels in the brain tissue were determined according to the method of Fukushima and Nixon (19) with slight modifications.

In the putamen of Cases 1 and 2, BP concentrations were markedly reduced as compared with mean BP levels in the young and elderly controls, respectively (Fig. 3). Concentrations of NP in the putamen of Cases 1 and 2 were also substantially lower than mean NP levels in the young and elderly controls, respectively (Fig. 4). The mean BP level in the elderly controls was lower than the young controls, whereas the mean NP level in the elderly controls was higher than the young controls. In both cases, the magnitude of reduction of BP

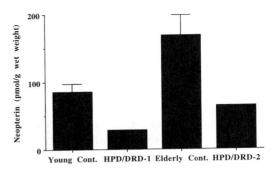

FIG. 4. The total neopterin (NP) levels in the putamen of hereditary progressive dystonia/dopa-responsive dystonia Cases 1 and 2 (HPD/DRD-1, HPD/DRD-2), and the mean ($\pm$SE) NP levels in the putamen of three young and three elderly controls (Young Cont., Elderly Cont.)

was more severe than that of NP. In Case 1, the BP and NP values were decreased to 17% and 34% of the young controls. In Case 2, the concentration of BP was reduced to 15% of the elderly controls, and that of NP was reduced to 38%. As mentioned above, NP in CSF may reflect the GCH activity in the brain, and in the HPD/DRD patients, the mean CSF NP level was reduced to 37% of the age-matched controls (see Fig. 2). This percentage was compatible with those of the NP concentrations in the putamen of Cases 1 and 2.

Because HPD/DRD patients are heterozygotes for mutations in the GCH gene, NP levels in the brain and CSF were expected to be reduced to about 50% of control values. In adult heterozygous mice obtained by targeted disruption of the TH gene, however, levels of TH activity were decreased to 38% of wild-type mice in both whole brain and adrenal glands (50). Levine and associates (53) have reported that, in lymphoblastoid cell lines detected from HPD/DRD patients and asymptomatic carriers, levels of the GCH activity were 20% to 50% of normal controls. These results, including our NP data in the HPD/DRD brain and CSF, suggest that the GCH activity in HPD/DRD is reduced to approximately 30% to 40% of age-matched controls due to congenital partial

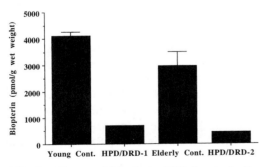

FIG. 3. The total biopterin (BP) levels in the putamen of hereditary progressive dystonia/dopa-responsive dystonia Cases 1 and 2 (HPD/ DRD-1, HPD/DRD-2), and the mean ($\pm$SE) BP levels in the putamen of three young and three elderly controls (Young Cont., Elderly Cont.).

GCH deficiency. Such a degree of reduction of the GCH activity in the liver appears to be sufficient to provide the usual BH_4 requirement of phenylalanine hydroxylase, but not sufficient to tolerate the phenylalanine loading test. Therefore, although HPD/DRD patients never have hyperphenylalaninemia, they usually show slow clearance of phenylalanine from plasma after the loading test (37).

The more severe depletion of BP than NP observed in the HPD/DRD putamen suggests that there may be a combination of mildly decreased nigrostriatal dopaminergic terminals due to abnormal development (either insufficient arborization or greater than normal retraction) and the congenital GCH deficiency. Because BP is highly concentrated in the putamen and localized in the nigrostriatal dopaminergic terminals (15,19,52,54,82), even a mild reduction of the terminal tree (either incomplete establishment or excessive regression) may result in the decrease of putaminal BP. In contrast, because the brain distribution of NP is not parallel with BP and relatively homogeneous (82), and NP usually leaks out of the cells and easily diffuses (97,98), putaminal NP content may not be significantly influenced by the terminal reduction owing to abnormal development. Rajput and coworkers (81) reported that, in the putamen of Case 1, the binding of [^{3}H]GBR 12935 to the DA transporter was at the lower end of control range. Sawle and colleagues (83) analyzed FD-PET scanning in HPD/DRD patients and, in contrast to normal putaminal FD uptake observed by Snow et al. (89), they found moderately but significantly decreased mean putaminal FD uptake in their patients. Various trophic agents (including DA) have been suggested to be crucial for dopaminergic neuronal development and function (12,14), and BH_4 itself might have such a trophic-factor-like activity. Before discovery of the GCH gene as a causative gene for HPD/DRD, Hornykiewicz (33) speculated that an inborn or developmental abnormality of a trophic factor may be involved in etiopathology of HPD/DRD. Recently, Kang et al. (Chapter 32 of this volume) found that BH_4 stabilizes TH protein and increases its half-life

following *in vivo* grafting of nonneuronal cells, in which both GCH and TH genes are expressed, into the denervated rat striatum.

As described above, HPD/DRD Case 2 had no mutations in the coding region (including the splicing junctions) of the GCH gene by DNA sequencing of all the exons, whereas Case 1 showed the nonsense mutation in exon 1 of this gene (27). However, neither the magnitude of reduction relative to the age-matched controls of BP nor that of NP in Case 1 differed from those in Case 2. These biochemical findings suggest that there is no quantitative difference in terms of BH_4 synthesis in the putamen between HPD/DRD patients with and without mutations in the coding region of the GCH gene. Similarly, Ichinose et al. (39,40) reported that there was no difference of GCH activity levels in PHA-stimulated mononuclear cells between HPD/DRD patients having mutations in the translated portion of the GCH gene and those not having the mutation.

MOLECULAR AND BIOCHEMICAL DIAGNOSTIC APPROACH TO HPD/DRD

Because the clinical differentiation between HPD/DRD and early-onset parkinsonism with dystonia (EOP-D) (22) is difficult (especially in the early course of the disorder), we previously examined the GCH gene in EOP-D patients whose age at onset was 6 and 8 years (27). We could find no mutations in any of the exons and the splicing junctions of the GCH gene in these two patients. We have also examined the TH gene in these patients, and could not detect the mutations (Gln 381 Lys and Leu 205 Pro) reported by Lüdecke et al. (60,61) in this gene (unpublished data). Although clinical features of EOP-D are relatively homogeneous, pathologic findings of EOP-D are known to be heterogeneous and not identical to typical Lewy body PD pathology (22,27,64,65,91,102,103, 104). Recently, microsatellite polymorphism analyses in some Japanese EOP-D families (AR trait) have suggested the linkage on chromosome 6q (H. Matsumine, personal communication, 1996). Bandmann et al. (3) analyzed the GCH gene in 29 parkinsonian patients (including familial patients) and four autopsied brains with clinical diagnosis of PD but without pathologic features. No mutations in the GCH gene were also identified in these parkinsonian cases. Very recently, genetic markers on chromosome 4q21-q23 have shown linkage to an autosomal-dominant PD phenotype (80).

Because there have been no common mutations of the GCH gene in HPD/DRD patients (see Table 1), complete sequencing of all of the exons is necessary to detect a possible mutation in each clinically suspected HPD/DRD patient. Furthermore, even if this is conducted, mutations in the translated portion of this gene would not be found in approximately 40% to 50% of patients with HPD/DRD (4,39,40). In these patients, who have no mutations in the coding region of the GCH gene, the effort to detect a significant mutation in noncoding promoter or intronic region of the GCH gene (38, 73,94,101) is needed. This makes the screening of the GCH gene time-consuming, and thus the present DNA testing for HPD/DRD is not suitable for routine clinical practice.

Ichinose and associates (40,41) measured GCH activity in PHA-stimulated mononuclear blood cells in HPD/DRD and early-onset parkinsonian patients, and found decreased activity in HPD/DRD and normal activity in early-onset parkinsonism. As mentioned, however, it has been shown that responses to different enzyme stimulations (including PHA) in lymphoblastoid cell lines detected from HPD/DRD patients and controls were not constant (53, Chaper 29 of this volume). Hyland et al. (37) demonstrated usefulness of phenylalanine loading test for the diagnosis of HPD/DRD; however, this was not confirmed in another study (11). In contrast to these diagnostic tools, to our knowledge, there have been no negative reports on the results of CSF NP analysis (reduced NP concentrations) in HPD/DRD patients (see Table 2). Data of CSF in an obligate carrier also showed a considerable reduction of NP (90). Bandmann et al. (4) measured CSF NP concentrations in an HPD/DRD family, and found decreased NP levels in family members with a mutation of the GCH gene but not in a member without the mutation (CSF BP levels were not measured). The measurement of CSF NP concentration has been shown to be useful for

the differential diagnoses among HPD/DRD (decreased), EOP-D or PD (normal), and PTPS deficiency (increased) (6,22,25,27,85). Moreover, we have confirmed substantial decreases of putaminal NP levels in HPD/DRD Cases 1 and 2. Thus, decreased CSF NP content (compared with age-matched controls, see Fig. 2) appears to have value as a biochemical marker for HPD/ DRD.

CONCLUSIONS

The accumulated molecular and biochemical evidence suggests the following.

1. Among HPD/DRD families, no single mutation of the GCH gene has been detected in more than one family, and approximately 40% to 50% of families have no mutations in the coding region (including the splicing junctions) of this gene. Thus, the present genetic testing for HPD/DRD is unlikely to be suitable for routine clinical practice.
2. In the putamen of HPD/DRD patients, both BP and NP concentrations are decreased to less than 50% of age-matched controls, findings which can be explained by a reduction of GCH activity due to congenital partial GCH deficiency.
3. The cause of HPD/DRD is a substantial reduction of brain BH_4 synthesis.
4. There appears to be no quantitative difference in terms of putaminal BH_4 synthesis (compared with age-matched controls) between typical HPD/DRD patients with and without mutations in the coding region of the GCH gene.
5. Measurement of CSF NP content is useful for the diagnosis of HPD/DRD.

ACKNOWLEDGMENTS

We wish to thank L. W. Morris, L. J. Chang, and K. S. Shannak for their technical support.

NOTE ADDED IN PROOF

Since submission of this manuscript, we have found the mutant GCH mRNA with skipping of the entire exon 4 due to defective splicing and the wild-type mRNA in Family 2 (21a).

REFERENCES

1. Aqeel AA, Ozand PT, Gascon G, et al. Biopterin-dependent hyperphenylalaninemia due to deficiency of 6-pyruvoyl tetrahydropterin synthase. *Neurology* 1991;41:730–737.

2. Ashida A, Owada M, Hatakeyama K. A missense mutation (A to G) of 6-pyruvoyltetrahydropterin synthase in tetrahydrobiopterin-deficient form of hyperphenylalaninemia. *Genomics* 1994;24:408–410.

3. Bandmann O, Daniel S, Marsden CD, Wood NW, Harding AE. The GTP-cyclohydrolase I gene in atypical parkinsonian patients. *J Neurol Sci* 1996;141: 27–32.

4. Bandmann O, Nygaard TG, Surtees R, Marsden CD, Wood NW, Harding AE. Dopa-responsive dystonia in British patients: new mutations of GTP-cyclohydrolase I gene and evidence for genetic heterogeneity. *Hum Mol Genet* 1996;5:403–406.

5. Bernheimer H, Birkmayer W, Hornykiewicz O, Jellinger K, Seitelberger F. Brain dopamine and the syndromes of Parkinson and Huntington. *J Neurol Sci* 1973;20:415–455.

6. Blau N, Barnes I, Dhondt JL. International database of tetrahydrobiopterin deficiencies. *J Inher Metab Dis* 1996;19:8–14.

7. Blau N, Ichinose H, Nagatsu T, Heizmann CW, Zacchello F, Burlina B. A missense mutation in a patient with guanosine triphosphate cyclohydrolase I deficiency missed in the newborn screening program. *J Pediatr* 1995;126:401–405.

8. Blau N, Joller P, Atarés M, Cardesa-Garcia J, Niederwieser A. Increase of GTP cyclohydrolase I activity in mononuclear blood cells by stimulation: detection of heterozygotes of GTP cyclohydrolase I deficiency. *Clin Chim Acta* 1985;148:47–52.

9. Brenneman AR, Kaufman S. The role of tetrahydropteridines in the enzymatic conversion of tyrosine to 3,4-dihydroxyphenylalanine. *Biochem Biophys Res Commun* 1964;17:177–183.

10. Bressman SB, Leon D, Kramer PL, et al. Dystonia in Ashkenazi Jews; clinical characterization of a founder mutation. *Ann Neurol* 1994;36:771–777.

11. Brique S, Dhondt JL, Destée A. Hepatic activity of GTP cyclohydrolase I is not limited in dopa-responsive dystonia disease. *Mov Disord* 1996;11[Suppl 1]:221.

12. Casper D. Growth factors and dopaminergic neurons. In: Stone TW, ed. *CNS neurotransmitters and neuromodulators dopamine.* Boca Raton, Florida: CRC Press, 1996: 131–163.

13. Dhondt JL, Farriaux JP, Boudha A, et al. Neonatal hyperphenylalaninemia presumably caused by guanosine triphosphate-cyclohydrolase deficiency. *J Pediatr* 1985;106:954–956.

14. Du X, Iacovitti L. Synergy between growth factors and transmitters required for catecholamine differentiation in brain neurons. *J Neurosci* 1995;15:5420–5427.

15. Duch DS, Bowers SW, Woolf JH, Nichol CA. Biopterin cofactor biosynthesis: GTP cyclohydrolase, neopterin and biopterin in tissues and body fluids of mammalian species. *Life Sci* 1984;35:1895–1901.

16. Fink JK, Barton N, Cohen W, Lovenberg W, Burns RS, Hallett M. Dystonia with marked diurnal variation associated with biopterin deficiency. *Neurology* 1988;38:707–711.

17. Fletcher NA, Holt IJ, Harding AE, Nygaard TG, Mallet J, Marsden CD. Tyrosine hydroxylase and levodopa responsive dystonia. *J Neurol Neurosurg Psychiatry* 1989;52:112–114.

18. Fujita S, Shintaku H. The pathogenesis of hereditary progressive dystonia with marked diurnal fluctuation (HPD) and a metabolic abnormality of pteridines. *Kushiro J Med* 1990;2:64–67.

19. Fukushima T, Nixon JC. Analysis of reduced forms of biopterin in biological tissues and fluids. *Anal Biochem* 1980;102:176–188.

20. Furukawa Y, Kondo T, Nishi K, et al. Total biopterin and neopterin levels in the ventricular CSF of patients with Parkinson's disease. In: Nagatsu T, Fisher A, Yoshida M, eds. *Basic, clinical, and therapeutic aspects of Alzheimer's and Parkinson's diseases, Vol 2.* New York: Plenum Press, 1990:49–52.

21. Furukawa Y, Kondo T, Nishi K, Yokochi F, Narabayashi H. Total biopterin levels in the ventricular CSF of patients with Parkinson's disease; a comparison between akineto-rigid and tremor types. *J Neurol Sci* 1991;103:232–237.

21a. Furukawa Y, Lang AE, Trugman JM, et al. Gender-related penetrance and de novo GTP-cyclohydrolase I gene mutations in dopa-reponsive dystonia. *Neurology* 1998;50:1015–1020.

22. Furukawa Y, Mizuno Y, Narabayashi H. Early-onset parkinsonism with dystonia; clinical and biochemical differences from hereditary progressive dystonia or dopa-responsive dystonia. *Adv Neurol* 1996; 69:327–337.

23. Furukawa Y, Mizuno Y, Nishi K, Narabayashi H. A clue to the pathogenesis of dopa-responsive dystonia. *Ann Neurol* 1995;37:139–140.

24. Furukawa Y, Nishi K, Kondo T, Mizuno Y, Narabayashi H. Juvenile parkinsonism; ventricular CSF biopterin levels and clinical features. *J Neurol Sci* 1992;108:207–213.

25. Furukawa Y, Nishi K, Kondo T, Mizuno Y, Narabayashi H. CSF biopterin levels and clinical features of patients with juvenile parkinsonism. *Adv Neurol* 1993;60:562–567.

26. Furukawa Y, Nishi K, Kondo T, Tanabe K, Mizuno Y. Significance of CSF total neopterin and biopterin in inflammatory neurological diseases. *J Neurol Sci* 1992;111:65–72.

27. Furukawa Y, Shimadzu M, Rajput AH, et al. GTP-cyclohydrolase I gene mutations in hereditary progressive and dopa-responsive dystonia. *Ann Neurol* 1996; 39:609–617.

28. Graeber MB, Kupke KG, Müller U. Delineation of the dystonia-parkinsonism syndrome locus in Xq13. *Proc Natl Acad Sci USA* 1992;89:8245–8248.

29. Hanihara T, Inoue K, Kawanishi C, et al. 6-Pyruvoyltetrahydropterin synthase deficiency presenting generalized dystonia with diurnal fluctuation of symptoms; a clinical and molecular study. *Mov Disord* 1997; 12: 408–411.

30. Heberlein I, Vieregge P, Steinberger D, Wauschkuhn B, Nitschke M, Müller U. A new family with dopa-responsive dystonia and linkage mapping to chromosome 14q; dopa-responsive neuropsychology. *Ann Neurol* 1995;38:300.

31. Hirano M, Tamaru Y, Ito H, Matsumoto S, Imai T, Ueno S. Mutant GTP cyclohydrolase I mRNA levels contribute to dopa-responsive dystonia onset. *Ann Neurol* 1996;40:796–798.

32. Hirano M, Tamaru Y, Nagai Y, Ito H, Imai T, Ueno S. Exon skipping caused by a base substitution at a splice site in the GTP cyclohydrolase I gene in a Japanese family with hereditary progressive dystonia/dopa-responsive dystonia. *Biochem Biophys Res Commun* 1995;213:645–651.

33. Hornykiewicz O. Striatal dopamine in dopa-responsive dystonia: comparison with idiopathic Parkinson's disease and other dopamine-dependent disorders. In: Segawa M, Nomura Y, eds. *Age-related dopamine-dependent disorders*. Basel: Karger, 1995:101–108.

34. Howells DW, Smith I, Hyland K. Estimation of tetrahydrobiopterin and other pterins in cerebrospinal fluid using reverse-phase high-performance liquid chromatography. *J Chromatogr* 1986; 381:285–294.

35. Howells DW, Smith I, Hyland K. Dihydroneopterin and CNS infections. *Lancet* 1987;2:686–687.

36. Hyland K, Surtees RAH, Heales SJR, Bowron A, Howells DW, Smith I. Cerebrospinal fluid concentrations of pterins and metabolites of serotonin and dopamine in a pediatric reference population. *Pediatr Res* 1993;34:10–14.

37. Hyland K, Trugman JM, Rost-Ruffner E, et al. Abnormal phenylalanine metabolism in dopa-responsive dystonia: a possible diagnostic test. *Neurology* 1996;46[Suppl 1]:A273.

38. Ichinose H, Ohye T, Matsuda Y, et al. Characterization of mouse and human GTP cyclohydrolase I genes; mutations in patients with GTP cyclohydrolase I deficiency. *J Biol Chem* 1995;270:10062–10071.

39. Ichinose H, Ohye T, Segawa M, et al. GTP cyclohydrolase I gene in hereditary progressive dystonia with marked diurnal fluctuation. *Neurosci Lett* 1995;196: 5–8.

40. Ichinose H, Ohye T, Takahashi E, et al. Hereditary progressive dystonia with marked diurnal fluctuation caused by mutations in the GTP cyclohydrolase I gene. *Nat Genet* 1994;8:236–242.

41. Ichinose H, Ohye T, Yokochi M, Fujita K, Nagatsu T. GTP cyclohydrolase I activity in mononuclear blood cells in juvenile parkinsonism. *Neurosci Lett* 1995; 190:140–142.

42. Ichiyama A, Nakamura S, Nishizuka Y, Hayaishi O. Enzymic studies on the biosynthesis of serotonin in mammalian brain. *J Biol Chem* 1970;245:1699–1709.

43. Imamura T, Okano Y, Sawada Y, et al. A missense mutation of 6-pyruvoyl-tetrahydropterin synthase deficiency in Japanese. *Pteridines* 1994;5:31.

44. Kaufman S. The structure of the phenylalanine-hydroxylation cofactor. *Proc Natl Acad Sci USA* 1963; 50:1085–1093.

45. Kettler R, Bartholini G, Pletscher A. In vivo enhancement of tyrosine hydroxylation in rat striatum by tetrahydrobiopterin. *Nature* 1974;249:476–478.

46. Kish SJ, Shannak K, Hornykiewicz O. Uneven pattern of dopamine loss in the striatum of patients with idiopathic Parkinson's disease. *N Engl J Med* 1988; 318:876–880.

47. Kish SJ, Shannak K, Rajput A, Deck JHN, Hornykiewicz O. Aging produces a specific pattern of striatal dopamine loss: implications for the etiology of idiopathic Parkinson's disease. *J Neurochem* 1992; 58:642–648.

48. Kluge C, Brecevic L, Heizmann CW, Blau N, Thöny B. Chromosomal localization, genomic structure and characterization of the human gene and a retropseudogene for 6-pyruvoyltetrahydropterin synthase. *Eur J Biochem* 1996;240:477–484.

49. Knappskog PM, Flatmark T, Mallet J, Lüdecke B, Bartholomé K. Recessively inherited L-DOPA-responsive dystonia caused by a point mutation (Q381K) in the tyrosine hydroxylase gene. *Human Mol Genet* 1995;4:1209–1212.

50. Kobayashi K, Morita S, Sawada H, et al. Targeted disruption of the tyrosine hydroxylase locus results in severe catecholamine depletion and perinatal lethality in mice. *J Biol Chem* 1995;270:27235–27243.

51. Kwiatkowski DJ, Nygarrd TG, Schuback DE, et al. Identification of highly polymorphic microsatellite VNTR within the argininosuccinate synthetase locus: exclusion of the dystonia gene on 9q32-34 as the cause of dopa-responsive dystonia in a large kindred. *Am J Hum Genet* 1991;48:121–128.

52. Levine RA, Kuhn DM, Lovenberg W. The regional distribution of hydroxylase cofactor in rat brain. *J Neurochem* 1979;32:1575–1578.

53. Levine RA, Bezin L, Flam MD, et al. Lymphoblast GTP cyclohydrolase I activity in dopa-responsive dystonia. *Soc Neurosci Abstr* 1996;22:229.

54. Levine RA, Miller LP, Lovenberg W. Tetrahydrobiopterin in striatum; localization in dopamine nerve terminals and role in catecholamine synthesis. *Science* 1981;214:919–921.

55. LeWitt PA, Miller LP, Levine RA, et al. Tetrahydrobiopterin in dystonia; identification of abnormal metabolism and therapeutic trials. *Neurology* 1986;36: 760–764.

56. LeWitt PA, Miller LP, Newman RP, et al. Tyrosine hydroxylase cofactor (tetrahydrobiopterin) in parkinsonism. *Adv Neurol* 1984;40:459–462.

57. Liu TT, Hsiao KJ. Identification of a common 6-pyruvoyl-tetrahydropterin synthase mutation at codon 87 in Chinese phenylketonuria caused by tetrahydrobiopterin synthesis deficiency. *Hum Genet* 1996;98:313–316.

58. Lovenberg W, Jequier E, Sjoerdsma A. Tryptophan hydroxylation: measurement in pineal gland, brainstem and carcinoid tumor. *Science* 1967;155:217–219.

59. Lovenberg W, Levine RA, Robinson DS, Ebert M, Williams AC, Calne DB. Hydroxylase cofactor activity in cerebrospinal fluid of normal subjects and patients with Parkinson's disease. *Science* 1979;204: 624–626.

60. Lüdecke B, Dworniczak B, Bartholomé K. A point mutation in the tyrosine hydroxylase gene associated with Segawa's syndrome. *Hum Genet* 1995;95:123–125.

61. Lüdecke B, Knappskog PM, Clayton PT, et al. Recessively inherited L-DOPA-responsive parkinsonism in infancy caused by a point mutation (L205P) in the tyrosine hydroxylase gene. *Hum Mol Genet* 1996;5: 1023–1028.

62. Maier J, Witter K, Gütlich M, Ziegler I, Werner T, Ninnemann H. Homology cloning of GTP-cyclohy-

drolase I from various unrelated eukaryotes by reverse-transcription polymerase chain reaction using a general set of degenerate primers. *Biochem Biophys Res Commun* 1995;212:705–711.

63. Miwa S, Watanabe Y, Hayaishi O. 6R-L-erythro-5,6,7,8-tetrahydrobiopterin as a regulator of dopamine and serotonin biosynthesis in the rat brain. *Arch Biochem Biophys* 1985;239:234–241.

64. Miyasaka H, Mori H, Saikawa T, et al. Neurological CPC 41: A 78-year-old man with young onset parkinsonism and sudden death. *Brain Nerve* 1996;48:487–495.

65. Mori H, Kondo T, Matsumine H, Yokochi M, Mizuno Y. Dopa-responsive juvenile parkinsonism without Lewy bodies. *Mov Disord* 1996;11[Suppl 1]:172.

66. Mount SM. A catalogue of splice junction sequences. *Nucleic Acids Res* 1982;10:459–472.

67. Nagatsu T, Levitt M, Udenfriend S. Tyrosine hydroxylase: the initial step in norepinephrine biosynthesis. *J Biol Chem* 1964;239:2910–2917.

68. Nagatsu T, Yamaguchi T, Kato T, et al. Biopterin in human brain and urine from controls and parkinsonian patients; application of a new radioimmunoassay. *Clin Chim Acta* 1981;109:305–311.

69. Nar H, Huber R, Meining W, Schmid C, Weinkauf S, Bacher A. Atomic structure of GTP cyclohydrolase I. *Structure* 1995;3:459–466.

70. Nar H, Huber R, Auerbach G, et al. Active site topology and reaction mechanism of GTP cyclohydrolase I. *Proc Natl Acad Sci USA* 1995;92:12120–12125.

71. Naylor EW, Ennis D, Davidson AGF, Wong LTK, Applegarth DA, Niederwieser A. Guanosine triphosphate cyclohydrolase I deficiency: early diagnosis by routine urine pteridine screening. *Pediatrics* 1987;79:374–378.

72. Niederwieser A, Blau N, Wang M, Joller P, Atarés M, Cardesa-Garcia J. GTP-cyclohydrolase I deficiency, a new enzyme defect causing hyperphenylalaninemia with neopterin, biopterin, dopamine, and serotonin deficiencies and muscular hypotonia. *Eur J Pediatr* 1984;141:208–214.

73. Nomura T, Ohtsuki M, Matsui S, et al. Isolation of a full-length cDNA clone for human GTP cyclohydrolase I type 1 from pheochromocytoma. *J Neural Transm [Gen Sect]* 1995;101:237–242.

74. Nyberg P, Nordberg A, Wester P, Winblad B. Dopaminergic deficiency is more pronounced in putamen than in nucleus caudatus in Parkinson's disease. *Neurochem Pathol* 1983;1:193–202.

75. Nygaard TG, Duvoisin RC. Hereditary dystonia-parkinsonism syndrome of juvenile onset. *Neurology* 1986;36:1424–1428.

76. Nygaard TG. Dopa-responsive dystonia. In: Tsui JKC, Calne DB, eds. *Neurological disease and therapy. Vol. 39. Handbook of dystonia.* New York: Marcel Dekker, 1995:213–226.

77. Nygaard TG, Marsden CD, Duvoisin RC. Dopa-responsive dystonia. *Adv Neurol* 1988;50:377–384.

78. Nygaard TG, Wilhelmsen KC, Risch NJ, et al. Linkage mapping of dopa-responsive dystonia (DRD) to chromosome 14q. *Nat Genet* 1993;5:386–391.

79. Oppliger T, Thöny B, Nar H, et al. Structural and functional consequences of mutations in 6-pyruvoyl-tetrahydropterin synthase causing hyperphenylala-ninemia in humans. *J Biol Chem* 1995;279:29498–29506.

80. Polymeropoulos MH, Higgins JJ, Golbe LI, et al. Mapping of a gene for Parkinson's disease to chromosome 4q21-q23. *Science* 1996;274:1197–1199.

81. Rajput AH, Gibb WRG, Zhong XH, et al. Dopa-responsive dystonia; pathological and biochemical observations in a case. *Ann Neurol* 1994;35:396–402.

82. Sawada M, Hirata Y, Arai H, Iizuka R, Nagatsu T. Tyrosine hydroxylase, tryptophan hydroxylase, biopterin, and neopterin in the brains of normal controls and patients with senile dementia of Alzheimer type. *J Neurochem* 1987;48:760–764.

83. Sawle GV, Leenders KL, Brooks DJ, et al. Dopa-responsive dystonia: [^{18}F]dopa positron emission tomography. *Ann Neurol* 1991;30:24–30.

84. Schuback D, Kramer P, Ozelius L, et al. Dopamine beta-hydroxylase gene excluded in four subtypes of hereditary dystonia. *Hum Genet* 1991;87:311–316.

85. Scriver CR, Kaufman S, Eisensmith RC, Woo SLC. The hyperphenylalaninemias. In: Scriver CR, Beaudet AL, Sly WS, Valle D, eds. *The metabolic and molecular bases of inherited disease.* 7th ed. New York: McGraw-Hill, 1995:1015–1075.

86. Segawa M, Hosaka A, Miyagawa F, Nomura Y, Imai H. Hereditary progressive dystonia with marked diurnal fluctuation. *Adv Neurol* 1976;14:215–233.

87. Segawa M, Nomura Y, Tanaka S, et al. Hereditary progressive dystonia with marked diurnal fluctuation; consideration on its pathophysiology based on the characteristics of clinical and polysomnographical findings. *Adv Neurol* 1988;50:367–376.

88. Shintaku H. Early diagnosis of 6-pyruvoyl-tetrahydropterin synthase deficiency. *Pteridines* 1994;5:18–27.

89. Snow BJ, Nygaard TG, Takahashi H, Calne DB. Positron emission tomographic studies of dopa-responsive dystonia and early-onset idiopathic parkinsonism. *Ann Neurol* 1993;34:733–738.

90. Takahashi H, Levine RA, Galloway MP, Snow BJ, Calne DB, Nygaard TG. Biochemical and fluorodopa positron emission tomographic findings in an asymptomatic carrier of the gene for dopa-responsive dystonia. *Ann Neurol* 1994;35:354–356.

91. Takahashi H, Ohama E, Suzuki S, et al. Familial juvenile parkinsonism; clinical and pathologic study in a family. *Neurology* 1994;44:437–441.

92. Tanaka H, Endo K, Tsuji S, et al. The gene for hereditary progressive dystonia with marked diurnal fluctuation maps to chromosome 14q. *Ann Neurol* 1995;37:405–408.

93. Tanaka K, Yoneda M, Nakajima T, Miyatake T, Owada M. Dihydrobiopterin synthesis defect; an adult with diurnal fluctuation of symptoms. *Neurology* 1987;37:519–522.

94. Togari A, Ichinose H, Matsumoto S, Fujita K, Nagatsu T. Multiple mRNA forms of human GTP cyclohydrolase I. *Biochem Biophys Res Commun* 1992;187:359–365.

95. Tsuji S, Tanaka H, Miyatake T, Ginns EI, Nomura Y, Segawa M. Linkage analysis of hereditary progressive dystonia to the tyrosine hydroxylase gene locus. In: Segawa M, ed. *Hereditary progressive dystonia with marked diurnal fluctuation.* New York: Parthenon, 1993:107–114.

96. Ueno S, Hirano M, Tamaru Y, Imai T, Kawamura J. Three novel mutations in the GTP cyclohydrolase I gene in 3 Japanese families with dopa-responsive dystonia. *Ann Neurol* 1996;40:537.

97. Wachter H, Fuchs D, Hausen A, Reibnegger G, Werner ER. Neopterin as marker for activation of cellular immunity; immunologic basis and clinical application. *Adv Clin Chem* 1989;27:81–141.

98. Werner ER, Werner-Felmayer G, Wachter H. Tetrahydrobiopterin and cytokines. *Proc Soc Exp Biol Med* 1993;203:1–12.

99. Williams A, Eldridge R, Levine R, Lovenberg W, Paulson G. Low CSF hydroxylase cofactor (tetrahydrobiopterin) levels in inherited dystonia. *Lancet* 1979;2:410–411.

100. Williams AC, Levine RA, Chase TN, Lovenberg W, Calne DB. CSF hydroxylase cofactor levels in some neurological diseases. *J Neurol Neurosurg Psychiatry* 1980;43:735–738.

101. Witter K, Werner T, Blusch JH, et al. Cloning, sequencing and functional studies of the gene encoding human GTP cyclohydrolase I. *Gene* 1996;171:285–290.

102. Yamamura Y, Arihiro K, Kohriyama T, Nakamura S. Early-onset parkinsonism with diurnal fluctuation; clinical and pathological studies. *Clin Neurol* 1993; 33:491–496.

103. Yokochi M. Juvenile parkinsonism and other dopa-responsive syndromes. In: Segawa M, Nomura Y, eds. *Age-related dopamine-dependent disorders*. Basel: Karger, 1995:25–35.

104. Yokochi M, Narabayashi H, Iizuka R, Nagatsu T. Juvenile parkinsonism; some clinical, pharmacological, and neuropathological aspects. *Adv Neurol* 1984;40: 407–413.

Dystonia 3: Advances in Neurology, Vol. 78,
edited by S. Fahn, C. D. Marsden, and M. DeLong.
Lippincott–Raven Publishers, Philadelphia © 1998.

28

Atypical Presentations of Dopa-Responsive Dystonia

Oliver Bandmann, Charles David Marsden, and Nicholas W. Wood

University Department of Clinical Neurology, Institute of Neurology, London WC1N 3BG, United Kingdom.

THE CLASSIC PRESENTATION OF DOPA-RESPONSIVE DYSTONIA

Dopa-responsive dystonia (DRD) has only been recognized as a new and distinct clinical entity since Segawa described this condition in a series of Japanese patients in the early 1970s (39). Earlier descriptions of what is now called DRD do, however, exist and the earliest description in the English literature dates back to a case presentation at the National Hospital, Queen Square, London (3,7). The patient presented is in many ways typical for the classic presentation of DRD: A girl (DRD is more common among females) presented at age 7 (the typical age of presentation) with walking problems (the most common complaint). The patient was considerably worse toward the latter part of the day (indicating the classic feature of diurnal fluctuation) and her left leg was more severely affected than the right (reflecting the recognized side preference to the left). She also had fine tremor in both hands (postural tremor with higher frequency of 8 to 10 Hz rather than the slower parkinsonian rest tremor of 4 to 6 Hz is typical for DRD) and a "somewhat expressionless" face as well as "somewhat clumsy" fine finger movements were noted (the dystonia is often accompanied by some parkinsonian features). The most striking feature, however, was her excellent response to

anticholinergics. The patient was followed up and was later put on L-dopa, again, with an excellent response (28).

From the beginning there was the hint that there may be a genetic cause for this illness in that two other members of this particular family suffered from similar problems. In 1994, Ichinose et al. (15) identified the GTP-cyclohydrolase gene (GCH-I) as the first causative gene for DRD and a Phe234Ser mutation of the GCH-I gene has now also been found in this original patient, 49 years after her initial presentation at the National Hospital, Queen Square ("family Sm" in Reference 2). Unfortunately, this first patient shared an experience with many later patients: She was initially diagnosed as suffering from a hysterical illness. DRD is an eminently treatable condition and it is thus crucial to be aware of atypical presentations of this disorder.

DOPA-RESPONSIVE DYSTONIA PRESENTING AS CEREBRAL PALSY

DRD presenting in early infancy is particularly important to diagnose, as it may be difficult to distinguish from cerebral palsy. To illustrate this presentation, the first case of genetically confirmed DRD presenting in this way ("family Hu" in Reference 2), will be described in some detail.

The patient is a 9-year-old Caucasian boy of nonconsanguineous parents. The mother's pregnancy was unremarkable and he was born at term with a normal birth weight and good APGAR values. There were no perinatal complications, in particular birth asphyxia or jaundice. He was initially a floppy baby, but no other abnormalities were present; he fed well from the beginning and developed head control at the age of 3 months. At 8 months his parents noted his inability to sit unsupported or to roll over. He lost the previously acquired head control and was now noted to be slow at feeding. He was never able to walk unaided. His muscle tone gradually increased and at 16 months he was diagnosed as suffering from athetoid cerebral palsy.

At 29 months, he was formally assessed by a clinical medical officer and his mental age was estimated to be 7.8 months. His test result illustrates the limitations of standard test batteries in the assessment of children with severe motor problems. It is understandable that he did poorly on the locomotor scale, since he was still unable to sit unaided and could only stand when held up. However, he also obtained poor ratings on the personal social-scale, as his motor problems prevented him from being able to play or obey simple commands.

At that time it was clear that he also had severe problems with his speech; he was only able to say a few short words as a result of the dystonia affecting his mouth and tongue. His inability to speak was also misinterpreted as an inability to identify simple objects.

At age 4 1/2 years, he was only able to use 30 to 50 short words. At age 6 1/2 years it was noted that he was always considerably better in the morning. Detailed neurologic examination revealed pronounced spasm of his mouth and difficulty in moving his tongue. Rigidity and marked distal dystonia in an asymmetric pattern in all limbs was noted. His deep tendon reflexes were normal. For the first time the possible diagnosis of a progressive dystonia rather than athetoid cerebral palsy was made.

His family history is of interest in that a half-sister started toe-walking at age 7 and gradually developed a stiff-legged inverted gait. Ini-

tially, a diagnosis of hereditary spastic paraplegia was made. A few months after the correct diagnosis was made in her brother, she was also put on L-dopa and has made a virtually complete recovery since then. Another sister has an identical illness to her brother's, except that she is 10 years older and thus has had longer term difficulties and resultant problems.

Extensive investigations including magnetic resonance imaging (MRI) scan and neurophysiology were normal. Examination of his cerebrospinal fluid (CSF) revealed low neopterin levels, and a heterozygote Lys224 Arg mutation in exon 6 of the GCH I coding region was found (2).

He was put on slowly increasing doses of L-dopa and has shown a dramatic recovery. His speech has become fluent, he has regained head and trunk control, and his dexterity has improved. He now walks unaided and takes great delight in outdoor activities such as football.

Previously, Nygaard et al. (33) have described a series of five children presenting in infancy, with a delay in early motor milestones, or in early childhood with combinations of pyramidal and extrapyramidal signs in conjunction with normal cognitive function. Three had apparently sporadic disease; the other two were siblings with an affected paternal grandmother. Other reports of DRD misdiagnosed as cerebral palsy clearly differ in that the children were normal until age 5 and only then developed the classic walking problems due to dystonia of the lower limbs (5).

Delayed-onset progressive dystonia due to perinatal or early childhood anoxia has been reported (6). However cerebral palsy typically causes a nonprogressive motor impairment and it is difficult to understand why perinatal asphyxia should have led to dystonia with delayed onset in the particular patients of the above-mentioned series. Interestingly, 40% of these patients with delayed-onset dystonia after a static encephalopathy showed marked or excellent response to treatment with anticholinergics, but none of them were put on L-dopa. So far, neither biochemical studies investigating possible disturbances of the BH4 pathway nor sequence analysis of GCH-I have been published in these cases.

DOPA-RESPONSIVE DYSTONIA PRESENTING WITH GENERALIZED IDIOPATHIC TORSION DYSTONIA

The most common presenting complaint in DRD is equinovarus posturing of the foot or gait disturbance, and gait or balance problems continue to cause the greatest disability later in the course of the illness. However, in most cases dystonia also spreads to other parts of the body, leading to symptomatic arm involvement as well as to axial involvement, manifested by torticollis, scoliosis or increased lumbar lordosis. The time to generalization varies from less than 1 year to 10 years (31).

Patients with generalized DRD are not infrequently initially misdiagnosed as suffering from idiopathic torsion dystonia (ITD). Childhood onset as well as onset in the foot or leg are characteristic features of both ITD and DRD and therefore not necessarily helpful in the differentiation between these disorders (24,31). It is thus important to search for a history of diurnal variation, a classic, but not invariable feature of DRD. Careful clinical examination may also provide helpful clues in the differentiation between these two dystonic syndromes: A degree of rigidity, bradykinesia, and hyperreflexia is frequently seen in DRD, but they are not present in ITD.

Although patients with DRD as well as some patients with ITD improve following treatment with anticholinergics, the response tends to be excellent and sustained with only small doses of anticholinergics in DRD (31) but variable and frequently only poorly sustained in ITD. Jarman et al. (17) have analysed the GCH-I gene in 7 patients diagnosed as suffering from ITD with a good and sustained response to anticholinergics. Mutations in GCH-I were found in two of these patients. Interestingly, diurnal fluctuation was only present in one of them (17). DRD should thus be considered in the differential diagnosis of all patients with generalized dystonia and good response to anticholinergics, even in the absence of diurnal variation.

It is also of interest that four of the seven selected patients had a positive family history for dystonia. However, the two patients with proven mutations were apparently sporadic, emphasizing the markedly reduced penetrance of this disorder. Moreover, these two patients also responded to the considerably smaller doses of anticholinergics than the other patients in this group. One of the DRD patients was shown to have a second mutation on his paternal allele. The significance of this second mutation is unclear as it has been found in one of 210 control chromosomes. Possible explanations include true compound heterozygosity leading to a relatively severe (generalized) phenotype or chance association between a pathogenic mutation and a rare, nonpathogenic polymorphism.

DOPA-RESPONSIVE DYSTONIA PRESENTING WITH FOCAL DYSTONIA

As mentioned above, DRD leads to generalized dystonia in the majority (at least 75%) of cases (31). Although onset with dystonia in the lower limbs is the most frequent presentation, DRD may occasionally start in the arms or with torticollis (31,43) before involving other parts of the body or indeed remain as a focal dystonia. A member of a large North American family with DRD suffered from isolated spasmodic dysphonia for 37 years before he was put on L-dopa. He is an obligate gene carrier since his daughter is definitely affected with DRD. However, his spasmodic dysphonia did not improve on L-dopa (31). Another member of the same family suffered from writer's cramp, but his response to L-dopa has not been reported and a deceased member of that family may have suffered from isolated blepharospasm (29). A further sporadic patient with isolated torticollis was initially thought to show complete response to L-dopa, but a few years later his torticollis reappeared despite continued therapy (31). Therefore, it seems likely that this was a case of torticollis with temporary spontaneous remission (16), which happened to coincide with the start of the L-dopa treatment.

However, one of our patients with an identified mutation of the GCH-I gene has continued to demonstrate isolated focal dystonia with good response to L-dopa ("family Ha" in Reference 2). She came to medical attention after her child developed classic DRD affecting the lower limbs. The mother then reported that she had to stop playing classic guitar in her 30s because of guitarist's cramp. She remained asymptomatic for several years until this focal action-induced dystonia became a constant feature, affecting any fine manipulation involving the hand, such as writing or sewing. Sometimes, particularly in stressful social situations, the hand would also assume an abnormal posture at rest. On L-dopa treatment, she showed considerable improvement such that her handwriting was now normal and no dystonic postures were seen on examination, although she was still unable to play the guitar. In two reported cases of combined foot dystonia and writer's cramp, the foot dystonia alone responded in one patient whereas both dystonic features resolved in the other (8,30). Response to L-dopa thus appears to be less predictable in DRD patients with focal dystonia. Focal presentation of this disorder is certainly rare. However, the above examples show that DRD should nevertheless be considered in the differential diagnosis in patients with focal dystonia and a positive family history for generalized dystonia.

DOPA-RESPONSIVE DYSTONIA PRESENTING WITH PARKINSONISM

Rather than producing dystonia of the lower limbs in childhood, DRD may manifest with an akinetic-rigid parkinsonian syndrome in middle and old age (14). Nygaard et al. (32) reported a family in which five family members had dystonia of the lower limbs and another three members, unaffected by dystonia, developed parkinsonism after the age of 50. The latter three patients had onset with unilateral rest-tremor, later developing hypomimia, bradykinesia, and rigidity as well as a stiff or shuffling gait. None of these patients had been exposed to neuroleptics and there was no diurnal fluctuation in their symptoms. In contrast, the severity of symptoms in three of the family

members with dystonia worsened toward the evening and was related to exertion in the other two. In a large series of 21 families with DRD, seven out of 50 (14%) first-degree relatives older than 40 years of age were found to have definite parkinsonism (30). This frequency is far higher than the general population prevalence of Parkinson's disease (PD), which is 0.6% after the age of 40 years (38). Although some of these patients initially developed dystonic symptoms such as foot dystonia in childhood or writer's cramp later in life, others were similar to the patients described above with parkinsonism as the first presenting feature. Dystonia preceding the onset of akinetic rigid features can also be seen in PD and is thus not a helpful feature in the differential diagnosis (32,35).

Although age of onset, symptoms, and signs are similar in the adulthood-onset akinetic rigid presentation of DRD and PD, there are three marked differences between these two conditions. First, all patients with the akinetic-rigid presentation of DRD so far described have other family members who also suffer from extrapyramidal disorders such as dystonia or parkinsonism. It is, however, not clear whether the positive family history in all these cases is a real phenomenon or due to ascertainment bias. Although familial PD seems to be more common than previously thought (19) the majority of patients with PD are sporadic and do not have a positive family history of other neurologic disorders (23). Second, patients with the akinetic-rigid presentation of DRD continue to respond well to small doses of L-dopa for a long period of time without developing motor side effects such as on-off fluctuations or dyskinesias (32). This excellent response to L-dopa resembles the good long-term response to L-dopa in childhood-onset cases of DRD (31). Initially, L-dopa also produces a stable motor response in patients with PD (23). Unfortunately, this "levodopa honeymoon" (36) does not tend to last and at least one-half of the patients with PD begin to manifest motor fluctuations within the first 5 years of treatment (25). Finally, the only postmortem examination of a patient with DRD revealed a normal cell count in the substantia nigra without gliosis (37). No abnormal intraneuronal inclusions such as Lewy bodies or neurofibrillary tangles were detected and there was no neuronal immunostaining with ubiquitin. In contrast, the histopathologic diagnosis of PD is based on the detection of pars compacta nigral cell loss of at least 60% with Lewy bodies in the surviving nerve cells (13).

We thus considered the possibility that some of our patients with a clinical diagnosis of PD actually suffered from the akinetic-rigid presentation of DRD due to mutations in the GCH-I gene rather than Lewy-body PD. Twenty-nine parkinsonian patients were selected who shared at least one feature with the akinetic-rigid presentation of DRD, but did not have a positive family history for DRD. Twenty-three patients had at least one living relative who also suffered from an akinetic-rigid syndrome; two patients had an abnormally mild course of their parkinsonism in that they continue to respond well to L-dopa for more than 10 years with no motor fluctuations. DNA was also analysed from four brain samples of patients who were clinically diagnosed as suffering from PD, but did not show any pathologic changes at postmortem. In all 29 patients the entire coding region of the GCH-I gene was sequenced. The sequence was normal in all cases examined. The absence of mutations in any of these cases makes an involvement of the GCH-I gene in parkinsonian patients without a positive family history of classic, childhood-onset DRD unlikely (1).

OTHER POSSIBLE PRESENTATIONS OF DOPA-RESPONSIVE DYSTONIA

Persistent responsiveness to L-dopa has been observed in adult patients with hemidystonia (own observations) or isolated dystonic tremor (N. Fletcher, personal communication) as well as in infants with dystonic spasms (L. Carr, personal communication) or oculogyric crisis. However, biochemical or genetic confirmation of a defect in the BH_4 synthetic pathway is so far lacking in these patients and their dystonia may thus be due to a different cause such as an unidentified neurodegenerative process or other metabolic disturbances.

DOPA-RESPONSIVENESS IN SECONDARY DYSTONIA

Rarely, secondary dystonia may mimic DRD. Peppard et al. (34) described a patient with neuroacanthocytosis who developed dystonia of his right foot at age 16. This was followed by generalized akinetic-rigid features. Both the dystonia as well as the parkinsonism responded well to dopaminergic treatment: The patient was reported to walk normally and resumed employment for the first time in 4 years. It was suggested that his illness resembled DRD in that his deficits disappeared during sleep and became worse during the course of the day. However, both worsening during the day as well as absence of extrapyramidal deficits during sleep can be seen in various extrapyramidal disorders (see below) and neither the extent of the diurnal variation nor the duration of the response to L-dopa treatment was documented. In a further report, "progressive dystonia with marked diurnal variation" was reported in an Indian girl who had previously suffered from tuberculous meningitis. However, the patient responded only partially to L-dopa in that she remained severely affected in the evening despite treatment. She is thus likely to have developed symptomatic dystonia following her meningitis (30).

Fletcher et al. (12) reported an interesting series of three patients with childhood-onset symptomatic dystonia and marked response to L-dopa treatment. Additional features such as cognitive impairment or eye movement abnormalities clearly differentiate them from classic cases of DRD. However, the authors rightly emphasize the importance of a therapeutic trial with L-dopa in such cases, regardless of whether a satisfying diagnosis has been reached or not. This point is further emphasized by occasional reports of improvement of symptomatic dystonia on L-dopa treatment in patients with an established diagnosis of diseases as different as Leigh's disease or metachromatic leukodystrophy (27).

Patients with atypical phenylketonuria due to autosomal-recessively inherited, complete deficiency of GCH-I or other enzymes in the synthetic pathway of BH_4 may sometimes have dystonia responding to L-dopa as part of their generalized illness. However, these patients typically present in infancy with a median age of onset at 4 to 5 months. Common symptoms include mental retardation, convulsions (grand mal or myoclonic attacks), disturbances of tone and posture, drowsiness, irritability, and recurrent hypothermia without infection (4). Not infrequently, microcephaly can be seen (4). The clinical picture may be dominated by abnormal movements such as paroxysmal tremor and orofacial dyskinesia (9). Rarely, problems only manifest at a later stage: Tanaka et al. (40) reported a patient who was normal until age 10 when he developed difficulty with walking. On examination at age 14, mental retardation, dysarthria, and increased tone was found. Biochemical analysis proved a defect of the second enzyme in the synthetic pathway of BH_4, 6-pyruvoyl tetrahydropterin synthase (40). Abnormally high phenylalanine levels in blood and urine should help in the differential diagnosis of these cases (4).

DRD has also been reported in two sibs with autosomal-recessively inherited tyrosine hydroxylase deficiency (18,21). However, clinical details of these patients are lacking. An infant with an identified mutation in the tyrosine hydroxylase gene presented not only with akinetic-rigid features but also with ptosis, indicating additional involvement of the sympathetic nervous system, as well as trunk hypotonia and myoclonic jerks (22). This has not been described in classic DRD due to GCH-I deficiency. Wevers et al. (41) reported a series of four unrelated children with biochemical evidence for tyrosine hydroxylase deficiency. The children were 11 to 38 months old and presented with severe motor retardation and an apparent spastic tetraparesis combined with hypokinesia and axial hypotonia after the

first months of life. All of them showed considerable improvement on L-dopa (41).

CLINICAL AND INVESTIGATORY DIFFICULTIES IN THE DIAGNOSIS OF DOPA-RESPONSIVE DYSTONIA

The clinical diagnosis of DRD should be straightforward in classic cases with prominent dystonia of the lower limbs and marked diurnal variation as well as worsening of the symptoms after exercise. It will be further facilitated by the presence of some parkinsonian features such as rigidity and bradykinesia. The almost pathognomonic dramatic relief of the dystonia after the initiation of L-dopa and the continuing response to this drug will secure the diagnosis in such cases.

However, there are several "red herrings" in the diagnosis of DRD: At least 20% of all patients have pathologically brisk deep tendon jerks and the frequently presented "striatal toe" may be misinterpreted as a positive Babinski sign, potentially leading to the false assumption of upper motor neuron damage and thus facilitating the errant diagnosis of cerebral palsy or hereditary spastic paraplegia. In addition, evidence of cognitive impairment in children should be viewed with caution, as many of the measurements rely heavily on motor skills for an overall assessment. Resolution of these deficits can result in a complete reevaluation of previous conclusions before therapy.

Diurnal variation is neither specific for DRD nor invariably present. Its absence has been reported in 25% of all cases and varies widely in the remaining cases (31). Furthermore, patients with ITD may also report some diurnal variation as well as sleep benefit and worsening after exercise (30). Worsening toward the evening has also been described in isolated cranial dystonia (26).

It is crucial not to expect a "magic cure" on the first small dose of L-dopa in all patients with DRD. This seems to be especially the case in patients with very early onset of the disease. In the patient described above who first developed problems at the age of 6 months, improvement was limited at the beginning, but has now continued for more than 2 years. A delayed response to treatment may also be seen in adults and once the decision has been made that a patient warrants a trial of L-dopa, he or she should then be put on a reasonably high dose for a sufficiently long period (i.e., 400 mg L-dopa/carbidopa for the first 4 weeks and 600 mg for the second 4 weeks).

No long-term follow-up studies have documented L-dopa treatment motor side effects such as dyskinesias or on-off fluctuation, which one can frequently see in late-stage PD (25). However, at the beginning of the therapy hyperkinesias are not uncommon and should thus not be considered as evidence against the diagnosis of DRD (31).

A clinically suspected diagnosis of DRD can be supported by low CSF levels of the neurotransmitter metabolite homovanillic acid (HVA) as well as reduced CSF levels of neopterin and BH_4 and the detection of a mutation in the GCH-I gene. Indeed, low levels of BH_4 were a recognized feature in patients with DRD well before GCH-I, the rate-limiting enzyme in the synthesis of BH_4, was identified as the first causative gene for this disorder (11,20). However, neither CSF analysis of BH_4 levels nor the genetic analysis of the GCH-I gene are necessarily diagnostic in every case of DRD: Low levels of BH_4 have also been described in other basal ganglia disorders and are thus not specific for DRD (42) and mutations in the coding region of GCH-I cannot be found in all cases of DRD (2). This may be due to mutations in the regulatory regions of GCH-I or caused by an involvement of other genes. Low CSF levels of HVA with normal amounts of BH_4 and neopterin are characteristic for tyrosine hydroxylase deficiency (22), which may also cause DRD (see above).

Further diagnostic help may be gained from the phenylalanine loading test (see also Chapter 30 of this volume). A combined approach, using both biochemical as well as genetic investigations, is thus most likely to achieve diagnostic clarity in atypical cases. Imaging studies with single photon emission computed tomography may be of further help, since the integrity of the nigrostriatal dopamine transporters (characteristic for DRD) can be demonstrated with this method (see Chapter 31 of this volume).

CONCLUSION

The identification of GCH-I as the first causative gene for DRD has fueled the interest in this disorder and allowed the genetic confirmation of DRD in patients with previously not recognized presentations. Although still a rare disease, it is clear from the above discussion that there is a growing list of disorders in which a response to L-dopa should be sought. Moreover, it is worth noting that treatment, even after many years of illness, is still a worthwhile venture and we would urge increased vigilance for potential cases of DRD. Further work should therefore concentrate on the investigation of other possible presentations of this disorder such as cases with isolated exercise-induced dystonia.

ACKNOWLEDGMENTS

Financial support of the Deutsche Forschungsgemeinschaft (DFG) and the Dystonia Society, UK, is gratefully acknowledged.

REFERENCES

1. Bandmann O, Daniel S, Marsden CD, Wood NW, Harding AE. The GTP-cyclohydrolase I gene in atypical parkinsonian patients: a clinico-genetic study. *J Neurol Sci* 1996;141:27–32.
2. Bandmann O, Nygaard T, Surtees T, Marsden CD, Wood NW, Harding AE. Dopa-responsive dystonia in British patients: new mutations of the GTP-cyclohydrolase I gene and evidence for genetic heterogeneity. *Hum Mol Genet* 1996;5:403–406.
3. Beck D. Dystonia musculorum deformans with another case in the same family. *Proc R Soc Med* 1947;40:551–552.
4. Blau N, Thöny B, Heizmann CW, Dhondt J-L. Tetrahydrobiopterin deficiency: from phenotype to genotype. *Pteridines* 1993;4:1–10.
5. Boyd K, Patterson V. Dopa-responsive dystonia: a treatable condition misdiagnosed as cerebral palsy. *BMJ* 1989;298:10–11.

6. Burke R, Fahn S, Gold S. Delayed-onset dystonia in patients with "static" encephalopathy. *J Neurol Neurosurg Psychiatry* 1980;43:789–797.

7. Corner B. Dystonia musculorum deformans in siblings. Treated with Artane (trihexyphenidyl). *Proc R Soc Med* 1952;45:451–452.

8. Deonna T, Ferreira A. Idiopathic fluctuating dystonia: a case of foot dystonia and writer's cramp responsive to L-dopa. *Dev Med Child Neurol* 1985;27:819–821.

9. Factor SA, Coni RJ, Cowger M, Rosenblum EL. Paroxysmal tremor and orofacial dyskinesia secondary to a biopterin synthesis defect. *Neurology* 1991; 41:930–932.

10. Fahn S. High dosage anticholinergic therapy in dystonia. *Neurology* 1982;33:1255–1261.

11. Fink J, Barton N, Cohen W, Lovenberg W, Burns R, Hallett M. Dystonia associated with marked diurnal variation associated with biopterin deficiency. *Neurology* 1988;38:707–711.

12. Fletcher N, Thompson P, Scadding J, Marsden C. Successful treatment of childhood onset symptomatic dystonia with levodopa. *J Neurol Neurosurg Psychiatry* 1993;56:865–867.

13. Gibb W, Lees A. Pathological clues to the cause of Parkinson's disease. In: Marsden C, Fahn S, eds. *Movement disorders 3*. London: Butterworth Heinemann, 1994:147–166.

14. Harwood G, Hierons R, Fletcher NA, Marsden CD. Lessons from a remarkable family with dopa-responsive dystonia. *J Neurol Neurosurg Psychiatry* 1994; 57:460–463.

15. Ichinose H, Ohye T, Takahashi E, et al. Hereditary progressive dystonia with marked diurnal fluctuation caused by mutations in the GTP cyclohydrolase I gene. *Nat Genet* 1994;8:236–242.

16. Jahanshahi M, Marion M-H, Marsden C. Natural history of adult-onset idiopathic torticollis. *Arch Neurol* 1990;47:548–552.

17. Jarman PR, Bandmann O, Marsden CD, Harding AE, Wood NW. GTP cyclohydrolase I mutations in patients with dystonia responsive to anticholinergic drugs *J.Neurol Neurosurg Psychiatry* 1997; 63:304–308.

18. Knappskog P, Flatmark T, Mallet J, Luedecke B, Bartholome K. Recessively inherited L-dopa-responsive dystonia caused by a point mutation (381K) in the tyrosine hydroxylase gene. *Hum Mol Genet* 1995;4:1209–1212.

19. Lazzarini A, Myers R, Zimmermann T, et al. A clinical genetic study of Parkinson's disease: evidence for dominant transmission. *Neurology* 1994;44:499–506.

20. LeWitt P, Miller L, Levine R, et al. Tetrahydrobiopterin in dystonia: identification of abnormal metabolism and therapeutic trial. *Neurology* 1986;36: 760–764.

21. Luedecke B, Dworniczak B, Bartholome K. A point mutation in the tyrosine hydroxylase gene associated with Segawa's syndrome. *Hum Genet* 1995;95:123–125.

22. Luedecke B, Knappskog P, Clayton P, et al. Recessively inherited L-DOPA-responsive parkinsonism in infancy caused by a point mutation (L205P) in the tyrosine hydroxylase gene. *Hum Mol Genet* 1996;5: 1023–1028.

23. Marsden CD. Parkinson's disease. *J Neurol Neurosurg Psychiatry* 1994;57:672–681.

24. Marsden CD, Harrison M. Idiopathic torsion dystonia (dystonia musculorum deformans): a review of forty-two patients. *Brain* 1974;97:793–810.

25. Marsden CD, Parkes J. "On-Off" effects in patients with Parkinson's disease. *Lancet* 1976;1:292–296.

26. Montagna P, Procaccianti G, Lugaresi A, Zuconi M, Lugaresi E. Diurnal variability in cranial dystonia. *Mov Disord* 1990;5:44–46.

27. Nordenbo A, Tonnesen T. A variant of metachromatic leucodystrophy in a patient suffering from another congenital degenerative neurological disorder. *Acta Neurol Scan* 1985;71:31–36.

28. Nygaard T, Marsden C, Duvoisin R. Dopa-responsive dystonia. *Adv Neurol* 1988;50:377–384.

29. Nygaard T, Trugman J, Yebenes J, Fahn S. Dopa-responsive dystonia: the spectrum of clinical manifestations in a large North American family. *Neurology* 1990;40:66–69.

30. Nygaard T. Dopa-responsive dystonia. *Adv Neurol* 1993;60:577–585.

31. Nygaard T, Marsden C, Fahn S. Dopa-responsive dystonia: long term treatment response and prognosis. *Neurology* 1991;41:174–181.

32. Nygaard T, Takahashi H, Heiman G, Snow B, Fahn S, Calne D. Long-term treatment response and fluordopa positron emission tomographic scanning of parkinsonism in a family with dopa-responsive dystonia. *Ann Neurol* 1992;32:603–608.

33. Nygaard T, Waran S, Levine R, Naini A, Chutorian A. Dopa-responsive dystonia simulating cerebral palsy. *Pediatr Neurol* 1994;11:236–240.

34. Peppard R, Lu C, Chu N-S, Teal P, Martin W, Calne D. Parkinsonism with neuroacanthocytosis. *Can J Neurol Sci* 1990;17:298–301.

35. Poewe W, Lees A, Stern G. Dystonia in Parkinson's disease: clinical and pharmacological features. *Ann Neurol* 1988;23:73–78.

36. Quinn N. Drug treatment of Parkinson's disease. *BMJ* 1995;310:575–579.

37. Rajput A, Gibb W, Zhong X, et al. Dopa-responsive dystonia: pathological and biochemical observations in a case. *Ann Neurol* 1994;35:396–402.

38. Schoenberg B, Anderson D, Haerer A. Prevalence of Parkinson's disease in the biracial population of Copiah County. *Neurology* 1985;35:841–845.

39. Segawa M, Hosaka A, Miyagawa F, Nomura Y, Imai H. Hereditary progressive dystonia with marked diurnal fluctuation. *Adv Neurol* 1976;14:215–233.

40. Tanaka K, Yoneda M, Nakajima T, Miyatake T, Owada M. Dihydrobiopterin synthesis defect: an adult with diurnal fluctuation of symptoms. *Neurology* 1987;37: 519–522.

41. Wevers RA, de Rijk-van Andel, Jansen MJT, Gabreels FJM, Smeitink JAM. Tyrosine hydroxylase deficiency: clinical presentation, biochemistry and treatment in four Dutch cases. *J Inher Metab Dis* 1996;19 (S1):7.

42. Williams A, Levine R, Chase T, Lovenberg W, Calne C. CSF hydroxylase cofactor levels in some neurological diseases. *J Neurol Neurosurg Psychiatry* 1980;43: 735–738.

43. Yebenes J, Moskowitz C, Fahn S, Saint Hillaire M. Long-term treatment with levodopa in a family with autosomal dominant torsion dystonia. *Adv Neurol* 1988;50:577–585.

Dystonia 3: Advances in Neurology, Vol. 78,
edited by S. Fahn, C. D. Marsden, and M. DeLong.
Lippincott–Raven Publishers, Philadelphia © 1998.

29

Tetrahydrobiopterin Metabolism and GTP Cyclohydrolase I Mutations in L-Dopa-Responsive Dystonia

*Laurent Bezin, *Panagiotis Z. Anastasiadis, †Torbjoern G. Nygaard, and *‡§Robert A. Levine

*William T. Gossett Neurology Laboratories, Henry Ford Hospital, Detroit, Michigan 48202; †Department of Neurology, Columbia University, New York, New York 10032, ‡Detroit Veterans Administration Medical Center, Detroit, Michigan 48202; and §Department of Psychiatry and Behavioral Neurosciences, Wayne State University, Detroit, Michigan 48202.

INTRODUCTION AND BACKGROUND

Early studies on pigments in butterfly wings led to the discovery of pterins (35) (from the Greek *pteron* for wing). The first biologic role for tetrahydrobiopterin (BH_4) discovered in humans was as the endogenous cofactor for phenylalanine hydroxylase in liver (43). BH_4 was subsequently identified as an essential cofactor for tyrosine hydroxylase (TH) and tryptophan hydroxylase (TPH), the rate-limiting enzymes in dopamine and serotonin synthesis. Beyond its key role in the synthesis of these biogenic amines, it is now known that BH_4 is also a cofactor for nitric oxide synthase (NOS) in the production of nitric oxide.

The metabolism of BH_4 and its *de novo* biosynthetic pathway are shown in Fig. 1. Efforts to understand the role of BH_4 biosynthesis in regulating brain biogenic amine metabolism were aided by discoveries (11,44,68) that certain forms of phenylketonuria in newborns (called atypical) were caused by a liver deficiency of BH_4 (and not phenylalanine hydroxylase).

Several recessively inherited deficiencies in the enzymes responsible for BH_4 biosynthesis have been recognized and cause "atypical phenylketonuria." The initial and rate-limiting enzyme in BH_4 synthesis, GTP cyclohydrolase I (GCH1), catalyzes the formation of dihydroneopterin triphosphate (NH_2TP) from GTP, and its expression is known to be defective in some cases of this disease (14,67). Mutations in 6-pyruvoyl-tetrahydropterin (6-PPH_4) synthase, the second enzyme in BH_4 biosynthesis (69), leads to high circulating neopterin and low biopterin levels. Although no sepiapterin reductase (SR) deficiencies have yet been detected in disease, the cloning of rat and human SR cDNAs (19,53) may allow detection of such deficiencies.

A salvage pathway for BH_4 synthesis exists in cells (66), but is not normally active (Fig. 2). The salvage pathway enables the elevation of intracellular BH_4 levels by converting exogenous sepiapterin or dihydrobiopterin to BH_4. This pathway can be utilized experimentally in cell culture to raise intracellular BH_4 levels.

More recently, we have defined other roles for BH_4 in cellular metabolism that include the enhancement of cell proliferation by BH_4, the requirement of intracellular BH_4 for growth factor enhancement of cell proliferation, and the involvement of BH_4 as a mediator of apop-

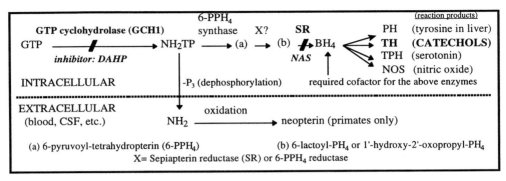

FIG. 1. *De novo* BH_4 biosynthetic pathway from GTP, and BH_4 metabolism.

tosis (programmed cell death). This chapter will review basic BH_4 metabolism and its involvement in neurologic diseases, additional roles for BH_4 in cell biology, and the effect of altered BH_4 metabolism in dopa-responsive dystonia (DRD).

Regulation of BH_4 Biosynthesis

Initial studies examined BH_4 biosynthesis in the periphery; however, with the elucidation of this pathway, recent studies have focused on its regulation and its role in the central nervous system. The catecholamine depleter, reserpine, elevates GCH1 activity and BH_4 levels in adrenal (1) and GCH1 mRNA in CNS aminergic neurons (32). The production of interferon-γ (IFN-γ) as a result of immune system activation elevates GCH1 activity and intracellular BH_4 levels in macrophages (88). GCH1 activity and mRNA, and BH_4 synthesis are also increased by IFN-γ in lymphocytes (77) and rat C6 glioma (20). The activities of other BH_4 biosynthetic enzymes under these activating conditions are usually unaltered.

The discovery of the GCH1 feedback regulatory protein (29,59), which complexes with the enzyme, explains how BH_4 accomplishes feedback inhibition (16) and how phenylalanine loading in humans stimulates GCH1 activity (48,60); BH_4 facilitates the binding of this feedback regulatory protein to GCH1, whereas phenylalanine promotes its dissociation from GCH1. Of the BH_4 biosynthetic enzymes, GCH1 has received the most attention due to its importance in controlling intracellular BH_4 levels, and its resultant influence on catecholamine and nitric oxide synthesis. However, BH_4 biosynthesis in humans is distinct from nonprimates in that neopterin appears in tissues and fluids as a result of accumulation of dihydroneopterin triphosphate and subsequent dephosphorylation and oxidation; this suggests that the enzymes after dihydroneopterin triphosphate, 6-PPH$_4$ synthase, and sepiapterin reductase may also play a role in regulating human BH_4 biosynthesis.

Regulation of Catecholamine and Nitric Oxide Synthesis by BH_4

Experiments both *in vivo* (62) and *in vitro* (2,18,40,49,75,76) have shown that BH_4 administration leads to an increase in TH activity

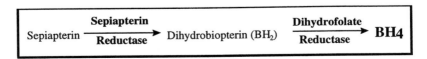

FIG. 2. Salvage pathway to BH_4 synthesis.

(45,62) and catecholamines and their metabolites in brain (62) and PC12 cells (6,7). An inhibitor of GCH1, 2,4-diamino-6-hydroxypyrimidine (DAHP), reduces brain BH_4 levels, which results in diminished catecholamine synthesis (83). Inhibition of GCH1 in PC12 cells reduces BH_4 levels and catecholamine synthesis in a dose-dependent manner (17). Catecholamine synthesis is elevated by exogenous BH_4, presumably by stimulating TH molecules that are subsaturated with respect to BH_4 (52). In the absence of exogenous BH_4, the short-term elevation of TH activity by phosphorylation occurs as a result of a reduction in the K_m of TH for BH_4. Because phosphorylation of TH does not alter its V_{max}, this mechanism is physiologically relevant because the intracellular concentration of BH_4 in catecholamine neurons is subsaturating for nonphosphorylated TH (4,52,56,92).

Inhibition of GCH1 and BH_4 biosynthesis by DAHP has also been shown to block the elevation of nitric oxide synthesis in many cell types (73,82). Binding of BH_4 to NOS is required for catalytic activity, although BH_4 is thought not to serve as an electron donor (28). It is presumed that synthesis of new BH_4 molecules is required for the catalytic activity of newly synthesized NOS to produce elevated nitric oxide levels. Thus, BH_4 plays a critical role in the rate of production and availability of both catecholamines and NO.

BH_4 Metabolism in Cell Proliferation, Apoptosis, and Neurodegeneration

BH_4 levels are significantly decreased in cerebrospinal fluid (CSF) of patients with Parkinson's disease (51). It is still not known whether the reduction of BH_4 simply reflects the loss of nigrostriatal DA cells in Parkinson's disease or whether BH_4 plays an active role in the neurodegenerative process. It has been shown in Parkinson's disease that DA neurons in the substantia nigra pars compacta die by apoptosis (9,63), and our recent studies have implicated BH_4 in mediating apoptosis when catecholamine cells are deprived of trophic support (manuscript submitted). Indeed, loss of trophic support over time is hypothesized to

play a role in several neurologic diseases, including Alzheimer's disease (78) and Parkinson's disease; neurotrophin therapy may be a viable approach in neurodegenerative diseases (81). A major focus in studies on the pathogenesis of Parkinson's disease is the formation of reactive oxygen species causing oxidative damage to nigrostriatal DA neurons (42). BH_4 and catecholamine metabolism may induce apoptosis by the formation of H_2O_2 (21) and oxygen free radical species (41,87), respectively. L-dopa therapy has been proposed to damage DA neurons in Parkinson's disease by elevating the formation of hydroxyl radical (80). Reactive oxygen species formed from dopamine catabolism can cause apoptotic cell death in PC12 cells (86) and cultured sympathetic neurons (93). There is also evidence in Parkinson's disease for the potential involvement of peroxynitrite, which can be formed from nitric oxide in neurons and glial cells in the nigrostriatal system (36). BH_4 itself is capable of degrading and liberating superoxide, which can oxidize nitric oxide to form peroxynitrite (58). The role of nitric oxide metabolism in apoptosis of PC12 cells is not clear; the nitric oxide-peroxynitrite pathway has been implicated to cause apoptosis in some studies (22,85), and delay the onset of apoptosis in another study (24). Clearly, further investigations are required to resolve the differing reports on nitric oxide metabolism in apoptosis.

Apoptosis is characterized by autolysis of DNA, nuclear condensation, and cell membrane blebbing (34). The homeostatic regulation of multicellular environments involves a balance among cell proliferation, growth arrest and differentiation, and eventual cell death. It has recently been demonstrated that BH_4 is mitogenic in rat PC12 cells and C6 gliomas (7). Further, the mitogenic effects of nerve growth factor and epidermal growth factor on undifferentiated PC12 cells absolutely requires the elevation of BH_4 biosynthesis (5). The connection between the mitogenic potential of BH_4 and apoptosis is relevant when one considers that differentiated neurons deprived of proper trophic support may initiate an inappropriate and fatal attempt to reenter the cell cycle (25);

any impetus for neuronal reentry in the cell cycle at an inappropriate time may initiate apoptosis. Indeed, we have recently shown that raising intracellular BH_4 levels during withdrawal of trophic support (nerve growth factor) in differentiated catecholamine neuron-like PC12 cells enhances apoptosis (manuscript submitted).

BH$_4$ Metabolism and Dopa-Responsive Dystonia

An alteration in BH_4 metabolism in dystonia was first suggested in 1979 when decreased CSF levels of BH_4 were detected in the affected members of one family (89,90); the importance of this was later confirmed (26,54). Reduced BH_4 levels in dystonia were ultimately shown to indicate the presence of DRD (65). A hallmark of DRD is that patients benefit from low doses of L-dopa (70). The locus of DRD, inherited as an autosomal-dominant trait, has been mapped to chromosome 14q (72). DRD was then found to be related to mutations in the gene for GCH1 (39). Mutations in the gene for GCH1 have been associated with DRD in numerous Japanese (27,31,38,39) and non-Japanese (10,27) families. The mutation identified in each of these families was unique; no mutation has been identified in about 30% of the families despite evidence of defective GCH1 enzyme function. These patients with no coding region mutations are phenotypically the same as individuals with recognized GCH1 mutations. Patients with clinically similar phenotypes have been suggested to exhibit autosomal-recessive deficiencies in TH (46,57) and 6-pyruvoyl-tetrahydropterin synthase (26,84).

DETECTION OF GCH1 DYSFUNCTION IN DOPA-RESPONSIVE DYSTONIA

Our studies in DRD were designed to develop an accurate diagnostic test for GCH1 dysfunction and further the understanding of dysfunctional GCH1 causing DRD. This is especially important because DRD can be misdiagnosed as cerebral palsy (71), which means that there are many more potential DRD pa-

tients that can be treated successfully. It has been reported that abnormally increased plasma phenylalanine levels several hours after phenylalanine loading in patients can be used to diagnose DRD (37). However, this test cannot identify if GCH1 or other enzymes are responsible for this abnormal clearance. Thus, an *in vitro* diagnostic test that identifies dysfunctional GCH1 or other BH_4 biosynthetic enzymes would be useful.

Mutational analysis seems inappropriate for routine diagnostic purposes because of its labor-intensive nature and that it will produce false positives in those patients lacking mutations in the coding region or in another related and as yet unidentified gene. Therefore, measuring GCH1 activity appears to be the best alternative for definitively identifying GCH1 dysfunction in the etiology of DRD. In this regard, Ichinose and coworkers (39) detected less *in vitro* GCH1 activity in monocytes from DRD patients stimulated with phytohemagglutinin (PHA) than controls. The measurement of GCH1 activity in monocytes poses a potential problem. Monocyte GCH1 activity cannot be detected under basal conditions and must be measured after cells are stimulated with PHA (39). In a control patient with an inability to induce the GCH1 gene in response to inducing agents such as PHA, a false positive for DRD associated with GCH1 dysfunction would be generated. Thus, we investigated whether SV40-transformed lymphocytes (lymphoblasts) could be used to measure GCH1 activity under basal conditions to identify carriers of GCH1 dysfunction in DRD. We measured the content of endogenous neopterin (the major byproduct of GCH1 activity) as a reflection of *in vivo* GCH1 activity in lymphoblasts derived from members of a four-generation family affected by DRD (13). We have also examined the effects of IFN-γ plus lipopolysaccharide (LPS), interleukin-2 (IL-2) plus LPS, or PHA stimulation on lymphoblast neopterin content. The activity of sepiapterin reductase, the final BH_4 biosynthetic enzyme, was assayed to reveal the specificity of lymphoblast neopterin measurement as a marker for DRD associated with GCH1 dysfunction.

Patient Samples

Eleven individuals in the four-generation family exhibit different phenotypes, including:

1. Four females, each from different generations, expressing DRD symptoms and carrying the great-grandmaternal chromosome 14 that leads to GCH1 dysfunction;
2. One asymptomatic female carrying the gene for GCH1 dysfunction;
3. One male having a nonconservative mutation in exon 6 of the GCH1 coding region for which he was asymptomatic; he is related only by marriage to an affected female, and their daughter exhibited the most severe phenotype of all affected members;
4. Six unaffected male noncarriers.

The combination of the exon 6 mutation with the dysfunctional GCH1 in the maternal line has caused expression of a more severe phenotype in the daughter than occurs in the other affected females. Lymphocytes from carriers and noncarriers were SV40-transformed to stable lymphoblasts lines and cultured as previously described (8).

Lymphoblast Treatments

In untreated conditions, media was changed each 24 hours and cells were harvested 24 hours after the last media change. When cells were treated with IFN-γ plus LPS, IL-2 plus LPS, or PHA, they were stabilized (as described above) for 48 hours before initiation of treatment. For IL-2 plus IFN-γ, we treated lymphoblasts for 72 hours, which had previously been shown to induce GCH1 activity in transformed human lymphocytes (91). All experiments have been done at least in duplicate. In each series of experiments, each cell line was seeded in duplicate or triplicate.

Assays

Total neopterin was measured in 90 μl of supernatant from extracts of ~3.6 $\times 10^6$ lymphoblasts (after dephosphorylation of NH_2TP and subsequent oxidation of NH_2). Supernatants were exposed to alkaline phosphatase to form dihydroneopterin from the dephosphorylation of NH_2TP, which was followed by acid iodine oxidation of dihydroneopterin to produce neopterin (15). Neopterin was measured by high pressure liquid chromatography (HPLC). In certain experiments, *in vitro* GCH1 activity was measured in 50 μl of supernatant derived from lymphoblast extracts (~2 $\times 10^6$ lymphoblasts) by monitoring the conversion of GTP (1 mM) to dihydroneopterin triphosphate (NH_2TP) at maximum velocity (15). The activity of sepiapterin reductase was measured in 40 μl of supernatant (~1.6 $\times 10^6$ lymphoblasts) under saturating cosubstrate conditions as described previously (50).

DNA Sequencing

Genomic DNA from all available family members was sequenced for the six exons of GCH1 by standard techniques using primers published by Ichinose et al. (39). All exons were sequenced in both directions. The resulting sequences were compared with published GCH1 sequence data (GenBank accession numbers U15256-15259).

Major Findings

We were able to measure endogenous neopterin in all lymphoblast extracts under basal and GCH1 induction conditions. When attempting to measure GCH1 activity *in vitro* under basal or cytokine treatment conditions, all neopterin detected was present at the start of the assay and represented *in vivo* GCH1 activity. Thus, our measures of endogenous neopterin reflect *in vivo* GCH1 activity, since 2 mM DAHP treatment of cultured cells eliminated intracellular neopterin at 48 hours. An advantage of this assay is that all components of the GCH1 assay are examined, so any alteration in the expression and induction of GCH1 that changes *in vivo* activity can be detected.

All DRD patients and the asymptomatic carrier had lymphoblast neopterin levels significantly less than noncarriers. There was no overlap between these groups, and the carrier with the highest neopterin level was well below the noncarrier with the lowest neopterin level. The specificity of the measure of decreased GCH1 function in DRD was indicated because carriers were not distinguished from noncarriers by the measurement of sepiapterin reductase activity. Thus, the measurement of neopterin content in lymphoblast cultured under basal conditions appears to be a viable method for detecting carriers of dysfunctional GCH1 associated with DRD.

No lymphoblast lines from the carriers of great-grandmaternal chromosome 14 exhibited elevated neopterin levels following treatment with either IFN-γ plus LPS, IFN-γ plus IL-2, or PHA after 48 hours. Although we expected all noncarriers to have higher neopterin levels to due to stimulation of *in vivo* GCH1 activity by these treatments, this was not uniformly the case. In response to IFN-γ plus LPS, only two of the four noncarriers tested exhibited an increase in lymphoblast neopterin content. We then tested the same four noncarriers for lymphoblast stimulation by PHA for 48 hours. In this case, the two noncarriers who exhibited elevated lymphoblast neopterin by IFN-γ plus LPS did not respond to PHA. Equally unexpected was that the two noncarriers that did not respond to IFN-γ plus LPS exhibited significantly higher lymphoblast neopterin content. Thus, there is not a uniform response of control patients to treatments that are traditionally thought to induce GCH1 activity. If this same phenomenon occurs in lymphocytes, then a lack of GCH1 activity in lymphocytes from asymptomatic patients measured under stimulation conditions may yield false positives for DRD due to a lack of GCH1 induction (GCH1 activity is not detectable in lymphocytes cultured in basal conditions). This points to the potential importance of assaying enzyme activity in unstimulated cells to distinguish carriers from noncarriers of dysfunctional GCH1. It is also possible that certain cases of DRD where no coding region mutations exist are caused by dysfunctional induction of GCH1.

In sequencing the GCH1 gene, [a 1 base deletion in exon 2] was detected in the first three generations of women affected with DRD. There was a nonconservative heterozygous T->C mutation in exon 6 from the youngest female and her father, which caused a methionine to be replaced by threonine at amino acid 221 in GCH1. The exon 6 mutation did not cause obvious GCH1 dysfunction in the father, because neopterin levels were the same as other controls and neopterin levels could be induced. This demonstrates that not all GCH1 coding region mutations significantly affect GCH1 activity. Since his daughter, who inherited the DRD-related GCH1 defect from her symptomatic mother, exhibited the most severe phenotype (13), it appears that defects affecting both copies of the GCH1 gene may lead to greater neurologic dysfunction.

While it has been shown that patients with essentially identical phenotypes as our patients exhibit coding region mutations (39), some other dysfunction in GCH1 expression must be invoked to explain why some DRD patients with no coding region mutations exhibit dysfunctional GCH1. Perhaps all of the induction mechanisms for GCH1 expression are disabled in DRD with associated dysfunctional GCH1. However, this cannot account for the asymptomatic carrier of dysfunctional GCH1; clearly, further studies are required to understand fully the extent to which dysfunctional GCH1 causes the symptoms of DRD.

SUMMARY

Our studies have shown that BH_4 can under certain conditions exhibit mitogenic actions on dividing catecholamine cells. Furthermore, the mitogenic actions of nerve growth factor and epidermal growth factor are dependent on and mediated by intracellular BH_4. Because growth factors are important in defining and maintaining neuronal phenotype in development, alterations in BH_4 metabolism in DRD may reduce the degree of expression of catecholamine neuronal character in development. In conditions of trophic support withdrawal, the intracellular

BH$_4$ that supports critical functions in normal neuronal metabolism switches to accelerating apoptotic cell death. It may be possible to protect catecholamine neurons from death in diseases where apoptosis of catecholamine neurons has been observed, such as Parkinson's disease.

In DRD associated with dysfunctional GCH1, we have shown the importance of assessing GCH1 activity in lymphoblasts under basal conditions rather than after stimulation of GCH1 expression. The endogenous level of neopterin, which directly reflects the intracellular activity of GCH1, can be measured reliably in unstimulated lymphoblasts and is a potential marker for carriers of dysfunctional GCH1 associated with DRD. The establishment of these immortalized lymphoblasts will enable in-depth analysis of pedigrees containing a larger number of generations. They also represent a system whereby other factors involved in the *in vivo* expression of GCH1 can be analyzed. Cultured lymphoblasts will be of value for examining other potential defects at different enzymatic steps in BH$_4$ metabolism in neurologic diseases, including DRD.

ACKNOWLEDGMENT

This work was supported, in part, by a grant from the Dystonia Medical Research Foundation (RAL) and NIH NS 32035 (TGN).

REFERENCES

1. Abou-Donia MM, Viveros OH. Tetrahydrobiopterin increases in adrenal medulla and cortex: a factor in the regulation of tyrosine hydroxylase. *Proc Natl Acad Sci USA* 1981;78:2703–2706.
2. Abou-Donia MM, Zimmerman TP, Nichol CA, Viveros OH. Tetrahydrobiopterin synthesis and the role of the cofactor in the regulation of tyrosine hydroxylase in adrenomedullary chromaffin cells. *Biochem Clin Aspects Pteridines* 1985;4:221–236.
3. Allsopp TE, Wyatt S, Paterson HF, Davies AM. The proto-oncogene bcl-2 can selectively rescue neurotropic factor-dependent neurons from apoptosis. *Cell* 1993;73:295–307.
4. Ames MM, Lerner P, Lovenberg W. *J Biol Chem* 1978; 253:27–31.
5. Anastasiadis PZ, Bezin L, Imerman BA, Kuhn DM, Louie MC, Levine RA. Tetrahydrobiopterin as a medi-
6. Anastasiadis PZ, Kuhn DM, Levine RA. Tetrahydrobiopterin uptake in rat brain synaptosomes, cultured PC12 cells, and rat striatum. *Brain Res* 1994;665:77–84.
7. Anastasiadis PZ, States JC, Imerman BA, Louie MC, Kuhn DM, Levine RA. Mitogenic effects of tetrahydrobiopterin in PC12 cells. *Mol Pharmacol* 1996;49: 149–155.
8. Anderson MA, Gusella JF. Use of cyclosporin A in establishing Epstein-Barr virus-transformed human lymphoblastoid cell lines. *In Vitro* 1984;29:856–858.
9. Anglade P, Vyas S, Javoy-Agid F, et al. Apoptosis and autophagy in nigral neurons of patients with Parkinson's disease. *Histol Histopathol* 1997; 12:603–610.
10. Bandmann O, Nygaard TG, Surtees R, Marsden CD, Wood NW, Harding AE. Dopa-responsive dystonia in British patients: new mutations of the GTP-cyclohydrolase I gene and evidence for genetic heterogeneity. *Hum Mol Genet* 1996;5:403–406.
11. Bartholome K, Byrd DJ. L-Dopa and 5-hydroxytryptophan therapy in phenylketonuria with normal phenylalanine-hydroxylase activity. Lancet 1975;2:1042–1043.
12. Batistatou A, Greene LA. Internucleosomal DNA cleavage and neuronal cell survival/death. *J Cell Biol* 1993;122:523–532.
13. Bebin EM, Fryberg JS, Trugman JM. Dopa-responsive dystonia (DRD) presenting in the first year of life. *Neurology* 1995;45:184.
14. Blau N, Ichinose H, Nagatsu T, Heizmann CW, Zacchello F, Burlina AB. A missense mutation in a patient with guanosine triphosphate cyclohydrolase I deficiency missed in the newborn screening program. *J Pediatr* 1995;126:401–405.
15. Blau N, Niederwieser A. Guanosine triphosphate cyclohydrolase I assay in human and rat liver using high-performance liquid chromatography of neopterin phosphates and guanine nucleotides. *Anal Biochem* 1983;128:446–452.
16. Blau N, Niederwieser A. GTP-cyclohydrolases: a review. *J Clin Chem Clin Biochem* 1985;23:169–176.
17. Brautigam M, Dreesen R, Herken H. Tetrahydrobiopterin and total biopterin content of neuroblastoma (N1E-115,N2A) and pheochromocytoma (PC-12) clones and the dependence of catecholamine synthesis on tetrahydrobiopterin concentration in PC-12 cells. *J Neurochem* 1984;42:390–396.
18. Brautigam M, Pfleiderer W. Effects of tetrahydropterins on DOPA production in vitro and in vivo. In: Curtius H-C, Blau N, Levine RA, eds. *Unconjugated pterins and related biogenic amines.* Berlin, New York: Walter de Gruyter, 1987:359–366.
19. Citron BA, Milstien S, Gutierrez JC, Levine RA, Yanak BL, Kaufman S. Isolation and expression of rat liver sepiapterin reductase cDNA. *Proc Natl Acad Sci USA* 1990;87:6436–6440.
20. D'Sa C, Hirayama K, West A, Hahn M, Zhu M, Kapatos G. Tetrahydrobiopterin biosynthesis in C6 glioma cells: induction of GTP cyclohydrolase I gene expression by lipopolysaccharide and cytokine treatment. *Mol Brain Res* 1996;41:105–110.
21. Davis MD, Kaufman S. Products of the tyrosine-dependent oxidation of tetrahydrobiopterin by rat liver

phenylalanine hydroxylase. *Arch Biochem Biophys* 1993;304:9–16.

22. Estevez AG, Radi R, Barbeito L, Shin JT, Thompson JA, Beckman JS. Peroxynitrite-induced cytotoxicity in PC12 cells: evidence for an apoptotic mechanism differentially modulated by neurotrophic factors. *J Neurochem* 1995;65:1543–1550.

23. Evan G, Harrington E, Fanidi A, Land H, Amati B, Bennett M. Integrated control of cell proliferation and cell death by the c-myc oncogene [Review]. Philos Trans R Soc London B Biol Sci 1994;345:269–275.

24. Farinelli SE, Park DS, Greene LA. Nitric oxide delays the death of trophic factor-deprived PC12 cells and sympathetic neurons by a cGMP-mediated mechanism. *J Neurosci* 1996;16:2325–2334.

25. Ferrari G, Greene LA. Proliferative inhibition by dominant-negative Ras rescues naive and neuronally differentiated PC12 cells from apoptotic death. *EMBO J* 1994;13:5922–5928.

26. Fink JK, Barton N, Cohen W, Lovenberg W, Burns RS, Hallett M. Dystonia with marked diurnal variation associated with biopterin deficiency. *Neurology* 1988;38:707–711.

27. Furukawa Y, Shimadzu M, Rajput AH, et al. GTP-cyclohydrolase I gene mutations in hereditary progressive and dopa-responsive dystonia. *Ann Neurol* 1996; 39:609–617.

28. Giovanelli J, Campos KL, Kaufman S. Tetrahydrobiopterin, a cofactor for rat cerebellar nitric oxide synthase, does not function as a reactant in the oxygenation of arginine. *Proc Natl Acad Sci USA* 1991;88: 7091–7095.

29. Harada T, Kagamiyama H, Hatakeyama K. Feedback regulation mechanisms for the control of GTP cyclohydrolase I activity. *Science* 1993;260:1507–1510.

30. Hermeking H, Eick D. Mediation of c-myc-induced apoptosis by p53. *Science* 1994;265:2091–2093.

31. Harano M, Tamaru Y, Nagai Y, Ito H, Imai T, Ueno S. Exon skipping caused by a base substitution at a splice site in the GTP cyclohydrolase I gene in a Japanese family with hereditary progressive dystonia dopa responsive dystonia. *Biochem Biophys Res Commun* 1995;213:645–651.

32. Hirayama K, Lentz SI, Kapatos G. Tetrahydrobiopterin cofactor biosynthesis: GTP cyclohydrolase I mRNA expression in rat brain and superior cervical ganglia. *J Neurochem* 1993;61:1006–1014.

33. Hockenbery DM, Oltvai ZN, Yin XM, Milliman CL, Korsmeyer SJ. Bcl-2 functions in an antioxidant pathway to prevent apoptosis. *Cell* 1993;75:241–251.

34. Hoffman B, Liebermann DA. Molecular controls of apoptosis: differentiation/growth arrest primary response genes, proto-oncogenes, and tumor suppressor genes as positive & negative modulators. *Oncogene* 1994;9:1807–1812.

35. Hopkins FG. Yellow pigments in butterflies. *Nature* 1989;40:355.

36. Hunot S, Boissiere F, Faucheux B, et al. Nitric oxide synthase and neuronal vulnerability in Parkinson's disease. *Neuroscience* 1996;72:355–363.

37. Hyland K, Fryburg JS, Wilson WG, et al. Oral phenylalanine loading in dopa-responsive dystonia: a possible diagnostic test. *Neurology* 1997; 48:1290–1297.

38. Ichinose H, Ohye T, Segawa M, et al. GTP cyclohydrolase I gene in hereditary progressive dystonia with marked diurnal fluctuation. *Neurosci Lett* 1995;196:5–8.

39. Ichinose H, Ohye T, Takahashi E, et al. Hereditary progressive dystonia with marked diurnal fluctuation caused by mutations in the GTP cyclohydrolase I gene. *Nat Genet* 1994;8:236–242.

40. Iuvone PM, Reinhard JR Jr, Abou-Donia MM, Viveros OH, Nichol CA. Stimulation of retinal dopamine biosynthesis in vivo by exogenous tetrahydrobiopterin: relationship to tyrosine hydroxylase activation. *Brain Res* 1985;359:392–396.

41. Jenner P, Dexter DT, Sian J, Schapira AH, Marsden CD. Oxidative stress as a cause of nigral cell death in Parkinson's disease and incidental Lewy body disease. The Royal Kings and Queens Parkinson's Disease Research Group [Review]. *Ann Neurol* 1992;32[Suppl]: S82–S87.

42. Jenner P, Olanow CW. Oxidative stress and the pathogenesis of Parkinson's disease. *Neurology* 1996;47: S161–S170.

43. Kaufman S. The structure of the phenylalanine-hydroxylation cofactor. *Proc Natl Acad Sci USA* 1963; 50:1085–1093.

44. Kaufman S, Holtzman NA, Milstien S, Butler I, Krumhotz A. Phenylketonuria due to a deficiency of dihyropteridine reductase. *N Engl J Med* 1975;293: 785–790.

45. Kettler R, Bartholini G, Pletscher A. *In vivo* enhancement of tyrosine hydroxylation in rat striatum by tetrahydrobiopterin. *Nature* 1974;249:476–478.

46. Knappskog PM, Flatmark T, Mallet J, Ludecke B, Bartholome K. Recessively inherited L-DOPA-responsive dystonia caused by a point mutation (Q381K) in the tyrosine hydroxylase gene. *Hum Mol Genet* 1995; 4:1209–1212.

47. Korsmeyer SJ, Yin XM, Oltvai ZN, Veis-Novack DJ, Linette GP. Reactive oxygen species and the regulation of cell death by the Bcl-2 gene family. *Biochim Biophys Acta* 1995;1271:63–66.

48. Leeming RJ, Blair JA, Green A, Raine DN. Biopertin derivatives in normal and phenyl ketonuric patients after oral loads of L-phenylalanine, L-tyrosine, and L-tryptophan. *Arch Dis Child* 1976;51:771–777.

49. Levine RA. In: Cooper BA, Whitehead VM, eds. *Tetrahydrobiopterin and the regulation of catecholamine synthesis in bovine adrenal medullary chromaffin cells.* Berlin, New York: Walter de Gruyter & Co, 1986;373–376.

50. Levine RA, Kapatos G, Kaufman S, Milstien S. Immunological evidence for the requirement of sepiapterin reductase for tetrahydrobiopterin biosynthesis in brain. *J Neurochem* 1990;54:1218–1224.

51. Levine RA, Kuhn DM, Lovenberg W. The regional distribution of hydroxylase cofactor in rat brain. *J Neurochem* 1979;32:1575–1578.

52. Levine RA, Miller LP, Lovenberg W. Tetrahydrobiopterin in striatum: localization in dopamine nerve terminals and role in catecholamine synthesis. *Science* 1981;214:919–921.

53. Levine RA, Solus JF, Goustin AS, et al. Isolation of a putative cDNA encoding human brain sepiaptrin reductase. In: Blau N, Curtius HC, Levine RA, Cotton RGH, eds. *Pterins and biogenic amines in neurology, pediatrics, and immunology.* Grosse Pointe: Lake shore Publishing, 1991:81–88.

54. LeWitt PA, Miller LP, Levine RA, et al. Tetrahydro-biopterin in dystonia: identification of abnormal metabolism and therapeutic trials. *Neurology* 1986;36: 760–764.

55. Lopes UG, Erhardt P, Yao R, Cooper GM. p53-dependent induction of apoptosis by proteasome inhibitors . *J Biol Chem* 1997;272:12893– 12896.

56. Lovenberg W, Bruckwick E, Hanbauer I. ATP, cyclic AMP, and magnesium increase the affinity of rat striatal tyrosine hydroxylase for its cofactor. *Proc Natl Acad Sci USA* 1975;72:2955–2958.

57. Ludecke B, Dworniczak B, Bartholome K. A point mutation in the tyrosine hydroxylase gene associated with Segawa's syndrome. *Hum Genet* 1995;95:123–125.

58. Mayer B, Klatt P, Werners ER, Schmidt K. Kinetics and mechanism of tetrahydrobiopterin-induced oxidation of nitric oxide. *J Biol Chem* 1995;270:655–659.

59. Milstien S, Jaffe H, Kowlessur D, Bonner TI. Purification and cloning of the GTP cyclohydrolase I feedback regulatory protein, GFRP. *J Biol Chem* 1996;271: 19743–19751.

60. Milstien S, Kaufman S. Regulation of biopterin biosynthesis in the rat. In: Blair JA, ed. *Chemistry and biology of pteridines*. 1993 Plenum Press, NY.

61. Miura M, Zhu H, Rotello R, Hartwieg E, Yuan J. Induction of apoptosis in fibroblasts by IL-1 beta-converting enzyme, a mammalian homolog of the *C. elegans* cell death gene ced-3. *Cell* 1993;75:653.

62. Miwa S, Watanabe Y, Hayaishi O. 6R-L-erythro-5,6, 7,8-tetrahydrobiopterin as a regulator of dopamine and serotonin biosynthesis in the rat brain. *Arch Biochem Biophys* 1985;239:234–241.

63. Mochizuki H, Goto K, Mori H, Mizuno Y. Histochemical detection of apoptosis in Parkinson's disease. *J Neurol Sci* 1996;137:120–123.

64. Motoyama N, Wang F, Roth KA, et al. Massive cell death of immature hematopoietic cells and neurons in Bcl-x-deficient mice. *Science* 1995;267:1506–1510.

65. Naini AB, Nygaard TG, Hirsch O, et al. Cerebrospinal fluid biopterin in disorders causing juvenile dystonia-parkinsonism. *Neurology* 1995;45:430.

66. Nichol CA, Lee CL, Edelstein MP, Chao JY, Duch DS. Biosynthesis of tetrahydrobiopterin by *de novo* and salvage pathways in adrenal medulla extracts, mammalian cell cultures, and rat brain *in vivo*. *Proc Natl Acad Sci USA* 1983;80:1546–1550.

67. Niederwieser A, Blau N, Wang M, Joller P, Atares M, Cardesa-Garcia J. GTP cyclohydrolase I deficiency, a new enzyme defect causing hyperphenylalaninemia with neopterin, biopterin, dopamine, and serotonin deficiencies and muscular hyptonia. *Eur J Pediatr* 1984; 141:208–214.

68. Niederwieser A, Curtius HC, Wang M, Leupold D. Atypical phenylketonuria with defective biopterin metabolism. Monotherapy with tetrahydrobiopterin or sepiapterin, screening und study of biosynthesis in man. *Eur J Pediatr* 1982;138:110–112.

69. Niederwieser A, Shintaku H, Leimbacher W, et al. "Peripheral" tetrahydrobiopterin deficiency with hyperphenylalaninaemia due to incomplete 6-pyruvoyl tetrahydropterin synthase deficiency or heterozygosity. *Eur J Pediatr* 1987;146:228–232.

70. Nygaard TG, Marsden CD, Duvoisin RC. Dopa-responsive dystonia [Review]. *Adv Neurol* 1988;50: 377–384.

71. Nygaard TG, Waran SP, Levine RA, Naini AB, Chutorian AM. Dopa-responsive dystonia simulating cerebral palsy. *Pediatr Neurol* 1994;11:236–240.

72. Nygaard TG, Wilhelmsen KC, Risch NJ, et al. Linkage mapping of dopa-responsive dystonia (DRD) to chromosome 14q. *Nature* 1993;5:386–391.

73. Oddis CV, Finkel MS. NF-kappaB and GTP cyclohydrolase regulate cytokine-induced nitric oxide production by cardiac myocytes. *Am J Physiol Heart Circ Physiol* 1996;270:H1864–H1868.

74. Oltvai Z, Millman C, Korsmeyer S. Bcl-2 heterodimerizes in vivo with a conserved homolog, bax, that accelerates programed cell death. *Cell* 1993;74:609.

75. Patrick RL, Barchas JD. Dopamine synthesis in rat brain striatal synaptosomes II: Dibutyryl cyclic adenosine 3′:5′-monophosphoric acid and 6-methyltetrahydropterine-induced synthesis increases without an increase in endogenous dopamine release. *J Pharmacol Exp Ther* 1976;197:97–104.

76. Sawada M, Sugimoto T, Matsuura S, Nagatsu T. (6R)-tetrahydrobiopterin increases the activity of tryptophan hydroxylase in rat raphe slices. *J Neurochem* 1986;47:1544–1547.

77. Schott K, Gutlich M, Ziegler I. Induction of GTP-cyclohydrolase I mRNA expression by lectin activation and interferon-gamma treatment in human cells associated with the immune response. *J Cell Physiol* 1993; 156:12–16.

78. Scott SA, Crutcher KA. Nerve growth factor and Alzheimer's disease. *Rev Neurosci* 1994;5:179–211.

79. Selvakumaran M, Lin HK, Sjin RT, Reed JC, Lieberman DA, Hoffman B. The novel primary response gene MyD1180
and the proto-oncogenes myb, myc, and bcl-2 modulate transforming growth factor beta 1-induced apoptosis of myeloid leukemia cells. *Mol Cell Biol* 1994;14:2352–2360.

80. Smith TS, Parker WD Jr, Bennett JP Jr. L-dopa increases nigral production of hydroxyl radicals in vivo: potential L-dopa toxicity? *Neuroreport* 1994;5:1009–1011.

81. Snider WD, Johnson EM Jr. Neurotrophic molecules. *Ann Neurol* 1989;26:489–506.

82. Sung YJ, Hotchkiss JH, Dietert RR. 2,4-Diamino-6-hydroxypyrimidine, an inhibitor of GTP cyclohydrolase I, suppresses nitric oxide production by chicken macrophages. *Int J Immunopharmacol* 1994;16: 101–108.

83. Suzuki S, Watanabe Y, Tsubokura S, Kagamiyama H, Hayaishi O. Decrease in tetrahydrobiopterin content and neurotransmitter amine biosynthesis in rat brain by an inhibitor of guanosine triphosphate cyclohydrolase. *Brain Res* 1988;446:1–10.

84. Tanaka K, Yoneda M, Nakajima T, Miyatake T, Owada M. Dihydrobiopterin synthesis defect: an adult with diurnal fluctuation of symptoms. *Neurology* 1987;37: 519–522.

85. Troy CM, Shelanski ML. Down-regulation of copper/zinc superoxide dismutase causes apoptotic death in PC12 neuronal cells. *Proc Natl Acad Sci USA* 1994;91:6384–6387.

86. Velez-Pardo C, Jimenez Del Rio M, Verschueren H, Ebinger G, Vauquelin G. Dopamine and iron induce apoptosis in PC12 cells. *Pharmacol Toxicol* 1997;80:76–84.

87. Walkinshaw G, Waters CM. Induction of apoptosis in

catecholaminergic PC12 cells by L-DOPA. Implications for the treatment of Parkinson's disease. *J Clin Invest* 1995;95:2458–2464.

88. Werner ER, Werner-Felmayer G, Fuchs D, et al. Tetrahydrobiopterin biosynthetic activities in human macrophages, fibroblasts, THP-1, and T24 cells. *J Biol Chem* 1990;265:3189–3192.

89. Williams AC, Eldridge R, Levine RA, Lovenberg W, Paulson G. Low CSF hydroxylase cofactor (tetrahydrobiopterin) levels in inherited dystonia. *Lancet* 1979;8139:410–411.

90. Williams AC, Levine RA, Chase TN, Lovenberg W, Calne DB. CFS hydroxylase cofactor levels in some

neurological diseases. *J Neurol Neurosurg Psychiatry* 1980;43:735–738.

91. Ziegler I, Schott K, Lubbert M, Herrmann F, Schwulera U, Bacher A. Control of tetrahydrobiopterin synthesis in T lymphocytes by synergistic action of interferon-gamma and interleukin-2. *J Biol Chem* 1990;265:17026–17030.

92. Zigmond RE. A comparison of the long-term and short-term regulations of tyrosine hydroxylase activity. *J Physiol (Paris)* 1988;83:267–271.

93. Zilkha-Falb R, Ziv I, Nardi N, Offen D, Melamed E, Barzilai A. Monoamine-induced apoptotic neuronal cell death. *Cell Mol Neurobiol* 1997;17:101–118.

Dystonia 3: Advances in Neurology, Vol. 78,
edited by S. Fahn, C. D. Marsden, and M. DeLong.
Lippincott–Raven Publishers, Philadelphia © 1998.

30

Defects of Biopterin Metabolism and Biogenic Amine Biosynthesis: Clinical, Diagnostic, and Therapeutic Aspects

*†Keith Hyland, *Lauren A. Arnold, and ‡Joel M. Trugman

*Kimberly H. Courtwright and Joseph W. Summers Institute of Metabolic Disease, Dallas, Texas 75226; †Department of Neurology, University of Texas Southwestern Medical Center, Dallas, Texas 75235; and ‡Department of Neurology, University of Virginia School of Medicine, Charlottesville, Virginia 22908.

Dopa-responsive dystonia (DRD), an autosomal-dominant condition, has recently been associated with mutations in the gene for GTP cyclohydrolase I (20). This is the first and rate-limiting enzyme involved in the synthesis of tetrahydrobiopterin (BH_4), the obligatory cofactor for the synthesis of serotonin and the catecholamine neurotransmitters (Fig. 1). Autosomal recessively inherited defects in BH_4 metabolism have also been recognized (7,14, 23,31,32). Deficiencies of GTP cyclohydrolase I and 6-pyruvoyltetrahydropterin synthase decrease the rate of BH_4 biosynthesis, whereas defects of pterin-4a-carbinolamine dehydratase and dihydropteridine reductase affect the rate at which the cofactor is recycled back to its active form following oxidation in the hydroxylase reactions (Fig. 1). In addition to these disorders of BH_4 metabolism, autosomal recessively inherited defects of tyrosine hydroxylase (TH) (24,27) and aromatic L-amino acid decarboxylase (AADC) (19,28) also lead to severe monoamine neurotransmitter deficiency within the central nervous system. Although all of these disorders are associated with defective monoamine biosynthesis, the clinical features differ and the type of treatment depends on the site of the metabolic block.

CLINICAL FEATURES

Dopa-Responsive Dystonia

DRD normally presents as a dystonic gait disorder with mean age of onset around 6 years; however, the spectrum of clinical manifestations is broad (34,40). A diurnal variation in symptoms is common (34,40). Some children have presented in the first 2 years of life with developmental motor delay (35,40), whereas in some older children, prominent upper motor neuron findings, including spastic diplegia, have led to the misdiagnosis of cerebral palsy (4,10,35). Because of the reduced penetrance some carriers remain asymptomatic, whereas others present with parkinsonian features in later life. The primary defects of TH have also been referred to as DRD as these infants have responded to levodopa therapy (24,27). Unfortunately the clinical features of this condition have not yet been clearly documented.

Other Defects of Tetrahydrobiopterin Metabolism

The recessively inherited defects of BH_4 metabolism present within the first 2 to 8 months of life with a mixture of fairly nonspe-

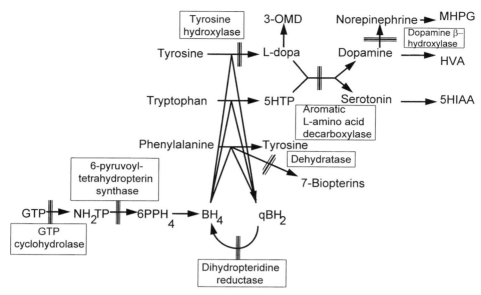

FIG. 1. Defects of tetrahydrobiopterin metabolism and biogenic amine biosynthesis. Boxed headings and triple bars indicate the sites of known inborn errors of metabolism. GTP, guanosine triphosphate; NH_2TP, dihydroneopterin triphosphate; $6PPH_4$, 6-pyruvoyltetrahydropterin; BH_4, tetrahydrobiopterin; qBH_2, quinonoid dihydrobiopterin; dehydratase, pterin-4a-carbinolamine dehydratase; 3-OMD, 3-*O* methyldopa; L-dopa, levodopa; 5HTP, 5-hydroxytryptophan; MHPG, 3-methoxy-4-hydroxyphenylglycol; HVA, homovanillic acid; 5HIAA, 5-hydroxyindoleacetic acid.

cific neurologic symptoms that normally include hypokinesis, distal chorea, myoclonic epilepsy, temperature disturbance, and hypersalivation. These can be associated with mental retardation, microcephaly, developmental delay, pinpoint pupils, excessive irritability, convulsions, oculogyric crises, hyper- or hypotonia, and swallowing difficulties. Untreated, the infants slowly develop a more easily recognizable parkinsonian-type syndrome with hypokinesis, drooling, swallowing difficulty, sweating, pinpoint pupils, oculogyric spasms, truncal hypotonia, increased limb tone, and blank facies, which is found together with myoclonus, chorea, and brisk tendon jerks. Infantile spasms, grand mal fits, and hyperpyrexia may also be present (14,41). Dystonia is not a prominent feature of the recessively inherited disorders of BH_4 metabolism, although it has occasionally been reported (9,44). As well as these "typical" disorders of BH_4 metabolism, there are "atypical" forms in which the central nervous system seems

to be unaffected and neurologic signs are absent (2).

An insidious deficiency of folate may occur in dihydropteridine reductase deficiency (23,42) and if not recognized it can lead to devastating changes within the central nervous system. Brain lesions consist of multifocal, perivascular demyelination in the subcortical white matter accompanied by perivascular, microcalcification that is also present in the basal ganglia (26,42, 43). The folate deficiency is thought to arise as a result of competitive inhibition of dihydrofolate reductase and 5,10-methylenetetrahydrofolate reductase by the 7,8- and quinonoid dihydrobiopterins that accumulate due to the absence of dihydropteridine reductase activity (30,42).

Aromatic L-Amino Acid Decarboxylase Deficiency

The authors are aware of five cases of AADC deficiency and the clinical features in many respects resemble those of the recessive BH_4 disorders (19,28; unpublished information). Presentation has been between 2 and 6 months of age and symptoms have included generalized hypotonia, developmental delay, oculogyric crises, irritability, feeding difficulties, hypokinesia, poor head control, fine chorea of the distal limbs, temperature instability, ptosis, excessive sweating, and dystonia. Some diurnal variation of symptoms has also been present.

Dopamine β-Hydroxylase Deficiency

Dopamine β-hydroxylase deficiency has only been diagnosed in adults who have presented with severe orthostatic hypotension and noradrenergic failure. There is no evidence of other neurologic defects, either central or peripheral. Retrospective evaluations have exposed difficulties in the perinatal period, including ptosis, delayed eye opening, hypotension, hypothermia, and hypoglycemia (37).

DIAGNOSIS

The procedures required for the diagnosis of the "typical" autosomal recessively inherited defects of BH_4 metabolism have been adequately reviewed previously (3,17,33). Briefly, as BH_4 is required for the hydroxylation of phenylalanine in the liver, infants are detected at newborn screening due to the presence of hyperphenylalaninemia. Examination of the urine pterin pattern (biopterin and its precursor, neopterin) together with measurement of dihydropteridine reductase activity in blood permit the precise location of the defect to be defined and allow these conditions to be distinguished from primary defects affecting phenylalanine hydroxylase (17,33) (Fig. 2). In the "typical" defects, BH_4 metabolism is also compromised within the central nervous system. There is a similar abnormal pattern of biopterin and neopterin in cerebrospinal fluid (CSF) and the low levels of BH_4 in the brain impair the synthesis of serotonin and the catecholamines. This is reflected by decreased levels of 5-hydroxyindoleacetic acid (5-HIAA), homovanillic acid (HVA), and 3-methoxy-4-hydroxyphenylglycol (MHPG) in CSF (5) (Fig. 1).

In the "atypical" defects of BH_4 metabolism, the central nervous system does not seem to be involved. Infants are still detected at neonatal

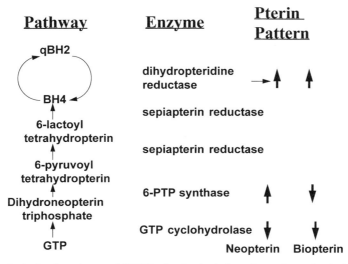

FIG. 2. Pattern of pterins in urine and CSF in the typical disorders of tetrahydrobiopterin metabolism. Samples are first oxidized to convert all reduced pterins to the fully oxidized state and then the total oxidized biopterin and oxidized neopterin are measured by HPLC with fluorescence detection (26,33) ↑, increased levels; ↓, decreased levels; →, normal levels; 6-PTP synthase, 6-pyruvoyltetrahydropterin synthase.

screening because of hyperphenylalaninemia and an abnormal urine pterin pattern. However, the CSF biopterin and neopterin levels are normal as are the concentrations of the neurotransmitter metabolites.

The diagnosis of DRD, TH deficiency, or AADC deficiency cannot be accomplished by simple basal metabolite analysis in peripheral fluids. Initial suspicion for DRD may be made on clinical grounds in the patients that present with dystonic gait disorder in childhood, but more mildly affected individuals and the early-onset forms can present a confusing clinical picture. Similarly the early clinical features of TH and AADC deficiency are nonspecific. In-

dications toward the individual diagnoses can, however, be made by examination of neurotransmitter metabolite and BH_4 and neopterin profiles in CSF. Figure 3 demonstrates the approach taken in our laboratory. The methodology requires analysis of CSF using high-performance liquid chromatography with electrochemical and fluorescence detection (12,15). Each sample is analyzed for neurotransmitter metabolites and pterins. Follow-up tests are then performed as appropriate in order to confirm a diagnosis. It is important that metabolite values be compared with age-related reference ranges as there is a rapid drop in CSF monoamine metabolite and BH_4 concentrations during

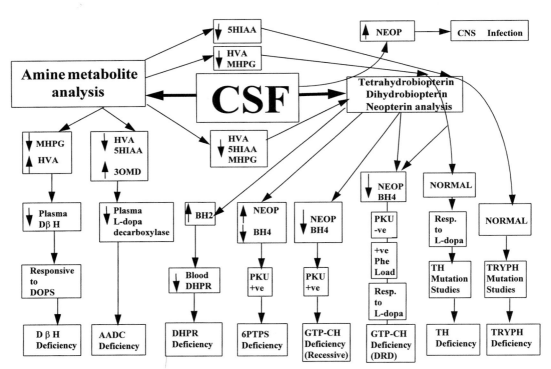

FIG. 3. Diagnostic flow chart. Each CSF sample is analyzed for biogenic amine metabolites and pterins. The HPLC technique used for pterin analysis allows direct measurement of tetrahydrobiopterin, dihydrobiopterin (which accumulates in dihydropteridine reductase deficiency), and neopterin (11,12,30,32). MHPG, 3-methoxy-4-hydroxyphenylglycol; HVA, homovanillic acid; DβH, dopamine β-hydroxylase; DOPS, dihydroxyphenylserine; 5HIAA, 5-hydroxyindoleacetic acid; 3OMD, 3-O-methyldopa; AADC, aromatic L-amino acid decarboxylase; BH2, 7,8-dihydrobiopterin; DHPR, dihydropteridine reductase; NEOP, neopterin; BH_4, tetrahydrobiopterin; PKU, phenylketonuria; GTP-CH, GTP cyclohydrolase; TH, tyrosine hydroxylase; TRYPH, tryptophan hydroxylase.

the first few years of life (18). CSF must also be collected in a standardized fashion as there is a rostrocaudal gradient of neurotransmitter metabolites in CSF (25). Handling of specimens is also critical because the neurotransmitter metabolites and the pterins are labile. CSF for the analysis of pterins should be collected into a separate tube containing antioxidants (11) and all samples should be frozen immediately following collection and stored below $-70°C$ at all times prior to analysis.

Decreased MHPG with increased HVA and normal 5-HIAA, BH_4, and neopterin levels suggests DβH deficiency. Additional evidence can be obtained by measurement of plasma catecholamine profiles in conjunction with physiologic tests of autonomic function (37,38). There are absent or very low levels of plasma norepinephrine, epinephrine and their metabolites, dopamine concentrations are five- to tenfold elevated, and there is a two- to threefold increase in L-dopa. A finding of low DβH activity in plasma is suggestive of DβH deficiency but is not totally diagnostic because 5% of the normal population have low or zero plasma DβH activity (8). A correction of the orthostatic hypotension by dihydroxyphenylserine confirms the diagnosis. This compound is decarboxylated by AADC to yield norepinephrine in noradrenergic neurons (1,29).

Greatly decreased levels of HVA, MHPG, and 5-HIAA, associated with large elevations of 3-*O*-methyldopa (3-OMD) and normal levels of BH_4 and neopterin are the characteristic pattern seen in AADC deficiency (19). There are also elevations of levodopa and 5-hydroxytryptophan in CSF (19). Confirmation of the diagnosis is achieved by measurement of AADC activity in plasma. All cases so far detected have had less than 5% of normal activity.

Decreased levels of HVA, 5-HIAA, and MHPG in the presence of normal concentrations of 3-OMD are usually associated with defects in BH_4 metabolism. It is important to ensure that there are no gross changes in brain anatomy as lesions within the brain, particularly in the basal ganglia, can also lead to decreased levels of all the metabolites.

Normally, diagnosis of a defect in BH_4 metabolism will be made because of hyperphenylalaninemia; however, occasionally an infant will "slip through" the neonatal screening system and will present with severe neurologic symptoms after 2 months of age. We are also aware of a child with GTP cyclohydrolase deficiency who did not become hyperphenylalaninemic until 5 years of age (unpublished observation). The pterin profiles in CSF in the defects of BH_4 metabolism are similar to those seen in urine (Fig. 2). Plasma phenylalanine concentrations should always be determined after finding abnormal pterin profiles in CSF.

Decreased concentrations of both BH_4 and neopterin point to a defect in GTP cyclohydrolase. The autosomal recessively inherited form of this disease also leads to hyperphenylalaninemia, whereas the autosomal dominant form (DRD) does not. We have recently demonstrated that a peripheral defect in phenylalanine metabolism can be exposed in DRD by stressing the phenylalanine hydroxylase system by administration of an oral phenylalanine load (16,45). This simple test can identify both symptomatic patients and asymptomatic carriers of this disease. Compared with controls, plasma phenylalanine levels rise to a higher level, and tyrosine and biopterin concentrations do not rise appropriately following the phenylalanine loading. Confirmation of the diagnosis of DRD can be established by finding a response to low-dose levodopa, demonstration of low activity of GTP cyclohydrolase in transformed lymphoblasts, and by identification of mutations in the GTP cyclohydrolase gene (20).

The concentration of HVA in CSF from patients with DRD is consistently low whereas 5-HIAA concentrations can be normal or even elevated. Confusion could therefore arise between GTP cyclohydrolase-associated DRD and TH deficiency if only neurotransmitter metabolites were measured, because TH deficiency also leads to reduced levels of HVA in CSF in the absence of any changes in 5-HIAA. Distinction between the two conditions is accomplished following the analysis of pterins, because BH_4 and neopterin profiles in CSF are normal in TH deficiency, whereas the levels have been low in all the cases of DRD where they have been measured (34). Currently, identification of mutations in the gene for TH is the only way to confirm a diagnosis of TH deficiency, because there is no easily accessible source of this enzyme that can be used for kinetic studies. It is possible that this might be accomplished in the future using cultured keratinocytes because these cells contain TH mRNA (6) and are reported to have TH activity (36).

A decrease in the concentration of 5-HIAA in CSF in the presence of normal levels of HVA, MHPG, BH_4, and neopterin would suggest an isolated deficiency of tryptophan hydroxylase. Such a defect, which only affects serotonin metabolism, has yet to be described. A secondary tryptophan hydroxylase deficiency occurs in the defects of BH_4 metabolism, suggesting that primary mutations affecting tryptophan hydroxylase would not be lethal. It is therefore likely that an isolated defect in tryptophan hydroxylase does exist, but as yet we do not recognize the neurologic profile that would accompany such a deficiency.

Analysis of CSF pterins in children with undiagnosed neurologic disease has an additional benefit outside of its use in the diagnosis of monoamine defects. Neopterin is released from macrophages following stimulation by interferon gamma (13). An elevation of this pterin in CSF therefore acts as a nonspecific marker indicating that the immune system has been stimulated within the central nervous system. As such, measurement of CSF neopterin can provide information as to whether neurologic symptoms may be related to an infectious process or some other condition that affects the central nervous system immune system status.

TREATMENT

The management of the autosomal recessively inherited abnormalities of BH_4 metabolism requires correction of the hyperphenylalaninemia in all cases, correction of the monoamine neurotransmitter deficiency in the typical forms of the disease, and prevention of the onset of folate deficiency within the central nervous system in dihydropteridine reductase deficiency.

Correction of hyperphenylalaninemia in GTP cyclohydrolase deficiency, 6-pyruvoyltetrahydropterin synthase deficiency, and pterin-4a-carbinolamine dehydratase deficiency can be achieved by administration of small doses of BH_4 (2 to 4 mg/kg/day). The use of BH_4 is generally not feasible for the treatment of hyperphenylalaninemia in dihydropteridine reductase deficiency as large doses are required in the absence of this recycling enzyme (22). Unfortunately, BH_4 does not cross the blood–brain barrier easily; the central nervous system monoamine deficiency is therefore corrected by administration of levodopa and 5-hydroxytryptophan in conjunction with carbidopa to inhibit the peripheral decarboxylation of these monoamine precursors. The mean concentrations (mg/kg/day) that have been used are as follows: levodopa 8.9, carbidopa 1.0 and 5-hydroxytryptophan 6.0; however, the dose required in each individual patient varies considerably ranging from 1.7 to 20 for levodopa, 0.8 to 12 for 5-hydroxytryptophan, and 0.2 to 2.5 for carbidopa. The initial dose tried should be low and should be gradually increased over a few weeks to the optimum. This optimum dose is established by the measurement of neurotransmitter metabolites in CSF, assessment of improvement or disappearance of neurologic symptoms when they exist, and by balancing these criteria with any side effects that may arise due to the therapy.

The central folate deficiency that arises in some cases of dihydropteridine reductase deficiency can lead to rapid neurologic deterioration despite good control of plasma phenylalanine and treatment of the neurotransmitter deficiency with precursor therapy (42). Treatment with folinic acid is therefore recommended. A dose of 12.5 mg/day together with the above therapy has prevented neurologic damage in at least one patient (21) and has been beneficial in many others (39,42).

Treatment of DRD only requires administration of levodopa and carbidopa. Again therapy should commence with small doses and the correct therapeutic dose be established by titration. Patients with TH deficiency are also reported to respond to levodopa but again full details of the use of this therapy have not been published.

Treatment of AADC deficiency requires a different approach because it is not possible to stimulate monoamine synthesis by precursor administration. A trial with high-dose pyridoxyl phosphate should always be attempted because AADC is a vitamin-B_6-requiring enzyme. Treatment, which commenced at the age of 10 months in the index cases of the disease (19), consisted of bromocriptine (dopamine agonist, 2.5 mg b.i.d.), tranylcypromine (nonselective monoamine oxidase inhibitor, 4 mg b.i.d.), and pyridoxine (100 mg b.i.d.) in combination. Therapy led to a marked clinical and biochemical improvement. At the age of 7 years, the children are walking well but show a mild mental retardation with a more strongly retarded speech development. Two older children, in whom therapy was started after 4 years of age, have been treated with similar medications with only minor clinical improvement (28; unpublished observation).

The treatment of choice in DβH deficiency is L-threo-3,4-dihydroxyphenylserine, 250 to 500 mg, twice daily, which leads to a modest rise in blood pressure and sustained relief of the orthostatic hypotension (1,29).

CONCLUSIONS

Autosomal recessively inherited defects of BH_4 metabolism were recognized over 20 years ago because of the associated hyperphenylalaninemia that is detected during newborn screening. Unfortunately, the other inherited conditions affecting biogenic amine biosynthesis cannot readily be detected by the usual screening methodologies (urine organic acids, plasma amino acids, etc.). The spectrum of neurologic signs in these disorders is broad, appears generally to be nonspecific, and because of the relatively few number of patients described, is still evolving. It is therefore important that the neurologist consider a neurotransmitter defect in patients who have been labeled as having "undiagnosed neurologic disease" and that CSF be collected for analysis. When interpreting monoamine metabolite profiles found in CSF, it should be remembered that monoamine metabolism can be altered by mechanisms other than primary defects of the enzymes required for their biosynthesis. Disruption of any of the multitude of different mechanisms that regulate neurotransmitter synthesis, degradation, release, re-uptake, and overall turnover should also be considered if unusual profiles are found.

REFERENCES

1. Biaggioni I, Robertson D. Endogenous restoration of noradrenaline by precursor therapy in dopamine-beta-hydroxylase deficiency. *Lancet* 1987;2:1170–1172.
2. Blau N, Dhondt J-L. Tetrahydrobiopterin deficiency and an international database of patients. In: Ayling JE, Nair MG, Baugh CM, eds. *Chemistry and biology of pteridines and folates.* New York, London: Plenum Press, 1993:255–261.
3. Blau N, Kierat L, Heizmann CW, Endres W, Giudici T, Wang M. Screening for tetrahydrobiopterin deficiency in newborns using dried filter paper. *J Inher Metab Dis* 1992;15:402–404.
4. Boyd K, Patterson V. Dopa responsive dystonia: a treatable condition misdiagnosed as cerebral palsy. *BMJ* 1989;298:1019–1020.
5. Butler IJ, Koslow SH, Krumholz A, Holtzman NA, Kaufman S. A disorder of biogenic amines in dihydropteridine reductase deficiency. *Ann Neurol* 1978;3:224–230.
6. Chang YT, Mues G, Pittelkow MR, Hyland K. Cultured human keratinocytes as a peripheral source of mRNA for tyrosine hydroxylase and aromatic L-amino acid decarboxylase. *J Inherit Metab Dis* 1996;19:239–242.
7. Curtius H-Ch, Adler C, Rebrin I, Heizmann C, Ghisla S. 7-substituted pterins: formation during phenylalanine hydroxylation in the absence of dehydratase. *Biochem Biophys Res Commun* 1990;172:1060–1066.
8. Dunnette J, Weinshilbourn RM. Inheritance of low immunoreactive human plasma dopamine hydroxylase. *J Clin Invest* 1977;60:1080–1087.
9. Fink JK, Barton N, Cohen W, Lovenberg W, Burns RS, Hallett M. Dystonia with marked diurnal variation associated with biopterin deficiency. *Neurology* 1988;38:707–711.
10. Fink JK, Filling-Katz MR, Barton NW, Macrae PR, Hallett M, Cohen WE. Treatable dystonia presenting as spastic cerebral palsy. *Pediatrics* 1988;82:137–138.
11. Howells DW, Hyland K. Direct analysis of tetrahydrobiopterin in cerebrospinal fluid by high-performance liquid chromatography with redox electrochemistry: prevention of autoxidation during storage and analysis. *Clin Chim Acta* 1987;167:23–30.
12. Howells DW, Smith I, Hyland K. Estimation of tetrahydrobiopterin and other pterins in cerebrospinal

fluid using reversed-phase high-performance liquid chromatography with electrochemical and fluorescence detection. *J Chromatogr* 1986;381:285–294.

13. Huber C, Batchelor JR, Fuchs D, et al. Immune response-associated production of neopterin. Release from macrophages primarily under control of interferon-gamma. *J Exp Med* 1984;160:310–316.

14. Hyland K. Abnormalities of biogenic amine metabolism. *J Inherit Metab Dis* 1993;16:6–690.

15. Hyland K, Clayton PT. Aromatic L-amino acid decarboxylase deficiency: diagnostic methodology. *Clin Chem* 1992;38:2405–2410.

16. Hyland K, Fryburg JS, Wilson WG, et al. Oral phenylalanine loading in dopa-responsive dystonia: a possible diagnostic test. *Neurology* 1997;48:1290–1297.

17. Hyland K, Howells DW. Analysis and clinical significance of pterins. *J Chromatogr* 1988;429:95–121.

18. Hyland K, Surtees RAH, Heales SJR, Bowron A, Howells DW, Smith I. Cerebrospinal fluid concentrations of pterins and metabolites of serotonin and dopamine in a pediatric reference population. *Pediatr Res* 1993;34:10–14.

19. Hyland K, Surtees RAH, Rodeck C, Clayton PT. Aromatic L-amino acid decarboxylase deficiency: clinical features, diagnosis and treatment of a new inborn error of neurotransmitter amine synthesis. *Neurology* 1992; 42:980–1988.

20. Ichinose H, Ohye T, Takahashi EI, et al. Hereditary progressive dystonia with marked diurnal fluctuation caused by mutations in the GTP cyclohydrolase I gene. *Nat Genet* 1994;8:236–242.

21. Irons M, Levy HL, O'Flynn E, et al. Folinic acid therapy in treatment of dihydropteridine reductase deficiency. *J Pediatr* 1987;110:61–67.

22. Kaufman S. Unsolved problems in diagnosis and therapy of hyperphenylalaninemia caused by defects in tetrahydrobiopterin metabolism. *J Pediatr* 1986;109: 572–578.

23. Kaufman S, Holtzman NA, Milstein S, Butler IJ, Krumholz A. Phenylketonuria due to deficiency of dihydropteridine reductase. *N Engl J Med* 1975;293: 785–790.

24. Knappskog PM, Flatmark T, Mallet J, Lüdecke B, Bartholomé K. Recessively inherited L-dopa-responsive dystonia caused by a point mutation (Q381K) in the tyrosine hydroxylase gene. *Hum Mol Genet* 1995; 4:1209–1212.

25. Kruesi MJP, Swedo SE, Hamburger SD, Potter WZ, Rapoport JL. Concentration gradient of monoamine metabolites in children and adolescents. *Biol Psychiatry* 1988;24:507–524.

26. Longhi R, Valsasina R, Buttè C, Paccanelli S, Riva A, Giovannini M. Cranial computerized tomography in dihydropteridine reductase deficiency. *J Inherit Metab Dis* 1985;8:109–112.

27. Lüdecke B, Dworniczak B, Bartholomé K. A point mutation in the tyrosine hydroxylase gene associated with Segawa's syndrome. *Hum Genet* 1995;93:123–125.

28. Maller A, Hyland K, Milstien S, Biaggioni I, Butler IJ. Aromatic L-amino acid decarboxylase deficiency: clinical features, diagnosis and treatment of a second family. *J Child Neurol* 1997;12:349–356.

29. Man in't Veld AJ, Boomsma F, van den Meiracker AH, Schalekamp MADH. Effect of an unnatural noradrenaline precursor on sympathetic control and orthostatic hypotension in dopamine β-hydroxylase deficiency. *Lancet* 1987;2:1172–1175.

30. Matthews RG, Kaufman S. Characterization of the dihydropterin reductase activity of pig liver methylenetetrahydrofolate reductase. *J Biol Chem* 1980;255: 6014–6017.

31. Niederwieser A, Blau N, Wang M, Joller P, Ataré M, Cardesa-Garcia J. GTP cyclohydrolase I deficiency, a new enzyme defect causing hyperphenylalaninemia with neopterin, biopterin, dopamine and serotonin deficiencies and muscular hypotonia. *Eur J Pediatr* 1984;141:208–214.

32. Niederwieser A, Leimbacher W, Curtius H.Ch, Ponzone A, Rey F, Leupold D. Atypical phenylketonuria with "dihydrobiopterin synthetase" deficiency: absence of phosphate-eliminating enzyme activity demonstrated in liver. *Eur J Pediatr* 1985;144:13–16.

33. Niederwieser A, Staudenmann W, Wetzel E. Automated HPLC of pterins with or without column switching. In: Wachter H, Curtius H.Ch. Pfleiderer W, eds. *Biochemical and clinical aspects of pteridines.* Vol. 1. Berlin: de Gruyter, 1982:81–102.

34. Nygaard TG. Dopa-responsive dystonia. Delineation of the clinical syndrome and clues to pathogenesis. *Adv Neurol* 1993;60:577–585.

35. Nygaard TG, Waren SP, Levine RA, Naini AB, Chutorian AM. Dopa-responsive dystonia simulating cerebral palsy. *Pediatr Neurol* 1994;11:236–240.

36. Ramchand CN, Clark AE, Ramchand R, Hemmings GP. Cultured human keratinocytes as a model for studying the dopamine metabolism in schizophrenia. *Med Hypotheses* 1995;44:53–57.

37. Robertson D, Haile V, Perry SH, Robertson RM, Phillips JA, Biaggioni I. Dopamine β-hydroxylase deficiency. A genetic disorder of cardiovascular regulation. *Hypertension* 1991;18:1–8.

38. Robertson D, Mosqueda-Garcia R, Robertson RM, Biaggioni I. Chronic hypotension. In the shadow of hypertension. *Am J Hypertens* 1992;5:200S–205S.

39. Scriver CD, Kaufman S, Woo SLC. The hyperphenylalaninemias. In: Scriver CR, Baudet AL, Sly WS, Valle D, eds. *The metabolic basis of inherited disease.* New York: McGraw Hill, 1989:495–546.

40. Segawa M, Hosaka A, Miyagawa F, et al. Hereditary progressive dystonia with marked diurnal fluctuation. *Adv Neurol* 1976;14:215–233.

41. Smith I. Disorders of tetrahydrobiopterin metabolism. In: Fernandes J, Saudubray JM, Tada K, eds. *Inborn metabolic disease.* Heidelberg: Springer-Verlag, 1990: 183–187.

42. Smith I, Hyland K, Kendall B, Leeming R. Clinical role of pteridine therapy in tetrahydrobiopterin deficiency. *J Inherit Metab Dis* 1985;8[Suppl 1]:39–45.

43. Tada K, Narisawa K, Arai N, Ogasawara Y, Ishizawa S. A sibling case of hyperphenylalaninemia due to deficiency of dihydropteridine reductase: biochemical and pathological findings. *Tohoku J Exp Med* 1980;132:123–131.

44. Tanaka K, Yoneda M, Nakajima T, Miyatake T, Owada I. Dihydrobiopterin synthesis defect: an adult with diurnal fluctuations of symptoms. *Neurology* 1987;37:519–522.

45. Trugman JM, Hyland K, Fryburg JS, et al. Peripheral biopterin defect in dopa-responsive dystonia demonstrated with a phenylalanine load test. *Mov Disord* 1995;10:698.

Dystonia 3: Advances in Neurology, Vol. 78,
edited by S. Fahn, C. D. Marsden, and M. DeLong.
Lippincott–Raven Publishers, Philadelphia © 1998.

31

Dopa-Responsive Dystonia: A Syndrome of Selective Nigrostriatal Dopamine Deficiency

*Beom S. Jeon, †Jae-Min Jeong, ‡Sung-Sup Park, and †Myung-Chul Lee

*Departments of *Neurology, †Nuclear Medicine, and ‡Clinical Pathology, College of Medicine,
Seoul National University, Seoul National University Hospital, Seoul 110-744, Korea.*

The diagnosis of dopa-responsive dystonia (DRD) is clinical. The usual features are childhood-onset foot dystonia and parkinsonism. However, the clinical features are broad, and are not specific enough to make a confirmatory diagnosis (reviewed in References 20 and 27). The dramatic and sustained L-dopa response can confirm the diagnosis, however, it requires a long-term follow-up. Recent studies in molecular genetics and biochemistry have been very helpful in understanding the pathogenesis, and in making the diagnosis. However, there are limitations in making the diagnosis by molecular genetic and biochemical studies. Genetic defects in the synthetic pathway of dopamine have been uncovered as a cause for DRD. Mutations were discovered in the GTP cyclohydrolase-1 (GCH-1) (1,2,10,14,18) and tyrosine hydroxylase (TH) genes (23). The mutation sites in the GCH-1 gene are multiple, each known family having distinct mutations. Therefore, it is necessary to fully sequence the entire gene to detect possible mutations. Furthermore, a mutation in the TH gene was found in an autosomal-recessive DRD family (23). Therefore, it is difficult to diagnose DRD by mutation studies. This point is further underscored by reports that no mutations were found in some DRD cases (1,18). Neopterin is a degradation product of dihydroneopterin triphosphate, which is the first intermediate in the biosynthesis of tetrahydrobiopterin (BH_4) from GTP (Fig. 1). Dihydroneopterin triphosphate is formed from GTP by GCH-1. Therefore, cerebrospinal fluid (CSF) neopterin reflects the activity of GCH-1. CSF neopterin was decreased in DRD (9,10). However, CSF neopterin will be normal in DRD from mutations in the TH gene.

There are several difficulties in making an accurate clinical diagnosis of DRD. The broad clinical spectrum of DRD is one difficulty. There have been cases of DRD mimicking cerebral palsy (4,30), and adult-onset parkinsonism (35). Differential diagnosis from juvenile Parkinson's disease (JPD) can be a particular challenge (reviewed in Reference 20). Both conditions present with early-onset parkinsonism and dystonia. Diurnal fluctuation and early L-dopa response do not differentiate the two. Both are familial in a high percentage of the patients. The critical clinical difference between these two conditions is long-term L-dopa benefit and motor complications (27,29). Clinical differentiation from JPD is often difficult without long-term follow-up. There are reports of DRD that were later shown to be JPD based on the appearance of motor fluctuation and dyskinesia (27–29. See review in Reference 20). As the prognosis is very different in DRD and JPD, clinical distinction becomes very important.

The differences in long-term L-dopa benefit and prognosis in these two conditions are due

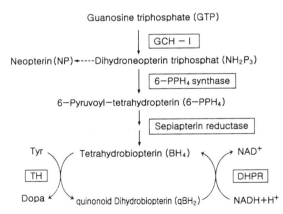

FIG. 1. The biosynthetic pathway of tetrahydrobiopterin (BH_4) from guanosine triphosphate (GTP). GTP cyclohydrolase-1 (GCH-1) is an initial and rate-limiting step in the synthesis of BH_4. BH_4 is a cofactor of tyrosine hydroxylase (TH), which is a rate-limiting enzyme in the dopamine synthesis. Therefore, decrease in GCH-1 activity results in decreased dopamine synthesis.

to underlying neuropathologic differences. Pathologic studies in JPD show that there is degenerative neuronal loss and Lewy bodies in the substantia nigra (11,31), whereas there is no nigral cell loss in DRD (32). (Even though reported as DRD, the case of Olsson et al. (31) is believed to be JPD. The patient showed dyskinesia and motor fluctuation. L-dopa needed to be increased, and did not completely reverse her motor deficits. There was extreme loss of melanotic nerve cells and pronounced gliosis in the substantia nigra. Some remaining neurons showed Lewy bodies.)

Dopamine transporter (DAT) is a protein located in the dopaminergic nerve terminals. DAT imaging measures the density of DAT in the striatum, and thus examines the integrity of the nigrostriatal dopaminergic nerve terminals. DAT imaging has proved to be a reliable and sensitive test for PD (8,19), where there is a degenerative loss of the nigral cells and decrease in DAT (37).

[^{123}I] [(1R)-2β-carbomethoxy-3β-(4-iodophenyl)tropane] ([^{123}I]-β-CIT) is a ligand for the DAT, and was found to be a useful marker for dopamine neurons that degenerate in PD

(5,19,24,34). Therefore, we performed [^{123}I]-β-CIT single photon emission computerized tomography (SPECT) in clinically diagnosed DRD, PD, and JPD, and examined whether the DAT measured by *in vivo* nuclear imaging study will differentiate DRD from PD and JPD. We then studied mutations in the candidate gene GCH-1 and measured CSF neopterin to further support the diagnosis of DRD and examine the role of DAT study.

PATIENTS

Since 1986, we have followed nine (eight from two families and one sporadic) DRD patients. Diagnosis of DRD was made by the history of early-onset dystonia, parkinsonism, diurnal fluctuation, and marked L-dopa benefit without dopa-related complications during follow-up. Clinical summary is in Table 1. The pedigrees are shown in Fig. 2. Among nine cases of DRD, four familial (two from each family, arrowed in Fig. 2) and one sporadic case were studied using [^{123}I]-β-CIT SPECT. The ages ranged from 19 to 30 years (mean = 23.6). Numbered members in the pedigree are the ones who were examined and had a gene study done. Members who are not numbered do not have any neurologic symptoms by history. CSF neopterin was measured in four patients (three underlined members in the pedigree and the sporadic case). (Gene study confirmed asymptomatic carriers are shaded in the pedigree.)

METHODS AND RESULTS

[^{123}I]-β-CIT Single Photon Emission Computed Tomography Study

The detailed methods of [^{123}I]-β-CIT SPECT and data analysis are described elsewhere (21,22). After intravenous 10 mci [^{123}I]-β-CIT, scans were done at 18 hours after injection using a double-headed SPECT camera (Prism 2000, Picker International Inc., Cleveland, Ohio, USA). Reconstructed images were used to identify the brain anatomy and measure the radioactivity. Specific striatal binding was estimated by

TABLE 1. Clinical summary of patients

	Age/sex (yr)	Onset (yr)	Initial symptom	Additional features	L-dopa (mg)[a]	Wearing off
Patient 1 (K II-2)	42/F	12	Both toe hyperflexion	Walking difficulty, antecollis, trunk tilt, speech difficulty, masked face, left hand tremor, left hemiparesis, both feet equinus, striatal toes, bradykinesia, increased DTRs, postural instability	250	2 d
Patient 2 (K II-3)	30/F	7	Left foot dystonia	Left hand tremor, left elbow flexion on walking, left hand fisting, torticollis, scoliosis, fatigue, bradykinesia, postural and rest tremor, trunk tilt on walking	100	36 hr
Patient 3, 4 (K II-4, 5)	24/F	11	Right foot inversion	Trunk anteflexion, both hand fisting, left arm dystonia, writing difficulty, both hand postural tremor	100	2–3 d
Patient 5 (K III-1)	6/F	1	Walking difficulty with tip-toeing	Poor balance, impaired hand dexterity, both feet equinovarus, scoliosis, increased DTRs	100	3 d
Patient 6 (C III-2)	24/F	12	Left foot equinovarus	Writing and walking difficulty, torticollis, left foot equinovarus, both leg spasticity, scoliosis, fatigue, bradykinesia, postural instability	200	2 d
Patient 7 (C III-4)	19/F	9	Left foot equinovarus	Torticollis, fatigue, dysarthria, writing and walking difficulty, tremor in both hands, both feet equinovarus, both hand fisting, striatal toe on left, leg weakness, increased DTRs	100	2 d
Patient 8 (C III-6)	6/F	1	Walking difficulty	Difficulty with writing and piano-playing, left hemiparesis, left hand fisting, increased DTRs, spastic wide-based gait	100	3 d
Patient 9	21/F	10	Left foot dragging	Twisting of body and neck, walking and writing difficulty, parkinsonism	100	3d

[a]L-Dopa was given with L-aromatic amino acid-decarboxylase inhibitors.

Family K

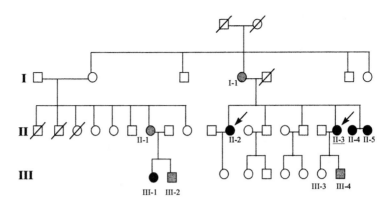

Family C

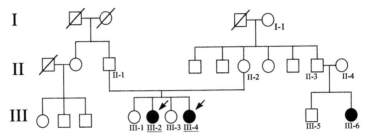

FIG. 2. Pedigrees of DRD families K and C. Affected members were all females, and are shown in closed circles. Asymptomatic gene carriers confirmed by the gene study are shown in shades. Family members who were examined and had a gene study done are numbered. Arrowed are the ones who had the [^{123}I]-β-CIT SPECT study done. Underlined are the ones who had the neopterin study done.

subtracting occipital counts/pixel/minute from striatal counts/pixel/minute. Fifteen healthy volunteers and six PD patients served as controls. Five patients were in the Hoehn-Yahr stage 1, and one was in stage 2. A 17 1/2 year-old girl with JPD was also studied.

In normal controls, [^{123}I]-β-CIT binding was very high in the striatal region and low in other areas including occipital areas (Fig. 3A). In the PD and JPD patients, [^{123}I]-β-CIT binding was severely decreased in the striatal region most marked in the caudal part (Fig. 3B and C). [^{123}I]-β-CIT binding was normal in DRD (Fig.

3D). The specific striatal:occipital (S/O) ratio was 6.22 ± 1.32 (mean $\pm$SD) in normal controls ($N = 15$), 8.15 ± 0.90 in DRD ($N = 5$), and 3.78 ± 0.65 in PD ($N = 6$). In the JPD patient, the S/O ratio was 2.46. Figure 4 summarizes the results of the S/O ratios in these four groups. The S/O ratios in DRD were within the normal range, and clearly higher than those of PD without overlap. The JPD patient showed a very low S/O ratio in the PD range. The mean S/O ratio of DRD was higher than that of normal controls ($p < 0.01$), suggesting that DAT is upregulated in DRD (perhaps to economize dopamine).

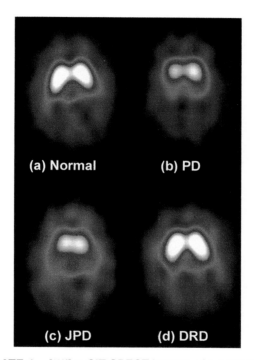

COLOR PLATE 1. [¹²³I]-β-CIT SPECT images of a normal control, PD, JPD, and DRD. [¹²³I]-β-CIT binding is very high in the striatum in this 20-year-old normal control (**a**) and 30-year-old DRD (**d**), whereas it is markedly decreased in the 42-year-old PD (**b**) and 17-year-old JPD (**c**).

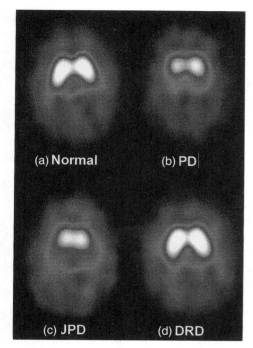

FIG. 3. [^{123}I]-β-CIT SPECT images of a normal control, PD, JPD, and DRD. [^{123}I]-β-CIT binding is very high in the striatum in this 20-year-old normal control **(A)** and 30-year-old DRD **(D)**, whereas it is markedly decreased in the 42-year-old PD **(B)** and 17-year-old JPD **(C)**.

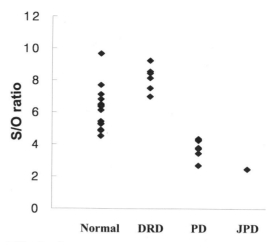

FIG. 4. Summary result of the [^{123}I]-β-CIT specific striatal:occipital binding ratios (S/O ratios) in the normal control, DRD, PD, and JPD. The ranges of the S/O ratios in the normal control (*N* = 15) and DRD (*N* = 5) are similar. All the S/O ratios in PD (*N* = 6) are below the ranges of normal control and DRD without overlap. The S/O ratio in JPD (*N* = 1) is even lower in the PD range.

Gene Study

Genomic DNA was studied for mutations in the GCH-1 gene using the method modified from Ichinose et al. (18). A novel nonsense mutation at codon position 114 (TCH->TGA) in exon I of the GCH-1 gene was found in Family K. This mutation results in a substitution of serine residue with a termination codon [Ser^{114}Ter]. The patients were heterozygous in terms of this mutation. The mutation was found in all symptomatic and some asymptomatic members (K I-1, II-1, III-2,4) (shaded in the pedigree). In Family C and the sporadic case, mutations were not found in the exons of the GCH-1 gene.

Cerebrospinal Fluid Neopterin

CSF neopterin was below 1 pmol/ml when measured in the four DRD patients. In the disease control with parkinsonism or dystonia from causes other than DRD, neopterin levels ranged from 2 to 5 pmol/ml (mean = 3 pmol/ml).

DISCUSSION

Based on the history of early-onset dystonia, parkinsonism, diurnal fluctuation, and marked L-dopa benefit without dopa-related complications during long-term treatment, the clinical diagnosis of DRD is firm. Normal striatal DAT on [^{123}I]-β-CIT SPECT, an evidence for normal dopaminergic innervation and nondegenerative basis of parkinsonism and dystonia, support our clinical diagnosis of DRD. Demonstration of a mutation and decreased CSF neopterin lends further support. Family K II-2 was considered somewhat unusual in that she took more L-dopa (250 mg/day with benserazide) than usual DRD and had vague aches after 12 hours of medication withdrawal. However, examination performed 48 hours after drug withdrawal did not show any motor deficit so that there was no objective evidence of wearing off.

Our data demonstrate that [123I]-β-CIT SPECT clearly distinguishes PD from normal controls. A single case of JPD showed severely decreased DAT in the lower PD range, consistent with the data that there is nigral cell loss in JPD, and with the suggestion that JPD is on a spectrum with PD. Our data that the striatal DAT is normal in DRD when measured *in vivo* by [123I]-β-CIT SPECT, is consistent with our prediction based on lack of nigral cell loss, and *in vitro* measurement (32).

There has been diagnostic difficulty in reliably distinguishing DRD from JPD, as shown by reports of DRD that were later shown to be JPD based on later appearance of motor fluctuation and dyskinesia (27–29,31). Instructive examples would be a case of Olsson et al. (31) and case 7 of "atypical DRD" in Sawle et al. (33). Sawle's case 7 closely resembled DRD early in the illness, and was reported as such (6,12). However, the dose of L-dopa needed to be increased, and fluctuation and dyskinesia appeared during follow-up. Fluorodopa positron emission tomography (PET) study showed a major reduction of fluorodopa uptake, which was clearly different from other DRD cases. Thus, the PET study established the diagnosis of JPD. The fluorodopa PET study examines a complex of decarboxylation, vesicular uptake, and storage of fluorodopa. As DAT imaging directly measures the DAT density, it provides more pertinent information in this clinical setting. PET scanners are not available in many centers. However, DAT imaging can be done on the SPECT scanners, and therefore is more accessible.

Molecular genetic confirmation or exclusion of the diagnosis is difficult due to the facts that (a) there are no common mutations in the GCH-1 gene, (b) mutations are not found in the GCH-1 gene in some clinical DRD cases, and (c) mutations may be found in the TH gene. Furthermore, reports that the defects in dihydropteridine reductase (DHPR) (26) and 6-pyruvoyl-tetrahydropterin synthase (6-PPH$_4$ synthase) (7,13,36), two other enzymes in BH$_4$ metabolism (Fig. 1), may present with dystonia responsive to L-dopa, make it possible that genes other than GCH-1 and TH may be found to cause DRD. Absence of mutations will not be able to exclude DRD. CSF neopterin will detect DRD from mutations in the GCH-1 gene, but not from mutations in other candidate genes, such as TH.

Even though direct measurement of GCH-1 activity was not done, the mutation [Ser^{114}Ter] in Family K is believed to be functionally significant. CSF neopterin in one of this Family (K II-3) was low. As neopterin reflects the activity of GCH-1, we consider it as an indirect evidence of low GCH-1 activity. The mutation in the GCH-1 gene in the affected members was heterozygous, consistent with autosomal-dominant inheritance. Based on the pedigree, Family K I-1, II-1 are obligate carriers, which is proven correct by the gene study. Penetrance is lower than 50% in this pedigree. Both tested male members in the family had mutations, but did not have symptoms, showing sex-related penetrance. It is to be noted that the same mutation caused two different phenotypes in this family: classic childhood-onset dystonia-parkinsonism and cerebral palsy.

In Family C and the sporadic case, low CSF neopterin level suggests low activity of the GCH-1 enzyme. Absence of mutation in the exons of the GCH-1 gene suggests that mutations lie outside the exons. Whether and how mutations in nonexonal sites of the gene affect enzyme activity is a very interesting question. Possibilities include pathologic alternative splicing due to mutation of donor acceptor sites, alternative polyadenylation of mRNA, and posttranslational differences. A study showed that mutant mRNA level was important for phenotypic variability among cases with a known mutation (14). Therefore, measurement of mRNA level may give a clue as to its mechanism in cases with presumed nonexonal mutations. Whatever the mechanism might be, it makes the molecular genetic diagnosis more difficult, again emphasizing the need for other means of supporting the clinical diagnosis.

Phenylalanine is metabolized into tyrosine by phenylalanine hydroxylase in the liver and kidney. BH$_4$ is a cofactor for phenylalanine hydroxylase. Patients with autosomal-recessive defects in BH$_4$ biosynthesis present with hyperphenylalaninemia (3). Although DRD has a defect in synthesis of BH$_4$, there are no known DRD patients who have hyperphenylalaninemia. However, when phenylalanine was orally loaded in DRD patients, blood phenylalanine level increased to a higher level than in normal controls, with slow clearance of phenylalanine from blood and decreased production of tyrosine (16). This abnormality was corrected by pretreatment with BH$_4$. The data indicate that patients with DRD have sufficient systemic BH$_4$ store to metabolize normal intake of phenylalanine, but insufficient BH$_4$ store and synthetic capacity to metabolize a high phenylalanine load. The test may be useful in metabolically screening DRD patients, and in diagnosing DRD when mutation is not demonstrable. However, it should be noted that phenylalanine load test is abnormal in defects of BH$_4$ biosynthesis other than GCH-1. The test has not been done in DRD patients with TH mutation. Quality control of the test has been difficult in our hands.

CONCLUSION

The concept and definition of Segawa's disease or DRD has been clinical. However, the broad clinical spectrum and nonspecific nature of the clinical features make the clinical definition less useful. The dramatic and sustained L-dopa response can confirm the diagnosis; however, it requires a long-term follow-up. The genetic definition and diagnosis of DRD are neither simple nor practical for reasons discussed above. There will be cases of DRD that meet every clinical definition and cannot be confirmed by genetic study.

Therefore, we propose the definition of DRD as a syndrome of selective nigrostriatal dopamine deficiency caused by genetic defects in the dopamine synthetic pathway without nigral cell loss. This definition assumes all the known clinical, biochemical, genetic, and pathologic information on DRD. It covers all

the typical and atypical presentations of DRD with proven mutations, and allows a diagnosis of DRD without requiring the demonstration of gene mutations, which is not practical, and may not be possible in some cases. Homozygous defects in GCH-1, DHPR, and 6-PPH$_4$ synthase can cause dystonia, but also cause other neurologic deficits such as mental retardation and seizures as well (7,13,15,26,36), therefore are excluded by the definition. This definition excludes JPD and other degenerative disorders that have neuronal loss in the nigra. DAT imaging will provide the needed information of nigral integrity. Our definition of DRD is not only simple but also practical, needing only clinical information and DAT imaging.

We further propose the term DRD-plus, defined as inherited metabolic disorders that have features of DRD and those features that are not seen in DRD as well (Table 2) (20,21). Homozygous defects in GCH-1, DHPR, and 6-PPH synthase are examples of DRD-plus. L-Aromatic amino acid decarboxylase (AADC) deficiency is another example of DRD-plus. The reported twins had developmental delay, generalized hypotonia, and oculogyric crises (17), which can all be seen in early-onset DRD. They showed diurnal fluctuation (Dr. Blair Ford, personal communication), which was thought to be characteristic for Segawa's disease (20). However, the twins had features of autonomic instability, which is not seen in DRD. Laboratory investigation showed decrease in both catecholamines and serotonin. In addition to the differences in clinical presentations, L-dopa response is another hallmark in distinguishing DRD and DRD-plus. We regard marked L-dopa response as an essential feature of DRD. L-dopa only partially reversed neurologic deficits in DHPR and 6-PPH$_4$ synthase deficiency, and dopamine receptor agonist was partially effective in AADC deficiency. Our concept of DRD and DRD-plus gives insights into the pathophysiology, the framework for clinical and laboratory investigation and therapeutic intervention.

DRD offers us a unique opportunity to know what occurs when there is a striatal dopamine deficiency. PD has similar degree and

TABLE 2. *Differential diagnosis of DRD and related disorders*

	ITD[a]	JPD	DRD	DRD-plus[b]
Symptoms and signs				
Motor symptoms				
Dystonia	+	+/−	+	+/−
Parkinsonism	−	+	+/−	−[e]
Nonmotor symptoms[c]	−	−	−	+
Systemic symptoms[d]	−	−	−	+
Laboratory tests				
Fluorodopa PET	Normal	Abnormal	Normal[f]	Normal[g]
Dopamine transporter imaging	Normal	Abnormal	Normal[h]	Normal[f]
CSF neopterin	Normal	Mild decrease	Marked decrease[f]	Abnormal[i]
Phenylalanine loading test	Normal[g]	Normal[g]	Abnormal[f]	Abnormal[j]
L-dopa response				
Dose	Large	Small[k]	Small	Large
Response degree	Minimal	Good	Marked	Partial
Long-term complication	Absent	Frequent	Absent	Absent[g]

[a]Idiopathic torsion dystonia (may include several genetically distinct subtypes such as Dyt1).

[b]Currently, includes homozygous defects in GCH-I, DHPR, 6-PPH$_4$ synthase, and AADC.

[c]Mental retardation, seizures, autonomic instability, lethargy, irritability, hypersalivation, microcephaly. Sensory complaints without objective sensory loss is not included.

[d]Physical retardation, rash, eczema, pneumonia, sudden death.

[e]Not recorded, but expected to be present in some.

[f]No data on DRD due to TH mutation.

[g]No data yet. Based on prediction.

[h]Our data suggest that dopamine transporter may be upregulated in DRD.

[i]Increased in DHPR and 6-PPH$_4$ synthase deficiency. Decreased in homozygous GCH-1 deficiency. Expected to be normal in AADC deficiency.

[j]No data in AADC deficiency.

[k]Need increase with time.

Modified from ref. 20, with permission.

rostrocaudal pattern of changes in dopamine and its metabolites. Even though the different age distribution does not allow us a direct comparison, there are conspicuous differences in some features, such as dementia and depression. The neuropathologic and neurobiochemical substrates for cognitive decline in PD have been debated. One of the simple questions is whether pure nigral pathology with striatal dopamine deficiency is sufficient or whether an extranigral involvement is needed to cause dementia. As the decrease in striatal dopamine in DRD is comparable to that of PD, it is unlikely that decrease in striatal dopamine alone causes dementia. Likewise, depression in PD is unlikely to be caused by decrease in striatal dopamine alone, but needs involvement of other parts of the brain as well. Further investigation with detailed clinical evaluation and studies in the other neurotransmitter systems are needed.

ACKNOWLEDGMENTS

This study was in part supported by the Korea Science Foundation (95-0403-96-3). B.J. is a Houston M. Merritt Fellow at Columbia University at the time of writing. The authors would like to acknowledge that the gene analysis was done with generous help of Dr. Segawa and Dr. Tsuji in Japan. We also would like to thank Dr. Paul Greene and Rev. Peregrine L. Murphy for reading the manuscript and giving thoughtful suggestions. We deeply appreciate the active cooperation of the patients, chief residents of the Department of Neurology, and other participants in the study.

ADDENDUM

A case report that DAT is normal in DRD was published recently (25).

REFERENCES

1. Bandmann O, Daniel S, Marsden CD, Wood NW, Harding AE. The GTP-cyclohydrolase I gene in atypical parkinsonian patients: a clinico-genetic study. *J Neurol Sci* 1996;5:27–32.
2. Beyer K, Lao-Villadoniga JI, Vecino-Bilbao B, Cacabelos R, de La Fluente-Fernandez R. A novel point mutation in the GTP cyclohydrolase I gene in a Spanish family with hereditary progressive and dopa-responsive dystonia. *J Neurol Neurosurg Psychiatry* 1997;62:420–421.
3. Blau N, Barnes I, Dhondt JL. International database of tetrahydrobiopterin deficiencies. *J Inherit Metab Dis* 1996;19:8–14.
4. Boyd K, Patterson V. Dopa responsive dystonia: a treatable condition misdiagnosed as cerebral palsy. *BMJ* 1989;298:1019–1020.
5. Brucke T, Asenbaum S, Pozzera A, et al. Dopaminergic cell loss in Parkinson's disease quantified with [^{123}I]-β-CIT and SPECT correlates with clinical findings. *Mov Disord* 1994;9[Suppl 1]:120(abst).
6. Deonna T. Dopa-sensitive progressive dystonia of childhood with fluctuations of symptoms—Segawa syndrome and possible variants. Results of a collaborative study of the European Federation of Child Neurology Societies (EFCNS). *Neuropediatrics* 1986; 17:81–85.
7. Fink JK, Barton N, Cohen W, Lovenberg W, Burns RS, Hallett M. Dystonia with marked diurnal variation associated with biopterin deficiency. *Neurology* 1988; 38:707–711.
8. Frost JJ, Rosier AJ, Reich SG, et al. Positron emission tomographic imaging of the dopamine transporter with 11C-WIN 35,428 reveals marked declines in mild Parkinson's disease. *Ann Neurol* 1993;34:423–431.
9. Furukawa Y, Mizuno Y, Narabayashi H. Early-onset parkinsonism with dystonia: clinical and biochemical differences from hereditary progressive dystonia or DOPA-responsive dystonia. *Adv Neurol* 1996;69: 327–337.
10. Furukawa Y, Shimadzu M, Rajput AH, et al. GTP-cyclohydrolase I gene mutations in hereditary progressive and dopa-responsive dystonia. *Ann Neurol* 1996;39:609–617.
11. Gibb WRG, Narabayashi H, Yokochi M, Iizuka R, Lees AJ. New pathologic observations in juvenile onset parkinsonism with dystonia. *Neurology* 1991;41: 820–822.
12. Gordon N. Fluctuating dystonia and allied syndromes *Neuropediatrics* 1982;13:152–154.
13. Hanihara T, Inoue K, Kawanishi C, et al. 6-pyruvoyl-tetrahydropterin synthase deficiency with generalized dystonia and diurnal fluctuation of symptoms: a clinical and molecular study. *Mov Disord* 1997;12:408–411.
14. Hirano M, Tamaru Y, Ito H, Matsumoto S, Imai T, Ueno S. Mutant GTP cyclohydrolase I mRNA level contribute to dopa-responsive dystonia onset. *Ann Neurol* 1996;40:796–798.
15. Hyland K. Other biopterin deficient diseases. *Mov Disord* 1997;12[3,Suppl]:35–36(abst).
16. Hyland K, Fryburg JS, Wilson WG, et al. Oral phenylalanine loading in dopa-responsive dystonia: a possible diagnostic test. *Neurology* 1997;48:1290–1297.
17. Hyland K, Surtees RAH, Rodeck C, Clayton PT. Aromatic L-amino acid decarboxylase deficiency: clinical features, diagnosis, and treatment of a new inborn error of neurotransmitter amine synthesis. *Neurology* 1992;42:1980–1988.
18. Ichinose H, Ohye T, Takahashi E, et al. Hereditary progressive dystonia with marked diurnal fluctuation caused by mutations in the GTP cyclohydrolase I gene. *Nat Genet* 1994;8:236–242.
19. Innis RB, Seibyl JP, Scanley BE, et al. Single photon emission computed tomographic imaging demonstrates loss of striatal dopamine transporters in Parkinson disease. *Proc Natl Acad Sci USA* 1993;90:11965–11969.
20. Jeon BS. Dopa-responsive dystonia: a syndrome of selective nigrostriatal dopaminergic deficiency. *J Korean Med Sci* 1997;12:269–279.
21. Jeon BS, Jeong JM, Park SS, et al. Dopamine transporter density measured by [^{123}I]-β-CIT SPECT is normal in dopa-responsive dystonia. *Ann Neurol* 1998 *(in press)*.
22. Jeon BS, Kim JM, Jeong JM, et al. Dopamine transporter imaging with [^{123}I]-β-CIT demonstrates presynaptic nigrostriatal dopaminergic damage. *J Neurol Neurosurg Psychiatry* 1998 *(in press)*.
23. Ludecke B, Dworniczak B, Batholome K. A point mutation in the tyrosine hydroxylase gene associated with Segawa's syndrome. *Hum Genet* 1995;95:123–125.
24. Marek KL, Seibyl JP, Zoghbi SS, et al. [^{123}I]-β-CIT/SPECT imaging demonstrates bilateral loss of dopamine transporters in hemi-Parkinson's disease. *Neurology* 1996;46:231–237.
25. Naumann M, Pirker W, Reiners K, Lange K, Becker G, Brucke T. [^{123}I]-β-CIT single-photon emission tomography in dopa-responsive dystonia. *Mov Disord* 1997;12:448–451.
26. Nomura Y, Uetake K, Hagiwara Y, et al. Dystonia responding to levodopa and failure in biopterin metabolism. *Mov Disord* 1997;12[3 Suppl]:38(abst).
27. Nygaard TG. Dopa-responsive dystonia: delineation of the clinical syndrome and clues to pathogenesis. *Adv Neurol* 1993;60:577–585.
28. Nygaard TG, Marsden CD, Duvoisin RC. Dopa-responsive dystonia. *Adv Neurol* 1988;50:377–384.
29. Nygaard TG, Marsden CD, Fahn S. Dopa-responsive dystonia: long-term treatment response and prognosis. *Neurology* 1991;41:174–181.

Dystonia 3: Advances in Neurology, Vol. 78,
edited by S. Fahn, C. D. Marsden, and M. DeLong.
Lippincott–Raven Publishers, Philadelphia © 1998.

32

The Effect of GTP Cyclohydrolase-1 on Tyrosine Hydroxylase Expression: Implications in DOPA-responsive Dystonia

*†Un Jung Kang, *Craig Bencsics, *Stephen Wachtel, and †Robert Lew

*Departments of *Neurology and †Physiological and Pharmacological Sciences,
University of Chicago, Chicago, Illinois 60637.*

The discovery of mutations in the GTP cyclo-hydrolase-1 (GCH-1) gene in patients with dopa-responsive dystonia (DRD) (4) is a major breakthrough in our understanding of the disorder. The candidate gene approach in discovering the genetic defect has paid off in this case whereas such an approach has often failed in many other conditions due to our lack of understanding about the pathophysiology of the diseases investigated. GCH-1 is the first and rate-limiting step of tetrahydrobiopterin (BH_4) synthesis (10). BH_4 is an essential cofactor for the biochemical function of amino acid hydroxylases such as phenylalanine hydroxylase (PAH), tyrosine hydroxylase (TH), and tryptophan hydroxylase (TPH). The deficiency of BH_4 has been amply demonstrated in patients with DRD (2,9). The lack of BH_4 accounts for the inactivity of TH in producing L-DOPA and subsequent loss of dopamine. In addition, there are several pieces of evidence from both autopsy studies of patients with DRD (12) and experimental studies in animals (3) that indicate a role of BH_4 in TH expression aside from its role as a biochemical cofactor. In this chapter, we describe our preliminary data from grafting studies demonstrating a role of BH_4 in stabilization of TH protein, and review evidence in the literature that supports our hypothesis that BH_4 affects TH expression.

To specifically address whether the presence of BH_4 can stabilize the TH protein, we utilized nonneuronal cells to express TH with and without GCH-1. In our previous study (1), TH-immunoreactive cells were more prominent in primary fibroblast grafts expressing both TH and GCH-1 than in grafts with TH alone when placed in the denervated striatum of rats. Subsequently we also noted that the difference became greater over time *in vivo*. To further characterize the differences in expression of TH transgenes in these grafts, two groups of rats were grafted with either PFTH or PFTHGC cells for semiquantitation of mRNA levels and protein expression.

METHODS

We used primary fibroblast cells (PF) from Fischer 344 rats and genetically modified them with retrovirus vectors expressing TH and GCH-1. The cells expressing TH alone (PFTH) showed TH activity by enzymatic assay, but did not produce L-DOPA spontaneously in culture. Addition of BH_4 in the culture media was necessary for L-DOPA production by PFTH cells. The cells expressing both TH and GCH-1 (PFTHGC) produced L-DOPA spontaneously in culture. The details of the methods to generate genetically modified cells were described previously (1).

Animals were grafted with either PF, PFTH, or PFTHGC cells and were transcardially perfused with PBS, 4 days after grafting. Brains were removed and 10-μm sections were cut with a cryostat and mounted on slides coated with a 0.01% solution of polylysine. The sections were then fixed for 5 minutes with 4% paraformaldehyde and stored at 4°C in 100% ethanol. The sections were air dried before being used for *in situ* hybridization. A parallel group of animals were processed for immunohistochemistry as described previously (1).

Probes for the *in situ* hybridization were generated specific for the sense strand of human TH type 2 (hTH-2) message (5′CATGGTAA-GAGGGCAGTCCCCG3′) and for the antisense strand of hTH-2 (5′CGGGGACTGCCCTCT-TACCATG3′). Two pmoles of oligonucleotides were labeled with 25 units of terminal transferase in a reaction containing 50 μCi ^{33}P-labeled ATP. The reaction was initiated by the addition of oligonucleotides and incubated at 37°C for 1 hour. After the incubation, the reaction was terminated with ice-cold terminal transferase buffer. The labeled oligonucleotide was separated from unincorporated ^{33}P-ATP by applying the mixture to G-50 sephadex spin column and centrifuging the mixture at 1,500 g for 4 to 5 minutes. The labeled probe was then quantified by scintillation counting.

Sections were hybridized with 90 μl (220,000 cpms) of probe per section and covered with parafilm. Covered hybridization sections were placed in a humidified chamber for 18 to 19 hours at 37°C. The hybridization solution contained 50% formamide, 4 × SSC, 10% dextran sulfate, 5 × Denhardt's, 200 mg/ml acid-alkali-cleaved salmon sperm DNA, 100 mg/ml long-chain polyadenylic acid, 25 mM sodium phosphate, pH 7.0 1 mM sodium pyrophosphate in addition to the probe. After hybridization, parafilm covers were gently removed in 2 × SSC and tissue sections were washed with 2 × SSC (1 × SSC is 0.15 M NaCl and 0.015 M sodium citrate) at room temperature for 30 minutes, 0.5 × SSC at 37°C for 60 minutes, and 0.1 × SSC at 37°C for 60 minutes. After the sections were washed, they were dehydrated with 70%, 95%, and 100% ethanol for 5 minutes, 95% ethanol for 5 minutes each. Dried sections were exposed to Kodak film for 1 to 2 weeks and developed. The differences in intensity of the signal were quantified by first scanning the images and then analyzing the optical densities using NIH Image 1.60 software.

RESULTS

Immunohistochemistry for TH showed more TH-immunoreactive cells in PFTHGC grafts than in PFTH grafts (Fig. 1). TH-positive cells were counted in every fourth section through the grafts (a total of ten sections from each rat, $n = 4$). The number of TH-immunoreactive cells in PFTHGC grafts were about eight times that in PFTH grafts ($p < 0.05$; Fig. 2). The sur-

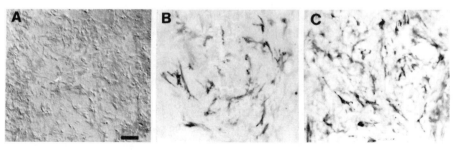

FIG. 1. Immunostaining of grafts with polyclonal antibody against TH. **A:** Unmodified primary fibroblast cells. Nomarski optics were used to visualize the unstained control cells. **B:** Fibroblasts transduced with TH. **C:** Fibroblasts doubly transduced with TH and GCH-1. The scale bar represents 100 μm.

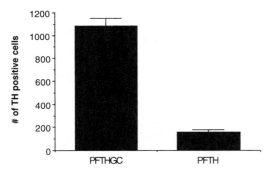

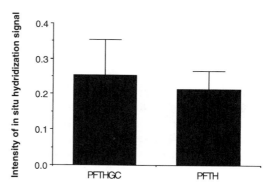

FIG. 2. Semiquantitative assessment of the TH-positive cells in genetically modified fibroblast grafts. The cell counts in PFTHGC (primary fibroblasts grafts expressing both TH and GCH-1) and PFTH (primary fibroblast grafts with TH) were performed as described in methods. The data show means and standard errors of means.

FIG. 4. Semiquantitative assessment of the mRNA levels. Quantitation of the *in situ* hybridization signals in PFTHGC (primary fibroblast grafts expressing both TH and GCH-1) and PFTH (primary fibroblast grafts with TH) were performed by densitometry as described in Methods. The data show means and standard errors of means.

vival of the PF, PFTH, and PFTHGC cells after grafting and total size of the grafts were comparable to previous studies (1). To see if the discordance was present at the transcript level, TH mRNA was detected by *in situ* hybridization using a radiolabeled probe specific for hTH-2 (Fig. 3). The TH mRNA levels were estimated from the hybridization signals in the sections containing PFTH and PFTHGC grafts (a total of three planes from each rat, $n = 3$). The density of signals in the two groups was not significantly different (Fig. 4).

DISCUSSION

Several lines of evidence in the literature have implicated an effect of BH_4 on TH expression. An autopsy study from patients with DRD showed that TH protein is decreased in both the putamen and the caudate by Western blot analysis as well as by TH activity levels. However, TH protein levels did not change in the substantia nigra (SN) of DRD patients. In addition, immunohistochemistry showed nor-

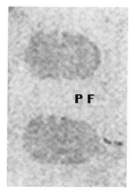
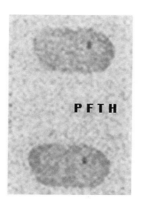
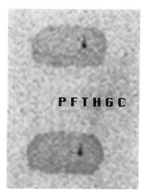

FIG. 3. *In situ* hybridization signals for TH mRNA in grafts. Two representative coronal sections containing striatal grafts from each group are shown. PF is unmodified primary fibroblast cells, PFTH is fibroblasts expressing TH, and PFTHGC is fibroblasts expressing both TH and GCH-1.

mal TH-positive cells in the SN and TH-positive fibers in the nigrostriatal bundle. The binding of GBR 12935 to the dopamine transporter was normal in the caudate and the putamen, indicating normal terminal structures of dopaminergic neurons (12). Positron emission tomography (PET) studies using binding of the dopamine uptake site ligand [^{123}I](1R)-2β-carbomethosy-3β-(4-ioodo-phenyl)tropane as an index of dopaminergic terminals also indicated that the terminals were not significantly affected in DRD patients compared with controls (5). The reason for the decrease in the level of TH protein in the terminals but not in the cell bodies is not obvious. Some authors have postulated an effect of BH$_4$ deficiency and lack of dopamine production on the development of dopaminergic neurons and their axonal aborizations (12). However, the relative preservation of dopamine transporters suggests that the terminal structures are likely to be intact, and thus there is a selective loss of TH protein in the terminals. One might speculate a defect in transport of TH protein from the cell bodies to the terminals as the cause. Alternatively, TH protein may be unstable in the absence of BH$_4$, and therefore maintenance of the TH levels in the terminals may be more dependent on the stability of protein because the cell bodies are more readily replenished by newly synthesized TH.

More recent studies in hph-1 mice that have a deficiency in GCH-1 also show that the activities and levels of TH in the striatum are significantly decreased whereas aromatic L-amino acid decarboxylase (AADC) is unchanged, again suggesting a specific effect of BH$_4$ deficiency on TH expression (3). Furthermore when BH$_4$ was administered in a sufficient amount to restore the level of BH$_4$ in the brain, serotonin and dopamine levels were not restored. This is consistent with the fact that there is a reduction in the enzyme protein levels as well as reduction in the cofactor, BH$_4$. A similar reduction of PAH, but not AADC was noted in the liver. Whether the changes in the steady-state levels of PAH and TH occur at the level of transcription of RNA messages, RNA stability, rate of translation of protein from

RNA, or stability of protein cannot be deduced from the these data.

Interesting clues about stability of TH protein expression come from basic studies attempting to express TH in nonneuronal cells. TH has been used as the major enzyme necessary to produce a genetically modified cell that can produce L-DOPA or dopamine. Wu and Cepko (15) compared the half-life of TH in PC12 cells, where TH is expressed endogenously, to that in NIH-3T3 cells with exogenous TH. The difference in half-life of TH in these two cell lines was striking. In PC12 cells, the half-life of TH was 20 hours but it was only 3 hours in NIH-3T3 cells. Wu and Cepko (15) pointed out that this may reflect differences between neuronal and nonneuronal cellular environment, but clues as to mechanism have been elusive. Likewise, the *in vivo* expression of TH protein in genetically modified nonneuronal cells has been particularly short-lived compared with other transgenes such as AADC or neurotrophic factors (6).

Our finding that the expression of TH protein is enhanced in primary fibroblast grafts when GCH-1 is added to produce BH$_4$ suggests that BH$_4$ may be the main factor responsible for the TH protein stability in PC12 cells. Because we have used nonneuronal cells to express TH with and without GCH-1, we can attribute the difference in TH expression to this single gene. Although retroviral transduction results in integration of the transgenes at random sites, and the integration sites may affect the transcription of the transgenes, such variation is unlikely to explain the difference in expression that we have observed. First, the primary fibroblast cells are bulk populations representing mixtures of cells with different integration sites. Second, PFTHGC cells were derived from PFTH cells. Therefore, even if there was a predilection for particular integration sites, the status of the TH gene should be the same in both cells, the only difference being the integration of the GCH-1 gene in PFTHGC cells. Third, mRNA levels were similar in both groups, and the difference seems to be at the level of protein. All these point to a role of BH$_4$ in stability of TH protein.

It is interesting that BH_4 has also been shown to be involved in the formation and stabilization of the dimeric complex of nitric oxide synthase (NOS) (7). This stabilization leads to increased activity of NOS. Similarly, dopamine has been shown to prolong the enzymatic stability of the TH molecules, while it kinetically inhibits the enzymatic activity (11). Dopamine binds TH molecule through the active site Fe^{2+} molecules at histidine residues 331 and 336 near the C-terminal end of TH (13). TH molecules form tetramers through interaction at the C-terminal 20 amino acids that appear to have leucine zipper motif (14). However, the mechanism for stabilization of TH protein by BH_4 is unknown. It should also be pointed out that the studies of stability of NOS and TH mentioned above addressed the stability of the enzymatic activities, which may be different from the turnover of immunoreactive protein levels that we discussed in the context of DRD. Stability of enzymatic activity reflects the pool of protein that still retains the enzymatic function, whereas examination of immunoreactive proteins may include molecules that are not active but have preserved antigenic components. There have been very few studies in the literature that address the aspects of TH protein turnover (8).

Although the preliminary data we present provide interesting insights into the possible mechanism of the effect of BH_4 in TH expression, the precise mechanism of BH_4 effect needs to be explored further. *In vitro* studies examining the relative levels of TH transcripts and proteins in clonal cells are necessary to confirm the tantalizing evidence from bulk populations of primary cells described above. In addition, studies directly examining synthesis rate versus degradation rate of mRNA and protein are necessary to pinpoint the mechanism of action by BH_4. For example, additional confirmation of the BH_4 effect may be obtained by inhibition of the synthesis of BH_4 in neuronal cells such as PC12 cells and demonstrating that the half-life of TH protein is reduced to that seen in fibroblast cells.

In conclusion, expression of neural genes in a nonneuronal environment provided us an opportunity to address the biology of neural proteins from a new perspective. Changes in TH expression can be attributed to the effect of a single gene, GCH-1 expressed in fibroblast cells. The hypothesized role of BH_4 in TH stability has both a practical implication in designing gene therapy for Parkinson's disease and an implication in understanding the biological principles underlying the pathophysiology of DRD.

ACKNOWLEDGMENTS

This research was supported by Dystonia Medical Research Foundation, R29 NS32080, Parkinson's Disease Foundation Junior Faculty Award, the H.G. and Catharine Lieneman Memorial Fund of United Parkinson Foundation, National Parkinson Foundation, and Brain Research Foundation. CB was supported by T32 NS07113, and SRW by T32 DA07255.

We thank Lewis Seiden for his support.

REFERENCES

1. Bencsics C, Wachtel SR, Milstien S, Hatakeyama K, Becker JB, Kang UJ. Double transduction with GTP cyclohydrolase I and tyrosine hydroxylase is necessary for spontaneous synthesis of L-DOPA by primary fibroblasts. *J Neurosci* 1996;16:4449–4456.
2. Furukawa Y, Mizuno Y, Nishi K, Narabayashi H. A clue to the pathogenesis of dopa-responsive dystonia. *Ann Neurol* 1995;37:139–140.
3. Hyland K, Gunasekera RS, Engle T, Arnold LA. Tetrahydrobiopterin and biogenic amine metabolism in the *hph-1* mouse. *J Neurochem* 1996;67:752–759.
4. Ichinose H, Ohye T, Takahashi E, et al. Hereditary progressive dystonia with marked diurnal fluctuation caused by mutations in the GTP cyclohydrolase 1 gene. *Nat Genet* 1994;8:236–209.
5. Jeon BS, Chung J-M, Lee M-C. This volume chap. 31.
6. Kang UJ. Genetic modification of cells with retrovirus vectors for grafting into the central nervous system. In: Kaplitt MG, Loewy AD, eds. *Viral vectors: gene therapy and neuroscience applications.* San Diego: Academic Press, 1995:211–237.
7. Klatt P, Schmidt K, Lehner D, Glatter O, Bachinger HP, Mayer B. Structural analysis of porcine brain nitric oxide synthase reveals a role for tetrahydrobiopterin and L-arginine in the formation of an SDS-resistant dimer. *EMBO J* 1995;14:3687–3695.
8. Kumer SC, Vrana KE. Intricate regulation of tyrosine hydroxylase activity and gene expression. *J Neurochem* 1996;67:443–462.

9. LeWitt PA, Miller LP, Levine RA, et al. Tetrahydro-biopterin in dystonia: identification of abnormal metabolism and therapeutic trials. *Neurology* 1986;36:760–764.

10. Nagatsu T. Biopterin cofactor and monoamine-synthesizing monooxygenases. *Neurochem Int* 1983;5:27–38.

11. Okuno S, Fujisawa H. Conversion of tyrosine hydroxylase to stable and inactive form by the end products. *J Neurochem* 1991;57:53–60.

12. Rajput AH, Gibb WRG, Zhong XH, et al. Dopa-responsive dystonia: pathological and biochemical observations in a case. *Ann Neurol* 1994;35:396–402.

13. Ramsey AJ, Daubner SC, Ehrlich JI, Fitzpatrick PF. Identification of iron ligands in tyrosine hydroxylase by mutagenesis of conserved histidinyl residues. *Protein Sci* 1995;4:2082–2086.

14. Vrana KE, Walker SJ, Rucker P, Liu X. A carboxyl terminal leucine zipper is required for tyrosine hydroxylase tetramer formation. *J Neurochem* 1994;63:2014–2020.

15. Wu DK, Cepko CL. The stability of endogenous tyrosine hydroxylase protein in PC-12 cells differs from that expressed in mouse fibroblasts by gene transfer. *J Neurochem* 1994;62:863–872.

Dystonia 3: Advances in Neurology, Vol. 78,
edited by S. Fahn, C. D. Marsden, and M. DeLong.
Lippincott–Raven Publishers, Philadelphia © 1998.

33

Inherited Myoclonus-Dystonia Syndrome

Thomas Gasser

*Department of Neurology, Klinikum Großhadern, Ludwig-Maxmilians-University,
München 81377, Germany.*

INTRODUCTION

The clinical diagnosis and classification of movement disorders is based on the observation and description of the abnormal movements. These movements are defined phenomenologically by their speed, duration, and their topical and temporal distribution.

Dystonia, for example, is defined as "a syndrome of sustained involuntary muscle contractions frequently causing repetitive or twisting movements or abnormal postures" (7). Although this definition of dystonia emphasizes the fact that the movement is often sustained at the peak of the excursion, it is important to realize that movements in dystonia may be extremely variable in speed, and in fact, are more often rapid than slow (6). *Myoclonus,* on the other hand, describes a brief, rapid, shock-like, involuntary, usually insuppressable movement (8).

However, the occurrence of different types of abnormal movements in a single patient, concurrently or sequentially during the course of a disease, may complicate diagnostic classification, and this appears to be the rule, rather than the exception, for many disorders. For example, patients with inherited primary generalized torsion dystonia linked to chromosome 9q34 frequently exhibit quick, jerky movements in addition to dystonia, which meet all the phenomenologic criteria of myoclonus. The disorder is then usually classified according to the *predominant* abnormal movement observed.

The Problem of Terminology: Essential Myoclonus, Myoclonic Dystonia, or Dystonic Myoclonus?

Classification may become very difficult in familial disorders, in which different family members are presumed to suffer from the same genetic disease, but exhibit a different spectrum of abnormal movements. This is the case in several published pedigrees in which affecteds show various combinations of myoclonus and dystonia, a problem that has led to considerable confusion in the terminology. This subject has been elegantly reviewed by Quinn et al. (27,29).

In patients and families in whom myoclonic movements are the most prominent manifestation of the disease the term *(hereditary) essential myoclonus* (in earlier publications also "paramyoclonus multiplex" or "essential myoclonia") has been used (3,5,9,16,22,26,37). Quinn and Marsden (28) noted that in many of these patients dystonic movements coexist with myoclonus, although less conspicuously, and used the term *myoclonic dystonia.* However, this designation had also been used to describe patients in whom primary torsion dystonia was the most likely diagnosis and who also exhibited rapid, brief muscle jerks in addition to dystonia (24). In order to differentiate these two groups of patients, it was Quinn and co-workers again who suggested the term *inherited dystonia with lightning jerks responsive to alcohol* (28) and later *dystonic myoclonus* (27) for the former.

There are arguments in favor of each of these terms, but neither seems to be ideal, mostly because it is still uncertain if the described families actually represent a nosologic entity and what in fact is the underlying movement abnormality. As a consequence of the discussion at the Third International Dystonia Symposium, held in Miami, Florida, October 9–11, 1996, it shall be suggested here to use the more neutral term *inherited myoclonus-dystonia syndrome* to designate an autosomal-dominant disorder characterized by myoclonus or dystonia or frequently a combination of both without other signs of neurologic dysfunction.

Clinical, electrophysiologic, and genetic findings in families who fit this definition will be reviewed in this chapter. The question whether all these families represent a single genetic disorder will only be answered when the responsible gene(s) are mapped and cloned.

HISTORICAL REVIEW

Essential Myoclonus

The first description of a patient with a myoclonic syndrome without evidence of additional neurologic dysfunction (which therefore has been called "essential" myoclonus) is now generally attributed to Nikolaus Friedreich, Professor at the University of Heidelberg (11).

In Friedreich's patient, subtle, rapid, involuntary movements affecting all parts of the body appeared at the age of 45 years after what is described as a "frightening experience." This patient had no known family history of abnormal movements. Symptoms were most prominent at rest and disappeared during action, and after "a few galvanisations," the patient had a complete remission. Friedreich concluded that what he had observed was a hitherto undescribed disorder that was distinct from epilepsy and from chorea (St. Vitus dance), the two important differential diagnoses known at Friedreich's time. He called the condition "Paramyoklonus multiplex" and the abbreviated term *myoclonus* has since become widely used for this type of movement (14).

Myoclonic movements can occur in a large number of neurologic disorders ("symptomatic" or "secondary" myoclonus), and only a minority can be labeled as "essential" (1). More than 100 years after Friedreich's account, Bressman and Fahn (2) reviewed 15 of their patients who were diagnosed as essential myoclonus (i.e., patients in whom myoclonic jerks were the sole neurologic abnormality and etiology was unknown). Thirteen of them had no family history of a movement disorder, only one had a family history of myoclonus, and another patient had a family history of tremor. There was a wide range in age of onset (2 to 64 years) and there was marked heterogeneity in the clinical appearance of myoclonus. It is therefore very likely that essential myoclonus, as defined here, is a heterogeneous group of conditions.

Myoclonic Dystonia

The term *myoclonic dystonia* was introduced by Dawidenkow, a Russian neurologist who at that time published in German. He described a patient with tonic muscle spasms of the trunk and neck with superimposed rapid muscle twitches involving the face, neck, arms, and trunk. The disorder became apparent at the age of 45, and one sister was similarly affected (4). Dawidenkow thought that recessive inheritance was most likely in this disease, and he differentiated the condition from Oppenheim's dystonia (now *primary generalized dystonia*), on the basis of the late age at onset and the fact that his patients, by contrast with most patients affected with Oppenheim's disease, were non-Jewish. From his detailed description, it is likely that the index patient suffered from adult-onset segmental dystonia with severe axial involvement and retrocollis, with superimposed rapid myoclonic jerks, a condition that today would most likely be classified within the spectrum of primary torsion dystonia.

Obeso and coworkers (24) used the term *myoclonic dystonia* again (referring to Dawidenkow's description) to emphasize the fact that myoclonic jerks may be prominent in otherwise typical primary torsion dystonia. They described 14 patients with detailed information on electromyographic (EMG) and electroencephalographic (EEG) recordings. Age at onset was variable, all patients in this series were sporadic, and all fulfilled the diagnostic criteria for primary torsion dystonia. In addition to dystonic movements and postures, which were prominent in all patients, they showed brief contractions in the proximal muscles more than the distal ones, associated with EMG bursts of 50 to 250 milliseconds in duration. In a number of patients, both dystonia and myoclonus involved the same muscles, but in the majority dystonia was more prominent within the proximal muscles of the neck and shoulder, whereas myoclonus was seen more distally. Myoclonic jerks were provoked or exacerbated by action.

In Dawidenkow's and Obeso's patients, the basic clinical condition appears to be that of primary torsion dystonia, on which myoclonic jerks are superimposed. These patients are correctly described as suffering from *myoclonic dystonia,* as the adjective *myoclonic* modifies the noun, dystonia, which specifies the basic underlying disorder, namely dystonia, but there is no good reason to separate these patients from other patients with primary dystonia.

AUTOSOMAL-DOMINANT MYOCLONUS-DYSTONIA SYNDROME (PREVIOUSLY CALLED PARAMYOCLONUS MULTIPLEX OR HEREDITARY ESSENTIAL MYOCLONUS, OR MYOCLONIC DYSTONIA)

Over the years, several families have been described with a rare inherited disorder with a variable combination of myoclonus and dystonia. All these families had an apparently autosomal-dominant mode of inheritance and also shared other characteristics, so that Mahloudji and Pikielny, based on their own observations and a brief review of the literature, suggested diagnostic criteria for this condition (22) (see Table 1).

The following summary of the spectrum of clinical features is based on the description of 19 families reported in 14 publications in the

TABLE 1. *Diagnostic criteria, set forth by Mahloudji and Pikielny (22), for "hereditary essential myoclonus," with modifications, printed in bold italics, in order to incorporate more recent observations in this syndrome*

1. Onset of myoclonus *usually* in the first or second decade of life; *mild dystonic features are observed in some affecteds in addition to myoclonus and may rarely be the only manifestation of the disorder*
2. Males and females *(equally?)* affected
3. A benign cause, often variable, but compatible with an active life of normal span
4. Autosomal-dominant mode of inheritance with variable severity, *and incomplete penetrance*
5. Absence of other neurologic signs such as dementia, ataxia, or seizures
6. Normal EEG, *normal SSEP*

literature. These families were chosen because of the completeness of the clinical description and because it was felt by the author that it is possible that these families actually represent a single disorder. The clinical characteristics are summarized in Table 2. Based on the synopsis of these family descriptions, the criteria by Mahloudji and Pikielny shall be modified (Table 1).

Clinical Features

Myoclonus

In the majority of affecteds from all families, myoclonic movements are the most prominent clinical feature. The distribution of the jerks is variable, but most frequently they are described to affect predominantly the proximal muscles, the shoulders, arms, neck, and trunk, rarely the face and the legs. Focal, segmental, multifocal, and generalized distribution of myoclonus has been described. Jerks may occur synchronously or asynchronously in different muscle groups, usually in an asymmetric fashion. Myoclonus is usually markedly exacerbated by voluntary movements or occurs on action only. It is also worsened when the patients are anxious and fatigued.

Quinn and coworkers noted that the jerks are usually extremely rapid ("lightning-like"), but burst discharges recorded by surface EMG range from 30 milliseconds to 1.5 seconds in duration, with a continuous spectrum of burst lengths in-between (27). In several reports it is mentioned that single or repetitive jerks can be precipitated by sudden loud noises, but jerking in response to tactile stimuli appears to be rare and has been mentioned in one family only (17).

Fahn and Sjaastad commented on a waxing and waning character of jerky movements in their family (9) in the form of an "oscillatory" myoclonus. This had been documented electromyographically in an earlier description of this family (34), but has not been mentioned in other families.

Dystonia

Quinn and Marsden (28) described patients from six families and noted that in addition to myoclonus, they also displayed abnormal movements with prolonged muscle spasms or abnormal postures characteristic of torsion dystonia. Reviewing the literature, they concluded that at least some of the affecteds in almost all families who had been described under the name of "hereditary essential myoclonus" also had some dystonic features (29).

For example, one patient in the family of the Mahloudji and Pikielny study was described as having a tendency to hold his head to the right (22), and several patients in the family described by Przuntek and Muhr (26) had "phasic torticollis" in addition to myoclonus. The association of dystonic and myoclonic movements has also been observed in other families that have been described more recently. In the families described by Kurlan et al. (17), Kyllerman et al. (18), Fahn and Sjaastad (9), and Gasser et al. (12), most had myoclonic jerks, but some also had mild dystonia in addition to myoclonus, mainly torticollis or writer's cramp. In a few patients, dystonia was the sole sign of the disease (see Table 2).

Other Abnormal Movements in Families with Myoclonus-Dystonia Syndrome

Postural tremor, associated with rhythmic burst discharges on EMG, have been noted par-ticularly in the family described by Korten et al. (16). In some of their patients, periods of rhythmic discharges alternated with phases of arrhythmic jerks that were either asynchronous and multifocal, or bilaterally synchronous and generalized. Three patients had tremor only. The particular phenotype appears to be age related as patients with tremor usually developed symptoms during adult life, whereas myoclonus appeared during childhood or adolescence, as in other described families (see Table 1). Postural tremor has also been noted occasionally in affecteds from other families (9,17,31).

A combination of myoclonic jerks and progressive cerebellar dysfunction has been described under the eponym of the Ramsay Hunt syndrome. Frank cerebellar dysfunction with ataxia and intention tremor is not seen in the families reviewed here, but mild dysmetria often cannot be excluded with confidence, as it may be impossible to separate mild dysmetria from myoclonic jerks during movements toward a target.

Response to Drugs and Alcohol

In most reports, response to a variety of drugs is described to be poor. A dramatic effect to the anticholinergic agent benztropine has been reported by Duvoisin (5), but this has not been found by others (27). Clonazepam has been found to be moderately effective by several authors. Other drugs that have been used with little success include 5-hydroxytryptophan, neuroleptics, and dopamine agonists. The alleviation of myoclonus upon ingestion of alcohol was particularly stressed by Quinn et al., but had also been noted earlier by Lindenmulder (21), Daube and Peters (3), and others. This seems to be a striking feature of the disorder in most, but not in all, patients. There may be a difference in response to alcohol even within individual families (9). A rebound worsening after a bout of drinking has also been described.

Age at Onset

In all reported families, age at onset in the majority of patients is in the first or second de-

TABLE 2. Main clinical features of published families with myoclonus and dystonia[a]

Family	Author	Year	n	Age at onset[b]	Symptoms (n)			Distribution	Stimulus sensitivity	Response to alcohol	Associated symptoms	Course
					mc	dys	mc/dys					
1	Lindenmulder	1993	5	<20	5		?	ue/n/t/f	n.m.	Positive ?	None	Stable
2	Biemond	1963	11	Juvenile	11			f/ue	n.m.	n.m.	None	Mild
3	Feldmann and Wieser	1964	4	11–14	4			n/ue/t/f	Noise	n.m.	Tremor (2)	Stable, partial improvement in some
4	Daube and Peters	1966	5	2–14	4		1	t/ue	Noise	Positive	Mild	Stable
			12	1–20	12			t/ue	Noise	Positive	Dysmetria	Stable, partial improvement in some
6	Mahloudji and Pikielny	1967	6	1.5–7 (3.6)	3		2	f/t/pa	n.m.	n.m.	None	
7	Korten et al.	1974	15	1–55	12			ue/t/n	n.m.	Positive	Tremor (7)	Stable
8	Przuntek and Muhr	1983	25	4–Adult	25		10	t/ue/n>f	n.m.	Positive	Tremor (7)	Slow progression in most, rapid progression, major disability in 2
9	Duvoisin	1984	3	5, 9, 1	1		2	ue/t	Noise	n.m.	None	Stable
10	Nutt and Bird	1984	3	3–~18	2		1	f/ue/t	no	Positive	Melanoma (2)	Slow progression or stable
11	Quinn et al.	1988	3	0–10	—		3	ue/n/t	n.m.	Positive	None	
12			1	Childhood	—	—	1	ue/t/n>f	n.m.	Positive	None	
13			1	3			1	ue/n	n.m.	Positive	None	
14			5	3–?	2		3	ue/t/n>f	n.m.	Positive	Melanoma (1)	
15			1	2			1	ue/n/t>f/le	n.m.	Positive	None	
16			2	8/?			2	ue/n/t	n.m.	n.a.		
17	Kurlan et al.	1988	7	6–18 (12)	2		5	t/n/ue	Noise (3) Touch (4)	Positive	Tremor (4)	Slow progression, then stable
18	Kyllerman et al.	1990	20	3–14	10	1	9	ue/n/t	n.m.	Positive	Tremor (3)	Slow progression, then stable
19	Fahn and Sjaastad	1991	15	9–60 (22, 6)	12		3	n/ue/t	n.m.	Positive in some	None	Slow progression, then stable, 2 remissions
3a[c]	Gasser et al.	1996	10	6–14 (8.7)	6	1	3	ue/t/n	n.m.	Positive	Tremor (1)	Stable

[a]These families have been published under the terms "paramyoclonus multiplex" (family 2), "familial myoclonia" (family 1) "(hereditary) essential myoclonus" (families 3–10, 19), "myoclonus and dystonia" (family 17), "myoclonic dystonia" (family 18, 3a) and "hereditary dystonia with lightning jerks responsive to alcohol" (families 11–16).
[b]Age at onset is given as range, with the mean in parentheses, if it can be calculated from the data available.
[c]The family described by Gasser et al. is an extension of the pedigree published by Feldmann and Wiesser and is therefore numbered as "3a."

n, number of affecteds; mc, myoclonus; dys, dystonia; f, face; n, neck; ue, upper extremities; t, trunk; le, lower extremities; n.m., not mentioned.

cade of life, although there were several adult-onset cases in the families described by Przuntek and Muhr (26) and by Fahn and Sjaastad (9). Mean age of onset in the families with sufficient data reported for calculation was between 3.6 and 22.6 years (see Table 2).

The sequence of appearance of dystonia and myoclonus in individual cases is also variable. In two of the patients described by Kyllerman et al., dystonia appeared in infancy, taking the form of hemidystonia with involvement of the leg. This symptom disappeared during childhood, to be replaced by myoclonic jerks. On the other hand, in the family described by Gasser et al. recently, one individual suffered from torticollis and writer's cramp only when he was examined at the age of 58. In an earlier description of this family (10), this individual is documented unequivocally as being affected with myoclonus.

Course of the Disease

The course of the disease is benign in the majority of cases. Remission of dystonia has been noted in the family described by Kyllerman et al. (19): In the two infants with leg-onset dystonia and hemidystonia, this symptom resolved by the time the children were about 5 years old, and they were left with myoclonus only. In another family, two living family members had a history compatible with myoclonus, but exhibited no abnormal movements on examination, so they were thought to represent permanent remissions (9).

Most frequently, the disease appears to be slowly progressive for a few years after onset and then stabilizes, fluctuates slightly over the years, or shows mild spontaneous improvement. Despite the embarrassment frequently caused by the abnormal movement, affecteds are able to lead a relatively normal and socially active life in the vast majority of cases.

The family first described by Feldmann and Wieser in 1964 has been reexamined recently, allowing for a 30-year follow-up examination (10,12). This observation confirmed earlier reports of the essentially nonprogressive nature

of the disorder with a slightly fluctuating course over the years.

However in the family studied by Przuntek and Muhr (26), there were at least two patients whose disease progressed within a few years so that they were unable to feed themselves. The secondary effects of chronic alcohol abuse, which is common when patients discover its beneficial effect on the abnormal movements, appear to be the most disruptive feature over the years.

Electrophysiology

Reports on electrophysiologic findings in patients with autosomal-dominant myoclonus-dystonia syndrome are relatively scarce.

Hallett (15) described a topical and temporal distribution of muscle contractions he called "ballistic movement overflow pattern" in two patients with "essential myoclonus" [who, based on his description, a positive family history, and a subsequent report by Quinn et al. (29) are likely to suffer from the condition under review here]. He observed sequential triphasic agonist-antagonist-agonist activation, as is seen during normal ballistic movements. However, muscle activity was not restricted to the muscles needed to move a particular joint, but tended to spread to adjacent muscles. This pattern was different from that observed in patients with epileptic myoclonus, who showed coactivation of antagonist muscle pairs (15).

However, this pattern has not been found consistently in all patients with this disorder. Quinn et al. (29) also reported on the electrophysiologic findings in their patients. They found the myoclonic jerks to be associated with EMG burst discharges ranging from 30 milliseconds to about 1.5 seconds, sometimes synchronous and symmetric, sometimes asynchronous and asymmetric. Bursts were sometimes limited to a single agonist, at other times co-contraction of agonist-antagonist pairs occurred. In some of their patients they saw the ballistic movement overflow pattern that had been described by Hallett earlier, but they saw co-contraction of antagonist muscles in others. They even reexamined a patient with the ballistic movement overflow pattern in Hallett's study; now this same patient showed a co-contraction pattern also. In conclusion, surface EMG documents the variability of the myoclonic jerks, but fails to detect a distinctive pattern.

In several studies, routine EEG and somatosensory evoked potential (SSEP) examinations were found to be completely normal (5,29,37). In particular, the abnormal enlargement of the cortical SEP seen in cortical reflex myoclonus has never been detected, and no jerk locked cortical spike can be found on back-averaged EEG (29). However, in four of ten patients studied with the latter technique, a generalized, symmetric, and synchronous cortical potential was detected, preceding the jerks by 25 to 70 milliseconds. These slow waves were negative in three patients and positive in one. Interestingly, the waves were similar in time-course and distribution to the terminal phase of the "Bereitschaftspotential" (29). They have been interpreted as an indication of the subcortical location of the generator of jerks.

Clinical Genetics

In all families described to date, transmission was compatible with autosomal-dominant inheritance. Whether sporadic cases with a similar clinical picture actually represent genetic cases, in whom family history is "masked" by reduced penetrance [as is the case, for example, in early-onset generalized dystonia in the Ashkenazi-Jewish population (25)] cannot be decided at this time.

Mahloudji and Pikielny emphasized that both males and females were equally affected by the disease. By contrast, in the family recently described by us, there was only one female affected as compared to ten males, although there was only a slight predominance of male at-risk individuals (12). An overrepresentation of male affecteds has also been noted in the family described by Przuntek and Muhr (26). This observation possibly reflects a variable penetrance of the mutation in males and females. The reverse finding, a higher penetrance in females as compared to males, has been reported for dopa-responsive dystonia (23).

Reduced penetrance was commented on in most published families. There are several documented cases of obligate carriers of the disease gene (based on the position in the pedigree, if autosomal-dominant inheritance is assumed), who lived to old age and never showed any abnormal movements.

Molecular Genetic Studies

The mapping and, in several cases, the identification of disease genes has helped in the classification of a number of inherited conditions. This has been the case for several forms of dystonia, such as early-onset generalized dystonia, dopa-responsive dystonia, and, very recently, some forms of focal dystonia (see Chapters 9, 10, 11, 20, and 34 of this volume; also Reference 20). Eventually, this type of study will also clarify if there is one or several inherited diseases causing the combination of myoclonus and dystonia described in this chapter, and whether some of the families described under different designations carry mutations in the same or in different genes.

To date, only a few molecular genetic studies have been published in families with inherited myoclonus-dystonia syndrome. Two studies examined regions carrying candidate genes for the disorder. Candidate genes are genes that can be hypothesized to play a role in the etiology of a disease, based on our knowledge of its pathophysiology. These candidate genes can either be analyzed directly, by sequencing the respective genes, or, if the location of the genes within the genome is known, this region can be investigated using polymorphic DNA markers surrounding the gene (Fig. 1).

Given the overlapping clinical spectrum of idiopathic torsion dystonia and myoclonic dystonia discussed above, an obvious candidate gene region is the region on chromosome 9q, which harbors the gene for primary early-onset generalized dystonia (DYT1). This region has been investigated by Wahlström and associates (35), who analyzed the large family described by Kyllerman et al. in 1990 (18). They found strongly negative two-point lod scores with several polymorphisms surrounding the DYT1

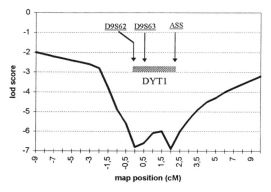

FIG. 1. Multipoint linkage analysis with DNA markers closely surrounding the DYT1 gene (the gene for early-onset primary torsion dystonia). The region containing the DYT1 gene is excluded (lod score < −.2).

region, excluding DYT1 as the disease gene in this family. This region has also been clearly excluded in a recently described large German family (12) (Fig. 1).

Several other candidate gene regions have been examined in the latter family. The molecular pathogenesis of inherited myoclonus is unknown, but it may be suspected that hyperexcitable neuronal circuits within the basal ganglia or the brainstem are involved. Therefore, inhibitory neurotransmitters or their receptors may well play a role and may be considered to be candidate genes. Neurotransmitter receptors are frequently composed of different receptor subunits, which are differentially expressed within different regions of the central nervous system. A mutation in one particular subunit could cause a highly selective disturbance of neuronal circuitry. In addition, the observed response to alcohol and benzodiazepines in inherited myoclonic disorders might point to an involvement of GABAergic transmission, as both components are thought to exert at least some of their effects via the GABA-receptor chloride channel complex. The glycine receptor may also be considered as a candidate gene, as another movement disorder that has some striking similarities with inherited myoclonus-dystonia is caused by mutations in the α-subunit of the glycine receptor: hyperekplexia, or startle dis-

ease (30,32,33). Fourteen of these candidate genes have been studied in the German pedigree (see Table 3), and all of them have been excluded (12).

Genome Screening

Preliminary results of a systematic screening of the entire genome have been published in abstract form by two groups. Wilhelmsen and associates (36) have excluded portions of the genome in the families described by Przuntek and Muhr (26) and that described by Fahn and Sjaastad (9). More than 90% of the genome has been excluded in the family described by Gasser and coworkers (12,13), but still no definitive proof for linkage with an autosomal locus was possible.

This could be due to the fact that the markers tested so far in these families have not been sufficiently informative, so true linkage has been missed. On the other hand, failure to discover linkage in spite of exhaustive screening of the genome could be due to more fundamen-

TABLE 3. *Map position of candidate genes evaluated in myoclonus-dystonia syndrome. Linkage to the genomic regions bearing these candidate genes has been excluded in a German family*

Gene	Localization
DYT1	9q34
GABA-A receptor	
α1 subunit	5q31-q35
α2 subunit	4p13-q11
α3 subunit	Xq28
α4 subunit	15q11.2-q12
α5 subunit	15q11.2-q12
α6 subunit	5q31-q35
β1 subunit	4q12
β2 subunit	5q31-q35
β3 subunit	15q11.2
γ1 subunit	4p12-q13
γ2 subunit	5q31
γ3 subunit	15q11.2-q12
δ subunit	1p
ρ1 subunit	6q14-21
ρ2 subunit	6q14-21
Glycine receptor	
α1 subunit	5q31
β subunit	Not mapped

tal problems of diagnostic accuracy, or the applicability of the genetic model used in the lod score calculations. Further studies in well-characterized families are needed.

CONCLUSION

This review of the published families with a syndrome of early-onset myoclonus, optional dystonia, and a generally benign course suggests that families that have been published under the names of "hereditary essential myoclonus," "myoclonic dystonia," or "hereditary dystonia with lightning jerks responsive to alcohol" may actually all suffer from a single genetic disorder, which is distinct from autosomal-dominant primary torsion dystonia. The diagnostic criteria set forth by Mahloudji and Pikielny in 1966 can still be regarded as valid, with the addition that dystonic movements may occur in some affecteds in addition to myoclonus and might even be the only sign of the disease in a small minority of patients.

Although myoclonus is certainly the defining abnormal movement in this disorder, myoclonic and dystonic movements may occur independently of each other in the same individual or in different individuals from the same family. It therefore appears most logical not to use one term as an adjective qualifying the other (as in "myoclonic dystonia" or "dystonic myoclonus"), but to use the more neutral and purely descriptive designation "inherited myoclonus-dystonia syndrome." The question whether all families with this phenotype actually represent a single monogenic disorder remains open until the causative gene(s) are mapped and cloned.

REFERENCES

1. Aigner BR, Mulder DW. Myoclonus. Clinical significance and approach to classification. *Arch Neurol* 1960;2:600–615.
2. Bressman S, Fahn S. Essential myoclonus. *Adv Neurol* 1986;43:287–294.
3. Daube JR, Peters HA. Hereditary essential myoclonus. *Arch Neurol* 1966;15:587–594.
4. Dawidenkow S. Auf hereditär-abiotrophischer Grundlage akut auftretende, regressierende und episodische Erkrankungen des Nervensystems und Bemerkungen

über die familiäre subakute, myoklonische Dystonie. *Z Ges Neurol Psych* 1926;104:596–622.
5. Duvoisin RC. Essential myoclonus: response to anticholinergic therapy. *Clin Neuropharmacol* 1984;7: 141–147.
6. Fahn S. The varied clinical expressions of dystonia. *Neurol Clin* 1984;2:541–553.
7. Fahn S, Marsden CD, Calne DB. Classification and investigation of dystonia. In: Marsden CD et al., eds. *Movement disorders 2.* London: Butterworths, 1987: 332–358.
8. Fahn S, Marsden CD, Van Woert MH. Definition and classification of myoclonus. *Adv Neurol* 1986;43: 1–5.
9. Fahn S, Sjaastad O. Hereditary essential myoclonus in a large Norwegian family. *Mov Disord* 1991;6:237–247.
10. Feldmann H, Wieser S. Klinische Studie zur essentiellen Myoklonie. *Arch Psych Z Ges Neurol* 1964; 205:555–570 (abst).
11. Friedreich N. Paramyoklonus multiplex. *Virchows Arch Path Anat* 1881;86:421–430.
12. Gasser T, Bereznai B, Müller B, et al. Linkage studies in alcohol-responsive myoclonic dystonia. *Mov Disord* 1996;12:363–370.
13. Gasser T, Oehlmann R, Bereznai B, et al. Genetic linkage studies in alcohol-responsive myoclonic dystonia. *J Neurol* 1996;243[Suppl 2]:S42.
14. Hallett M. Early history of myoclonus. *Adv Neurol* 1986;43:7–10.
15. Hallett M, Chadwick D, Marsden CD. Ballistic movement overflow myoclonus a form of essential myoclonus. *Brain* 1977;100:299–312.
16. Korten JJ, Notermans SL, Frenken CW, Gabreels FJ, Joosten EM. Familial essential myoclonus. *Brain* 1974;97:131–138.
17. Kurlan R, Behr J, Medved L, Shoulson I. Myoclonus and dystonia; a family study. *Adv Neurol* 1988;50: 385–389.
18. Kyllerman M, Forsgren L, Sanner G, Holmgren G, Wahlstrom J, Drugge U. Alcohol-responsive myoclonic dystonia in a large family: dominant inheritance and phenotypic variation. *Mov Disord* 1990;5: 270–279.
19. Kyllerman M, Sanner G, Forsgren L, Holmgren G, Wahlstrom J. Early onset dystonia decreasing with development. Case report of two children with familial myoclonic dystonia. *Brain Dev* 1993;15: 295–298.
20. Leube B, Rudnicki D, Ratzlaff T, Kessler KR, Benecke R, Auburger G. Idiopathic torsion dystonia: assignment of a gene to chromosome 18p in a German family with adult onset, autosomal dominant inheritance and purely focal distribution. *Hum Mol Genet* 1996;5:1673–1677.
21. Lindenmulder FG. Familial myoclonia occurring in three successive generations. *J Nerv Ment Dis* 1933; 77:489–492.
22. Mahloudji M, Pikielny RT. Hereditary essential myoclonus. *Brain* 1967;90:669–674.
23. Nygaard TG, Trugman JM, de Yebenes JG, Fahn S. Dopa-responsive disease: the spectrum of clinical manifestations in a large North American family. *Neurology* 1990;40:66–69.
24. Obeso JA, Rothwell JC, Lang AE, Marsden CD. Myoclonic dystonia. *Neurology* 1983;33:825–830.

25. Ozelius LJ, Kramer PL, de Leon D, et al. Strong allelic association between the torsion dystonia gene (DYT1) and loci on chromosome 9q34 in Ashkenazi Jews. Torsion dystonia genes in two populations confined to a small region on chromosome 9q32-34. *Am J Hum Genet* 1991;49:366–371.
26. Przuntek H, Muhr H. Essential familial myoclonus. *J Neurol* 1983;230:153–162.
27. Quinn NP. Essential myoclonus and myoclonic dystonia. *Mov Disord* 1996;11:119–124.
28. Quinn NP, Marsden CD. Dominantly inherited myoclonic dystonia with dramatic response to alcohol. *Neurology* 1984;34:236–237 (abst).
29. Quinn NP, Rothwell JC, Thompson PD. Marsden CD. Hereditary myoclonic dystonia, hereditary torsion dystonia and hereditary essential myoclonus: an area of confusion. *Adv Neurol* 1988;50:391–401.
30. Ryan SG, Sherman SL, Terry JC, Sparkes RS, Torres MC, Mackey RW. Startle disease, or hyperekplexia: response to clonazepam and assignment of the gene (STHE) to chromosome 5q by linkage analysis. *Ann Neurol* 1992;31:663–668.
31. Schaefer KP, Wieser S. Neurophysiologische Untersuchungen zur essentiellen Myoklonie. *Arch Psychiatr NervKrankh* 1964;205:572–590.
32. Shiang R, Ryan SG, Zhu YZ, et al. Mutational analysis of familial and sporadic hyperekplexia. *Ann Neurol* 1995;38:85–91.
33. Shiang R, Ryan SG, Zhu YZ, Hahn AF, O'Connell P, Wasmuth JJ. Mutations in the alpha 1 subunit of the inhibitory glycine receptor cause the dominant neurologic disorder, hyperekplexia. *Nat Genet* 1993;5:351–358.
34. Sjaastad O, Sulg I, Refsum S. Benign familial myoclonus-like movements, partly of early onset. *J Neural Transm Suppl* 1983;19:291–303.
35. Wahlstrom J, Ozelius L, Kramer P, et al. The gene for familial dystonia with myoclonic jerks responsive to alcohol is not located on the distal end of 9q. *Clin Genet* 1994;45:88–92.
36. Wilhelmsen KC, Nygaard T, Weeks DE, et al. Progress in genetic localization of the gene for hereditary essential myoclonus. *Mov Disord* 1994;9:132 (abst).
37. Zonda T, Szabo E. Hereditary essential myoclonus. *Hum Hered* 1979;29:348–350.

Dystonia 3: Advances in Neurology, Vol. 78,
edited by S. Fahn, C. D. Marsden, and M. DeLong.
Lippincott–Raven Publishers, Philadelphia © 1998.

34

Rapid-Onset Dystonia-Parkinsonism: A Report of Clinical, Biochemical, and Genetic Studies in Two Families

*Allison Brashear, †Ian J. Butler, ‡Laurie J. Ozelius, §Patricia L. Kramer,
*Martin R. Farlow, ‡Xandra O. Breakefield, and ‖William B. Dobyns

*Department of Neurology, Indiana University School of Medicine, Indianapolis, Indiana 46202;
†Department of Neurology, University of Texas Medical School-Houston, Houston, Texas 77030;
‡Molecular Neurogenetics Unit, Massachusetts General Hospital, Charlestown, Massachusetts 02129;
§ Department of Neurology, Oregon Health Sciences University, Portland, Oregon 97201;
‖Division of Pediatric Neurology, University of Minnesota, Minneapolis, Minnesota 55455.

Rapid-onset dystonia-parkinsonism (RDP) is a newly described autosomal-dominant movement disorder with a variable phenotype ranging from the classic presentation of abrupt onset over hours to days of combined dystonia and parkinsonism to mild writer's cramp (1, 2,4). Cumulative studies in two apparently unrelated midwestern families include the following:

1. Clinical descriptions of the typical RDP syndrome and the more mild phenotype of limb dystonia;
2. Cerebrospinal fluid (CSF) levels of the dopamine metabolite, homovanillic acid (HVA), in affected individuals, at-risk individuals (unaffected with a symptomatic parent or sibling), and asymptomatic gene carriers (AGCs) (unaffected with a symptomatic child);
3. Genetic linkage studies excluding RDP from the genomic region encoding for DYT1, the gene responsible for early idiopathic torsion dystonia (ITD) and the gene responsible for dopa-responsive dystonia (DRD).

We summarize the results of these studies and propose diagnostic criteria that exclude RDP from other dystonia and parkinsonian syndromes.

METHODS

Description of the Rapid-Onset Dystonia-Parkinsonism Syndrome

Typical Presentation

The typical form of RDP, as defined in ten affected patients, presents with sudden onset over hours to days of dystonic posturing of the limbs (arms more than legs), postural instability, bradykinesia (with greater involvement of the bulbar muscles), dysarthria, and dysphagia. Individuals are usually affected in the late teens to early 30s (age range 15 to 45 years), but onset of mild dystonia-parkinsonism has been reported by individuals as old as 58 years. Neurologic examination reveals slow, dysarthric speech with significant dysphagia, bradykinesia, dystonic spasms involving limbs, and an unsteady, slow gait with postural instability. The muscle stretch reflexes, plantar responses, and sensory examinations are normal. No abnormal eye movements, tremor, myoclonus, or dementia have been observed in these patients.

Affected individuals often report little progression over several years and are minimally responsive to carbidopa/levodopa or dopamine agonists.

Variable Phenotype of Rapid-Onset Dystonia-Parkinsonism

Four individuals in the first family (RDP-1) and three in the second (RDP-2) reported isolated mild limb dystonia involving the hand and/or foot. This may occur years before the abrupt onset of combined dystonia-parkinsonism or may remain unchanged. This focal dystonia is indistinguishable from idiopathic focal dystonia.

Clinical Descriptions

The First Family (RDP-1) Reported

In RDP-1 six individuals described sudden onset of classic RDP over several hours and four other individuals had subacute presentation of the complete syndrome over days to weeks (4). The age range of the individuals with rapid onset was 15 to 45 years compared to

a range of 15 to 25 years in those with slower onset. Several individuals reported abrupt onset of symptoms immediately after exposure to extreme heat, running long distances, or the stress of childbirth. Two others had intermittent limb dystonia indistinguishable from idiopathic focal dystonia. Subsequent studies of two newly affected individuals with mild limb dystonia and subtle parkinsonism at ages 58 and 23 years confirm the variable clinical presentation in RDP-1 (2). The 23-year-old patient had stable symptoms of mild limb cramping for 1 year. Then, 1 week after a fever he developed abrupt onset of bradykinesia, dysarthria, dysphagia, and worsening of dystonic spasms. The clinical summary of those affected in RDP-1 is listed in Table 1.

The Second Family (RDP-2)

Recently we described a second, apparently unrelated family with RDP-2 (1). Three of four individuals who developed the complete RDP symptom complex over hours reported stable, mild symptoms of limb dystonia (cramping of arms and legs with typing or walking, respec-

TABLE 1. *Clinical manifestations in RDP Family 1*

Pedigree number	II.2[a]	II.3[a]	II.4[a]	II.7[a]	II.8[a]	III.4[a,b]	III.6[a]
Sex	Male	Female	Female	Female	Male	Male	Male
Dystonia only							
Age at onset							
Site							
Rate							
Dystonia-parkinsonism							
Age at onset	45	25	29	58	15	35	17
Rate at onset	R	S	R	S	S	R	R
Progression	Slow	Slow	Slow	Slow	Slow	Non	Non
Time to stabilization	1 yr	< 1 mo	< 1 d	N/A	11 yr	< 1 d	< 1 d
Dystonia	+	+	+	+	+	+	+
Parkinsonism	+	+	+	+	+	+	+
Rating scales							
DMS	27	70	54	1	60	...	73
UPDRS	45	70	82	1	45	...	63
Severity scale	3	3	4	1	3	3	4
Brain MRI/CT			CT-NL	MRI-NL		MRI-NL	CT-NL

[a]Previously reported.
[b]Exam from medical records.
[c]Newly affected.
DMS, Dystonia Movement Scale; UPDRS, Unified Parkinson's Disease Rating Scale; +, present; ..., not known; N/A, not applicable; R, rapid; U, arms; L, legs; F, face including speech and swallowing; WC, writer's cramp; S, subacute; I, intermittent; CT-NL, brain CT normal; MRI-NL, brain MRI normal.

tively) for years before abrupt worsening of the dystonia, accompanied by new symptoms of parkinsonism with bradykinesia, dysarthria, dysphagia, and postural instability. A fourth individual, the child of an affected woman, suddenly developed the complete RDP symptom complex without preceding focal limb dystonia within minutes after feeling overheated. She later developed seizures that were easily controlled with divalproex sodium. She is the only individual in either family to develop seizures. Two of the four affected individuals were treated with carbidopa/levodopa with minimal clinical improvement. Magnetic resonance imaging (MRI) or computed tomography (CT) of the brain in all four affected individuals was normal. Neurologic examinations of two brothers and both parents of the three affected siblings were normal. Our discovery of a second family suggests that this disorder may be more commonly present in the general population than initially suspected. Our report suggests that RDP is not an isolated or private mutation unique to the first family. The clinical summary of the affected individuals in RDP-2 is listed in Table 2.

Summary of Clinical Studies to Date

To date 73 family members from family RDP-1 and eight from RDP-2 have been examined by our group. In RDP-1, we evaluated 11 individuals with dystonia-parkinsonism, presenting between the ages of 14 and 45 years with rapid onset of dystonia, bradykinesia, postural instability, and dysarthria; two individuals with mild dystonia-parkinsonism (one of whom suddenly worsened over hours); four with mild limb dystonia only; and two asymptomatic obligate gene carriers. In RDP-2 we have examined a total of eight individuals, four affected with the complete syndrome, two unaffected siblings, and the parents of the three affected siblings. The unaffected siblings and parents in RDP-2 with asymptomatic with normal neurologic examinations.

Rating Scales

The Dystonia Movement Scale (3) and the Unified Parkinson's Disease Rating Scale (8) have been used by our group in an attempt to quantitate the degree of dystonia and parkin-

III.7[a]	III.9[a]	III.14[a]	III.15[a]	III.19[c]	III.25[a]	IV.3[c]	IV.18[a]	IV.19[a]	IV.21[c]
Male	Male	Male	Male	Female	Male	Male	Male	Female	Male
...	14			11					15
WC	WC			WC					UL
I	I			I					S
N/A	27	N/A	21	N/A	16	23	16	14	N/A
	R		R		S	S	S	S	
	Non		Non		Slow	Rapid	Non	Non	
	< 1 d		< 1 mo		< 1 mo	< 7 d	< 1 mo	< 1 mo	
	+		+		+	+	+	+	
	+		+		+	+	+	+	
12	40	10	43	2	41	6	97	91	8
3	26	1	39	0	35	1	75	83	1
1	3	1	2	1	3	1	4	4	1
			MRI-NL		MRI-NL		MRI-NL	MRI-NL	

TABLE 2. *Clinical manifestations in RDP Family 2*

Pedigree number	II.2[a]	II.3[a]	II.5[a]	III.1[a]
Sex	Female	Female	Male	Female
Dystonia only				
Age at onset	18	18	18	None
Site	UL	UL	UL	None
Rate	Acute	Acute	Acute	N/A
Dystonia-parkinsonism				
Age at onset	22	23	20	12
Rate at onset	Acute	Acute	Acute	Acute
Progression	None	None	None	None
Time to stabilization	<1 d	2 d	<1 d	3 d
Site	FUL	FUL	FUL	FUL
Asymmetry	+	+	+	+
Rating Scales				
DMS	53	44	90	32
UPDRS	31	35	68	26
RDP Severity Scale	4	4	4	3
Brain MRI/CT	MRI-NL	MRI-NL	MRI-NL	MRI-NL

DMS, Dystonia Movement Scale; UPDRS, Unified Parkinson's Disease Rating Scale; +, present; U, arms; L, legs; F, face including speech and swallowing; MRI-NL, brain MRI normal; NA, not applicable.
[a]Previously reported.
From ref. 1, with permission.

sonism in RDP. Neither scale has adequately characterized this unique disease.

To describe the variable severity in RDP, we reported a severity scale based on the presence of parkinsonism and the ability to walk unassisted (2). The four-point scale assigns 0 to those unaffected; 1 to those having limb dystonia only, including writer's cramp; 2 to those affected in the face, arm, and neck and walking normally; 3 to those who are the same as 2 but affected in the legs and walk unassisted; and 4 to those who are the same as 3 but need a walker or use a wheelchair.

Cerebrospinal Fluid Studies

CSF analysis of HVA in affected, at-risk, and AGCs (by pedigree position) in both families confirms a deficit of the dopaminergic system. Together in both families we tested ten affected individuals with the complete RDP phenotype, two AGCs, and four at-risk individuals. HVA levels were at least one standard deviation below the mean in the two AGCs and six affected individuals from RDP-1 and in one affected person and two at risk from RDP-2. HVA levels increased with carbidopa/levodopa treatment in one of two treated affected individuals in

RDP-1, but the patient reported no symptomatic improvement. Although HVA levels were low, this did not predict the more severe clinical stages of the illness and were also observed in unaffected at-risk individuals, and AGCs. Based on our current findings, we propose that low HVA levels do not predict disease severity, but may be useful in identifying at-risk individuals for this illness.

Genetic Linkage Studies

Genetic linkage studies have been performed in both families to evaluate a possible role of the DYT1 gene located on chromosome 9q34, responsible for early-onset, generalized idiopathic torsion dystonia in Jewish and some non-Jewish families (6,7), as well as the gene responsible for dopa-responsive dystonia (DRD) located on chromosome 14q (5,9). In RDP-1 linkage analysis of three markers near the DYT1 gene showed several obligate recombinations (4). This excludes DYT1 as a candidate gene for RDP. There is no evidence for linkage to chromosome 14 in this family (2). In RDP-2 chromosome 9q markers are inconclusive because the family is too small and neither parent is clinically affected.

Proposed Diagnostic Criteria

We have proposed diagnostic criteria (1) listed in Table 3 to distinguish RDP from other more common dystonia-parkinsonism syndromes (1). A family history is required to distinguish the mild limb dystonia of RDP from idiopathic focal dystonia. Until further CSF studies are performed in those with writer's cramp and at-risk individuals we do not require low HVA levels to diagnosis RDP.

Pathogenesis

Neuropathologic studies are not yet available in an affected patient with RDP, so the pathogenesis remains undetermined. Many individuals in both families report the sudden onset or worsening of symptoms after a stressful event, such as running, childbirth, giving a speech, or fever. Because asymptomatic individuals have low CSF HVA levels, we assume that there must be another internal trigger other than low dopamine metabolite levels to initiate the cascade of biochemical changes leading abruptly to dystonia and parkinsonism. As patients with RDP quickly develop both dystonia and parkinsonism, the study of the internal trigger, possibly by functional neuroimaging of the central dopaminergic system, and comparing those with the typical classic syndrome to those at risk may provide further insights into the mechanism of both dystonia and Parkinson's disease.

ACKNOWLEDGMENTS

Dr. Ian J. Butler was supported in part by Clinical Research Center grant no. RR02558 at the University of Texas Medical School, Houston.

TABLE 3. *Diagnostic criteria*

Typical RDP
  Autosomal-dominant inheritance
  Sudden onset of combined dystonia and
    parkinsonism with stabilization in less than
    4 weeks
  Bulbar symptoms including dysarthria and
    dysphagia
  Bulbar and involvement in arms more than legs
  Moderate to no response to carbidopa/levodopa or
    dopamine agonists
  Normal brain CT or MRI
  Low CSF HVA levels[a]
Other spectrums of the RDP phenotype
  Family history of typical RDP
  Gradual or sudden onset of dystonia (± subtle
    parkinsonism)
  Moderate or no response to levodopa/carbidopa or
    dopamine agonists
  Normal brain CT or MRI
  Low CSF HVA levels

[a]Not required for diagnosis.
From ref. 1, with permission.

REFERENCES

1. Brashear A, DeLeon D, Bressman SB, et al. Rapid-onset dystonia-parkinsonism: in a second family. *Neurology* 1997;48:1066–1069.
2. Brashear A, Farlow MR, Butler IJ, et al. Variable phenotype of rapid-onset dystonia-parkinsonism. *Mov Disord* 1996;11:151–156.
3. Burke RE, Fahn S, Marsden CD, et al. Validity and reliability of a rating scale for the primary torsion dystonias. *Neurology* 1985;35:73–77.
4. Dobyns WB, Ozelius L, Kramer PL, et al. Rapid-onset dystonia-parkinsonism. *Neurology* 1993;43:2596–2602.
5. Ichinose H, Ohye T, Takahashi E, et al. Hereditary progressive dystonia with marked diurnal fluctuation caused by mutations in the GTP cyclohydrolase I gene. *Nat Genet* 1994;8:236–241.
6. Kramer PL, De Leon D, Ozelius L, et al. Dystonia gene in Ashkenazi Jewish population is located on chromosome 9q32-34. *Ann Neurol* 1990;27(2):114–120.
7. Kwiatkowski DJ, Ozelius L, Kramer PL, et al. Torsion dystonia genes in two populations confined to a small region on chromosome 9q32-34. *Am J Hum Genet* 1991;49:366–371.
8. Lang AE, Fahn S. Assessment of Parkinson's disease. In: Munsat TL, ed. *Quantification of neurologic deficit.* Boston: Butterworths, 1989:285–309.
9. Nygaard TG, Wilhelmsen KC, Risch NJ, et al. Linkage mapping of dopa-responsive dystonia (DRD) to chromosome. *Nat Genet* 1993;5:386–391.

Dystonia 3: Advances in Neurology, Vol. 78,
edited by S. Fahn, C. D. Marsden, and M. DeLong.
Lippincott–Raven Publishers, Philadelphia © 1998.

35

Molecular Genetic Analysis of Lubag

*Kirk C. Wilhelmsen, †Carol B. Moskowitz, ‡Daniel E. Weeks, †Michael Neystat, †Torbjoern G. Nygaard, *Lorraine Clark, †Muriel Dancoup, §Eufemio E. Sobrevega, ‖Raymond Rosales, ‖Gilberto L. Gamez, ¶Orlino Pacioles, **Martesio Perez, and †Stanley Fahn

*Department of Neurology, University of California, San Francisco, California, 94110; †Department of Neurology, Columbia University, New York, New York 10032; ‡Department of Human Genetics, University of Pittsburgh, Pittsburgh, Pennsylvania 15261; §Doctors Hospital, Iloilo City, Philippines; ‖University of Santo Tomas, Manila 1008, Philippines; ¶Ricardo Limso Medical Center, Devao City, Philippines; and **University of the Philippines, Manila, Philippines.*

Lubag (McKusick #314250) is a rare condition that was first recognized in the Philippines (9). Among Panay Island families with the disease, it is called by the Ilonggo name "lubag," when twisting movements (dystonia) are intermittent, "wa'eg" when twisting postures are sustained, or "sud-sud" (an onomatopoetic term denoting the sound of sandals slapping the pavement) when the gait is shuffling (a feature of parkinsonism). We refer to the clinical condition as Lubag, or X-linked dystonia-parkinsonism.

Lubag usually only affects men (12), with the earliest age of onset being 14 years of age. Young-onset patients tend to have focal dystonia that generalizes. In these cases parkinsonism may replace dystonic symptoms or may develop with persistent dystonia. Late-onset cases can present with parkinsonian features without dystonia. The parkinsonian features of Lubag are similar to those seen in idiopathic Parkinson's disease with the exception that resting tremor is rarely seen. It is therefore not surprising that the primary pathology is in the striatum (11).

Lubag has been unresponsive to pharmacologic intervention (unpublished observations). Dopaminergic agonists may cause a slight improvement in parkinsonian symptoms or induce dyskinesias. Anticholinergic drugs and benzodiazepines have had only a slight effect on dystonic symptoms. The failure of empirical pharmacologic intervention to symptomatically treat Lubag suggests that the best hope for the development of therapy may be based on an understanding of the etiology of the disease. The most direct approach to understanding the etiology of Lubag is through genetic analysis.

In a large Filipino family with a history of 16 affected men in six generations, we examined and did chromosome segregation analysis on eight affected men establishing linkage between Lubag and DNA markers that span the Xp11.22-Xq21.3 region (13) (Fig. 1). Similar analysis was done by Kupke et al. (7). Together these analyses indicate that the disease locus is in the Xq12-q21 region. The region identified by these family studies contains hundreds, and possibly thousands, of genes. Because there are few families with Lubag, and most are small, the ability to further localize the gene for Lubag by family chromosome segregation analysis is severely limited. Although several genes have been cloned strictly based on genetic data, most successful positional cloning projects have moved from a focus on linkage to a focus on genes based on either a candidate

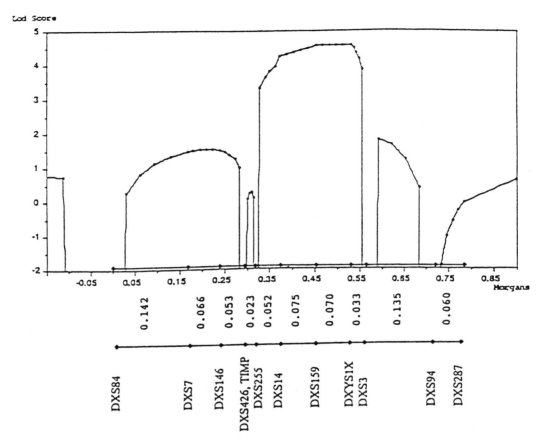

FIG. 1. Multipoint lod score analysis of a five-generation family with Lubag. The plot of the multipoint lod score indicates the most probable location for the disease gene relative to the genetic map shown below the graph. This analysis indicates that the disease susceptibility locus is in the region that contains the X chromosomal centromere between markers DXS255 and DXS3. The Kosambi map units are indicated below each interval. (From ref. 13, with permission.)

gene approach or analysis of chromosome rearrangements. All other successful positional cloning projects have relied on linkage disequilibrium to further localize disease genes after performing a family study (e.g., 5,6). Because Lubag does not appear to be due to chromosome rearrangements and a candidate gene is not obvious, we have sought evidence of linkage disequilibrium to further localize the disease gene and to enable its positional cloning.

LINKAGE DISEQUILIBRIUM

The Philippines comprise over 7,000 islands with an indigenous population of many differ-

ent ethnic groups. Lubag is prevalent among the Ilonggo language group in the Visayan islands group. The province of Capiz, on the island of Panay, is inhabited by this language group, which has the highest prevalence of Lubag in the Philippines (an estimated 1 in 4,000 men) (9). The restricted ethnic and geographic distribution of Lubag implies that the mutation causing it is very rare; a single mutation may account for most of the known cases of Lubag. If a founding mutation is responsible for most cases of Lubag, we would expect the frequencies of alleles for tightly linked markers in affected individuals to differ (be in disequilibrium) from the rest of the normal population. For these reasons, current efforts to localize the disease gene have focused on linkage disequilibrium analysis.

Linkage disequilibrium is expected to be greatest near the disease locus. However, this measurement is dependent on the population frequencies of the nearby marker allele with which a disease gene is associated. Thus, measures of linkage disequilibrium may not be greatest near the disease gene. The chi-square, Yule coefficient (14), and delta statistics (1) are different measures of linkage disequilibrium that give similar results.

Markers spanning over 4 cM (from DXS339 to DXS1002) show linkage disequilibrium with Lubag (Table 1). Several of these markers are outside of the region between our closest flanking linkage markers (DXS159-DXS441). Marker DXS453 is in greatest disequilibrium; the chi-square statistic observed for DXS453 is at least 25 standard deviations greater than the mean null distribution (assuming no linkage disequilibrium), as determined by stimulation

studies. The power of this association reflects the fact that the consensus allele for DXS453 was not observed in our Filipino control population on Panay Island (Table 2). Similarly, the consensus allele for NIMG9 was not found in the controls. Although the consensus alleles for DXS559, DXS986, and DXS56 are more frequent among index cases than the allele observed at DXS453, each is also relatively common in the control population. Thus, the high disequilibrium statistics for DXS453 should be interpreted with caution. In summary, disequilibrium has been detected between Lubag and several Xq13 polymorphisms (3,4); however, because linkage disequilibrium has been detected for markers across a large genetic region, the study provides little additional power in localizing the gene.

Single marker disequilibrium analysis ignores information contained in haplotypes. To appreciate how this approach can be used to localize disease genes, it is necessary to understand the scenario that leads to the observation

TABLE 1. *Allelic association with Lubag for selected markers*

Locus	Observed statistics			Simulated chi[a] distribution				FIBD[c] (%)
	Yule	delta	Chi[a]	Mean	SD	Max[b]	%[a]	
PGK1P	0.125	0.05	0.24	1.02	1.42	12.95	> 38	24
DXS159	0.224	0.02	0.28	1.99	2.32	18.75	> 33	58
DXS339	0.798	0.20	34.82	4.99	3.28	27.97	>100	53
NIMG7	0.481	0.17	14.59	6.05	2.84	19.27	> 99	55
NIMG9	1.000	0.26	39.18	7.04	2.84	26.44	>100	55
DXS453	1.000	0.29	108.20	7.07	3.98	30.90	>100	59
DXS559	0.912	0.26	29.07	6.14	2.90	25.09	>100	73
DXS441	0.627	0.22	33.57	7.06	3.34	25.10	>100	66
DXS56	0.833	0.24	24.40	6.08	2.74	21.14	>100	64
PGK1_a	0.478	0.15	6.78	2.01	2.02	17.11	> 94	64
PGK1_b	0.365	0.08	2.10	1.99	1.96	13.12	> 66	64
DXS986	0.818	0.17	26.04	12.17	3.70	30.83	> 99	64
DXS1002	0.556	0.19	8.12	3.05	1.99	23.37	> 97	33
DXYS1X	0.427	0.07	1.00	2.00	1.82	14.00	> 47	33
NIMG12	0.481	0.17	4.46	3.07	2.08	17.92	> 79	33

For this analysis, we typed 30 index cases with microsatellite loci from Xcen to Xq21.31 and calculated linkage disequilibrium statistics. Data for affected individuals are a subset of allele data presented in Fig. 2. The allele frequencies for normal individuals are shown in Table 2. We calculated chi-square statistics and also simulated 5,000 chi-square distributions under the null hypothesis of no association using the program ASSOC (Aravinda Chakravarti and Andrew Kompanek, personal communication). The Yule coefficient was calculated by pooling the alleles other than the allele most significantly associated for each marker. The absolute value of the Yule coefficient (14) takes on values between 0 (random association) and 1 (complete association) and does not depend on knowing the disease allele frequency. The delta statistics were calculated as previously described (1).

[a]Percentile rank of the observed chi[2] statistics in the simulated distribution.
[b]Maximum statistic observed in 5,000 simulations assuming the disease is not associated with the marker.
[c]Fraction of index case haplotypes presumed identical by descent.

TABLE 2. *Allele distribution among normal Filipinos from Panay Island*

Locus	\multicolumn{13}{c}{Alleles}													Total
	1	2	3	4	5	6	7	8	9	10	11	12	13	
PGK1P	14	38												52
DXS159	7	137	1											145
DXS339	32	4	11	26	68	0								141
NIMG7	10	28	1	4	2	0	3							48
NIMG9	1	17	0	3	4	1	23	1						50
DXS453	0	4	41	44	21	34	3	1						148
DXS559	8	1	10	5	4	2	8							38
DXS441	9	3	0	7	1	19	4	24						67
DXS56	13	6	9	10	1	0	3							42
PGK1_a[a]	1	3	5	5	4	3	0	2	2	1	7	7	2	42
PGK1_b[a]	54	50	1											105
DXS986	72	32	1											105
DXS1002	0	30	6	9										45
DXYS1X	2	65	4											71
NIMG12	1	10	7	2										20

[a]Adapted from ref. 3.

of linkage disequilibrium (Fig. 2). An ancestral founder is the ancestor of all individuals that possess the same mutation. However the most prevalent haplotype, the consensus haplotype, is not necessarily the same as the haplotype of the ancestral founder. A subset of individuals may be more closely related to each other than to the consensus haplotype but be the descendants of the individual with the consensus haplotype. The minimal haplotype common to all individuals with portions of the shared haplotype must contain the disease gene. The divergence of haplotypes from a consensus haplotype better predicts the locus of a disease gene than can linkage disequilibrium analysis.

HAPLOTYPE ANALYSIS

Obligate recombination events observed in chromosome segregation analysis of families localize the gene for Lubag to the 7.3 cM interval between DXS159 and DXS441 (Fig. 1) (7; Wilhelmsen et al., unpublished data). Because linkage disequilibrium exists for markers within and beyond these boundaries, we determined extended haplotypes for the 40 index cases using a set of ordered markers from DXS159 to DXS995 (Fig. 3). Further, we defined a consensus haplotype by starting with the markers in greatest linkage disequilibrium

and working outward. We defined three classes of haplotypes based on their relationship to the consensus haplotype: Class I haplotypes are identical with the consensus; Class II haplotypes have a contiguous set of marker alleles in common with the consensus haplotype alleles; and Class III haplotypes have no obvious relationship to the consensus haplotype. Because 73% of index case haplotypes are related to the consensus haplotype, we determined that in the population we sampled most patients with Lubag have the same mutation. Several index cases seem to have inherited large regions (>10 cM) of the same X chromosome, suggesting that these come from recently related families.

There is no known relationship between the families of index cases with Class I haplotypes. However, in most instances, index cases were unaware of family history beyond second-degree relatives. The apparent conservation of a large chromosomal region in these men suggests that they are closely related. This indicates that the measures of linkage disequilibrium in Table 1 most likely reflect the effects of linkage in both recent and distantly related individuals.

Inspection of Class II haplotypes indicates the potential for more refined localization of the gene for Lubag. We presume that our Class II haplotypes (Fig. 3) differ from the consensus

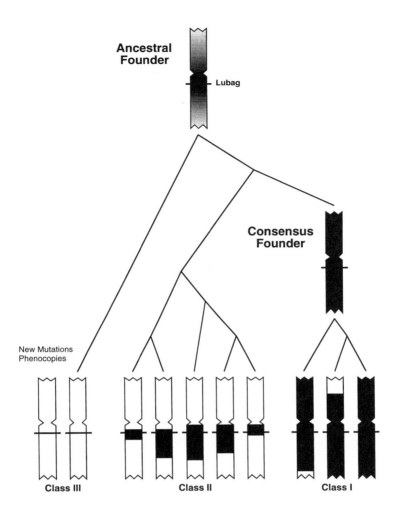

FIG. 2. Scenario for observing linkage disequilibrium. This figure shows a plausible scenario for the observation of linkage disequilibrium. In this figure only portions of a chromosome that contains a disease gene are shown. The ancestor with the original mutation, "the founding ancestor" is shown on the top of the page. The progeny are shown below and are connected by lines. One of the progeny of the founding ancestor, "the consensus founder," is the direct ancestor of a significant fraction of the index subjects with disease. The consensus founder's chromosome and the portion of this chromosome that has been inherited by index cases are filled in. The shading of the chromosome of the ancestral founder reflects that the haplotype of this individual cannot be completely determined. The index cases have been divided into classes by the same scheme as described in Fig. 3.

haplotype either because of meiotic recombination or mutation. The boundaries of divergence of individual haplotypes from the consensus haplotype may identify the location of the gene for Lubag. The haplotype in families 973 and 983 suggests that the gene for Lubag is telomeric to DXS7117. The haplotypes in families 973, 975, and 996 suggest that the gene for Lubag is centromeric to DXS1124. The haplotype analysis in these families appears to restrict the gene for Lubag to the interval between DXS7117 and DXS1124, an interval of

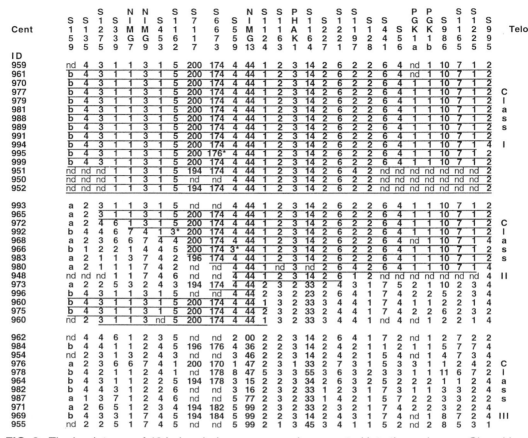

FIG. 3. The haplotypes of 40 Lubag index cases are shown sorted into three classes. Class I haplotypes have identical haplotypes for markers between DXS159 and DXS1225. The Class I haplotype is referred to in the text as the consensus haplotype. Class II haplotypes have a contiguous set of markers with alleles identical to the consensus haplotype. Putative segments of the consensus haplotype are underlined. Class III haplotypes have no apparent relationship to the consensus haplotype. The order of markers in this figure from left to right is Xcen to Xqter. * Indicates a putative mutation on the marker system; nd indicates that genotype data are not available.

approximately 1 million basepairs (data not shown). A similar analysis reaching similar conclusions with an independent group of Lubag patients was done by Graeber et al. (3).

Haplotype analysis enables the calculation of another statistic we call FIBD (fraction of index subjects that are presumed identical by descent) (Table 1), and reflects the location of the disease based on haplotype analysis. The FIBD is similar to a statistic that has been referred to as the P excess (2). The P excess attempts to estimate the fraction of index sub-

jects identical by descent by correcting for the estimate of subjects identical by state (individuals having the same allele without inheriting it from a common ancestor). Inspection of Fig. 3 shows that markers in the interval between DXS7117 and DXS1124 have the greatest FIBD and are the closest to the disease locus.

The identification of additional polymorphisms in this interval are needed to further localize the gene responsible for Lubag and clarify the boundaries for the region that must contain the mutation.

We presume that the Class III subjects are more distantly related to the consensus founder or have not inherited the same mutation from the ancestral founder. If the Class III subjects have in fact inherited the same mutation, then the identification of additional polymorphisms in the critical region will demonstrate a small region with a shared haplotype.

DISCUSSION

The localization of the disease gene for Lubag has been successively refined to smaller segments of the X chromosome by pedigree analysis, chromosome segregation studies in families, linkage disequilibrium analysis, and haplotype analysis. These analyses place the gene for Lubag in a region of less than 1 million basepairs, a size tractable for positional cloning. Our analysis suggests that haplotype analysis offers a powerful extension to single marker linkage disequilibrium mapping. The basis for linkage disequilibrium is easily illustrated in a population with a genetic disease arising from a single ancestor, the original founder (Fig. 2). In successive generations, a decreasing portion of the original founder's chromosome is inherited. Thus the chromosomal region (or haplotype) that is common to a collection of related individuals will contain the disease gene.

Haplotype analysis leads us to define a statistic that may be more useful than single marker linkage disequilibrium statistics. The property of the fraction of the index cases presumed identical by descent (FIBD, Table 1) should be maximal for markers near the disease gene locus. The FIBD will still be biased by sample clustering and fully reflects assumptions in haplotype analysis. The erroneous assumptions about presumed identity of alleles by descent will be discovered as the density of polymorphisms increases. Furthermore, a mutation in a marker system could lead to an erroneous conclusion. Thus, due to mutations, distantly related individuals may not in fact share alleles for a marker close to the gene for Lubag. Simple sequence repeat polymorphisms, as utilized here, have a nat-ural mutation rate estimated as 0.001 to 0.01/gamete (unpublished observation; 5,8,10). We have observed several genotypes that we presume to be different from the consensus founder due to mutations in the polymorphic system (Fig. 3).

Using a variation on the analysis reported by Hästbacka et al. (5) we can estimate that the gene mutation for Lubag occurred or was introduced into the population approximately 50 meiotic generations ago (1,000 to 2,000 years ago). Our estimate assumes that Lubag patients with Class III haplotypes are distant relatives of other Lubag patients in our study. If this assumption is correct, we would estimate that the closest meiotic recombination event in this collection of subjects will be 0.05 cM from the disease mutation. This rough calculation suggests that haplotype analysis can localize the disease gene to within 100 thousand basepairs, a region expected to contain one to three genes.

One of the caveats of using linkage disequilibrium analysis to localize a disease gene is that, ultimately, it may be difficult to determine whether a change in DNA sequence is causal or is a rare polymorphism found on the chromosome segment of the ancestral founder. In most positional cloning projects this problem is circumvented by identifying multiple mutations that produce the same phenotype. Because there appears to have been only one mutation responsible for Lubag in the Filipinos, it may ultimately be necessary to demonstrate how the mutation produces the disease. We will take this step as we attempt to understand the molecular basis of focal striatal degeneration that occurs in Lubag.

ACKNOWLEDGMENTS

The author is grateful to the patients with Lubag and to their families for their participation in this study; to the students and the faculty and students of the Iloilo medical school for supplying blood samples and assistance; to Dr. Eugenia Gamboa for logistical help; to Dr. Anthony Lang for supplying a blood sample from his patient; to Efthimia Pavlos, John Pica,

Matthew Higgins, and Rustituto Valetin for excellent technical assistance; and to Kamna Das for immortalization of the tissue culture lines.

This project was supported by the Parkinson's Disease Foundation, The Irving Foundation, The Dystonia Medical Research Foundation, and NIH grant R29NS31212.

REFERENCES

1. Chakravarti A, Buetow KH, Antonarakis SE, Waber PG, Boehm CD, Kazazian HH, Jr. Nonuniform recombination within the human beta-globin gene cluster. *Am J Hum Genet* 1984;36:1239–1258.

2. Devlin B, Risch N. A comparison of linkage disequilibrium measures for fine-scale mapping. *Genomics* 1995;29:311–322.

3. Graeber MB, Kupke KG, Muller U. Delineation of the dystonia-parkinsonism syndrome locus in Xq13. *Proc Natl Acad Sci USA* 1992;89:8245–8248.

4. Haberhausen G, Schmitt I, Köhler A, et al. Assignment of the dystonia-parkinsonism syndrome locus, DYT3, to a small region within a 1.8-Mb YAC contig of Xq13.1. *Am J Hum Genet* 1995;57:644–650.

5. Hästbacka J, delaChapelle A, Kaitila I, Sistonen P, Weaver A, Lander E. Linkage disequilibrium mapping in isolated founder populations: diastrophic dysplasia in Finland. *Nat Genet* 1992;2:204–211.

6. Kerem BS, Rommens JM, Buchanan JA, et al. Identification of the cystic fibrosis gene: genetic analysis. *Science* 1989;245:1073–1080.

7. Kupke KG, Lee LV, Muller U. Assignment of the X-linked torsion dystonia gene to Xq21 by linkage analysis. *Neurology* 1990;40:1438–1442.

8. Kwiatkowski DJ, Henske EP, Weimer K, Ozelius LJ, Gusella JF, Haines J. Construction of a GT polymorphism map of human 9q. *Genomics* 1992;12:229–240.

9. Lee LV, Pascasio FM, Fuentes FD, Viterbo GH. Torsion dystonia in Panay, Philippines. *Adv Neurol* 1976;14:137–151.

10. Straub RE, Speer MC, Luo Y, et al. A microsatellite genetic linkage map of human chromosome 18. *Genomics* 1993;15:48–56.

11. Waters CH, Faust PL, Powers J, et al. Neuropathology of lubag (x-linked dystonia parkinsonism). *Mov Disord* 1993;8:387–390.

12. Waters CH, Takahashi H, Wilhelmsen KC, et al. Phenotypic expression of x-linked dystonia-parkinsonism (lubag) in two women. *Neurology* 1993;43:1555–1558.

13. Wilhelmsen KC, Weeks DE, Nygaard TG, et al. Genetic mapping of "Lubag" (X-linked dystonia-parkinsonism) in a Filipino kindred to the pericentromeric region of the X chromosome. *Ann Neurol* 1991;29:124–131.

14. Yule GU. *An introduction to the theory of statistics* 14th ed. New York: Hafner Publishing, 1950.

Dystonia 3: Advances in Neurology, Vol. 78,
edited by S. Fahn, C. D. Marsden, and M. DeLong.
Lippincott–Raven Publishers, Philadelphia © 1998.

36

The Socioeconomic Implications of Dystonia

*Anthony G. Butler, †Philip O. F. Duffey, ‡Maurice R. Hawthorne,
and §Michael P. Barnes

*The Centre for Neurosciences, University of Newcastle-upon-Tyne, Hunters Moor Regional
Rehabilitation Centre, Newcastle-upon-Tyne, NE2 4NR, United Kingdom; †The School of Clinical
Neurosciences, The Medical School, University of Newcastle-upon-Tyne, Newcastle-upon-Tyne,
NE2 4HH, United Kingdom; ‡The ENT Department, The North Riding Infirmary, Middlesbrough,
Cleveland, TS1 5JE, United Kingdom; and §The Academic Unit of Neurological Rehabilitation,
University of Newcastle-upon-Tyne, Hunters Moor Regional Rehabilitation Centre, Newcastle-
upon-Tyne, NE2 4NR, United Kingdom.*

"Dystonia is not only a neurological movement disorder, it moves people socially and economically as well." This statement, made by the principal author in 1992, formed the thesis on which research into this previously unknown area of dystonia commenced in May 1993 in the northeast of England. Although there has been a great deal of research into the effect of disability in the United Kingdom (1,2,9,20,22, 24,27), very little is known about the implications that dystonia can have on the affected person and their families, apart from limited circulation articles in The Dystonia Society (TDS) newsletters in 1995 (6–8).

There has been some research into the psychosocial aspects of torticollis (12–19) but this is the first time that all types of dystonia have been included and that the economics have been specifically studied. The overall purpose of the research was designed to measure the quality of life of each patient, the severity and prevalence of dystonia in the United Kingdom, the implication the disease has had on the working life and environment of each patient, and how the patient is coping with the various personal, social, and family relationships caused by the onset and potential gradual deterioration of the disorder. This chapter will, however, only deal with how the disorder can move the affected person in relation to his or her social and economic position in society.

There are six million disabled people in the United Kingdom with at least one disability, of whom 400,000 are living in communal homes (3,23) and approximately one in every nine people in the United Kingdom is disabled in one form or another and one family in every six has a member who has a disability (22). The sense of isolation felt by most people with dystonia has never been measured and because the disorder is predominantly visual in presentation, a number of people with the disorder feel severe social and psychological pressure to remain hidden from public view. Social isolation in patients breeds a lack of diagnostic skill in family physicians, which in turn leads to non- or misdiagnosis and thus increases the isolation felt by most patients (Butler 1994, unpublished paper).

In social epidemiology, increasing attention is now given to attitudes, behavioral patterns, and more complex social processes in such nondemographic variables as social mobility, social isolation, and social stress, which play a prominent role in epidemiologic investigation (21). Other research has shown that the discrimination faced by disabled people in a society of "normal" people acts as a catalyst to the perpetuation of passivity and dependence among people with disabilities. A lack of facilities, and inadequate designs, ensure that they constantly face problems ranging from gaining access to a building to facing constant medical interventions, regardless of their value (1).

It has been argued that research needs to discover methods by which disabled people can achieve greater independence and an equal place in society, exercising freedom of choice for independent living as a right, rather than a privilege (2,24). Another aspect of controversy within the disabled population is the use of various terminology; in particular, the word "sufferer" is often used in literature designed for patient information. A small but significant number of subjects who were interviewed objected to the use of this "emotive" term with its connotations of "suffering" and "submissiveness." This was particularly interesting as one of the findings of this research has been the high number of subjects who displayed quite a remarkably positive attitude to life in general and their dystonia in particular, often despite severe physical disability and high levels of pain.

A number of other important questions were asked in the 40 months during which the fieldwork took place and the answers will help to identify various issues. These will substantially increase the working knowledge of various stakeholders, primarily The Dystonia Society, and through them, patients themselves. Other stakeholders include the small but important group of neurologists currently practicing throughout the United Kingdom, as well as general medical and family practitioners, who will be able to refer to this research as the definitive work on the subject to date.

IMPLEMENTATION STRATEGY

More than 600 subjects had their physical, medical, and social disability assessed and the clinical, psychological, and demographic profiles of each consenting person were measured. The fieldwork commenced in early 1993 and was divided into several distinct stages, which are briefly described as follows:

Stage 1: TDS Membership Files. Access to these files enabled the research team to identify all past and present members who had been diagnosed as having dystonia in the northeast. They were then invited to participate in the study by the local TDS NE Self-Help Group (SHG). This process commenced in January 1993 and is ongoing.

Stage 2: Cost Utility Analysis (CUA). Access to all patients who attended either the botulinum toxin clinic at the North Riding Infirmary (NRI) in Middlesbrough or the movement disorder clinic at Hunters Moor Regional Rehabilitation Centre (HMH) in Newcastle enabled the researchers to identify those patients diagnosed as having primary or secondary dystonic spasms. The CUA procedure commenced on May 5, 1993 and ended on June 30, 1994 resulting in a total of 199 patients being identified, plus 31 external controls, making a total of 230 people in that study (10,11).

Stage 3: Darlington Memorial Hospital (DMH) Neurology Clinic. Over a period of 20 visits from February 8 to August 8, 1995, all 665 patients who had attended the DMH neurology clinic from September 4, 1991 (when computer records commenced) to March 29, 1995 (when ICD-10 codes were introduced) were screened. A total of 24 cases of dystonic spasm were identified from the researcher's coding (ICD-9) of all 665 cases examined.

Stage 4: Other Neurology Clinics. A number of other regional and district hospitals in the region were visited during 1995 and 1996 with varying degrees of success regarding further identification of primary and secondary dystonic patients.

Stage 5: General Practitioners/Family Physicians. Liaison with the Family Health Services Authority (FHSA) established a database of 310 individual doctors practicing in County Durham and a series of GP Focus Groups established the best methodology for contacting and recruiting GPs into this research study, with limited success.

Stage 6: The Darlington Project. It had been decided that Darlington would be the subject of an intensive campaign in 1996 to establish the prevalence of dystonia within its known population. Further details of methodology are contained in Chapter 13 of this volume.

TABLE 1. *Year of patients' diagnoses*

1996	49	= the number of subjects diagnosed each year to date
1995	82	
1994	76	
1993	81	— Start of North East Dystonia Research Study
1992	62	— Commencement of Awareness Raising Campaigns
1991	52	
1990	40	— Formation of TDS—North East Self Help Groups
1989	30	— Start of botulinum toxin clinic at North Riding Infirmary
1988	13	
1987	11	— Start of botulinum toxin clinic at Hunters Moor Hospital
1986	7	
1985	8	
1984	7	
1983	8	— Formation of The Dystonia Society (TDS) in UK
1982	7	
1981	7	
1980	10	
1979	2	(There were 32 subjects diagnosed from 1937 to 1977, averaging less than 1 per year for
1978	6	40 years)

Mean	1990	Standard error	0.288	Median	1992	$n = 590$	
Mode	1995	Standard deviation	6.988	Variance	48.837		

DIAGNOSIS

Research has shown that in a survey of 705 people with dystonia in the United Kingdom; one-third take 5 years or more to diagnose, 37% said that at least one doctor had suggested that their condition was "all in the mind," and 32% had been referred at one time to a psychiatrist. A total of 66.7% of patients needed at least five consultations before diagnosis and 65.7% were misdiagnosed at some stage (5).

Because diagnosis seemed to be a major factor in getting sufficient numbers of people with dystonia available for research purposes, it was therefore decided in 1992 that an awareness-raising campaign would be run in conjunction with the local TDS SHGs. This has manifested itself in a number of seminars for medical professionals and a series of seven training videos made at Hunters Moor in Newcastle, as well as various radio and television broadcasts and newspaper articles being written over a 4-year period. All of this has helped to raise awareness of dystonia among the medical professionals and the general public, which has dramatically increased the number of diagnoses made, as shown in Table 1.

The sources from which the 641 subjects have been drawn are shown in Table 2. Interestingly

TABLE 2. *Sources of information*

Name of source/hospital and area	n	%
Hunters Moor Hospital, Newcastle	295	46.0
North Riding Infirmary, Middlesbrough	150	23.4
Patient registered at more than one hospital	38	5.9
Sunderland Eye Infirmary	38	5.9
Not registered at any clinic in the region (mainly from TDS membership sources)	26	4.1
ESD controls living outside the region	25	3.9
CUA controls living outside the region	18	2.8
Six small district hospitals in the region	15	2.3
Darlington Memorial Hospital	15	2.3
Newcastle General Hospital	15	2.3
Royal Victoria Infirmary, Newcastle	6	0.9
Total	641	100.0

4.1% of people are not registered at any clinic or hospital and this figure was originally 10.7%, before the research study started in 1993.

It could be argued that a figure of over 10% of subjects not being currently registered at any clinic or hospital was because these people had given up on the medical profession's ability to help them in any way. In fact, the words "given up," "doctors can't help," "they don't understand," and "they don't know about dystonia" were used on a significant number of occasions (qualitative data—content analysis) during the research.

GEOGRAPHIC AREA

Although the Epidemiology of Primary Dystonias (Chapter 13) restricted itself to the 2½ million population of the four northeastern Counties of England, this research had no such boundaries. Socioeconomic research makes no distinction between primary and secondary dystonias, because an abnormal posture or involuntary muscle spasm presents in exactly the same way in both cases. If the subjects are unemployed due to their dystonia, it does not matter if it was induced, genetically inherited, or idiopathic—they are still economically vulnerable.

Table 3 shows the geographic distribution of the subjects with some crude prevalence figures based on all forms of dystonic spasm within these populations (26).

The concentration on Darlington in 1996 has shown an even more dramatic increase in diagnosis and therefore the known prevalence of all forms of dystonia. Currently a total of 42 people display some form of dystonic spasm within the population of 101,766 in the Post Codes DL1, DL2, and DL3 (26); this gives a crude prevalence figure of 41.27 per 100,000 population for this town alone.

Table 3 shows the variation within the northern region as a whole. Although Durham, Cleveland and Tyne & Wear have approximately similar results, there is a distinct reduction in Northumberland, Cumbria, and North Yorkshire. Some of this can be explained by the fact that these three counties have a large geographic area with a small widely distributed rural population. However, the authors believe that the main explanation is due to the fact that awareness raising in these specific areas was carried out to a lesser degree of intensity than in the other more urban areas.

DISTRIBUTION OF THE STUDY POPULATION

Table 4 shows the study population of which two-thirds are female and over 50% are cur-

TABLE 3. *Geographic distribution of study population*

County	Post code	Number of subjects	Population (26)	Prevalence per 100,000
Durham	DH01–DH07			
	DL01–DL05			
	DL12–DL17			
	SR07–SR08			
	TS28–TS29	145	607,670	23.86
Cleveland	TS01–TS27	117	559,160	20.92
Tyne & Wear	NE01–NE21			
	NE25–NE40			
	SR01–SR06	229	1,131,015	20.25
Northumberland	NE22–NE24			
	NE41–NE71			
	TD12 & TD15	44	307,296	14.32
North Cumbria	CA01–CA28	52[a]		
South Cumbria	LA07–LA23	11[a]	492,067[a]	12.80[a]
North Yorkshire	DL06–DL11			
	YO21–YO22	10[a]	123,604[a]	8.09[a]
Other areas in the rest of United Kingdom		33[a]		
		Total = 641	2,605,141	22.53

[a]Not included in prevalence total.

TABLE 4. *Study population*

Age: *n* = 641
 Oldest: 91 yr on September 3, 1996, female with blepharospasm
 Youngest: 6 yr on May 13, 1996, female with crural dystonia
 Average age = 55.53 years

Gender	n	%	
Male	217	33.9	
Female	424	66.1	Ratio 1:1.95

Marital status: *n* = 516

Single	92	17.8
Married	296	57.4
Cohabiting	10	1.9
Separated	6	1.2
Divorced	38	7.4
Widowed	74	14.3

Etiology: *n* = 641

Primary (idiopathic)	466	72.7
Secondary (symptomatic)	169	26.4
Undiagnosed cause	6	0.9

Primary: *n* = 466

Idiopathic	442	94.8
Dopa-responsive	13	2.8
Paroxysmal	5	1.1
Myoclonic	6	1.3

rently married. The breakdown of primary etiology is also shown. The distribution of the dystonias is shown in Table 5. Hemifacial spasm is shown here as the socioeconomics were considered the same as if it were a focal dystonia.

TABLE 5. *Distribution*

	n	%
Focal dystonia (see below)	363	56.6
Hemifacial spasm	99	15.4
Generalized dystonia	59	9.2
Segmental dystonia (see below)	55	8.6
Multifocal dystonia	22	3.4
Hemidystonia	34	5.3
Others, undefined, undiagnosed	9	1.4

Focal dystonia: *n* = 363

Cervical	184	28.7
Blepharospasm	90	14.0
Spasmodic dysphonia	31	4.8
Writer's cramp	29	4.5
Peripheral (arm or leg)	22	3.4
Oromandibular/orofacial	7	0.1

Segmental dystonia: *n* = 55

Cranial (not including neck)	23	3.6
Craniocervical	19	3.0
Axial	5	0.8
Brachial	4	0.6
Crural	4	0.6

SOCIOECONOMIC METHODOLOGY

Social class can be defined in a number of different ways using a number of different classifications. A review of the common classifications of occupations in social classes used in empirical research in Britain (25) shows that only one meets the requirements of the current research into dystonia.

The six most common classifications used are:

1 = RG: The Registrar General's social class
2 = RG SEG: The Registrar General's socio-economic groups
3 = DE: Department of Employment classification
4 = FS: The Family Expenditure Survey
5 = NS: The National Survey of Health and Development
6 = MR: Market Research Categories

According to Reid (25) most commercial, social, advertising, and consumer research enterprises use the social grading of occupations, originating from the Institute of Practitioners in Advertising (MR). However, the only reason that this classification has been used in this research is that it is the only one in common usage that has the nonemployed category of retired, on disability benefit, income support, and other forms of allowance.

The categories are:

A: ***Professional.*** Defined as successful business persons (e.g., self-employed/manager/executive of large enterprise), higher professionals (e.g., bishop, surgeon, medical specialist, barrister, accountant), senior civil servants (above Principal) and local government officers (e.g., chief executive, treasurer, town clerk).

B: ***Managerial.*** Defined as senior, but not the very top, people in the same area of employment as category A.

C_1: ***White Collar Workers.*** Defined as small tradespeople, nonmanual, routine administrative, supervisory, and clerical.

C_2: ***Blue Collar Workers.*** Defined as skilled manual workers, at the top of their trade or skill.

D: ***Semiskilled and Unskilled Workers.*** Defined as all those people currently in work but not previously categorized.

E: *Unwaged.* Defined as those at the lowest levels of subsistence, including the retired, those on social security because of sickness or unemployment, and students.

By using these social gradings of occupations, this research has been able to give an insight into a number of different social and economic factors resulting in a large number of people with dystonia falling into the lowest category (i.e., being unemployed, prematurely retired, on incapacity benefit or income support). A total of 704 different variables producing 450,000 data sets were able to be measured and correlated giving previously unknown results that are too numerous and varied to be all detailed here.

Income has been derived from four different sources. First, all consenting subjects were interviewed at the earliest opportunity and all (then current) forms of income were noted and calculated to produce an annual income in £ sterling for the patient themselves. Where possible family or joint income was not shown, which resulted in a few individuals being shown with zero income. In some cases only the benefit title, not the level of subsidy was available.

Second, the published levels of state subsistence were used to calculate and confirm definite levels of income against subjective or unknown answers to previous questions. Third, a final questionnaire was sent out in 1996 to all subjects in the study asking if there had been any changes in the past years to income, employment, treatment, or attendance at a clinic or hospital and the results were correlated against previously obtained data.

Finally, the time between the original interview and the subsequent update was calculated for each person and where "no change" had been noted by the subject, an increase based on H. M. Government's published inflation figures was produced. The criteria used were:

The difference in time	Calculated inflation during that time
A.	
3.2 to 2.7 years	Income increased by 10%
2.6 to 1.6 years	Income increased by 7%
B.	
1.5 to 0.6 years	Income increased by 3%
0.5 to 0.0 years	Income increased by 0%

Because at least four fiscal year ends have passed where income tax and benefits are calculated from April 5th each year, there was an overlap and/or adjustment required for each individual case. The average increase over the period was 6.25%, however, a number of persons had a dramatic reduction in income and this is reflected in the results. A few had an increase above levels of inflation due to a promotion, a new job, or regaining employment having been previously unemployed. With very few exceptions, all subjects cooperated in this economic aspect of the research and the degree of participation is shown in Table 6 with 436 people (80.7%) participating and only 16.2% declining. All subjects also had their details included in the Epidemiological Survey of Dystonia (ESD).

RESULTS

Table 7 gives an excellent perspective on the way in which dystonia can move people over a period of time regarding their employment status. Although the number of deceased subjects increased by 16 throughout the period of the study, thus slightly skewing the results, there is a clear movement away from full-time employment to part-time and from all forms of employment to early retirement due to ill health.

TABLE 6. *Participation in the research study*

Category of subject	No.	%
Full participation	289	45.1
Part participation	130	20.3
Nonparticipation (min ESD only)	104	16.2
Died before interview	9	1.4
Died during the study	16	2.5
Died since the end of study	1	0.2
Full epidemiological data obtained (these subjects recruited in 1996)	92	14.3
Total	641	100.0

TABLE 7. *Employment status*

Employment status	When first interviewed (%)	By end of study (%)
Full-time employment	13.9	11.9
Part-time employment	7.4	8.3
Unemployed	7.8	5.3
Self-employed	3.1	0.8
Unwaged	10.0	8.7
Retired OAP	30.5	32.8
Retired ill health	11.8	14.0
On long-term sick	13.3	13.2
Deceased	2.2	4.5
Chi-square test results		
n	459	265
Chi-square	234.1348	163.2302
D.F.	8	8
Significance	$p < 0.001$	$p < 0.001$

Only 32.4% of the study population were either working or available for work at the start and this reduced to 25.5% over a 3-year period. As the statistical analysis by chi-square test shows $p < 0.001$, a direct correlation between employment status and social economic grouping (SEG) can be made.

Table 8 demonstrates very clearly that even though the SEG of the household as a whole is roughly the same as the national averages (25), there was higher weighting in SEG C_1 for the patient. This is due to the fact that 66.1% of the study population are female and the majority of female employment is often categorized as "White Collar Worker" or with "Clerical Status."

There is a definite movement downward in patient SEG status. Every category shows a reduction over time, except 70.2% of the study population start life in the lowest social and economic group (i.e., E—unwaged) and this increased to 72.8%. All correlations across the table by chi-square test come out as highly significant.

Perhaps more interesting are the results of comparing the patients' actual annual income on Table 9. Despite the fact that most incomes have risen by an average 6.25% over the period of the study, there is a universal diminution of income up to £15,000 ($24,300*) per year. One-half the study population have less than £6,000 ($9,720) to live on and only one-third have more than £8,000 ($12,960) per year.

In the band £3,000 to £7,000 ($4,860 to $11,340) there are up to 5.5% of patients who have had significant changes in their income downward and this at a time when they are already classed as one of the lowest income groups in U.K. society as a whole.

There is, however, some indication that recent improvements in treatment therapies are bearing fruit among the study population. A small but significant number of subjects remain in work as a direct result of botulinum toxin therapy, for example. A total of 19.6% of those patients in work had an average of 77.8%

---

*Exchange rates during November 1996 varied between 1.53 and 1.71, therefore $1.62 \times £$ = was selected as an appropriate rate for the US $.

TABLE 8. *Social economic groupings (SEG) of study population*

Social economic group	Patient's SEG		Highest SEG		National averages
	1993 (%)	1996 (%)	Patient (%)	Head of House (%)	
A: Professional	0.7	0.8	1.3	3.1	3%
B: Managerial	3.1	3.0	8.5	17.9	14%
C_1: White collar	14.6	12.5	38.9	22.1	22%
C_2: Blue collar	4.1	2.3	13.5	32.4	28%
D: Semiskilled/unskilled	5.2	4.2	21.6	19.7	18%
E: Unwaged	70.2	72.8	14.0	2.6	15%
Deceased	2.2	4.5	2.2	2.2	—
n	460	265	459	458	
Chi-square	1214.82	757.45	325.47	269.08	
D.F.	6	6	6	6	
Significance p	<0.001	<0.001	<0.001	<0.001	

TABLE 9. *Patients' income over time*

Annual income	n (in bands)	n	1993 (%)[a]	1996 (%)[a]	Difference
Up to £1,000			3.1	2.0	−1.1
£2,000	50	26	11.8	10.7	−1.1
£3,000			22.0	16.8	−5.2
£4,000	107	51	37.1	31.6	−5.5
£5,000			47.8	44.3	−3.5
£6,000	86	60	57.4	56.1	−1.3
£7,000			66.4	62.3	−4.1
£8,000	63	35	72.3	70.5	−1.8
£9,000			76.4	75.4	−1.0
£10,000	43	21	82.5	79.1	−3.4
£11,000			84.6	82.4	−2.2
£12,000	15	16	86.1	85.7	−0.4
£13,000			88.9	86.9	−2.0
£14,000	18	9	90.3	89.3	−1.0
£15,000			91.7	92.4	+0.5
£16,000	9	10	92.4	93.4	+1.0
£17,000			93.4	94.3	+0.9
£18,000	7	3	94.1	94.7	+0.6
£19,000			95.0	95.5	+0.5
£20,000	8	2	96.0	95.9	−0.1
£21,000			96.5	96.3	−0.2
£22,000			96.7	96.7	=
£23,000			96.9	97.5	+0.6
£24,000			97.2	—	
£25,000	9	5	98.1	—	
£26,000			—	98.0	
£27,000			98.3	98.6	+0.3
£28,000			98.6	—	
£30,000[b]	6	4	99.5	99.2	−0.3
£38,000[c]			99.8	—	
£39,000	2		100.0	—	
£42,000				99.6	
£43,000		2		100.0	
			Mean = £7,467.08	£7,406.58	−£527.19

Chi-square test results:

n	423	244
Chi-square	438.3499	237.5328
D.F.	12	12
Significance	$p < 0.001$	$p < 0.001$

[a]Percentages are shown as cumulative percentages of the whole study population.
[b]Rows £29k, £31k–£37k, and £40k–£41k were deleted—no data.
[c]No comparison is possible after income up to £30,000 per year.

time off work before the start of botulinum toxin therapy, whereas only 14.2% had to have an average 48.7% time off work after botulinum toxin therapy. However, the majority of the other subjects reap no direct economic benefit from any form of therapy or treatment.

A number of subjects (59.8%) were measured with moderate anxiety or depression and 8.8% had severe anxiety or depression. Over 60% had moderate pain or discomfort, with 21.8% experiencing severe pain or discomfort (4,10,11).

Treatments (generally) only stabilized the condition and made it bearable. Very few subjects found that any of the treatments worked sufficiently well to put them *back into work*. The point to be made here is not to get to the stage of *having to quit work*. The United Kingdom has a lower unemployment level currently than many of its European partners, but nevertheless having once had to opt out of the job market due to dystonic spasms, it is very difficult to get back into employment. There were many examples of this fact throughout the research and is borne out by the results in Table 7.

The majority of people with dystonia are aware of the so-called vicious circle syndrome. The subject starts with a minor muscular spasm; it is undiagnosed or they are told "it is all in your mind." They naturally get anxious and worried as it remains undiagnosed and they know the spasm is not in their imagination. Evidence from this research shows that anxiety and stress make dystonic spasms worse. The condition continues undiagnosed and effectively untreated, the anxiety and depression get worse, thus the intensity of spasm often increases, making a bad situation worse.

The most effective therapy is to break that circle by whatever means and the research has shown that treatment (of any kind) has a definite positive effect on social coping strategies.

MORTALITY

Death from dystonia is extremely rare with only a handful of reported cases worldwide. Although 26 people (4.1%) have died during the period of this study, the majority from natural causes from the ages of 57 to 88 from cancer, heart disease, and senility, there have been two deaths as an *indirect result* of dystonia.

A young man from a family of seven known generalized dystonia cases died of a drug overdose at the age of 21. He had turned to narcotics as his way of escaping the terrible onset of dystonia. He developed focal dystonia of a lower limb at the age of 16, in the same way as his grandmother, mother, uncle, and cousins. He knew the anticipated prognosis, having seen the severe effects on the rest of his family and therefore used drugs more and more heavily.

The second case involved a 31-year-old man who having developed torticollis found that, as his condition worsened, none of the therapies offered worked for him and, in a depressed state, he committed suicide.

CONCLUSION

Early diagnosis resulting in early treatment of most dystonic conditions has resulted in better and more effective results. Treatment of any kind has a definite positive effect on social coping strategies and this has been seen again and again as a direct result of the increased activity in the region.

Due to a combined effort between the local dystonia self-help groups and the medical professionals, a number of unique developments have taken place in the North East of England as a direct result of this research and its associated spinoffs.

An outreach dystonia nurse practitioner has been funded as part of the research program to administer botulinum toxin therapy in the patients' own homes and the effects and benefits will be measured over a 2-year period and compared to a group of matched patients who continue to receive therapy at their local clinic. Another clinic has had a dystonia counselor, who is a counseling psychologist, funded by the local self-help group but working closely with the medical professionals in the area. All of this increased awareness has seen the numbers of people with dystonia receiving botulinum toxin therapy steadily increase over the past 3 years at a rate of 2.6 new referrals per week.

There were a total of 17 different state benefits paid to subjects in the study that, when added to those with private occupational pension plans, meant that between 63.1% and 65.3% were receiving some benefit or allowance, 32.6% as a result of their dystonia.

Because there is a strong correlation between early onset meaning more severe the eventual condition, and late onset, resulting in a more focal dystonia, prognosis can now be better explained, and planned for, than in the past.

A final conclusion, however, is that if the medical professionals in any particular area are to develop and improve their treatment of dystonia, it can only be really effective with the help and support of the voluntary sector. The membership of TDS locally has increased by 118% since the start of the research, with 35.7% of the 641-member study group belonging to some form of voluntary sector charity. This has resulted in increased participation in, and support for, the local medical clinics and research facilities, which in turn leads to better and more effective treatment of those with dystonia, their carers, and families.

The research outlined in this chapter is just a small part of the ongoing development and it is hoped these other results will be analyzed and published for wider dissemination.

ACKNOWLEDGMENTS

The authors would like to acknowledge the contribution made by The Dystonia Society (TDS) in granting access to its membership and for the logistical and moral support without which this research would not have started. In addition, financial support has been received from Speywood Pharmaceuticals (U.K.) Ltd. (1993), the Northern and Yorkshire Regional Health Authority (1994), Allergan Ltd. (1996), as well as the charities Action for Disability in Newcastle (1994); Ear, Nose, Throat and Eye Research (ENTER) in Middlesbrough (1995); and the Research and Welfare Fund of TDS North East (1996).

Specific acknowledgment should go to Dr. Marjan Jahanshahi, Research Fellow at the Department of Clinical Neurosciences, the Institute of Neurology, for her support and advice, as well as to Robert Allchin, Consultant Ophthalmic Surgeon at Sunderland Eye Infirmary and Dr. P. J. B. Tilley, Consultant Neurologist at Darlington and Middlesbrough General Hospitals, for access to their patients.

Finally, the authors would like to thank all those subjects who have painstakingly completed the series of questionnaires and interviews over the 40 months during which the fieldwork was undertaken and particularly those who have done so, despite the often ever-present pain and debilitating effects of their own specific form of dystonic spasm.

REFERENCES

1. Barton L. *Disability and dependent living*. London: Falner Press, 1989.
2. Brisenden S. *Independent living and the medical model of disability*. Vol. 1. No. 2. Abingdon: Disability, Handicap and Society, 1986:173–178.
3. Central Statistical Office. *Annual Abstract of Statistics 1993*.
4. Dolan P, Gudex C, Kind P. *A social tariff for EuroQol: results from a UK general population survey*. Discussion Paper 138, Centre for Health Economics, University of York, 1995.
5. Dystonia Society. *Diagnostic Survey*. London, November 1992. Published in 1993 to Dystonia Society members.
6. Dystonia Society. *Newsletter*. Issue No. 19. Spring 1995:4–5.
7. Dystonia Society. *Newsletter*. Issue No. 20. Summer 1995:4–5.
8. Dystonia Society. *Newsletter*. Issue No. 21. Autumn 1995:5–6.
9. Etherington K. The Disabled Persons Act 1986: the need for counselling. *Br J Occup Ther* 1990;53:430–432.
10. Gudex CM, Hawthorne MR, Butler AG, Duffey POF. Measuring patient benefit from botulinum toxin in the treatment of dystonia—feasibility of cost utility analysis. *Pharmaco Economics* 1997;12:6;675–684.
11. Gudex CM, Hawthorne MR, Butler AG, Duffey POF. The effect of dystonia and botulinum toxin treatment on health-related quality of life (HRQoL). *Movement Disorders* 1998 (*in press*).
12. Jahanshahi M. Personality in torticollis: changes across time. *Person Individ Diff* 1990;11:355–363.
13. Jahanshahi M. Psychological factors and depression in torticollis. *J Psychosom Res* 1991;35:493–507.
14. Jahanshahi M, Marsden CD. Depression in torticollis: a controlled study. *Psych Med* 1988;18:925–933.
15. Jahanshahi M, Marsden CD. Personality in torticollis: a controlled study. *Psych Med* 1988;18:375–387.
16. Jahanshahi M, Marsden CD. Conversion "V" profiles in torticollis. *Behav Neurol* 1989;2:219–235.
17. Jahanshahi M, Marsden CD. A longitudinal follow-up study of depression, disability and body concept in torticollis. *Behav Neurol* 1990;3:233–246.
18. Jahanshahi M, Marsden CD. Body concept, disability and depression in patients with spasmodic torticollis. *Behav Neurol* 1990;3:117–131.
19. Jahanshahi M, Marsden CD. Psycho-social functioning before and after treatment of torticollis with botulinum toxin. *J Neurol Neurosurg Psychiatry* 1992;55:229–231.
20. Martin J, Meltzer H, Elliot D. *The prevalence of disability among adults*. London: HMSO. 1988, from OPCS report No. 1.
21. Mechanic D. *Medical sociology*. New York: Free Press, 1988.
22. O'Brien LG, McFetridge M. *Disability: the reason for improvements in local information systems*. Hastings: Burisa Newsletter. 1991, Dec. No. 101, 12–13.
23. Office of Population, Censuses and Surveys (OPCS). *Survey of disability in Great Britain*. Report No. 1, 1988.
24. Oliver M. *The politics of disablement*. Basingstoke, London: McMillan, 1990.
25. Reid I. *Social class differences in Britain*. Fontana Press, London: 3rd Edition. 1989.
26. Research and Intelligence Units of Cleveland, Cumbria, Durham, Northumberland and Tyne & Wear Councils. *Population statistics* as of 25th March 1993; updated by ONS. *Estimated residential population mid-1995* and by *Royal Mail population estimates for 1st July 1995*.
27. Wood P, Sainsbury S, Martin J, Piazza T. Researching disabilities, methodological issues. London: *Survey Methods Newsletter*. 1989, Autumn, 3–10.

Dystonia 3: Advances in Neurology, Vol. 78,
edited by S. Fahn, C. D. Marsden, and M. DeLong.
Lippincott–Raven Publishers, Philadelphia © 1998.

37

Summary and Conclusions

*Charles David Marsden and †Stanley Fahn

*University Department of Clinical Neurology, Institute of Neurology, London WC IN 3BG,
United Kingdom; and †Department of Neurology, Columbia-Presbyterian Medical Center,
New York, New York 10032.

The last 20 years have seen dramatic advances in our understanding of the condition known as torsion dystonia. If one scans the volumes of the First Dystonia Conference in 1976 and the Second in 1986 and then compares the data presented in three exciting days in Miami, October 1996, the pace of increased knowledge is easy to see.

THE CLASSIFICATION OF DYSTONIA

A major outcome of new knowledge has been a reappraisal of the classification of the etiology of the dystonias (see Chapter 1 of this volume). The original classification into primary or idiopathic versus secondary or symptomatic has been valuable, but now requires refinement. Idiopathic refers to unknown causes, but many of the primary dystonias now have an identified genetic cause. Accordingly, the new classification uses *primary dystonia* to include all conditions in which dystonia is the sole manifestation, including the various identified genetic abnormalities (see below). *Dystonia-plus* refers to neurochemical disorders in which there are neurologic features in addition to dystonia, such as parkinsonism. *Secondary dystonias* include those due mainly to environmental factors. *Heredodegenerative dystonia* includes the many conditions with known anatomic pathology that may cause dystonia.

THE PREVALENCE OF DYSTONIA

The exact prevalence of primary dystonia has always been uncertain. The study of Nutt et al., based on the records of the Mayo Clinic,

Rochester, Minnesota, suggested figures of 1 in 29,400 for generalized dystonia, and 1 in 3,400 for focal dystonia. We now have the results of a further community-based study in the northeast of England (see Chapter 13 of this volume). A number of complementary methods were employed to obtain as wide an ascertainment as possible. The figure that emerges for primary dystonia is about 1 in 7,000 of the population. As expected, adult-onset focal dystonia dominates, with blepharospasm and spasmodic torticollis being the most common. It is interesting that dopa-responsive dystonia accounted for some 10% of cases. If one adds patients with secondary symptomatic dystonia, those with drug-induced tardive dystonia, and those with athetoid cerebral palsy, this prevalence figure can probably be doubled and begins to approach that of multiple sclerosis. Dystonia thus is a common neurologic problem. Butler et al. (Chapter 36 of this volume) highlight the adverse social and economic effects of this illness.

THE GENETICS OF PRIMARY DYSTONIA

One of the most dramatic advances in the understanding of the primary dystonias has resulted from genetic discoveries. The localization of the DYT1 gene on chromosome 9q34 responsible for classic Oppenheim's dystonia has opened up the field (see Chapter 10 of this volume). Inheritance is dominant with 30% to 40% penetrance. What determines clinical expression of the disease is unknown. The DYT1 gene accounts for 90% or more of cases of primary dystonia in Ashkenazi Jews. The frequency of the gene in the New York Jewish population has been estimated to be 1 in 2,000, and of the disease to be 1 in 6,000. The phenotype of the DYT1 gene abnormality in this ethnic group has been clearly defined (see Chapter 9 of this volume). Onset is in childhood or before the age of about 28 years, and the legs and arms are most commonly affected. Generalization occurs in the majority. Haplotype analysis has established that this genetic abnormality arose from 350 years ago somewhere in Lithuania or Byelorussia as a founder effect, which then spread rapidly through the Ashkenazi Jewish population. Such haplotype analysis has enabled practical diagnosis of carriers and prenatal diagnosis in this population.

The DYT1 gene abnormality accounts for many cases of non-Jewish early-onset dystonia. However, other mutations also are responsible for a significant proportion of non-Jewish hereditary early-onset dystonia.

The DYT1 gene makes only a small contribution to adult-onset torsion dystonia and, apparently, negligible contribution to secondary dystonias such as tardive dystonia, postanoxic dystonia, and dystonias due to peripheral injuries.

The role of inheritance in the adult-onset focal and segmental primary dystonias is less clear. There are, however, a small number of families with adult-onset focal dystonia, in which the phenotype often breeds true for example, as hereditary spasmodic torticollis. Genetic abnormalities other than the DYT1 gene appear to be responsible for some adult-onset hereditary dystonias. Linkage to chromosome 8 has been established in two Mennonite families (DYT6), and to chromosome 18 in a German family (DYT7). There are other families in which the gene remains to be discovered, including the Australian family with whispering dysphonia (DYT4), a large Swedish family, the family with torticollis, tremor, and scoliosis described by Duane (see Chapter 12 of this volume), and perhaps the uncertain autosomal-recessive Spanish Gypsy families (DYT2).

Despite these major advances in genetic understanding through linkage studies, no single gene for primary dystonia has been identified, so far. There remains a huge gap between genetic linkage and the understanding of the true genetic abnormality and abnormal gene products responsible for the hereditary primary dystonias. No doubt this will be rectified in the next few years.

THE PATHOPHYSIOLOGY OF PRIMARY DYSTONIA

Much has been learned about the pathophysiology of dystonia from neurophysiologic and positron emission tomography studies in patients, and the investigation of animal models of dystonia, in particular levodopa-induced dystonia in monkeys.

An intriguing study is that by Eidelberg et al. (Chapter 14 of this volume) who investigated fluorodeoxyglucose metabolism in patients with DYT1 dystonia and asymptomatic carriers of the DYT1 gene. Clear abnormalities of covarying increased metabolism in the lentiform nucleus, cerebellum, and supplementary motor area were discovered in both groups. These abnormalities did not express themselves in the form of clinical symptoms in the carriers. The DYT1 gene is only about 30% penetrant, so it remains to be discovered why carriers do not have symptoms of the disease, and what additional factors trigger expression of the genetic abnormality in those who are affected.

Deoxyglucose metabolism in those with dystonia itself reveals interesting abnormalities of dissociation between lentiform and thalamic activity. These abnormalities can be interpreted in terms of increased drive in the direct striatopallidal pathway, inhibiting the internal segment of the globus pallidus (GPi).

Studies of the pattern of cortical activation on executing movement in patients with primary dystonia, using blood flow measurements, have revealed a fairly coherent picture (see Chapter 15 of this volume). When patients with generalized dystonia or focal arm dystonia try to execute repetitive hand movements, there is overactivity of the *planning centers* of the frontal lobe, in particular the anterior supplementary motor area, dorsolateral prefrontal cortex, and anterior premotor regions. There also is underactivity of the *motor executive areas* of the cortex, including the motor cortex itself, posterior supplementary motor area, and posterior lateral premotor regions. The explanation for this underactivity of the executive regions is uncertain.

At least a part of dystonia might reasonably be thought to be due to increased motor cortical drive to the brainstem and spinal cord motor machinery, to cause action dystonia and spontaneous dystonic muscle spasms, although this is not proven.

If there is increased motor output from the cortex to produce the dystonic spasms, metabolic underactivity may represent a reduction of some inhibitory input into the motor regions, or perhaps a reduction of interneuronal inhibitory cortical activity. Most if not all inputs from the thalamus and other regions of the cortex to the motor cortex are likely to be excitatory, so perhaps the latter explanation is correct.

Even though there is reduced motor cortical activation in metabolic studies, electrophysiology suggests that there is increased excitability of the motor cortex when tested by transcutaneous magnetic stimulation (see Chapter 2 of this volume; but also see Chapter 5 of this volume). Again this may point to a reduction of interneuronal inhibitory activity in the cortex leading to excess excitability. A range of neurophysiologic studies (see Chapter 2 of this volume) have identified abnormal interneuronal function in the brainstem and spinal cord in dystonia. Similar changes may also occur in the cerebral cortex.

How do these cortical changes arise? The overactivity of the anterior frontal planning network might well represent overactivity of input into these regions from thalamic nuclei Voa and Vop, which receive the major efferent output from the basal ganglia via GPi and substantia nigra pars reticulata.

Support for this notion comes from the analysis of levodopa-induced dystonia in *N*-methyl-4-phenyl-1,2,3,6-tetrahydropyridine (MPTP)-treated monkeys. Deoxyglucose studies suggest that there is indeed reduced Gpi activity, as a result of excessive drive in the direct (D1) striatopallidal pathway. Activity in the indirect pathway to GPe and subthalamus also is altered. In particular, there appears to be reduced subthalamic drive to GPi. Abnormal activity in the indirect pathway probably is important because of the first demonstration of reduced dopamine D_2 receptor binding in the striatum of patients with dystonia (see Chapter 17 of this volume).

The net effect of these changes in the direct and indirect striatopallidal pathways appear to be reduced or altered GPi inhibition of basal ganglia thalamic targets, with consequent increased thalamic drive to the premotor planning distributed network.

However, it is by no means clear how the changes in striatopallidal and pallidothalamic activity are different in chorea and dystonia. Chorea and dystonia are considered, for diagnostic purposes, to be different movement disorders. But the metabolic changes in the basal ganglia of levodopa-treated dyskinetic MPTP-intoxicated parkinsonian monkeys are similar in overall terms, although perhaps different in degree. Furthermore, chorea and dystonia are closely intertwined, often occurring together as "choreoathetosis." Indeed, patients with primary dystonia treated with high doses of anticholinergic drugs may be transformed from a dystonic phenotype into a picture of chorea, which returns to dystonia when the dose of anticholinergics is reduced. Much needs to be discovered to explain the differences and similarities between chorea and dystonia.

These predictions on basal ganglia functional changes from the monkey model of dystonia are, to some extent, now supported by direct observation of neuronal firing in the thalamus and medial globus pallidus at the time of stereotaxic surgery in patients with dystonia (see Chapters 4 and 21 of this volume).

GPi neuronal firing in dystonics shows reduced rates, increased receptive fields, and abnormal irregular burst or grouped patterns of discharge (see Chapter 21 of this volume). Therefore, GPi activity has now been proven to be abnormal in patients with dystonia. However, how these abnormalities of pallidal neuronal firing generate dystonia is unclear. It seems that the abnormal pattern of discharge may be more important than the absolute firing rate. It also remains mysterious as to why a medial pallidal lesion can improve dystonia, when the activity of this zone appears to be reduced by the disease itself. However, it may be best to remove a noisy machine and to do without it!

The reduction of GPi activity in dystonia would be predicted to lead to reduced inhibition of thalamic target regions. However, direct recording of single cells in Vop has not really confirmed this prediction (see Chapter 4 of this volume). Vop neurons in dystonics also appear to have reduced discharge rates, and there are many more sensory cells than normal. It also appears that the discharge in Vop actually is linked to dystonic muscle contraction. A similar pattern of reduced activity is found in the cerebellar projection zone in thalamus, namely nucleus Vim. Vim projections are distributed to the motor cortex itself, and it is likely that changes in cerebellar activity underlie some of the abnormalities of motor cortical function described above. The cerebellum has received little attention in metabolic studies but there is clear evidence for abnormality at least in the deoxyglucose investigation.

Another area that deserves attention is the impact of possible changes in descending pathways from basal ganglia to brainstem, in particular to pedunculopontine nucleus and to the other brainstem centers controlling posture and locomotion. These are highly likely to be abnormal in dystonia and, indeed, Eidelberg et al. (see Chapter 14 of this volume) have shown abnormal deoxyglucose activity in such brainstem regions. No doubt more attention will be paid to these descending pathways in future studies. Interestingly, in the MPTP parkinsonian monkey, a thalamic lesion in motor targets from basal ganglia can abolish levodopa-induced chorea, but does not affect levodopa-induced dystonia. This suggests that the descending projections to brainstem are critical for the manifestation of this drug-induced dystonia. In contrast, however, thalamic lesions can reduce dystonia in humans. This paradox may be due to the different siting of stereotaxic thalamotomy in patients with dystonia, but exactly why this should be so is uncertain.

THE TREATMENT OF PRIMARY DYSTONIA

Unfortunately, there have been no dramatic advances in the drug treatment of the primary dystonias. The best management remains a trial of levodopa, high-dose anticholinergics [trihexyphenidyl (Artane)] therapy, the second-line drugs such as baclofen, tetrabenazine etc. Studies in animal models suggest that drugs manipulating brain 5-hydroxytryptamine, opioid, and glutamatergic function may have a role in treating dystonia, but new drugs are urgently needed for clinical trials.

New methods of delivering established drugs are under investigation, in particular intrathecal infusion of baclofen (see Chapter 20 of this volume). In carefully selected patients with severe primary or symptomatic dystonia, intrathecal baclofen may be valuable, but the effect is unpredictable and not without complications.

Undoubtedly the use of botulinum toxin A has revolutionized the management of the focal dystonias and now is the treatment of choice for conditions such as blepharospasm, spasmodic dysphonia, spasmodic torticollis, and to some extent writer's and other occupational cramps (reviewed in Chapter 18 of this volume). The issue of emergence of neutralizing antibodies is of concern, and has prompted the development of other strains botulinum toxin (B and F), which may have a useful role.

Perhaps one of the most exciting therapeutic initiatives has been the reassessment of the role of stereotaxic surgery for dystonia (reviewed in Chapter 19 of this volume). This has been prompted by the dramatic reintroduction of stereotaxic posteroventral pallidotomy for Parkinson's disease, along with improved target localization and safety. In parallel there has been the development of chronic implanted electrostimulation of target sites in thalamus, globus pallidus, and subthalamus in Parkinson's disease. Reports posteroventral pallidotomy (see Chapters 21 and 22 of this volume) for dystonia are encouraging, but the number of patients so operated has been small and the best targets, methods, and patients will have to be established. The problem of adverse effects, especially on speech with bilateral lesions will have to be assessed, and the relative benefits of such surgery on limb dystonia (which may be good) versus axial dystonias (which may be poor) need to be discovered. Nevertheless, this avenue of treatment holds promise in severe cases of dystonia.

THE HEREDODEGENERATIVE DYSTONIAS

Among the heredodegenerative dystonia, of which there are many, two are worthy of comment. LUBAG (DYT3) is an X-linked form of dystonia-parkinsonism found in men from the Philippines; female carriers may be mildly affected. The pathologic substrate appears to be a curious form of striatal mosaicism (which has also been found in rare non-Filipino cases of symptomatic dystonia). The gene located at Xq13.1 is close to discovery, and the responsible region of the chromosome is being sequenced (see Chapter 35 of this volume). Rapid-onset dystonia-parkinsonism has been reported as an autosomal-dominant disorder in two families (see Chapter 34 of this volume) and is likely to be heredodegenerative, although brain magnetic resonance imaging is normal. Severe dystonia usually appears over hours to days in adolescents and adults (aged 14 to 58 years) and then stabilizes, although some may only have mild dystonia. There is no response to levodopa. There is no linkage to the DYT1 gene.

THE DYSTONIA-PLUS DYSTONIAS

Among the dystonia-plus syndromes, the syndrome of autosomal-dominant myoclonus dystonia is characterized by lightning myoclonic jerks, as well as dystonia, and frequently a beneficial response to alcohol. Linkage studies have excluded the DYT1 gene, but the exact locus has not been mapped (see

Chapter 33 of this volume). Whether this is related to the locus on chromosome 18 linked to adult-onset dystonia in the German family referred to above remains to be established.

Perhaps the most dramatic breakthrough in the field of dystonia has been the discovery that dopa-responsive dystonia (DRD) is due to mutations in the gene coding for the enzyme GTP cyclohydrolase I (GTP-CH1) on chromosome 14q22.1 (DYT5) (see Chapters 26 to 29 of this volume). Multiple mutations have been found, involving introns and exons, each family appearing to have a different mutation. DRD is inherited in autosomal-dominant manner and the gene appears 30% to 40% penetrant; the genetic abnormality is far more likely to express in women than men. Affected women tend to present in childhood and adolescence with gait dystonia and parkinsonism, whereas in men the condition may emerge as a parkinsonian syndrome in middle life. Atypical presentation in affected families also include "athetoid cerebral palsy," odd ataxias and falls, and an apparent spastic paraplegia (see Chapter 28 this volume).

GTP-CH1 is the first and rate-limiting step in the synthesis of tetrahydrobiopterin (BH_4) from guanosine triphosphate (GTP). BH_4 is an essential cofactor for the function of amino acid hydroxylases including tyrosine hydroxylase (TH), tryptophan hydroxylase, and phenylalanine hydroxylase (and nitric oxide synthase). Lack of BH_4 in DRD leads to failure of synthesis of L-DOPA from tyrosine and consequent failure of dopamine formation (see Chapter 27 of this volume). Treatment of patients with DRD with levodopa in small doses causes remarkable relief of symptoms with a stable long-term response.

Despite the extensive new knowledge of the genetic and biochemical background of DRD, many features of the illness remain unexplained. Why only 30% to 40% of gene carriers express the disease is unknown. The female preponderance of affected individuals hints at some hormonal or other factor necessary for expression of the genetic abnormality. Measurement of GTP-CH1 in peripheral tissues shows that those showing the disease have enzyme activity reduced to 30% to 40% of normal, but unaffected gene carriers showing no signs of the disease have a similar reduction (see Chapter 29 of this volume). Therefore some other factor must be responsible for expression of the genetic abnormality of GTP-CH1, but what this may be is unknown.

It seems clear that the nigrostriatal pathway is anatomically intact in DRD as judged by pathologic examination. Nigrostriatal terminal density also appears normal as indicated by binding of GBR 12935 to the dopamine transporter in caudate and putamen (see Chapter 27 of this volume), and by the binding of the dopamine uptake site ligand β-CIT on single photon emission computed tomography (SPECT) scanning in DRD patients in vivo (see Chapter 31 of this volume). Kang et al. (see Chapter 32 of this volume) have provided compelling evidence that BH_4 stabilizes TH protein and expression, which is decreased in striatum in DRD, and this may be important. BH_4 may also play a role in cell growth and cell survival.

Another mystery is why dopamine deficiency causes dystonia in DRD, along with elements of parkinsonism. The role of striatal dopamine in dystonia is complex. In DRD severe striatal dopamine depletion, especially in putamen, produces dystonia that is relieved by levodopa therapy. In Parkinson's disease, levodopa treatment causes dystonic dyskinesias, especially in "beginning and end-of-dose" diphasic dyskinesias, which disappear on reduction of levodopa dose. But patients with fluctuating advanced Parkinson's disease also develop "off-period" dystonia in the mornings or during the day when they become immobile; such "off-period" dystonias may also disappear after prolonged withdrawal of levodopa. It seems that dystonia may occur in these different conditions with low, high, or intermediate brain dopamine levels, a complex and unexplained relationship.

Finally, it has become apparent that aside from clinical autosomal-dominant DRD, there are rarer autosomal-recessive conditions interfering with dopamine synthesis, whether directly as in tyrosine hydroxylase deficiency, or indirectly via failure of BH_4 synthesis [e.g., 6-pyruvoyltetrahydropterin synthase (6-PTPS) deficiency, which leads to failure of conversion of dihydroneopterin triphosphate (the product of GTP-CH1 activity) to 6-pyruvoyltetrahydropterin; or dihydropteridine reductase (DHPR) deficiency, which recycles quinonoid dyhydrobiopterin to BH_4](see Chapters 30 and 26 of this volume). In general, these inherited conditions appear in early life with mental retardation, seizures, and a levodopa-responsive dystonic-parkinsonian syndrome reminiscent of DRD.

Hyland et al (Chapter 30) have presented a valuable algorithm for diagnosis of these and related metabolic conditions. A clue comes from finding a high blood phenylalanine level (which may be detected in routine screening of babies for phenylketonuria). A standard phenylalanine load test also may show failure of disposition of the amino acid. Cerebrospinal fluid (CSF) examination may reveal reduced levels of the monoamine neurotransmitter metabolites homovanillic acid (HVA) and 5-hydroxyindoleacetic acid (5-HIAA) reflecting depletion of brain dopamine and serotonin, respectively. CSF (and urinary) biopterin and neopterin levels are altered according to the specific metabolic defect.

CONCLUSIONS

The wealth of new data on dystonia presented at this meeting and in this volume is testimony to the effort of many individuals and teams dedicated to dystonia. It is hard to believe that a quarter of a century ago the problem was to convince many that dystonia was a neurologic disease. Now many dystonias are treatable, although sadly others remain a source of considerable disability. However, it is easy to see that the next accelerating phase of discovery will conquer the illness. Our thanks are due to the patients, their families, the Dystonia Medical Research Foundation in North America, their sister organizations elsewhere in the world, and to the National Institutes of Health for their help and encouragement.

Subject Index

Page numbers followed by *f* refer to figures and page numbers followed by *t* refer to tables.